METHODS IN DISEASE: INVESTIGATING THE GASTROINTESTINAL TRACT

METHODS IN DISEASE: INVESTIGATING THE GASTROINTESTINAL TRACT

Edited by

Victor R. Preedy
Ronald R. Watson

GMM

© 1998

GREENWICH MEDICAL MEDIA LTD
219 The Linen Hall
162-168 Regent Street
London
W1R 5TB

ISBN 1 900151 014

First Published 1998

British Library Cataloguing in Publication Data
A catalogue record for this book is available from the British Library.

Distributed worldwide by
Oxford University Press

Project Manager
Gavin Smith

Designed and Produced by
Derek Virtue, DataNet

Printed in Hong Kong by Dah Hua

CONTENTS

CHAPTER 14

CHAPTER 15

CHAPTER 16

CHAPTER 17

CHAPTER 18

CHAPTER 19

CHAPTER 20

CHAPTER 21

CHAPTER 29

CHAPTER 30

CHAPTER 31

CHAPTER 32

CHAPTER 33

INDEX

CONTRIBUTORS

Tor H Bark
Department of Surgery
Health Sciences Centre
SUNY Stonybrook
New York
USA

Jean-François Beaulieu
Department of Anatomy
and Cellular Biology
University of Sherbrooke
Sherbrooke, Québec
CANADA

Guido Biasco
Institute of Haematology
and Oncology
University of Bologna
Bologna
ITALY

Yamina Bouatrouss
Department of Anatomy and Cellular
Biology
University of Sherbrooke
Sherbrooke, Québec
CANADA

Barry J Campbell
Gastroenterology Research Group
University of Liverpool Department of
Medicine
Liverpool
UK

Romilda Cardin
Institute of Internal Medicine
University of Padua
Padua
ITALY

Roger Crane
Department of Clinical Biochemistry
King's College School of Medicine
and Dentistry
London
UK

Peter M Delaney
Department of Pharmacology
Monash University
Melbourne
AUSTRALIA

Lorenzo E Derchi
Institute of Radiology
University of Genoa
Genoa
ITALY

Sean P Devane
Department of Child Health
Kings College Hospital
London
UK

W Domschke
Department of Medicine
University of Münster
Münster
GERMANY

Hamish D Duncan
Department of Gastroenterology
New Cross Hospital
Wolverhampton
UK

Fabio Farinati
Institute of Internal Medicine
University of Padua
Padua
ITALY

Kazuhiko Fujiki
Division of Gastroenterology
Tokyo Medical and Dental University
Tokyo
JAPAN

Hideo Fukui
Drug Safety Research Laboratories
Takeda Chemical Industries Ltd
Osaka
JAPAN

Peter J Garlick
Department of Surgery
Health Sciences Centre
SUNY Stonybrook
New York
USA

Robert M Genta
Departments of Pathology
and Medicine
Baylor College of Medicine
Houston, Texas
USA

A Gillessen
Department of Gastroenterology
University Hospital Herne
Herne
GERMANY

George K Grimble
Addictive Behaviour Centre
The Roehampton Institute
London
UK

Peter W Hamilton
Department of Pathology
Queen's University of Belfast
Belfast
NORTHERN IRELAND

Dennis S Huang
Department of Pathology
Case Western Reserve University
Cleveland, Ohio
USA

Fen-Fang Huang
Department of Pathology
Case Western Reserve University
Cleveland, Ohio
USA

Tracy Karban
Department of Pathology
Case Western Reserve University
Cleveland, Ohio
USA

W K H Kauer
Department of Surgery
Klinikum rechts der Isar
Munich
GERMANY

Roger G King
Department of Pharmacology
Monash University
Melbourne
AUSTRALIA

Yukisato Kitamura
Second Department of Pathology
Tottori University, Faculty of Medicine
Yonago
JAPAN

S Komori
Department of Veterinary Science
Gifu University
Gifu
JAPAN

Motoharu Kondo
First Department of Medicine
Kyoto Prefectural University of
Medicine
Kyoto
JAPAN

Keith J Lindley
Gastroenterology Unit
Institute of Child Health
London
UK

Marìa C Lòpez
Division of Cellular Pathology
University of Cambridge
Cambridge
UK

S Mahé
INRA, Unit of Human Nutrition
and Physiology
Faculty of Science, Pharmaceuticals
& Biology
Paris
FRANCE

Luigi Maiuri
Department of Paediatrics
University Federico II of Naples
Naples
ITALY

Carlo Martinoli
Institute of Radiology
University of Genoa
Genoa
ITALY

Mary B Mazanec
Department of Pathology
Case Western Reserve University
Cleveland, Ohio
USA

Rachel Menon
Gastroenterology Unit
Institute of Child Health
London
UK

Ian S Menzies
Department of Clinical Biochemistry
King's College School of Medicine
and Dentistry
London
UK

Yuji Naito
First Department of Medicine
Kyoto Prefectural University
of Medicine
Kyoto
JAPAN

Shigemi Nakajima
Departments of Pathology
and Medicine
Baylor College of Medicine
Houston, Texas
USA

Ikuko Ogawa
Department of Histopathology
and Morbid Anatomy
Muhimbili University College
of Health Sciences
Dar es Salaam
TANZANIA

H Ohashi
Department of Veterinary Science
Gifu University
Gifu
JAPAN

Toshifumi Ohkusa
Division of Gastroenterology
Tokyo Medical and Dental
University
Tokyo
JAPAN

Glenn D Papworth
Department of Pharmacology
Monash University
Melbourne
AUSTRALIA

Jacques Poisson
Department of Anatomy
and Cellular Biology
University of Sherbrooke
Sherbrooke, Québec
CANADA

T Pohle
Department of Medicine
University of Münster
Münster
GERMANY

V R Preedy
Department of Clinical Biochemistry
King's College School of Medicine
and Dentistry
London
UK

Gordon B Proctor
Department of Oral Pathology
and Oral Medicine
King's College School of Medicine
and Dentistry
London
UK

K B Raja
Department of Clinical Biochemistry
King's College School of Medicine
and Dentistry
London
UK

Jonathan M Rhodes
Gastroenterology Research Group
University of Liverpool Department
of Medicine
Liverpool
UK

Marìa E Roux
Faculty of Pharmacy and Biochemistry
University of Buenos Aires
Buenos Aires
ARGENTINA

Ana Maria Segura
Departments of Pathology
and Medicine
Baylor College of Medicine
Houston, Texas
USA

Tarulata Shah
Department of Clinical Biochemistry
King's College School of Medicine
and Dentistry
London
UK

M Shahin
Department of Medicine
University of Münster
Münster
GERMANY

Deepak K Shori
Department of Oral Pathology
and Oral Medicine
King's College School of Medicine
and Dentistry
London
UK

Robert J Simpson
Department of Clinical Biochemistry
King's College School of Medicine
and Dentistry
London
UK

Harry Snady
Diplomate, American Board
of Gastroenterology
New York
USA

David I Soybel
Department of General and
Gastrointestinal Surgery
Brigham and Women's Hospital
Boston, Massachusetts
USA

H J Stein
Department of Surgery
Klinikum rechts der Isar
Munich
GERMANY

Tadashi Terada
Second Department of Pathology
Tottori University, Faculty of Medicine
Yonago
JAPAN

Hsin-Min Tsao
Department of Pathology
Case Western Reserve University
School of Medicine
Cleveland, Ohio
USA

Edda A M Vuhahula
Department of Histopathology
and Morbid Anatomy
Muhimbili University College
of Health Sciences
Dar es Salaam
TANZANIA

James Y Wang
Division of Gastroenterology
and Nutrition
University of Minnesota Medical
School
Minneapolis, Minnesota
USA

Ronald R Watson
University of Arizona School
of Medicine
Tucson, Arizona
USA

Kate E Williamson
Department of Pathology
Queen's University of Belfast
Belfast
NORTHERN IRELAND

Masao Yamamoto
Department of Anatomy
Hiroshima University School
of Medicine
Hiroshima
JAPAN

Masaki Yamamoto
Drug Safety Research Laboratories
Takeda Chemical Industries Ltd
Osaka
JAPAN

Toshikazu Yoshikawa
First Department of Medicine
Kyoto Prefectural University
of Medicine
Kyoto
JAPAN

PREFACE

The gastrointestinal tract is one of the most diverse mammalian systems, and even single regions contain cells of diverse physiology and function. It is thus not surprising that a variety of alterations arise in conditions of metabolic or cellular stress. At the very least, some of these transformations may be considered as adaptive (for example in response to starvation) and at the very worst, destructive (for example in necrosis due to toxins or cancer).

Ultimately, the clinician's aim is to reverse or ameliorate the adverse changes, but this can only be achieved with an understanding of the basic mechanisms responsible for the disease process. Thus, in simple terms, the function of this book is to provide a source of investigative techniques that can be applied to the gastrointestinal tract, from salivary gland secretion to cell turnover in the rectum. The techniques will be directly applicable to man, but their applications to animal studies are also discussed.

Finally, even though the reader is tempted to apply one of these techniques, it is important to remember that other methods described in this book will also be applicable to investigating pathological mechanisms. For example, changes in enterocyte turnover may have implications for permeability and protein turnover as well as indices of malabsorption and basement membrane structure. The reader is therefore encouraged to adopt a multi-faceted approach and this book is a useful tool to achieve these aims.

In this book, individual chapters contain detailed descriptions of the various techniques, as well as citations to other methods. An important feature of the book is the applicability of these procedures. Many techniques are described in relation to investigating a specific problem. This has the aim of placing the methodology in the context of relevant questions, thus indicating the usefulness of each procedure.

Victor R Preedy and Ronald R Watson
London and Tuscon
1998

1

Attention to methodology: Fundamental criteria for studies in gastroenterology

KB Raja, RJ Simpson, RR Watson and VR Preedy

In this book, a variety of techniques are described, including analytical subcellular fractionation, permeability, intestinal secretion, ambulatory pH monitoring, analysis of cytokine profiles, ion transport and motility measurements, to name just a few. However, it is important to note that following a set of protocols *per se* is no guarantee of unequivocal results. A number of problems can arise, which basically emphasizes that strict attention should be paid to the validity of the data generated. Most experimental scientists are familiar with routine methodological obstacles, such as water baths failing to attain a set temperature, the dispensing of inaccurate volumes by automatic pipettes, etc. However, in investigative pathology, each technique will have its own set of methodological limitations or danger areas where practical misfortune can arise. Many of the chapters in this book describe some of the specific difficulties pertaining to individual techniques. For example, in subcellular fractionation, steps are needed to prevent damage to organelles (due to mechanical disruption of membranes) or enzyme inactivation (as a consequence of excess heat generation). However, in the estimation of protein synthesis the problems are more conceptual. Thus, the development of the *flooding dose* method itself was a response to overcome problems that arose in the *constant infusion* technique, for example the inability to determine more precisely the specific radioactivity of the precursor pool in tissues with a high rate of protein turnover, such as the hepato-gastrointestinal tract.

It would be imprudent to list all the difficulties that could arise in the usage of the techniques described in this book. Instead, as an example, we have decided to concentrate on possible problems that can be encountered when using *in vitro/vivo* techniques for measuring intestinal nutrient absorption.

Intestinal transport processes have the capacity to adapt to physiological and/or pathophysiological demands. Alterations in the transport of solutes, which occurs via the transcellular or paracellular routes, can thus be brought about by events taking place in the lumen, in the epithelium itself or in the systemic blood supply to the epithelium. In order to investigate adequately the adaptive responses of the intestine one has to consider not only the mucosal dimensions (e.g. villous height, cell number) but also the functional characteristics of the enterocytes involved. However, measurement of the intestinal functional capacity within a living animal without any possible metabolic influences arising due to experimental manipulations, is technically a mammoth task!

In order to minimise the effects of luminal or corporeal factors on intestinal function, *in vitro* methods such as intestinal slices/fragments, everted sacs and brush-border membrane vesicles, are thus commonly employed to investigate the absorption of nutrients at the GI level. Although such studies have helped to elucidate important mechanisms, for example Na^+-dependent nutrient transport, and have contributed vastly to our current understanding of transport processes, one needs to critically evaluate the data before establishing how well the information relates to the physiological situation. One important aspect that needs addressing is whether the functional capacity of the intestinal tissue *in vitro* is analogous to the *in vivo* situation.

Tissue viability when performing *in vitro* studies, is commonly assessed by morphological (light and electron-microscopy) and/or biochemical (dye exclusion or release of intracellular enzymes/ components) studies. However, functional studies seldom consider the significance of the metabolic (energy) status of the tissue, even when investigating the kinetics of actively transported materials. The importance of metabolic status was highlighted in a study[1] which directly compared the rates of iron transport by mouse duodenum ascertained *in vitro* (intestinal fragments) and *in vivo* (in situ tied-off duodenal segment of anaesthetised animal). The study clearly demonstrated that duodenal ATP levels and nucleotide energy charge decline rapidly on simply removing the tissue from the animal. A further significant fall in the parameters ensued during preparation of the fragments. However, in addition to morphological observations at the electron microscopy level, metabolic viability of tissue was apparent by the recovery in both parameters following incubation of the fragments for a short period in oxygenated physiological media. Furthermore, the *in vitro* system exhibited similar quantitative and qualitative kinetics for iron transport to those *in vivo*, in both normal and experimental (i.e. hypoxia induced increase in iron absorption) animals.

The extrapolation of absorption rates to values obtained in anaesthetised acutely laporotomised animals (usually used as gold standard in transport studies) has however, recently been shown by Uhing and Kimura[2] to be subject to methodological limitations. These workers employed a dual-infusion technique for measuring glucose transport in rats implanted simultaneously with cannulas in the portal vein, the aorta and the GI tract. The absorption rates of 3-O-methyl-D-glucose, a non-metabolised glucose, was ascertained from the ratio of two isotopes in the aorta following infusion of radiolabelled solute into the GI tract, whilst the same solute labelled with a different isotope was simultaneously infused into the portal vein. Uhing and Kimura[2] demonstrated that glucose absorption in rats that had undergone the traditional surgical procedure (i.e. anaesthesia + laporotomy + loop perfusion) had markedly reduced absorption values as compared to the chronically cannulated, non-anaesthetised, non-restrained animals: Comparable absorption rates were not apparent until about 24h post-anaesthesia and laporotomy.[2] Furthermore, by determining the relative appearance of 3-O-methyl-D-glucose and of the passively transported marker, L-glucose (a non-metabolised stereoisomer of D-glucose), in the portal vein and aorta of the same animal (thus eliminating inter-animal variability), these workers were able to demonstrate that virtually all the glucose transport in their chronic experimental model was 'active', even at concentrations of upto 400 mM.[3] The contribution of passive transport was minimal and unaffected by anaesthesia and intestinal manipulation.[2,3] These findings of 'active' glucose transport are in agreement with *in vivo* studies carried out in humans,[4] under conditions in which anaethesia and intestinal manipulation was avoided. The data are however, in conflict with previous findings which demonstrated passive transport overhauling active transport even at lower glucose concentrations.[5-7] The discrepancies appear to have arisen potentially from the adverse effects of anaesthesia and of acute surgical bowel manipulation.

This elaborated example serves to illustrate that, not only the rates of absorption, but also the mechanism of absorption of the nutrient being studied could vary depending on the technique used, thus making the comparison to the *in vivo* physiological situation complicated.

The scientific method is an iterative process, with past results leading to new conceptual and technical advances which may render the earlier data or techniques obsolete. An essential part of this process however, is that the utmost attention is paid to the validity of any set of experimental data. If a scientist adheres to this principle, then future workers can build on the published findings, with confidence.

Many of the chapters in this book contain information on the steps needed to avoid artefactual results. The experimental scientist is thus advised to pay strict attention to these procedures.

References

1 Raja KB, Simpson RJ and Peters TJ Comparison of $^{59}Fe^{3+}$ uptake *in vitro* and *in vivo* by mouse duodenum. *Biochim Biophys Acta.* 1987; **901**: 52-60.

2. Uhing MR and Kimura RE The effect of surgical bowel manipulation and anaesthesia on intestinal glucose absorption in rats. *J Clin Invest* 1995; **95**: 2790-2798.

3. Uhing MR and Kimura RE Active transport of 3-O-methyl glucose by the small intestine in chronically catheterized rats. *J Clin Invest* 1995; **95**: 2799-2805

4. Fine KD, Santa AC, Porter JL and Fordtran JS Effect of D-glucose on intestinal permeability and its passive absorption in human small intestine *in vivo*. *Gastroenterology.* 1993; **105**: 1117-1125.

5. Debnam ES and Levin RJ An experimental method of identifying and quantifying the active transfer electrogenic component from the diffuse component during sugar absorption measured *in vivo*. *J Physiol.* 1975; **246**: 181-196.

6. Murakami E, Saito M and Suda M. Contribution of diffusive pathway in intestinal absorption of glucose in the rat under normal feeding condition. *Specialia* 1977; **15**: 1469-1470.

7. Westergaard H (Insulin modulates rat intestinal glucose transport: effect of hypoinsulinemia and hyperinsulinemia. *Am J Physiol* 1989; **256**: 9911-9918.

2

Measurement of protein synthesis in the gastrointestinal tract

Tor H Bark and Peter J Garlick

Summary

Protein synthesis is important for gastrointestinal tissues to maintain cell renewal and the production of intestinal hormones and immunoreactive proteins. Investigations of the pathophysiology of protein synthesis in intestinal disease have previously been restricted to studies *in vitro* or in animals. However, techniques using stable isotopes have now been developed to the stage where they can be employed to measure protein synthesis rates in tissues of human patients and volunteers. This article describes the theory and application to gastrointestinal tissues of the two most commonly employed methods for measuring protein synthesis rates in humans, the flooding method and the constant infusion method, and gives examples of their use.

Introduction

The gastrointestinal tract serves several important functions in the body. In addition to its digestive and absorptive functions, and the production of intestinal hormones and immunoreactive proteins, the gut also constitutes a selective barrier to a variety of potentially toxic substances in the intestinal lumen. To maintain these functions protein synthesis is an especially important metabolic process. Cell renewal and protein turnover rates are high in the gastrointestinal tract compared with other tissues. It has been calculated that 50-60 g of protein are synthesized in the intestine daily in an adult man, contributing about 15-20% of total body protein synthesis. This rapid cell and protein turnover may be associated with the intestinal vulnerability to medical treatments such as radiation or cytotoxic drug therapy. The importance of the intestinal barrier function has been emphasized in catabolic states such as trauma and sepsis. Translocation of enteric bacteria through a defect in the mucosal barrier layer is suspected of promoting multiple organ failure in severe stress.

The accumulation or loss of protein in organs such as the gastrointestinal tract can be achieved in various ways by changes in rates of synthesis and degradation of cell protein. Previous investigations of protein synthesis and degradation, known collectively as protein turnover, in states such as inflammatory bowel disease (IBD) have focused on protein turnover in the whole body, as available techniques for assessing whole body rates are relatively non-invasive. However, protein synthesis and protein degradation are complex and opposing processes, controlled by a variety of organ specific hormonal, chemical and physical signals. Therefore, it is important that rates of protein turnover can be measured in the intestinal tissues in order to understand the pathophysiology of disease in abdominal organs. This incentive has led to the development of methods for measuring gut protein synthesis in humans, mostly using stable isotopes, which have been used for example, to show that mucosal protein synthesis in the colon is increased during ulcerative colitis.[1] Changes in intestinal protein metabolism have also been related to gastrointestinal disturbances in clinical states of alcohol abuse.[2] Most studies on intestinal protein turnover have concentrated on outcome in terms of protein synthesis, as reliable direct methods for measuring protein degradation *in vivo* are less well documented. Therefore the aim of the present chapter is to describe techniques suitable for *in vivo* studies of protein synthesis in patients and human volunteers.

Rates of protein synthesis have been measured for many years in cells and animal tissues using radioactively labelled amino acids. However, since the introduction of stable isotopes for measuring protein and amino acid metabolism in 1939 by Schoenheimer, *et al*[3] labelling with stable isotopes has remained the method of choice for measuring both protein synthesis and degradation in human subjects. Stable isotopes have been very widely used for assessing rates of protein synthesis and degradation in the whole body,[4] but only in the last 10 to15 years have methods of measurement of stable isotopes been sufficiently sensitive to permit analysis on small samples of human tissues[5,6] Some stable isotopes commonly used in metabolic studies, and their more well known radioactive counterparts are shown in Table 2.1.

Table 2.1. – Isotopes of elements commonly used in metabolic research

Element	Normal	Stable	Radioactive
Hydrogen	^{1}H	^{2}H (0.015%)	^{3}H
Carbon	^{12}C	^{13}C (1.1%)	^{13}C
Nitrogen	^{14}N	^{15}N (0.37%)	–
Oxygen	^{16}O	^{18}O (0.2%)	–

The "Normal" isotope is the one occuring most abundantly in nature. "Stable" or "Heavy" isotopes also occur naturally, and their average natural abundance is shown in parentheses.

Methods

Theoretical aspects

The general procedure for measuring the rate of protein synthesis in a tissue is to administer an amino acid labelled with the chosen isotope into the bloodstream, and then to make measurements of the appearance of the isotope in tissue protein. The amount of label incorporated into protein can be measured directly by taking a sample of the tissue after a defined period of time, or it can be inferred from the disappearance of isotope from blood by measuring its arterio-venous difference. The other information that is needed is the average isotopic enrichment of the free amino acid that is being incorporated into protein (the precursor). The rate of protein synthesis is then calculated by the following equation:

$$FSR = E_p/E_f \times t$$

The FSR is the amount of protein that is synthesized per day expressed as the fraction of the protein in the tissue (units: %/d or %/h). E_p and E_f are the isotopic enrichments of the labelled amino acid in tissue protein and in the free amino acid precursor, respectively. The isotopic enrichment of a compound is defined as the proportion of the total molecules that are labelled with the tracer. In theory, the measurement of precursor enrichment should be obtained from the pool of amino acyl tRNA in the tissue. This measurement is difficult because of the extremely rapid rate of turnover of the amino acyl tRNA pool and its very small size which necessitates large tissue samples for analysis, so it is rarely used in practice. However, all techniques for measuring protein synthesis rates share the problem of identifying the proper precursor pool. Depending on how the labelled amino acid is administered, there can be large differences in enrichment between the free amino acid in the plasma and in the tissue, the two pools that are most readily available for analysis. When the label is given as a true tracer, i.e. in a very small amount so that metabolism cannot be disturbed, the intracellular enrichment may be 20% to 75% lower than the plasma.[7] This occurs because the precursor amino acid could be derived from a variety of sources (see Fig. 2.1), which might be highly labelled (e.g. directly from the plasma), unlabelled (e.g. from proteolysis) or intermediate in labelling (e.g. the general intracellular pool). As it is not clear which of these alternative pools is more appropriate for calculating protein synthesis rates, there has been an intense debate during recent years how best to make measurements of protein synthesis under different conditions. This debate has centered on two different methods of administering the labelled amino acid, by continuous infusion of a tracer amount or by injection of a large, non-tracer (flooding) amount.[5,6] These two approaches will be described in detail below.

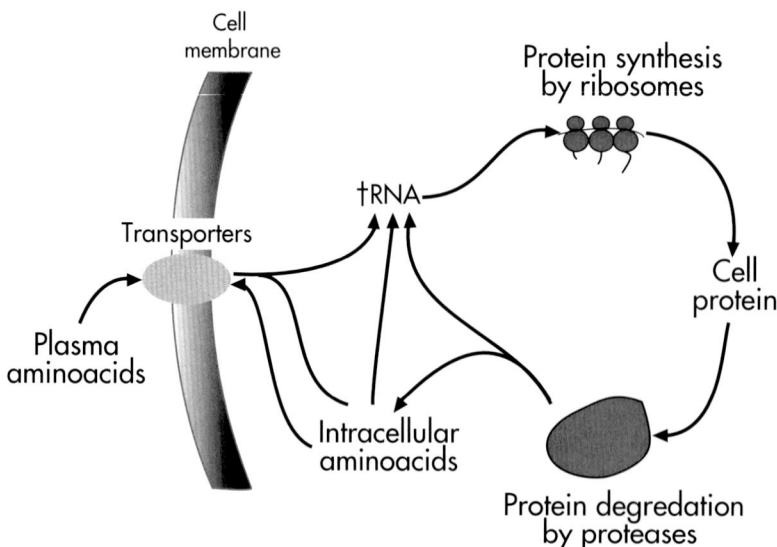

Figure 2.1 – The sources of amino acids for tRNA charging and protein synthesis.

Measurement of stable isotopes by mass spectrometry

As the stable isotopes are not radioactive, they cannot be measured by means of their radiation, and in general are measured by mass spectrometry. Two rather different types of instrument are in general use, depending on the application. A gas isotope ratio mass spectrometer (GIRMS) is used to determine the enrichment of a compound that is in gaseous form, usually as CO_2 (for ^{13}C or ^{18}O) or N_2 (for ^{15}N). Thus, the labelled compound must first be converted into this form by chemical means which might be either selective for a single atom in the molecule (e.g. conversion of a carboxyl group to CO_2) or non-selective (e.g. combustion). The gas is released into the mass spectrometer under high vacuum, where it is ionized by a stream of electrons and the masses distinguished by accelerating the molecules through a magnetic field.

The advantage of GIRMS is its ability to measure extremelylow levels of enrichment, but relatively large amounts of gas are required for analysis. This technique is usually used to assess the labelling of an amino acid in protein, which has low enrichment but is relatively abundant. With the newest generation of instruments, the limitation of sample size is much improved.

The second type of mass spectrometry is gas chromatography mass spectrometry (GCMS). With this procedure the labelled compound is first converted to a volatile derivative, by blocking polar groups such as $-NH_2$ or $-COOH$, which facilitates separation of the labelled compound on a gas chromatograph. The eluate from the GC is then led directly into a mass spectrometer where molecules are ionized by electrons (EI) or chemically (CI) before being separated according to their mass either electrostatically in a "quadrupole", or magnetically. The advantage of GCMS is that it requires very small amounts of sample, and can monitor several masses simultaneously, making multiple labelling experiments feasible. Typically, however, it requires high enrichment for accurate measurement. GCMS is therefore well suited for measurement of enrichment of free amino acids in plasma and tissues. When amino acids such as $[^{13}C]$leucine are used, both GIRMS and GCMS instruments are required to measure the protein and free amino acid respectively. However, with certain labelled amino acids (see $[^2H_5]$phenylalanine below), a modification of the GCMS technique can be used for measurements of

protein as well a free amino acid, so a relatively low-cost GCMS instrument is all that is required.[8] General descriptions of mass spectrometry and its applications to metabolism are available.[9-11]

Choice of labelled amino acid

In theory any amino acid can be used for measurement of protein synthesis rates. However, the amino acid chosen should be well distributed throughout body protein. It is not very important that the amino acid should not be degraded, which would result in the label being passed to other amino acids, as the mass spectrometric methods of analysis are sensitive enough to measure only the specific amino acid that is given. Commonly used labels are L-$[1-^{13}C]$ leucine, and L-$[^2H_5]$phenylalanine. Leucine is the amino acid used most often with constant infusion, although phenylalanine and valine have also been employed. Leucine was also used in initial investigations and validation of the flooding method in humans, but has now been superseded by phenylalanine, which is more easily measured by GCMS than leucine. With the methodological improvements referred to in the previous section, accurate measurements of low enrichment in samples of about 1 mg protein can be made.[8,12]

Measurement of protein synthesis by flooding with [²H₅]phenylalanine

Difficulties with measuring the true precursor enrichment when labelled amino acids are given in trace amounts led to the development of the flooding method, both in animal models and in human studies. In order to reduce the problem, Loftfield[13] suggested that a large dose of the unlabelled amino acid should be injected together with the label. This amount, often referred to as a flooding dose, would then dominate the small endogenous pool of unlabelled free amino acid and would facilitate equilibration between the various free amino acid pools. This is of particular importance when measuring protein synthesis in the gut. Due to the anatomical location of mucosal cells, the free amino acid in the gastrointestinal tract is derived from three possible sources, the blood, the lumen or from intracellular proteolysis. Injecting a large dose of amino acid reduces this problem by flooding the system with amino acid of uniform enrichment. Moreover, in the gastrointestinal tract the duration of measurements may be important, since synthesis of hormones and enzymes which are subsequently secreted, as well as the rapid turnover of mucosal proteins, will result in subsequent loss of label that has been incorporated into protein. The short period of measurement required by the flooding method minimizes these losses.

Experimental Protocol

To prepare the isotope for injection, 2 g of L-[^{2}H$_5$]phenylalanine are added to 1.0 L of 0.45% saline together with 18 g of unlabelled phenylalanine and dissolved with gentle warming and shaking. This makes a 2% solution of phenylalanine of 10% isotopic enrichment. This solution is filtered and heat sterilized, before storing in bags containing about 170 ml each, which are suitable for injection into a single subject at a dose of 45 mg/kg.

An intravenous line is established in each arm, one for injection, the other for sampling. First a base-line sample of blood is obtained from the sampling line before injection of isotope. The [^{2}H$_5$]phenylalanine is given intravenously into the injection line at a constant rate over a 10 min interval, starting at time zero. Blood samples are then taken at 5, 10, 15, 30, 45 and 60 min after starting the injection, to measure the enrichment of free phenylalanine in the plasma pool. Blood samples are initially kept on ice, to be centrifuged later and the plasma frozen for storage and GCMS analysis.

A tissue sample is taken at an accurately recorded time point between 30 and 60 min after the start of isotope injection. Samples from the gastrointestinal tract can be obtained by either perioperative biopsy or endoscopic sampling. Rapid subsequent handling of samples is important when studying protein synthesis rates to prevent continued incorporation of label into protein. Specimens should therefore be excised immediately and kept cold, or preferably put in liquid nitrogen. Specimens from solid organs like liver or spleen are usually frozen intact. Intestinal specimens may be frozen intact or refined using mucosal scraping or cell separation, in which case they must be kept cold. It is also advisable to add an inhibitor of protein synthesis such as cycloheximide[14] to all separation media to prevent continued incorporation of the isotope into protein during the isolation process. Tissue samples are then frozen in liquid N$_2$ and stored at -70°C.

Sample preparation.

Plasma for the determination of free phenylalanine enrichment is treated with an equal volume of 8% sulphosalicylic acid to precipitate protein, then centrifuged. The supernatant is purified by transferring to a cation exchange column (AG 50W - ×8, 100-200 mesh H$^+$ form), washing with water, then diluting with 1M NH$_4$OH. The eluate is then dried *in vacuo*.

A tissue specimen of about 50 mg is suitable for preparation, but the procedure for preparation can be modified for specimens down to 2 mg of tissue. After storage of samples, it is necessary to pulverize them prior to preparation for analysis by GCMS. For large samples (>50 mg) this is first done by grinding in a small mortar with liquid N$_2$, followed by precipitation of the protein with 3 ml of ice-cold 3% (wt/vol) perchloric acid (HClO$_4$). Smaller specimens can be placed in 1 ml HClO$_4$ and disrupted with a stirring rod. After vortex mixing, the samples are kept on ice for 10 min and then spun at 3000 rpm for 15 min. at 4°C to separate soluble free amino acids from the protein pellet. The supernatant is neutralized with KOH to precipitate KClO$_4$, kept on ice for 20 min to allow the precipitate to coalesce, and then spun at 3000 rpm for 15 min. The resulting supernatant is acidified with 1 M HCl to pH 5, then purified on small cation exchange columns (Biorad AG 50W-×8) and dried, as for plasma samples.

The protein pellet from the first spin is further washed twice with 3% HClO$_4$. The protein precipitate is dissolved in 0.3 M NaOH at 37°C for one hour and then reprecipitated with 40% HClO$_4$ to further enhance the protein washing procedure. The pellet is washed twice again in 3% HClO$_4$ before it is dissolved in 0.3 M NaOH (0.5 ml), mixed with 6 M HCl (5 ml) and hydrolyzed at 110°C for 24 hours. Before analysis, the samples are dried using a vacuum centrifugal evaporator.

Measurement of the isotopic enrichment of phenylalanine.

The enrichment of [^{2}H$_5$]phenylalanine in the dried samples of free amino acids from plasma and tissue homogenates is measured by GCMS under electron ionization and selective ion recording (EI-SIR). The procedure involves preparation of the tertiary-butyldimethylsilyl (t-BDMS) derivative[8,15,12] and measurement of the ions at mass-to-charge ratio (*m/z*) 336 and 341. The general details and theory of these procedures have been described by Wolfe.[9]

The enrichment of the phenylalanine in protein hydrolysates is measured by first converting the phenylalanine to phenethylamine with the enzyme tyrosine decarboxylase. The phenethylamine is then extracted by adding NaOH and shaking with diethyl ether. The ether layer is separated and added to a tube containing 0.1 ml of 0.1 M HCl, which is then evaporated to dryness in a stream of air. The sample is then reacted with heptafluorobutyric anhydride and the resulting heptafluorobutyryl derivative is measured by GCMS under EI-SIR. The ions monitored are m/z 106 and 109, rather than the expected m/z 104 and 109 which correspond to the unlabelled and labelled molecules respectively. The measurement at m/z 106 allows a larger amount of sample to be analysed without overloading the detectors, as the signal at m/z 106 is a small but fixed proportion of that at m/z 104. These procedures have been described in detail.[8,12]

Calculation

The FSR of protein (in %/d) is calculated from the formula:

$$FSR = 100 \times E_p / A_f$$

where E_p is the enrichment of phenylalanine in tissue protein at time t after isotope injection and A_f is the area under the curve for plasma phenylalanine enrichment versus time (expressed in days) between times zero and t.[16] If the experimental design includes a repeat measurement, then Ep will be the difference in enrichment in protein of two biopsies taken at times zero and t.

The enrichment of free phenylalanine in the tissue sample is used to check that 'flooding' has equalized the intracellular and plasma enrichments. If the tissue value is not at least 80% of the plasma value, either a larger dose of phenylalanine or a shorter period of measurement should be considered.

Constant infusion of [1-^{13}C]Leucine

The aim of the constant infusion method is to set up a steady state or plateau of labelling of the tracer amino acid in plasma and subsequently in all intracellular pools of the body.[17-19] Infusions lasting 4-12 h are usually primed with a bolus dose of the label to achieve a plateau more quickly. At the end of an infusion, a tissue sample is taken as with the flooding method. An obvious advantage of the constant infusion method is the possibility of making simultaneous determinations of whole body protein turnover, which also employ a constant infusion of [1-^{13}C]leucine.[4,20,21]

The first studies using constant infusion to assess tissue protein synthesis in humans involved measurement of muscle with [^{15}N]lysine[22] and of gastrointestinal tissues with [^{15}N]glycine.[23] Subsequently, most constant infusion studies have used [l-^{13}C]leucine, which is cheaper and easier to measure. The transamination product of leucine, α-ketoisocaproic acid (KIC), is often used in preference to plasma leucine to give an estimate of the precursor pool enrichment in muscle, since its enrichment was found to be similar to that of free leucine in muscle.[24] However, it is not advisable to use the KIC for non-muscle tissues such as the gut. As the KIC is made mainly in muscle, there is little reason to suppose that the KIC reflects the free leucine enrichment in gastrointestinal tissues. A recent study has shown that the enrichment of the tissue free leucine is better for calculating protein synthesis in duodenal mucosa then the plasma leucine or KIC.[25]

Experimental Protocol

The infusion solution is prepared by dissolving [l-^{13}C]leucine in 0.9% saline to the required concentration, without any additional unlabelled amino acid, followed by sterilization and storage. A suitable rate of infusion is 1.0 mg leucine per kg body weight per hour preceded by a priming dose of 1.0 mg per kg.[25] The tracer is administered into an arm vein over a period of between 4 and 6 h. Blood samples are taken from the opposite arm before starting infusion and at regular, usually hourly, intervals during the infusion. These are used to confirm that plateau labelling is maintained throughout the infusion. Tissue samples are obtained at the end of the infusion by the same procedures as those used with the flooding method, and are rapidly cooled in liquid N_2 and stored at -70°C.

Sample preparation and analysis

Blood samples for determination of the plasma isotopic enrichment are treated in the same way as for the flooding method. The tissue handling and preparation of protein hydrolysates are also the same as these for the flooding method. The isotopic enrichment of the free amino acid in plasma is measured by GCMS of the t-BDMS derivative under EI-SIR with monitoring of the ions at m/z 302 and 303.[15,26]

The enrichment of leucine in the protein hydrolysate is measured by GIRMS of CO_2 generated from the leucine. This is done either by decarboxylating the leucine with ninhydrin or by combusting the leucine to CO_2 in a special type of mass spectrometer known as a gas chromatography-combustion-gas isotope ratio mass spectrometer (GC-C-GIRMS). This instrument combines a GC to separate the amino acid, followed by a combustion furnace which feeds the CO_2 directly into the GIRMS. The technical details of these procedures have been described.[27]

Calculation

Rates of protein synthesis in %/day can be calculated by a similar formula to that used with the flooding method, i.e.

$$FSR = E_p /(E_f \times t)$$

where E_p is the enrichment of leucine in protein and E_f is the enrichment of the free leucine in the tissue sample, which is assumed to have remained constant over the full period of infusion. t is the duration of the infusion in days. However, there might be some uncertainty in the values for precursor enrichment during the period immediately following the priming dose and before a plateau is established. If it is possible to take 2 tissue samples, one at a time soon after the plateau is established and a second at the end of the infusion, the difference in enrichment of leucine in protein between these two samples (ΔE_p) can be used to calculate protein synthesis from the following formula:

$$FSR = 100 \, (\Delta E_p/(E_f \times t)$$

where E_f is the average leucine enrichment in the tissue and t is the time between tissue samples.

Arterio-Venous difference method

An alternative method for determining both the synthesis and the degradation of protein simultaneously

has also been used for the GI tract. The technique by which the net uptake or outflow of an amino acid is determined by measuring the arterial and venous concentrations and the blood flow rate has been used in metabolic studies for many years[28] However, if an isotopically labelled amino acid is simultaneously infused, the rates of synthesis and degradation of protein can also be determined.[29] Although this method avoids tissue biopsies, for measurement on the gut, placement of catheters in an artery and the portal vein limits its possibilities mainly to experimental animal models. However it has been used in humans to measure protein turnover in normal colon and in colonic tumours[30]

Application to animal studies

Both flooding and infusion have been widely used in animal studies. The flooding method in particular has been used successfully to measure protein synthesis in gastrointestinal tissues of a variety of animal species (e.g. rat,[7, 31] mouse,[32] sheep,[33] pig,[34] birds[35,36] and fish[37, 38]).

Results

Examples of studies of intestinal protein synthesis in man

The first published study of protein synthesis rates in human gastrointestinal tissue *in vivo* employed constant intravenous infusion of [^{15}N]glycine into cancer patients during 12-19 h immediately preceding surgery.[23] FSR values, determined for the tumor and

Table 2.2. — Rates of protein synthesis in human tissues

Normal tissues	FSR ± sem*	Pathological states	FSR ± sem*
Skeletal muscle [16]	1.95 ± 0.12	Muscle (3 days after surgery)[42]	0.91 ± 0.14
Heart [40]	5.2 ± 0.8	Liver (ulcerative colitis)[1]	35.4 ± 2.3
Liver [1]	20.7 ± 1.9	Colon (ulcerative colitis) [1]	24.7 ± 2.5
Colonic mucosa [1]	9.4 ± 1.2	Colon (villous adenoma) [1]	36.7 ± 2.5
Oesophagus [41]	28.2 ± 1.3	Colon (malignant tumor) [1]	21.7 ± 1.9
Stomach (antrum) [41]	43.9 ± 5.3	Oesophagus (Barrett's) [41]	23.1 ± 1.2
Stomach (fundus) [41]	47.0 ± 6.4		
Lymphocytes[14]	6.2 ± 0.4		

* Fractional synthesis rates and standard errors, measured by flooding with [^{2}H$_5$]phenylalanine or [1-^{13}C]leucine.

for adjacent normal tissue, were about 15%/d in both. Moreover, a significant correlation was demonstrated between rates in the tumor and in corresponding normal tissue. In a later study the same group measured rates in healthy gastrointestinal tissues, showing that intravenous hyperalimentation did not affect the values obtained.[39] The rates in the small intestine, duodenum and stomach were higher than those in liver and colon, and much higher than in the oesophagus.

More recently the flooding method, with either [1-13C]leucine or [2H5]phenylalanine, has also been employed to examine protein synthesis rates in human gastrointestinal tissues. Some of the results are shown in Table 2.2, together with values in a range of other tissues. It can be seen that in general, rates of protein synthesis in gastrointestinal tissues are much higher than those in other organs. Heys et al[1] injected a flooding amount of [1-13C]leucine into various groups of patients just before surgery began, then took samples during the operation. Rates of protein synthesis in liver were about twice as high as those in colonic mucosa. However, the rates in both tissues were much stimulated by the presence of inflammatory bowel disease. Similar results have been obtained from the small intestine with measurement by constant infusion,[43] showing an elevated rate of protein synthesis in the abnormal mucosa of patients with coeliac disease. The rates in tumours of the bowel, both malignancies and villous adenomas, were also higher than in healthy colonic mucosa. Changes in the rate of protein synthesis in malignant tumours have been used to indicate whether specific treatments altered the tumour growth rate.[23,44,45] For example, in patients who had been fed intravenously for 20 h before measurement, rates of tumour protein synthesis were elevated compared with those in patients who were fasted.[45] Moreover, the composition of the amino acid mixture given was also shown to be important: a solution enriched with branched chain amino acids did not stimulate the tumour as much as one containing a normal balanced mixture.[46] A similar conclusion was reached by measuring the expression of Proliferating Cell Nuclear Antigen, an independent marker of cell proliferation.[46] These results suggest not only that feeding stimulates the tumour, but also that tumour growth is dependent on the composition of the nutrients given. Changes in tumour protein synthesis with feeding have not, however, been detected when constant infusion of label was the method of measurement.[23,44]

Modern analytical techniques, either with GCMS for [2H5]phenylalanine or GC-C-GIRMS for [13C] leucine, are very sensitive and only require small samples of tissue for measurement. This is an advantage because the tissue can be sampled endoscopically. For example, Park et al[41] measured the synthesis rates in very small samples of mucosa taken endoscopically from the oesophagus and stomach after flooding with [2H5]phenylalanine. In patients with Barrett's disease, the mucosa of columnar lined oesophagus showed a lower rate of protein synthesis than that of healthy squamous lined oesophagus.[41]

Discussion

Reliable methods are now available for examining *in vivo* protein dynamics in the tissues of the human gastrointestinal tract. Hence studies in human volunteers and patients can now verify or replace those previously performed only in animal models. The techniques are relatively simple to perform, and the use of stable isotopes eliminates the potential radiation hazard associated with conventional use of radioisotopic labels. Relatively low-cost mass spectrometers are available for performing the analyses, and especially if [2H5]phenylalanine is employed, only one type of instrument (GCMS) is required. Also, the number of laboratories having mass spectrometry capability is increasing, and studies are frequently performed in collaboration with one of these centres. Instruments and analytical techniques are constantly being improved, broadening the range of possible investigations. In particular, the methods are becoming more sensitive, consequently requiring smaller samples of tissue for analysis. The value of this is that future studies will be less limited to measurements but on the mixed protein from the tissue, and will be able to examine specific cell types or individual proteins, thus bridging the gaps between whole organ physiology and cell and molecular biology.

References

1. Heys SD, Park KG, McNurlan MA, Keenan RA, Miller JD, Eremin O, Garlick PJ. Protein synthesis rates in colon and liver: stimulation by gastrointestinal pathologies. *Gut* 1992; **33**: 976-981.

2. Marway JS, Bonner A, Peters TJ, Preedy VR. Protein synthesis in the gastrointestinal tract and its modification by ethanol. In: Preedy VR, Watson RR, ed. *Alcohol and the Gastrointestinal Tract*. New York:CRC Press, 1996; 255-272.

3. Schoenheimer R, Ratner S, Rittenberg D. Studies in protein metabolism; metabolism of tyrosine. *J Biol Chem* 1939; **127**: 333-344.

4. Waterlow JC, Garlick PJ, Millward DJ. *Protein Turnover in Mammalian Tissues and in the Whole Body*. North Holland, Amsterdam. 1978.

5. Garlick PJ, McNurlan MA, Essén P, Wernerman J. Measurement of tissue protein synthesis rates *in vivo*: a critical analysis of contrasting methods. *Am J Physiol* 1994; **266**: E287-E297.

6. Rennie MJ, Smith K, Watt PW. Measurement of human tissue protein synthesis: an optimal approach. *Am J Physiol* 1994; **266**: E298-E307.

7. McNurlan MA, Tomkins AM, Garlick PJ. The effect of starvation on the rate of protein synthesis in rat liver and small intestine. *Biochem J* 1979; **178**: 373-379.

8. Calder AG, Anderson SE, Grant I, McNurlan MA, Garlick PJ. The determination of low d_5-phenylalanine enrichment (0.002-0.09 atom percent excess), after conversion to phenylethylamine, in relation to protein turnover studies by gas chromatography/mass spectrometry. *Rapid Comm Mass Spec* 1992; **6**: 421-424.

9. Wolfe RR. *Radioactive and Stable Isotope Tracers in Biomedicine (Principles and Practice of Kinetic Analysis.)* New York:Wiley-Liss, Inc. 1992.

10. Preston T, Slater C. Mass spectrometric analysis of stable-isotope-labelled amino acid tracers. *Proc Nutr Soc* 1994; **53**: 363-372.

11. Pacy PJ, Cheng KN, Thompson GN, Halliday D. Stable isotopes as tracers in clinical research. *Ann Nutr Metab* 1989; **33**: 65-78.

12. McNurlan MA, Essén P, Thorell A, Calder AG, Anderson SE, Ljungqvist O, Sandgren A, Grant I, Tjäder I, Ballmer PE, Wernereman J, Garlick PJ. Response of protein synthesis in human skeletal muscle to insulin: an investigation with L-[^{2}H$_5$]phenylalanine. *Am J Physiol* 1994; **267**: E102-E108.

13. Loftfield RB, Eigner EA. The time required for the synthesis of a ferritin molecule in rat liver. *J Biol Chem* 1958; **231**: 925-943.

14. Park KGM, Heys SD, McNurlan MA, Garlick PJ, Eremin O. (1994) Lymphocyte protein synthesis *in vivo*: a measure of activation. *Clin Sci* 1994; **86**: 671-675.

15. Calder AG, Smith A. Stable isotope ratio analysis of leucine and ketoisocaproic acid in blood plasma by gas chromatography/mass spectrometry. Use of the tertiary butyldimethylsilyl derivatives. *Rapid Commun Mass Spectrom* 1988; **2**: 14-16.

16. Garlick PJ, Wernerman J, McNurlan MA, Essén P, Lobley GE, Milne E, Calder AG, Vinnars E. Measurement of the rate of protein synthesis in muscle of postabsorptive young men by injection of a 'flooding dose' of [1-^{13}C]leucine. *Clin Sci* 1989; **77**: 329-336.

17. Loftfield RB, Harris A. Participation of free amino acids in protein synthesis. *J. Biol. Chem.* 1956; **219**: 151-159.

18. Waterlow J.C., Stephen JML. The effect of low protein diets on the turnover rates of serum, liver and muscle proteins in the rat measured by continuous infusion of L-[^{14}C]lysine. *Clin Sci Lond* 1968; **35**: 287- 305.

19. Garlick PJ, Millward DJ, James WPT. The diurnal response of muscle and liver protein synthesis *in vivo* in meal-fed rats. *Biochem J* 1973; **136**: 935-946.

20. James WPT, Sender PM, Garlick PJ, Waterlow JC. The choice of label and measurement technique in tracer studies in man. In *Dynamic Studies with Radioisotopes in Medicine*, 1974; **1**: 461-472. IAEA, Vienna.

21. Garlick PJ, McNurlan MA, Ballmer PE. Influence of dietary protein intake on whole-body protein turnover in humans. *Diabetes Care* 1991; **14**: 1189-1198.

22. Halliday D, McKeran RO. Measurement of muscle protein synthetic rate from serial muscle biopsies and total body protein turnover in man by continuous intravenous infusion of L-[1-^{15}N]lysine. *Clin Sci Mol Med* 1975; **49**: 581-590.

23. Mullen JL, Buzby GP, Gertner MH, Stein TP, Hargrove WC, Oram-Smith J, Rosato EF. Protein synthesis dynamics in human gastrointestinal malignancies. *Surgery* 1980; **87**: 331-338.

24. Matthews DE, Schwartz HP, Young RD, Motil KJ, Young VR. Relationship of plasma leucine and 1-ketoisocaproate during a L-[1-^{13}C]leucine infusion in man: a method for measuring human intracellular leucine tracer enrichment. *Metab Clin Exp* 1982; **31**: 1105-1112.

25. Nakshabendi IM, Obeidat W, Russell RI, Downie S, Smith K, Rennie MJ. Gut mucosal protein synthesis measured using intravenous and intragastric delivery of stable tracer amino acids. *Am. J. Physiol.* 1995; **269**: E996-999.

26. Schwenk WF, Berg PJ, Beaufrere B, Miles JM, Haymond MW. Use of *t*-butyldimethylsilylation in the gas chromatographic/mass spectrometric analysis of physiologic compounds found in plasma using electron-impact ionization. *Anal Biochem* 1984; **141**: 101-109.

27. Rennie MJ, Meier-Augenstein W, Watt PW, Patel A, Begley IS, Scrimgeour CM. Use of continuous- flow combustion MS in studies of human metabolism. *Biochem Soc Trans* 1996; **24**: 927-932.

28. Felig P. Amino acid metabolism in man. *Ann Rev Biochem* 1975; **44:** 933-955.

29. Gelfand RA, Barret EJ. Effect of physiologic hyperinsulinemia on skeletal muscle protein synthesis and breakdown in man. *J Clin Invest* 1987; **80:** 1-6.

30. Hagmüller E, Kollmar HB, Günther HJ, Holm E, Trede M. Protein metabolism in human colon carcinomas: *in vivo* investigations using a modified tracer technique with L-[1-^{13}C]Leucine. *Cancer Res* 1995; **55:** 1160-1167.

31. Garlick PJ, McNurlan MA, Preedy VR. A rapid and convenient technique for measuring the rate of protein synthesis in tissues by injection of [^{3}H]phenylalanine. *Biochem J* 1980; **192:** 719-723.

32. Bark TH, Garlick PJ, McNurlan MA, Lang CH. Increased protein synthesis after acute IGF-I infusion in mice is localized to muscle. *Clin Nutr* 1996; **15:** 16-17.

33. Southorn BG, Kelly JM, McBride BW. Phenylalanine flooding dose procedure is effective in measuring intestinal and liver protein synthesis in sheep. *J Nutr* 1992; **122:** 2398-2407.

34. Burrin DG, Shulman RJ, Reeds PJ, Davis TA, Gravitt KR. Porcine colostrum and milk stimulate visceral organ and skeletal muscle protein synthesis in neonatal piglets. *J Nutr* 1992; **122:** 1205-1213.

35. Muramatsu T, Coates ME, Hewitt D, Salter DN. The influence of the gut microflora on protein synthesis in liver and jejunal mucosa in chicks. *Br J Nutr* 1983; **49:** 453-462.

36. Murphy ME, Taruscio TG. Sparrows increase their rates of tissue and whole-body protein synthesis during the annual molt. *Comp Biochem Physiol* 1995; **111A:** 385-396.

37. Foster AR, Houlihan DF, Gray C, Medale F, Fauconneau B, Kaushik SJ, Le Bail PY. The effects of ovine growth hormone on protein turnover in rainbow trout. *Gen Comp Endocrinol* 1991; **82:** 111-120.

38. Lyndon AR, Houlihan DF, Hall SJ. The effect of short-term fasting and a single meal on protein synthesis and oxygen consumption in cod, Gadus morhua. *J Comp Physiol [B]* 1992; **162:** 209-15.

39. Stain TP, Mullen JL, Oram-Smith JC, Rosato EF, Wallace HW, Hargrove III WC. Relative rates of tumour, normal gut, liver, and fibrinogen protein synthesis in man. *Am J Physiol* 1978; **234:** E648-E652.

40. Park KGM, Heys SD, McKenzie J, Burns J, Eremin O, Garlick PJ. Comparison of protein synthesis rates in skeletal and heart muscle (Abstract). *J Roy Coll Surg Edinb* 1990; **35:** 121.

41. Park KGM, Thompson AM, Munro A, Langlois N, McNurlan MA, Eremin O, Garlick PJ. *in vivo* rates of mucosal protein synthesis in patients with Barrett's oesophagus. *Diseases of the Esophagus* 1994; **7:** 107-111.

42. Essén P, McNurlan MA, Sonnenfeld T, Milne E, Vinnars E, Wernerman J, Garlick PJ. Muscle protein synthesis after operation: the effects of intravenous nutrition. *Eur J Surg* 1993; **159:** 195-200.

43. Nakshabendi IM, Downie S, Russell RI, Rennie MJ. Increased rates of duodenal mucosal protein synthesis *in vivo* in patients with untreated coelia disease. *Gut* 1996; **39:** 176-179.

44. Shaw JH, Humberstone DA, Douglas RG, Koea J. Leucine kinetics in patients with benign disease, non-weight-losing cancer, and cancer cachexia: studies at the whole-body and tissue level and the response to nutritional support. *Surgery* 1991; **109:** 37-50.

45. Heys SD, Park KGM, McNurlan MA, Milne E, Eremin O, Wernerman J, Keenan RA, Garlick PJ. Stimulation of protein synthesis in human tumours by parenteral nutrition: evidence for modulation of tumour growth. *Br J Surg* 1991; **78:** 483-487.

46. McNurlan MA, Heys SD, Park KGM, Broom J, Brown DS, Eremin O, Garlick PJ. Tumour and host tissue responses to branched-chain amino acid supplementation of patients with cancer. *Clin Sci* 1994; **86:** 339-345.

3

Analytical subcellular fractionation

Tarulata Shah and Robert J Simpson

Summary

Analytical subcellular fractionation is a useful quantitative method for the investigation of tissue pathology and for the elucidation of fundamental mechanisms in cell biology. The method is based on homogenization and sucrose density gradient centrifugation to separate cellular organelles. Organelles are localized on the density gradient by assay of biochemical markers such as enzymes. Comparison of organelle profiles in diseased intestine with normal can provide useful data about pathological changes at cellular level. The technique is also useful in studies of intestinal absoptive mechanisms as the passage of nutrients such as iron through the enterocyte, can be followed.

Introduction

Analytical subcellular fractionation in combination with enzymatic microanalysis is a quantitative tool which can elucidate the causes of disease and pathological changes.[1] It can supplement qualitative morphological methods such as light and electron microscopy, by enabling analysis at the organelle level. Analytical subcellular fractionation is also useful in mechanistic studies of normal physiological and biochemical processes, e.g. the subcellular localization of specific proteins, lipids, carbohydrates or nucleic acids. In the intestine, studies of absorption of nutrients combined with subcellular fractionation can identify the absorption pathway of a nutrient.

Although studies on whole homogenates can indicate pathological changes, they are insensitive to early pathological events if these are restricted to a single region of the affected tissue, cell type or organelle. The extent of the pathological change may be obscured by the presence of a majority of normal organelles or different cell types in the homogenate. However, analytical subcellular fractionation provides a more precise indication of the target organelle and isolation of the organelle can give information on the possible pathogenesis of the disease. Despite limitations, the better defined the starting material, the more precise is the biochemical information obtained. When analytical subcellular fractionation is undertaken, using pathological tissue, it is assumed that the separation conditions will be identical with those used for the control (normal) tissue. It is therefore important to perform careful morphological analysis of the tissues studied.

Analytical subcellular fractionation usually involves the separation of organelles on the basis of size or density. The principles of separation of subcellular organelles are based on the time taken for a homogeneous population of particles of approximately equal densities to sediment at different rates in an applied field of centrifugal force, i.e. a gravitational field (g). Sedimentation is directly proportional to g, and inversely related to the density and the viscosity of the medium. Organelles are identified by marker enzyme assays.

This chapter describes the application of fractionation procedures to intestinal disease and experimental studies of intestinal iron absorption in animals and illustrates the pathological and mechanistic uses of the technique.

Methods

Highest grade chemicals are used (Merck Ltd, Lutterworth, Leics, UK or Sigma Chemical Co, Poole, Dorset, UK).

In vivo biopsies enable the use of very small quantities of tissue (at least 2 mg), avoid the problems of disintegration of tissue *post mortem* and allow studies to be performed while patients are still alive. Biopsy samples must be cooled immediately to prevent autolysis and processed rapidly. Preservation of tissue samples is best achieved by storing the biopsy intact in a small volume of buffered sucrose, e.g. 0.25 M sucrose containing 10 mM Tris-HCl, pH 7.4. Addition of chelating agents (1 mM EDTA) will minimize inactivation of enzymes.[2] Frozen tissue is usually considered unsuitable for analytical subcellular fractionation; however, rapid freezing techniques (e.g. liquid nitrogen) which preserve cell and organelle integrity may be appropriate.

Biopsy homogenization must break all cells but leave the organelles intact. The most commonly used homogenization methods involve the manually (Dounce) or mechanically (Potter) driven pestle and tube (Jencons Ltd, Leighton Buzzard, Herts. UK). The tight-fitting pestle is passed repeatedly to the bottom of the tube, forcing tissue/cells between the pestle and the side of the tube. The clearance between the pestle and tube is small enough to disrupt the cells but not to damage the organelles. It is important to prevent organelle damage and loss of enzyme activity caused by local heating during homogenization and this can be achieved by pre-cooling the pestle, tube and homogenization buffers. During homogenization

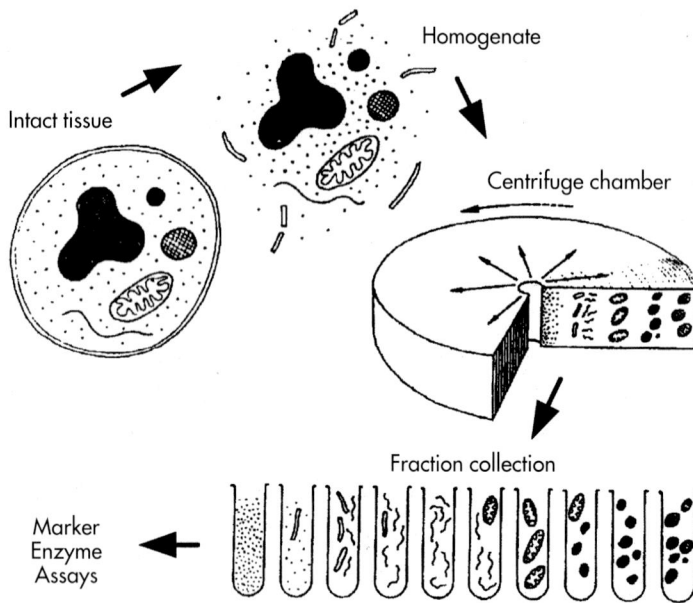

Figure 3.1 – Subcellular fractionation method.

the tube is cooled by packing ice around it and by employing slow disruption rates. The optimal number of passes with the pestle should be determined for each tissue under investigation as the rate of passage of pestle through the homogenate will vary between tissues as well as between personnel. When using glass homogenizers, careful attention must be paid to the wear of glass components as this leads to increased clearance between pestle and tube and changes in the effectiveness of homogenization over a series of experiments.

Analytical subcellular fractionation can also be carried out on post-nuclear supernatants. The use of whole homogenate could shorten the fractionation procedure and improve the integrity of the organelles recovered. However, this latter approach is disadvantaged by undisrupted cells and contamination due to erythrocytes which may overlap with other organelle marker enzyme peaks.

If only small amounts of tissue are available for study, the use of a shallow sucrose gradient to separate organelles of different sizes is preferred to lengthy fractionation procedures of differential pelleting. The specially designed small volume automatic zonal rotor of Beaufay allows rapid separation of organelles from biopsy tissue samples. The rotor and sucrose

gradient buffers are pre-cooled to 0-4°C before fractionation is commenced. This rotor is not commercially available but similar results have been reported with a commercially available vertical pocket rotor (Beckman Instruments Ltd, High Wycombe, Bucks. UK).[3,4]

Sample preparation

Jejunal biopsies are obtained with the Crosby capsule or the Debré multiple biopsy capsule from patients undergoing routine diagnostic biopsies for assessment of response to treatment.[5] The biopsy (approx. 10 mg) is homogenized in 2 ml of isotonic medium (0.25 M sucrose containing 1 mM EDTA, pH 7.4 and 22 mM ethanol, SVE medium) with 10 strokes of a loose-fitting (type A) pestle in a small Dounce homogenizer (Kontes Glass Co, Vineland, NJ, USA) and any undisrupted cells and nuclei are removed by low speed centrifugation at 800 g for 10 min.[5] The pellet is resuspended in 2 ml of SVE medium with three strokes of the type A pestle and centrifuged again. The supernatants are combined. The low-speed pellet, consisting of nuclei, large brush-border fragments and interstitial cells is resuspended in 2 ml of SVE medium with a tight-fitting (type B) pestle. All steps are carried out at 0-4°C. Fig. 3.1 shows the fractionation procedure.

Table 3.1 – Subcellular organelle marker enzymes

Organelle	Marker enzyme	EC number
Cytosol	Lactate dehydrogenase	1.1.1.27
Plasma membrane	5'-Nucleotidase	3.1.3.5
Endoplasmic reticulum	Neutral α-glucosidase	3.2.1.20
Mitochondria	Malate dehydrogenase	1.1.1.37
Lysosomes	N-Acetyl-β–glucosaminidase	3.2.1.30
Peroxisomes	Catalase	1.11.1.6
Nuclei	DNA	

Subcellular fractionation

The post-nuclear supernatant (3.5 ml) is layered onto a 30 ml sucrose gradient extending, linearly with respect to volume, from a density of 1.05 g/ml to 1.28 g/ml and resting on a 4 ml cushion of 1.32 g/ml in a specially constructed Beaufay zonal rotor. The rotor is run at 35000 rpm for 35 min at 0-4°C and after slowing to 8000 rpm the gradient is ejected from the rotor with high pressure nitrogen gas and a series of subcellular fractions are collected into pre-weighed tubes. Under high-speed sedimentation, organelles gravitate to their equilibrium densities. The weights and densities of these fractions are determined with an Abbe refractometer (Bellingham and Starley Ltd, London, UK) and reference to conversion tables.[6] All fractions are stored at -20°C provided the marker of interest is not cold labile. It is important to remember that some assays may require fresh (unfrozen) samples (e.g. DNA). The homogenate and 'gradient' fractions are then assayed for suitable marker enzymes using colorimetric, highly sensitive fluorimetric and radiometric assays. Details of enzyme assay conditions can be obtained from Peters.[5] Organelle marker enzymes are shown in Table 3.1. Automation of enzyme assays is desirable as large numbers of determinations must be made.[7]

Presentation of subcellular fractionation results

The distribution of organelle marker enzymes in sucrose density gradients for homogenates are shown as frequency-density histograms. The densities and weights of the fractions obtained after analytical subcellular fractionation are input to a computer program[8]. This calculates the frequency distribution of the enzyme activity as a function of the density span of that fraction. The soluble activity is the

activity remaining in the sample layer, pooled and plotted over the density region of 1.05-1.10 g/ml. The results are averaged by computer such that all histograms conform to the same density interval for statistical analysis. Once the distribution of organelles in the sucrose gradients is characterized by specific marker enzymes, it is possible to determine the localization of other cellular constituents.

Application to animal studies

Extensive use has been made of subcellular fractionation studies in animals. The following is a example. Adult male To-strain mice (6-8 weeks old) are used. Hypoxia is induced by placing mice in a hypobaric chamber at 0.5 atmospheres for 3 days with free access to food and water. Mice are anaesthetized with Hypnorm (Jansen Pharmaceutical Ltd, Oxford, Oxfordshire, UK - fentanyl citrate, 0.315 mg/ml/fluanisone, 10 mg/ml)/Hypnovel (Roche Products Ltd, Welwyn Garden City, Herts, UK). Radioactive iron as 0.1 ml of 0.1 mM ^{59}Fe(III)/ 0.2 mM nitrilotriacetate (NTA), in 20 mM HEPES-NaOH buffer (pH 7.2) containing 0.15 M NaCl is injected into a tied-off segment of duodenum and proximal jejunum. After 10 min incubation, the segment is removed, rinsed with 5 ml ice cold 0.15 M NaCl and the enterocytes are prepared. This is done by a modification of the vibration method of Levine & Weintraub.[9] Enterocytes are washed three times in ice-cold 10 mM HEPES-NaOH (pH 7.2)/0.15 M NaCl buffer. The enterocytes are homogenized on ice with 7 ml 0.25 M sucrose/ 10 mM HEPES-NaOH (pH 7.2) in a pre-cooled (0-4°C) Dounce homogenizer (Scientific, Millville, New Jersey, USA) with 10 strokes each of a loose and a tight-fitting pestle and the homogenate layered

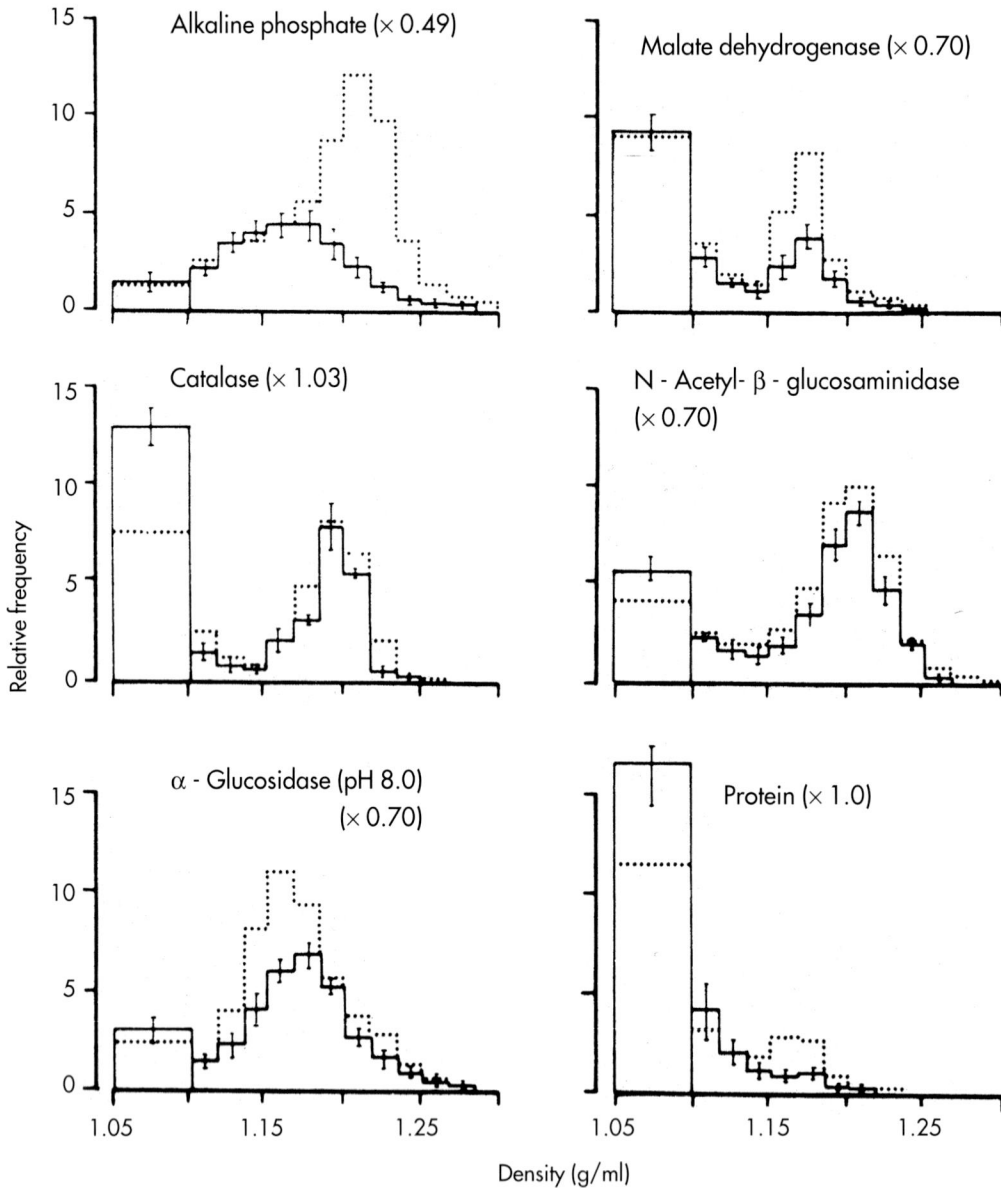

Figure 3.2 – Relative density histograms for marker enzymes. Isopycnic centrifugation of post-nuclear super-natant from jejunal biopsy homogenate from patients with treated coeliac disease showing subtotal villus atrophy. Frequency is defined as the fraction of total recovered activity present in the gradient fraction divided by the density span covered. Relative frequency is obtained by multiplying frequency data by relative specific enzyme activities (in parantheses) of homogenates of patients' biopsies (continuous lines) compared with those from control subjects (dotted lines). Activity present over the density range 1.05–1.10 g/ml represents enzyme in the sample layer and is presumed to reflect soluble activity. Percentage recoveries (± SD) for the enzymes were alkaline phosphatase, 74 ± 10 (n=5); malate dehydrogenase, 71 ± 6 (5); catalase, 108 ± 3 (3); N-acetyl-β-glucosaminidase, 79 ± 8 (3); α-glucosidase (pH 8.0), 108 ± 6 (5); protein, 81 ± 3 (4). Reproduced with permission from The Biochemical Society and Portland Press.[10]

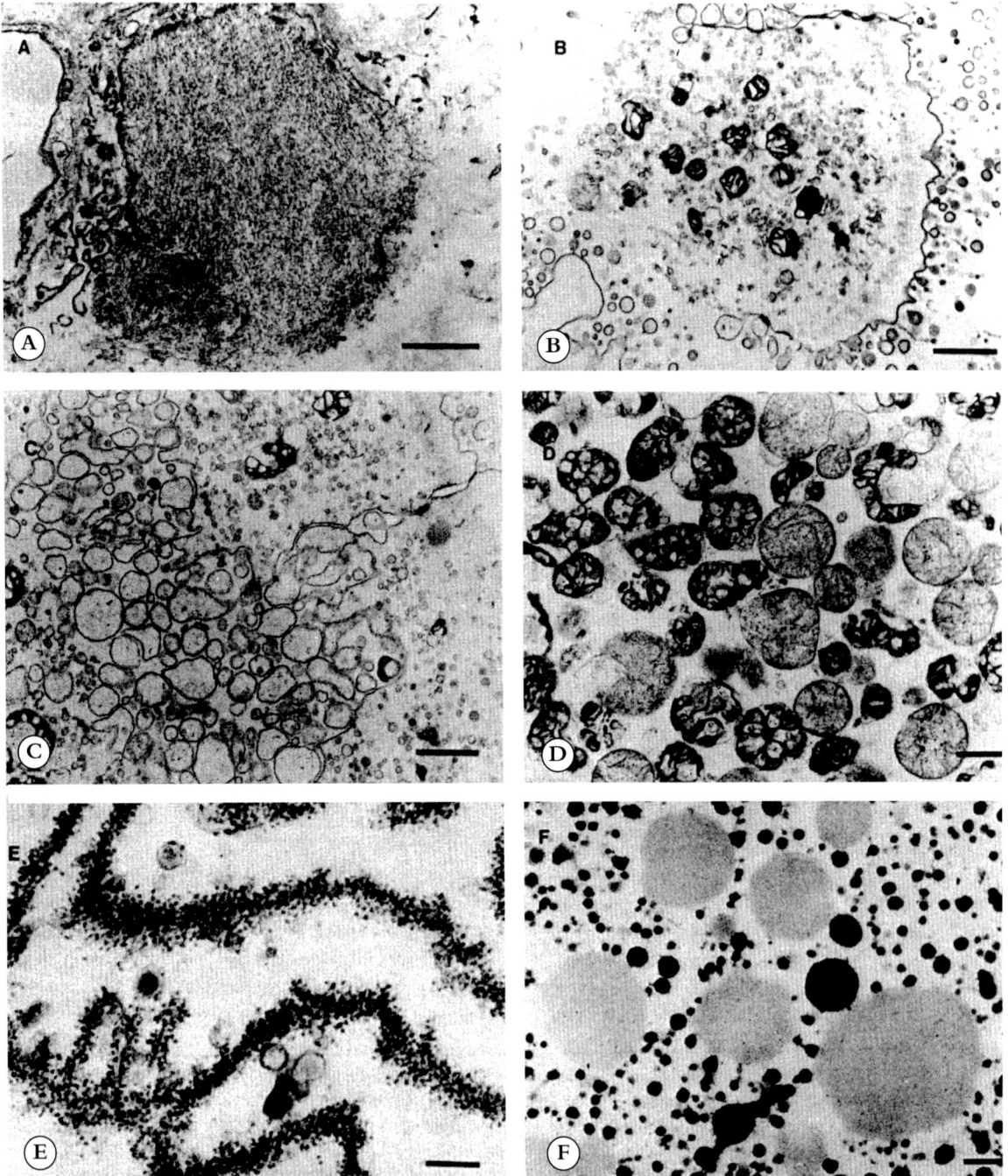

Figure 3.3 – Electron micrographs of sucrose density gradient fractions. Micrographs show density regions (g/ml) **A**, 1.25; **B**, 1.23; **C**, 1.20; **D**, 1.19; **E**, 1.10. Scale bars presented are: **A-C**, **E**, 1 μm, **D**, **F**, 0.5 μm. Reproduced with permission from Elsevier Science-NL.[18]

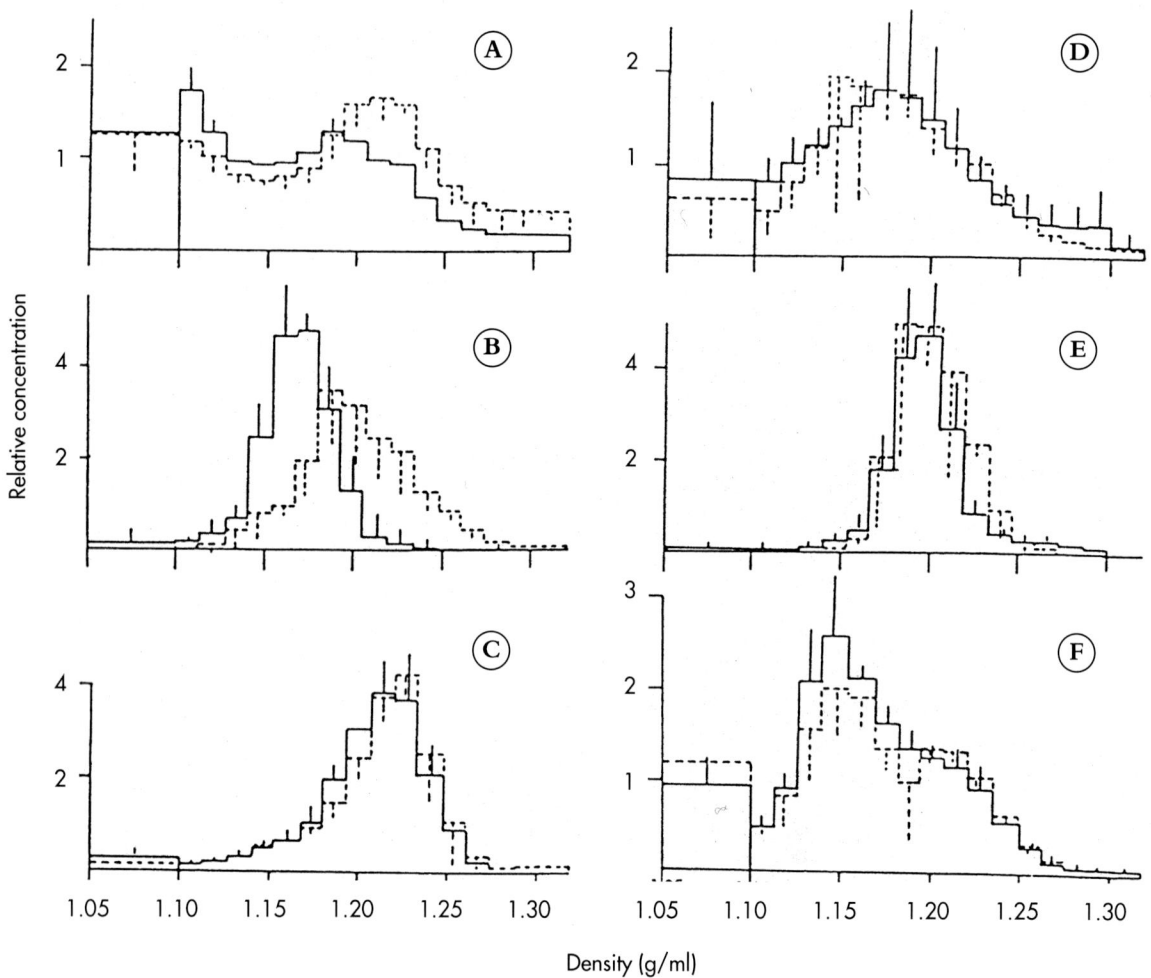

Figure 3.4 – Effect of digitonin treatment on subcellular distribution of ^{59}Fe and marker enzymes. Duodenal enterocytes isolated from hypoxic mice (3 days, 0.5 atmospheres) after *in vivo* incubation of tied loops with ^{59}FeNTA$_2$, were washed with 0.02 mg/ml digitonin and then three times in digitonin-free buffer prior to homogenization in 0.25 M sucrose. Distribution of ^{59}Fe or marker enzymes are shown for control experiments without digitonin treatment (continuous line) and digitonin-treated enterocytes (dashed line). **A**, ^{59}Fe; **B**, Na$^+$,K$^+$-ATPase (basolateral membrane); **C**, Zn^{2+}-resistant α-glucosidase (brush border membrane); **D**, N-acetyl-β–glucosaminidase (lysosomes); **E**, succinate dehydrogenase (mitochondria); **F**, Tris-resistant α-glucosidase (endoplasmic reticulum). Reproduced with permission from John Wiley and Sons Ltd.[9]

onto a density gradient and fractionated as described above. In addition to the organelle marker enzymes listed above, Zn-resistant α-glucosidase (EC 3.2.1.80, brush borders), Tris-resistant α-glucosidase (EC 3.2.1.80, endoplasmic reticulum) and Na$^+$,K$^+$-activated Mg^{2+}-ATPase (EC 3.6.1.3, basolateral membranes)[9] are assayed.

Results and discussion

Human jejunal biopsy fractionation

Fig. 3.2 is an example of the use of post-nuclear supernatant from jejunal biopsy homogenates as the starting material for gradient subcellular fractionation,[10,11] and shows the density gradient distributions and relative specific activities of marker enzymes in control and treated coeliac disease patients. The latter had only partially responded to treatment and they showed subtotal villus atrophy with a decrease in brush-border alkaline phosphatase activity. The brush-border markers showed the most striking changes in both treated and untreated (not shown) coeliac disease. Morphological studies have noted brush-border changes in coeliac disease,[12,13] however, the quantitative data from analytical subcellular fractionation highlights this effect. The soluble marker enzyme (lactate dehydrogenase, not shown) was within the normal range. The endoplasmic reticulum marker α-glucosidase suggests an increase in the density of this organelle. The change in β-glucosidase probably reflects an increase in rough relative to smooth endoplasmic reticulum.[14]

Application of subcellular fractionation to iron absorption

The use of subcellular fractionation to elucidate intestinal absorption pathways is well illustrated by studies on iron. These are based on *in vivo* labelling studies combined with subcellular fractionation of intestinal mucosa. Time course and/or pulse-chase labelling is used to identify sites which are stations on the absorptive pathway. Early work with rats dosed with ^{59}Fe attempted to identify organelles to which newly absorbed iron was bound. Rat duodenal mucosa has proved very difficult to fractionate, however, and data suggesting a mitochondrial localization were based on poorly resolved fractions.[15,16] A later study with guinea pigs was also interpreted as suggesting a mitochondrial localization.[17]

We have fractionated mouse duodenal mucosa, labelled with ^{59}Fe, by incubation in an *in vivo* tied-off gut segment.[18] Electron microscopy of particles from various regions of the sucrose gradient (Fig. 3.3) and organelle marker enzyme assays demonstrated that separation of organelles had been achieved.[18] The particulate distribution of iron demonstrated a peak at 1.18-1.20 g/ml. Time course studies and the use of mice with enhanced iron absorption, induced by previous exposure to hypoxia, suggested that this peak represented an important location for iron in the absorption pathway. The modal density and peak shape suggested a basolateral localization, however, this region of the gradient was congested with overlapping organelle peaks (lysosomes, endoplasmic reticulum and mitochondria) and an additional technique was used to confirm the basolateral membrane localization.

Digitonin is a plasma membrane perturbant used as a shift reagent in fractionation studies.[19] Fig. 3.4 shows the results of an experiment in which mouse duodenum was labelled *in vivo* with ^{59}Fe, then enterocytes were isolated by vibration.[9,18] The cells were incubated with digitonin and then washed and fractionated. Control enterocytes were fractionated without exposure to digitonin. It can be seen that digitonin shifts the density of both the ^{59}Fe peak and the basolateral marker enzyme Na$^+$/K$^+$-ATPase in the same direction while other organelle markers show distinct changes. This illustrates the value of shift reagents in confirming subcellular localization. In addition the basolateral localization for iron agrees with autoradiography studies.[20,21]

In general, subcellular fractionation for the localization of proteins or nucleic acids has been superseded by morphology-based techniques, such as immunocytochemistry and *in situ* hybridization. Preparative fractionation is, however, still important in providing purified membranes for studies of, for example, transport of small molecules.[22]

Acknowledgments

The authors thank Professor TJ Peters for helpful comments and Ms H Grindley, Dr K Osterloh and Dr S Snape for their contributions. This is a contribution from the King's College Centre for the Study of Metals in Biology and Medicine.

References

1. Peters TJ. Investigation of tissue organelles by a combination of analytical subcellular fractionation and enzymic microanalysis: a new approach to pathology. *J Clin Pathol* 1981; **34:** 1-12.

2. Peters TJ. Cell fractionation and purification: biopsy based methods. In: Masseyeff RF, Albert WH, Staines NA (Eds) *Cells and Tissues. Methods of Immunological Analysis,* vol 3. VCH, Weinheim, Germany, 1993; pp190-201.

3. Batt RM, Mann LC. Evaluation of preformed Percoll and reorientating sucrose density gradient centrifugation for the analytical subcellular fractionation of dog liver. *Res Vet Sci* 1983; **34:** 272-279.

4. Karmali A, Montague DJ, Holloway BR, Peters TJ. Comparative subcellular fractionation of control and cold-adapted rat brown and white adipose tissue with special reference to peroxisomal and mitochondrial distributions. *Cell Biochem Funct* 1984; **2:** 155-160.

5. Peters TJ. Analytical subcellular fractionation of jejunal biopsy specimens: methodology and characterisation of the organelles in normal tissue. *Clin Sci Mol Med* 1976; **51:** 557-574.

6. De Duve C, Berthet J, Beaufay H. Gradient centrifugation of cell particles - theory and applications. *Prog Biophys Biophysical Chem* 1959; **9:** 325-369.

7. Shah T, Heywood-Waddington D, Smith GD, Peters TJ. Automated enzymic, protein and DNA microanalysis of tissue biopsy samples and subcellular ractions. *Clin Chim Acta* 1984; **138:** 125-132.

8. Smith GO, Osterloh KRS, Peters TJ. Computational analysis of graidient distribution profiles. 1989 *Anal Biochem.* 1989; **160:**17-23.

9. Snape S, Simpson RJ, Peters TJ. Subcellular localization of recently absorbed iron in mouse duodenal enterocytes: identification of a basolateral membrane iron-binding site. *Cell Biochem Funct* 1990; **8:** 107-115.

10. Peters TJ, Jones PE, Wells G. Analytical subcellular fractionation of jejunal biopsy specimens: enzyme activities, organelle pathology and response to gluten withdrawal in patients with coeliac disease. *Clin Sci Mol Med* 1978; **55:** 285-292.

11. Peters TJ, Jones PE, Jenkins WJ, Wells G. Analytical subcellular fractionation of jejunal biopsy specimens: enzyme activities, organelle pathology and response to corticosteroids in patients with non-responsive coeliac disease. *Clin Sci Mol Med* 1978; **55:** 293-300.

12. Rubin W, Ross LL, Sleisenger MH, Weser E. An electron microscopic study of adult coeliac disease. *Lab Invest* 1966; **15:** 1720-1747.

13. Marsh MN, Brown AC, Swift J. The surface ultrastructure of the small intestinal mucosa of normal control human subjects and of patients with untreated and treated coeliac disease using the scanning electron microscope. In: Booth CC, Dowing RH (Eds) *Coeliac Disease.* Churchill Livingstone, Edinburgh, 1970, pp 26-44.

14. Tilleray J, Peters TJ. Analytical subcellular fractionation of microsomes from the liver of control and Gunn-strain rats. *Biochem Soc Trans* 1976; **4:** 248-250.

15. Huebers H, Huebers E, Simon J, Forth W. A method for preparing stable density gradients and their application for fractionation of intestinal mucosal cells. *Life Sci* 1971; **10:** 377-384.

16. Worwood M, Jacobs A. Subcellular distribution of ^{59}Fe in small intestinal mucosa: studies with normal, iron deficient and iron overloaded rats. *Br J Haematol* 1972; **22:** 265-272.

17. Hopkins JMP, Peters TJ. Subcellular distribution of radiolabelled iron during intestinal absorption in guinea-pig enterocytes with special reference to the mitochondrial localization of iron. *Clin Sci* 1979; **56:** 179-188.

18. Osterloh KRS, Snape S, Simpson RJ, Grindley H, Peters TJ. Subcellular distribution of recently absorbed iron and of transferrin in the mouse duodenal mucosa. *Biochim Biophys Acta* 1988; **969:** 166-175.

19. Smith GD, Peters TJ. Analytical subcellular fractionation of rat liver with special reference to the localisation of putative plasma membrane marker enzymes. *Eur J Biochem* 1980; **104:** 305-311.

20. Humphrys J, Walpole B, Worwood M. Intracellular iron transport in rat intestinal epithelium: biochemical and ultrastructural observations. *Br J Haematol* 1977; **36:** 209-217.

21. Bedard YC, Pinkerton PH, Simon GT. Radioautographic observations on iron absorption by the normal mouse duodenum. *Blood* 1971; **38:** 232-245.

22. Murer H, Biber J, Gmaj P, Stieger B. Cellular mechanisms in epithelial transport - advantages and disadvantages of studies with vesicles. *Mol Physiol* 1984; **6:** 55-82.

4

Intestinal perfusion techniques

George K Grimble and Hamish D Duncan

Introduction

This chapter will describe practical aspects of the design and use of perfusion tubes for investigating absorptive functions of the human small and large intestine. It is not an exhaustive review of the subject but is intended to help the investigator who wishes to attempt the technique. Intestinal perfusion techniques tend to be practised in few centres only and this reflects not only their particular gastroenterological research interests but also the fact that the technique is handed on from one researcher to the next. This chapter is an attempt to make the technique available to a wider audience in the hope that it will be more frequently used for investigating the absorptive function of the human intestine.

Design of jejunal perfusion tubes

Intubation tubes can have double-, triple- or even multi-lumens, and can be non-occlusive or occlusive (Fig. 4.1). An occlusive balloon is inflated to prevent endogenous secretions from more proximal segments contaminating the fluid in the area of bowel under study (test segment), as well as attempting to reduce reflux of the perfused solution. The test segment is between the infusion and aspiration ports and will encompass an indeterminate area of mucosa. It is assumed, when using simple two-lumen tubes (Fig. 4.1A), that uniform mixing of contents occurs, but the infused solution may reflux proximally, and proximal secretions may contaminate the perfusate.

The triple-lumen tube (Fig. 4.1B) was designed to take into account reflux of perfusate and contamination from endogenous secretions by aspirating from both distal ports. Perfusate and endogenous secretions mix in the proximal segment and by aspirating from both distal ports, allowance can be made for contamination. However, there may be variable water and solute absorption from the mixing segment which is difficult to account for. Sladen and Dawson[1] concluded from a comparative study that the double- and triple-segment tubes yielded no significant difference in measurement of water and electrolyte movements in the intestine. A proximal occluding balloon removes the need for a mixing segment (Fig. 4.1C), however it is very difficult to completely occlude a section of bowel and there can

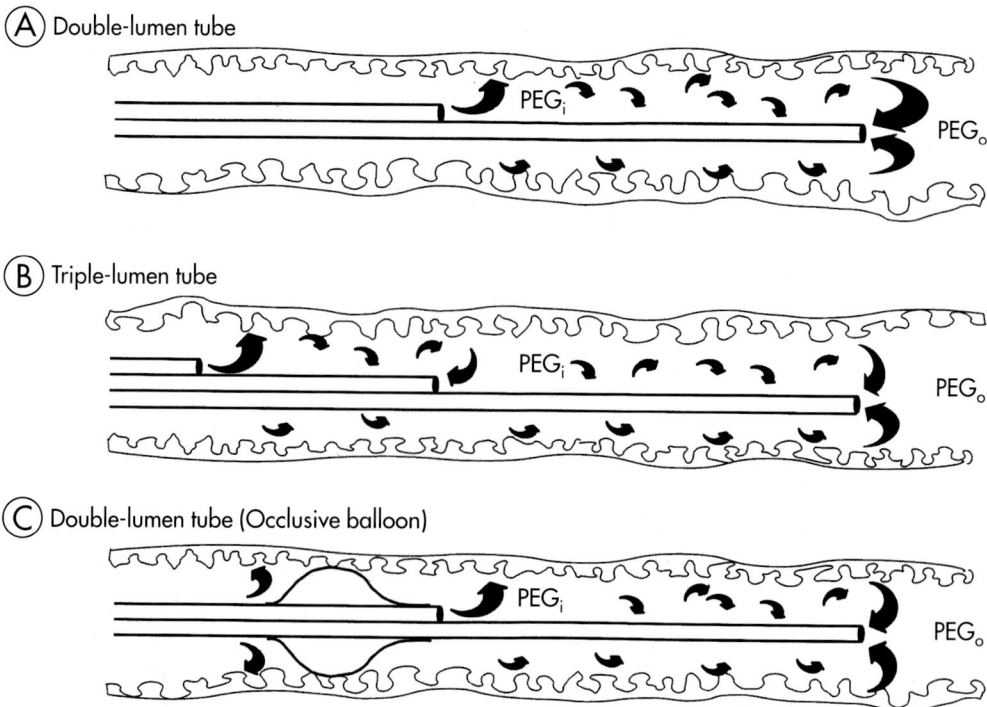

(A) Double-lumen tube

PEG_i PEG_o

(B) Triple-lumen tube

PEG_i PEG_o

(C) Double-lumen tube (Occlusive balloon)

PEG_i PEG_o

Figure 4.1 – Techniques of small-intestinal perfusion

still be some reflux and contamination from endogenous secretions. Balloons may stimulate peristalsis and induce hormone secretion and cause distortion of the bowel,[1] and thus interfere with or alter mucosal blood flow and motility.[2] Although an inflated balloon has been shown to reduce bowel motility[3] it does not affect absorption of sugars, sodium and water.[4] On balance, the occlusive balloon is a useful technique because it enables the investigator to measure the brush-border phase of digestion and absorption, free from the effects of luminal pancreatobiliary secretions.

Jejunal perfusion tube with occluded segment

Perfusion tubes can be constructed by any researcher with reasonable manual skills, from simple materials which are readily available. The widely used design of Sladen and Dawson[1] has been extensively refined at the Central Middlesex Hospital to the form shown in Figure 4.2.

It is important to use appropriate-sized tubes for each function. Thus the perfusion line need only be of sufficient size to allow perfusion solutions to be pumped with ease by a volumetric peristaltic pump, whereas it is important to use as large an aspiration line as possible to allow good siphonage. As shown in Figure 4.2 the perfusion line is 2.0 mm ID PVC tubing (3.0 mm OD, Portex Ltd Hythe, Kent) whilst the aspiration line is 2.5 mm ID PVC tubing (3.5 mm OD). Air lines of radio-opaque PVC (1.0mm ID, 2.0mm OD) allow the tube position to be determined prior to the start of the perfusion, by fluoroscopy.

The tube is formed by gluing a pre-positioned bundle of tubes together before ports are cut and balloons fitted. A convenient way to achieve this is with a wooden guide which can be made from a 2 metre length of 3-4 cm square-section hardwood in which a groove has been milled to the finished size of the perfusion tube. The bundle of tubes is laid in this groove without twisting or tension applied to any one tube in order to avoid the development of a 'set' or twist in the finished tube. The pre-assembled bundle of tubes can then be glued together by applying

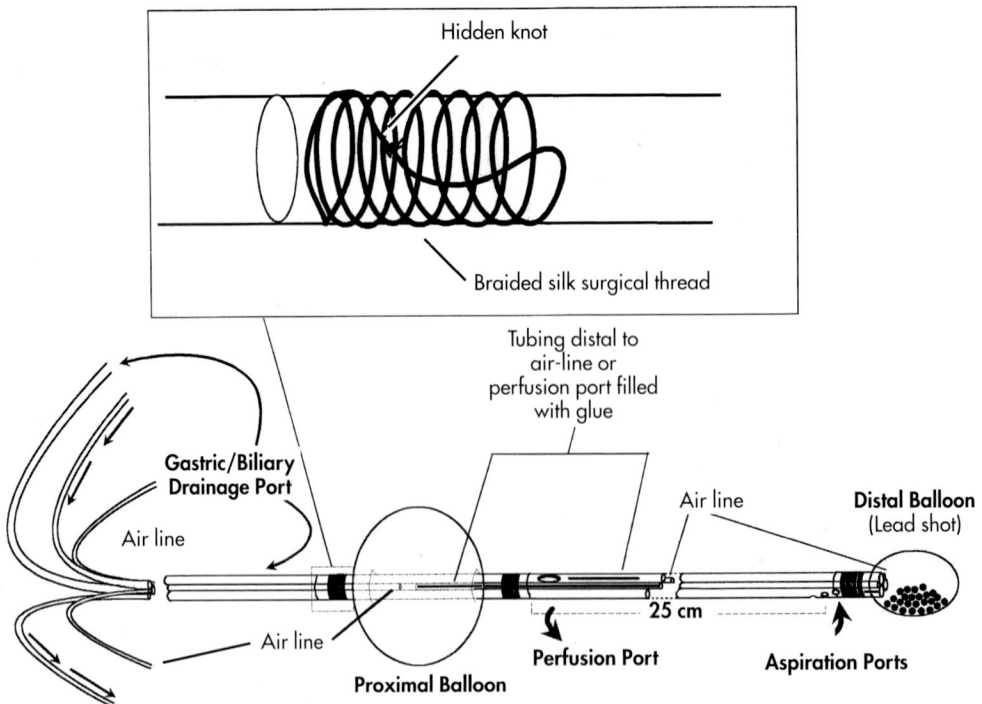

Figure 4.2 – Construction details of jejunal perfusion tube with occlusive balloon

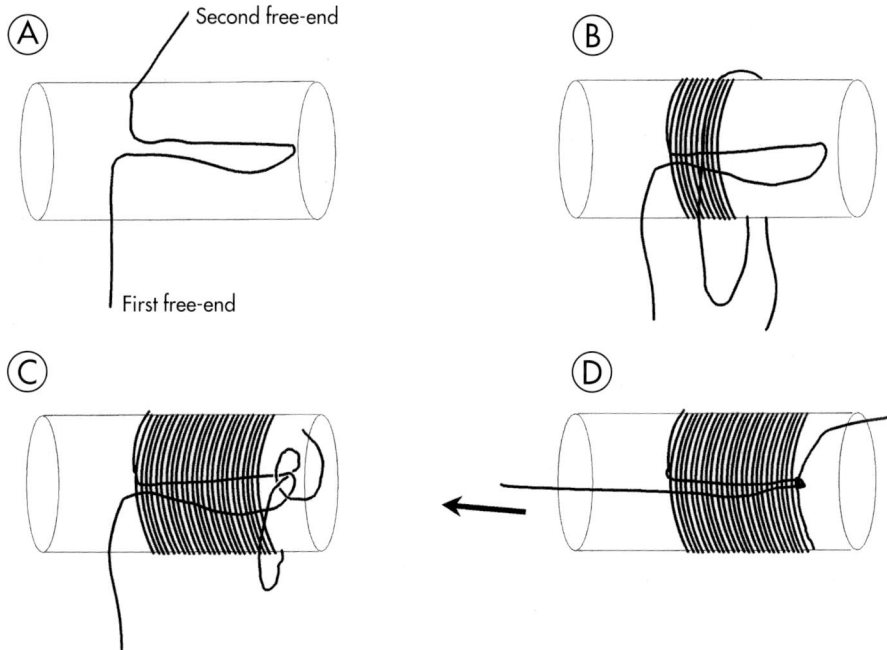

Figure 4.3 – Details of balloon fixing

tetrahydrofuran along the grooves in the tube bundle, with a pasteur pipette, and capillary flow ensures that the solvent reaches all points of contact between the individual tubes. Two applications are necessary and the tube can be handled after 30-40 minutes.

Perfusion and aspiration ports can be cut carefully in the tubing with a new scalpel blade or with a conchotone. It is important that ports have a smooth profile with no nicks and that it does not occupy more than half of the tubing circumference in order to minimise the risk of tube fracture as the tube is withdrawn from the subject. All sections of the tube distal to aspiration and perfusion ports can be blocked by PVC adhesive applied by syringe. The glue is made by dissolving short lengths of PVC tubing in a small volume of tetrahydrofuran.

Two types of balloons have been used. Until recently, stocks of purpose-made single-ended and double ended natural latex balloons (catalogue number DEB 2902 and SEB 2902) were available from Bibby Sterilin (Stone, Staffordshire, UK) but as an alternative, a condom or finger-end from a latex surgical glove can be used as a distal balloon. Thin-wall silicone rubber tubing of the same internal diameter as the outside diameter of the perfusion tube itself may

inflate sufficiently to act as a proximal balloon. The section of tube over which the balloon is fitted should be carefully sealed with tetrahydrofuran and built-up with PVC-glue to a smooth profile in order to avoid air-leaks along the joints between individual tubes. After the balloon has been fitted, a syringe with a blunt needle is used to introduce further PVC glue under the area which will form the seal and this is allowed to dry for 10-15 minutes. The balloon is then secured by use of braided silk surgical thread (Fig. 4.2, inset). Cotton and solid dissolving sutures are unsuitable because moisture and gastrointestinal enzymes lead to slackening of the thread tension or dissolution of the thread, respectively. The optimum method of securing the balloon is shown in Figure 4.2 (inset) and the method of achieving this is detailed in Figure 4.3. A loop of thread is laid along the axis of the tube (Fig. 4.3A) and is trapped by winding the thread along the seal of the balloon (Fig. 4.3B) until the second free-end of the thread can be knotted with the end of the loop (Fig. 4.3C). By pulling on the first free-end of the thread, the knot is pulled under the whipping (Fig. 4.3D) and the excess free-ends cut off. Very little tension need be applied to the 'whipping' and the final joint should be varnished with PVC-glue to render it waterproof.

The proximal end of each constituent tube should terminate in an appropriate fitting. The perfusion line can be attached to the silicone rubber peristaltic pump tubing by a double-ended male luer fitting. The air-line can be finished with a large-bore hypodermic needle (with the sharp end cut off) to which a three-way tap is attached. These are air-tight and allow the proximal or distal balloons to be maintained inflated.

Small intestine perfusion technique

Subjects are asked to fast from their previous evening meal and to abstain from drinking alcohol because this markedly impairs water and electrolyte absorption.[5] They are allowed a sip of water to aid swallowing of the perfusion tube and the oro-pharynx is anaesthetized using xylocaine 1% spray, following which the subject swallows the perfusion tube. The subject lays on their left side to help transpyloric passage of the tube, whereupon the terminal peristaltic balloon is inflated with 15 ml of air to aid distal movement of the tube. This process can be visualised by fluoroscopy and it is useful to place a tape marker on the portion of tube outside the subject, to give an idea of how far the tube has to move. Once the tube has passed the pylorus, the subject is free to move around and the tube is considered to be in position when the proximal port/occlusive balloon (Fig. 4.1) has reached the Ligament of Treitze. At this point, the subject is lain on their left side, the distal balloon is deflated, and the proximal balloon is inflated with 40-50 ml of air. Perfusion with 0.9% saline at 15 ml/min (37°C) can be started to wash out the perfusion segment. A 30 minute pre-perfusion period is usually sufficient to achieve this, the criteria of success being absence of bile pigment in the perfusion segment aspirate. Subsequently, test solutions can be perfused (at 15 ml/min) in randomised order using a 30 minute equilibration period before aspirates are collected over a 30 minute period for later analysis of ^{14}C-PEG, electrolytes and other solutes. At the end of the study, the proximal balloon is deflated and the tube is removed by applying gentle traction. The entire procedure can be performed within one day, it normally takes 2-3 hours for correct tube-placement to be achieved, and 5 solutions can be investigated if the pre-perfusion solution (0.9% saline) is replaced by a perfusion solution. Thus, total perfusion time will be 5 hours.

A skilled investigator and assistant can perform three successful jejunal perfusions simultaneously. With practice, technically successful perfusions can be achieved from 60% of intubations, but unforeseen events (eg. failure to obtain steady-state) tends to lower the overall success-rate to 40-50%. There are several factors which ensure success. Firstly, it is important to initiate adequate drainage of pancreatobiliary secretions via the port proximal to the occlusive balloon. Failure to do this will result in nausea and vomiting which will inevitably terminate the perfusion. When nutritional perfusion solutions are perfused, these secretions increase in volume and their viscosity may prevent adequate siphonage. Siphonage can be restarted by syringing warm saline back down the drainage port. Secondly, it is important to maintain adequate rates of siphonage from the perfused segment. Because solutions are being perfused at 15 ml/min, and ca. 30% of this will be absorbed, adequate siphonage normally occurs. It usually ceases because the port becomes occluded by the intestinal mucosal surface and change of position by the subject or gentle syringing with saline will generally restore flow. Thirdly, the technique is uncomfortable for the subject and every reasonable effort should be made to distract them from dwelling on this fact (e.g. television, books, newspapers, music). Finally, it is important to ensure that the balloons are in good condition before the subject swallows the tube. After perfusion, the tube is decontaminated by soaking for 30 minutes in suitable virucidal laboratory detergent (e.g. Decon) before thorough rinsing with water. No water should be allowed to enter the air lines and the outside of the balloon should be dried carefully before storage. Because latex degrades quite readily, we have found it necessary to change the balloons after 3-4 perfusions.

Large bowel perfusion techniques

Perfusion tube design

This steady-state perfusion technique is similar to that used by Bowling et al[6-8] which was derived from the technique used by Devroede and Phillips.[9] The method of construction is similar to that for jejunal perfusion tubes except that seven lengths of polyvinyl tubing of differing sized internal diameters ranging from 0.6-1.5 mm are used (Fig.4.4). The propulsive balloon at port 7 (Fig. 4.4 and Table 4.1) consists of a

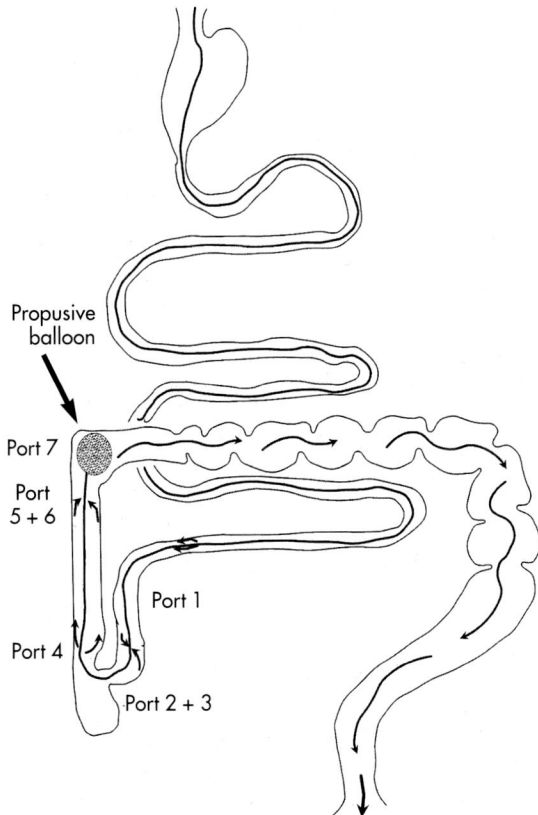

Propusive balloon

Port 7

Port 5 + 6

Port 1

Port 4

Port 2 + 3

Figure 4.4 – Schematic diagram of simultaneous ileal and colonic perfusion technique

latex balloon containing a mercury weight inside another latex balloon which can be inflated by injecting air into the proximal end of tube 7. Port side holes are cut into the distal ends of the remaining 6 tubes to enable either aspiration of bowel contents, insufflation of air or to infuse solutions into the bowel. The function of each of the tubes/ports is shown in Table 4.1.

Ileal/colonic perfusion technique

Subjects are asked to avoid alcohol or eating from a restaurant for at least 24 hours prior to the study and are fasted from midnight. Intubation is the same as for jejunal perfusion, but when the tip of the tube is in the antrum of the stomach, the volunteer is lain on their left hand side and the balloon inflated with 8 ml air, to aid passage through the pylorus. Once the tip has moved past the Ligament of Treitze, the balloon is inflated with a further 7ml of air and the subject is allowed to walk, sit or remain lying down until the distal end of the tube was situated just proximal to the hepatic flexure.

The fastest forward propulsion of the tube occurs when there is no slack coiled in the stomach. Fluoroscopic examination is used (infrequently) to visualise this process, coiling is minimised and only small lengths of tube need to be inserted, infrequently. Adequate radiation protection measures should be ensure that only the stomach is screened.

Table 4.1 – Function of the ports in a 7-lumen ileal/colonic perfusion

Tube/port	Function
1	Infusion of ^{3}H-PEG (in 0.9% NaCl) as non-absorbable marker into 20 cm segment of distal ileum
2	To insufflate air to aid aspiration of ileal contents at port 3
3	Aspiration of ileal contents 20 cm distal to port 1
4	Infusion of ^{14}C-PEG (in 0.9% NaCl) as non-absorbable marker into 40 cm segment of ascending colon
5	To insufflate air to aid aspiration of ileal contents at port 6
6	Aspiration port, 40 cm distal to port 4, at hepatic flexure
7	For inflation/deflation of propulsive balloon which aids tube passage through the small intestine

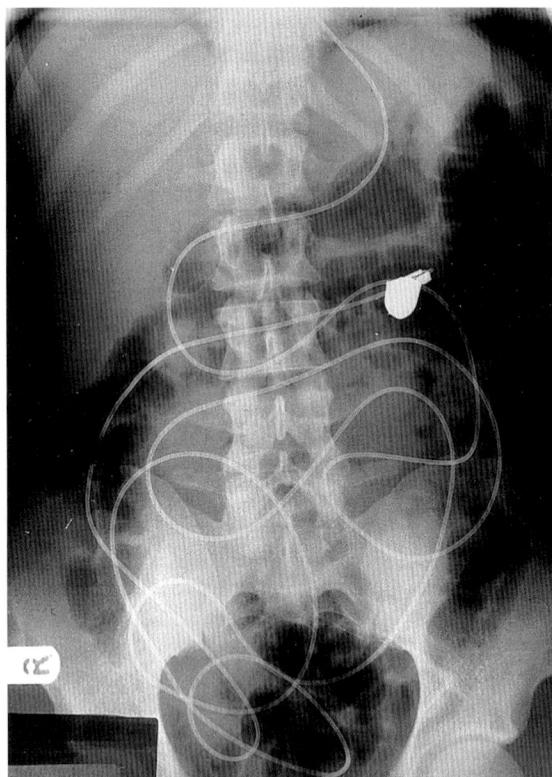

Figure 4.5 – X-ray of perfusion tube *in situ*

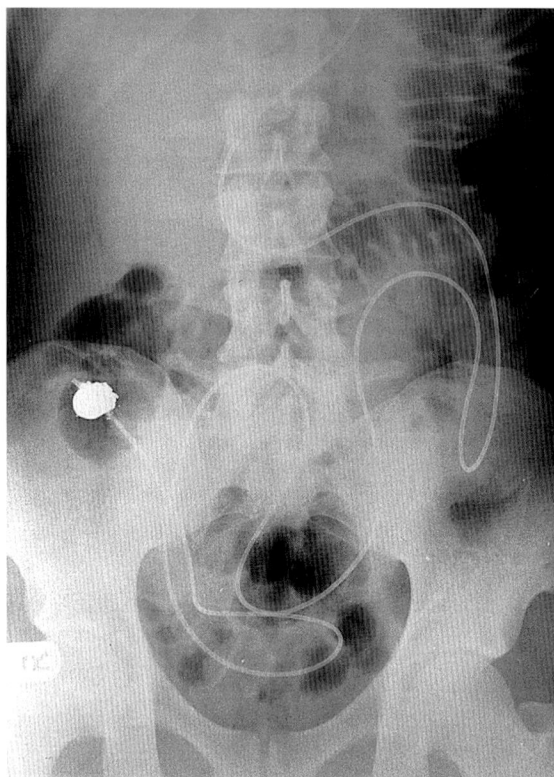

Figure 4.6 – X-ray of perfusion tube *in situ*

Occasionally the tip of the perfusion tube may proceed too far along the colon (Fig. 4.5), necessitating slow withdrawal of the tube until the tip is in the correct position (Fig. 4.6). Furthermore, the small bowel can 'concertina' over the tube (see Photo 1 & 2), which makes it difficult to assess accurately the length of perfusion tubing that is required to be inserted to reach the hepatic flexure, and may explain why estimates of *in vivo* length of the small bowel vary so much.[10]

Once in position, any coils of tube in the stomach are removed to prevent movement of the tube tip in the colon. The colon is perfused through port 4 (Fig. 4.4) with 0.9% saline (37°C) at 15 ml/min for at least two hours, to clear faeces. Simultaneously, 0.9% saline containing 0.5μCi/L ³H-PEG is perfused at 1 ml/min into the ileum via port 1 for at least 2 hours to achieve

a steady-state (see below). Thereafter, aspirates of terminal ileal fluid are collected every 20 minutes via port 3 for the rest of the study. As this technique uses discontinuous sampling (unlike the jejunal perfusion), the first 1 ml of aspirate corresponding to the dead-volume of the tube is discarded and subsequent fluid collected for analysis. Once the colon has been cleared of faeces, a 26 FG Riplex rectal tube (Rusch Incorporated, Buckinghamshire, UK) is inserted and taped to the buttocks. Thereafter, the isotonic perfusion solution (0.5μCi/L, ¹⁴CPEG, NaCl 120 mmol/l, KCl 5 mmol/l, NaHCO₃ 23 mmol/l) is perfused through port 4 at 10 ml/min and samples collected from port 6 and from rectal fluid. At the end of the study the position of the perfusion tube is checked fluoroscopically. The entire study takes two days since the tube is rarely in position until the evening of day 1 or even the morning of day 2.

Calculation of data and definition of a steady state

The two issues which affect the quality of the results and inferences which can be drawn from them is whether during the measurement period, water and solute transport remained steady or was in a transitional state and was being up- or downregulated. Secondly, the inherent variance of water flows and the variance inherent in analytical determinations may prevent the researcher from discerning whether a steady state has been achieved. The primary measurement which underpins all others is the relative change in concentration of the non-absorbable marker.

This should be an inert compound which is not absorbed and which is distributed evenly in aqueous and lipid phases of perfused solutions.[11] Polyvinylpyrrolidone and indocyanine green have both been investigated but suffer from problems of slow absorption and binding to intestinal mucus, respectively[12] and are thus unreliable. Phenol red can dissociate in solution rendering it lipophilic and thus absorbable. In contrast, polyethylene glycol is a hydrophillic-lipophilic polymer, unaffected by pH, whose high molecular weight limits its absorption.[13,14] In two colonic studies, complete recovery of PEG 4000 was obtained in subjects with normal mucosa and inflammatory bowel disease.[15] Thus PEG 4000 meets most criteria for an non-absorbable marker. Whilst it can be measured by a turbidimetric method, this is not ideal because accuracy is poor if samples had been frozen and then thawed.[16] We have found that an automated version of the assay had poor reproducibility (>±7%) and routinely use radiolabelled PEG 4000 as first described by Wingate and colleagues.[17] In order to prevent binding of labelled PEG to glassware and plastic sample tubes, 'cold' PEG 4000 should be added at a concentration of 2 g/L, a concentration which has been shown to have little effect on water absorption in the small intestine,[18] whereas higher concentrations exert a detectable osmotic effect.

In order to minimise the risk of radiation exposure to subjects, the amount of radiolabelled PEG 4000 administered should be kept as low as is consistent with the desired analytical accuracy and precision. Since a liquid scintillation counter detects random events, the precision of the determination will improve the more individual 'counts' are detected.

Thus, a total of 40,000 counts will yield an average which has a precision of ±2% and this is equivalent to counting a 1 ml aliquot of ^{14}C-PEG 4000 (1μCi/L) for 20 minutes, a 1 ml aliquot of ^{14}C-PEG 4000 (0.2μCi/L) for 100 minutes or a 2 ml aliquot of ^{14}C-PEG 4000 (0.1 μCi/L) for 100 minutes. Clearly, the latter case poses the least risk to the subject and will yield equally precise data. In colonic perfusions, the simultaneous use of ^{3}H-PEG 4000 and ^{14}C-PEG 4000 as markers for different segments posses its own problems. The isotope ^{14}C can be measured in the presence of ^{3}H with high accuracy and precision if the lower energy level of the detection window is set quite high to exclude any contribution from ^{3}H. However, ^{3}H can be counted in the presence of ^{14}C with high accuracy only if the proportion of ^{14}C which is being counted in the ^{3}H window is known. Although modern scintillation counters have programmes which take account of this and adjust it for the degree of quenching, for highest accuracy and precision, the lower efficiency of ^{3}H counting means that the concentration of ^{3}H in the aspirate should exceed that of ^{14}C by at least 2:1. We have used a Beckman scintillation counter (Model LS750, Beckman RIIC, High Wycombe, Bucks, UK) for several years because the method of quench correction (H-Number method) is robust and if plastic disposable mini-vials are used, is insensitive to solvent absorption into the walls of the tube unlike the sample-channels ratio method. This is important because intestinal aspirates can be highly coloured and this requires that the degree of colour quenching and efficiency of counting in double label studies (^{3}H-PEG/^{14}C-PEG) is accurately determined.

Careful inspection of the data will reveal whether a steady state has been obtained. The data shown in Table 4.2 is taken from a perfusion study which investigated the effect of chain-length of perfused peptides on nitrogen uptake in the perfused jejunum.[19] If $[PEG_i]$ is the ^{14}C PEG concentration in the perfusate and $[PEG_o]$ is the average ^{14}C PEG concentration in 3 successive aspirates and flow rate is 15 ml/min:-

$$Water\ movement\ (ml/min/25cm)= 900 \times [1-[PEG_i/PEG_o]]$$

In two separate experiments, for one perfused solution, average water movements were similar but in the case of perfusion 203, the variance of the estimate was 6.9%, in the case of perfusion 207 it was 79.9% and thus suggests that a steady-state had not been obtained. It is clear that if a variance of <10% in

Table 4.2 - Comparison of two perfusions which were apparently in a steady state

Solution	^{14}C PEG concentration (dpm/ml)	Water movement (ml/min/25cm perfused)
Perfusion 203		
Control (PEG$_i$)	2140.5	
Aspirate 1	2343.7	78.0
Aspirate 2	2375.3	89.0
Aspirate 2	2383.8	91.9
Average (PEG$_o$)	2367.6 ± 17.3 (CV 0.7%)	86.3 ± 6.0 (CV 6.9%)
Perfusion 207		
Control (PEG$_i$)	2351.1	
Aspirate 1	2403.3	19.55
Aspirate 2	2917.4	174.7
Average (PEG$_o$)	2660.4 ± 257.1 (CV 9.7%)	97.1 ± 77.6 (CV 79.9%)

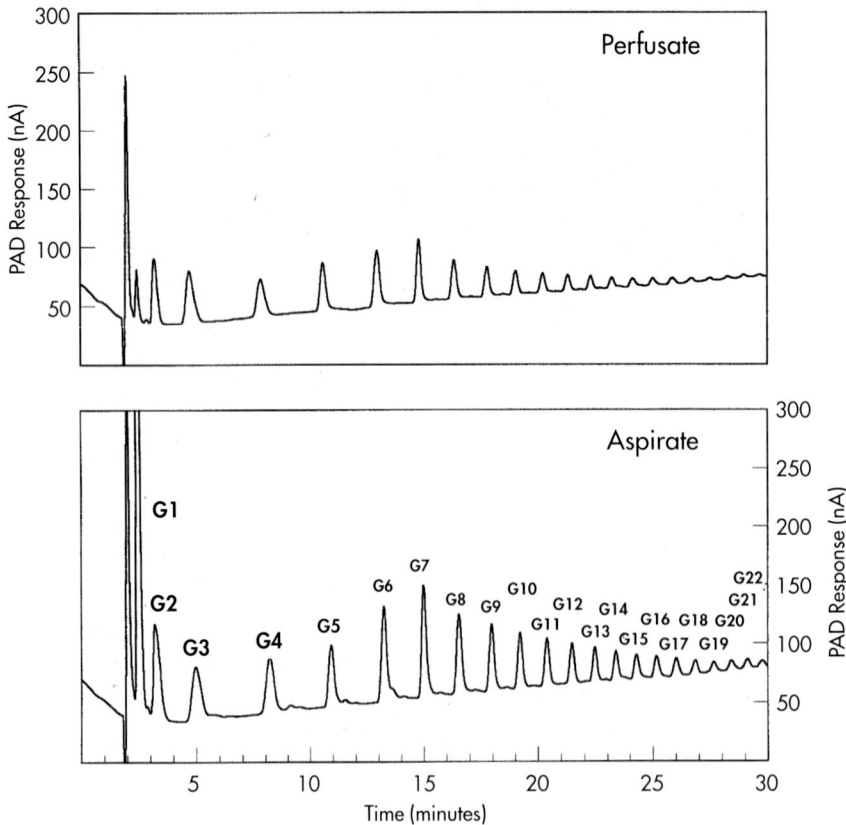

Figure 4.7 – High performance liquid chromatography of maltodextrin perfused in the human jejunum. A)Perfusate, B) Aspirate.

calculated water uptake is to be obtained, the coefficient of variation for PEG concentration in successive samples should not exceed 1.2%. On this basis, the data from Perfusion 207 should be discarded. Calculated rates of uptake of solutes are subject to added variance arising from the degree of precision of analytical methods.

Solutes whose uptake has been measured by jejunal perfusion in man

To date, the jejunal perfusion technique has been used to investigate the kinetics of uptake of numerous solutes such as glucose,[4,20] dibasic amino acids,[21-23] and dipeptides[24] (summarised in[25]). In addition, the technique has been used to determine the effect of maltodextrin polymer size on brush-border digestion and glucose assimilation.[26,27] Similar studies have defined the optimum chain-length of peptides from protein hydrolysates on nitrogen uptake in the jejunum.[19,28,29] An example of the utility of this method is shown in Figure 4.7. Complete enteral diets were perfused at 1/10th their normal concentration but at 15 ml/min with an occlusive balloon inflated. This corresponds to the load of nutrient administered during nasoenteral feeding. Anion-exchange HPLC with pulsed amperometric detection of perfusates and aspirates allowed the % disappearance rate of each glucose polymer species up to a chain-length of 27 glucose units, to be determined. As can be seen, above a chain-length of 5 units, the rate of disappearance of all polymers was similar, whilst there was little accumulation of free glucose.[30] This simple study provides confirmation that under these conditions, the rates of brush-border hydrolysis of glucose polymers and glucose uptake are matched and that hydrolysis probably rate limits glucose uptake.

Uptake of solutes and water in the large bowel

Several different methods have been used to investigate the absorptive and secretory function of the colon. Although the simplest method would be to compare the ileal effluent from ileostomies with that of normal stools,[31,32] excretion from ileostomies varies widely both intra- and inter-individually[32] because

of the extent of ileal resection, underlying residual disease, ileostomy dysfunction and changes in gastrointestinal motility following surgery.[33] Adaptive changes in small bowel absorption following colectomy[34] and increased mineralocorticoid secretion following ileostomy[35] may enhance absorption of sodium and water[36] in the remaining bowel. As an alternative, the use of bags containing hyperosmolar dextran has merit in that it can be collected with the faeces, but it is not clear whether the contents of the bag represent equilibration with the contents of the caecum, ascending colon, transverse colon or rectosigmoid lumen.[37]

Currently, therefore, the best method for measuring water and electrolyte movement at different sites in the colon is with perfusion tubes, the design of one such being shown in Figure 4.4. This design is a refinement of early tubes which consisted of a single lumen with a small rubber bag containing mercury attached to the distal end.[38,39] The procedure was lengthy (3-5 days) and subjects were fasted throughout. This tube was modified to a two-lumen design and finally a three lumen design[40] which was further modified so that the two proximal ports were separated by 20 cm,[41] the most proximal being used to continually aspirate ileal contents to minimise contamination of the infusion solution from the most distal port sited in the caecum. Perfusion studies in healthy subjects confirmed net absorption of water, sodium and chloride across the whole colon, whilst potassium was usually secreted.[42,43] Devroede and Phillips[44] developed a four lumen tube to enable continuous aspiration of ileal contents proximal to the caecal infusion point, to minimise ileal contamination and so attempt to reduce the error introduced by contamination of the perfusing solution. They observed reflux of colonic contents into the ileum and could not guarantee that all ileal fluid has been removed by continuous aspiration.

Several investigators attempted to study differences between right and left sides of the colon[38,45] and concluded that water, sodium and chloride absorption and potassium and bicarbonate secretion were greater on the right side of the colon. Devroede et al[44,46] extended these studies and used anatomical and radiological criteria to determine whether water and electrolyte movements were being measured in the caecum, transverse, descending colon or rectum. However, this approach can be criticised on several grounds, most notably that these regions were often poorly defined and that reflux may have affected the concentration non-absorbable marker in the aspirate.

The colonic perfusion method described in detail in this chapter was devised to study water and electrolyte movements in the ascending colon and the colon distal to the hepatic flexure.[7] The 7-lumen tube which could be used to assess colonic inflow, water and electrolyte movement in the ascending colon and in the colon distal to the hepatic flexure. The technique allowed reflux of ^{14}C-PEG labelled colonic contents into the ileum to be taken into account in the calculations and it was found that little occurred. The mean colonic inflow into the terminal ileum was found to be 2.0 ml/min in comparison with 1.0 ml/min from the study by Phillips and Giller.[40] Water and electrolyte movements derived from this method is compared with earlier studies in Table 4.3.

Validation of this method[7] therefore allowed it to be applied to the situation of nasogastric enteral feeding which is often accompanied by a high incidence of diarrhoea[47,48] which is strongly associated with antibiotic treatment. This may be caused by inhibition of carbohydrate fermentation in the colon, such that osmotic diarrhoea ensues.[48] However, in one perfusion study, intragastric feeding by nasogastric tube at low (1.4 kcal/min, 8.8 mgN/min) or high loads (4.2 kcal/min, 26.1 mgN/min) converted net absorption of water, sodium and chloride (see Table 4.3) into net secretion[8] whereas low load intraduodenal feeding had no effect. In subsequent studies, it was shown that this effect could be reversed by instilling short-chain fatty acids into the colon.[6] These products of luminal bacterial fermentation are potent stimulators of water and electrolyte uptake.[49,50] Most recently, it has been shown that when enteral diet was given as an oral bolus, there was no reduction in colonic motility which occurred when the diet was given as a bolus, intragastrically.[51] The reduction in motility was accompanied by diarrhoea in all cases. It is therefore possible that nasoenteral feeding predisposes to diarrhoea by reducing motility and by evoking a secretory state in proximal and distal colon. The combination of these two factors may be sufficient to overwhelm the ability of the colon to handle point loads of water, a maximum capacity of 500 ml.[52]

Conclusions

The use of intestinal perfusion techniques in man has yielded much useful information which could not easily be obtained by other methods. The techniques are often arduous and require a high level of skill and dedication on the part of the investigator (and subject) and it may take some time to collect sufficient data to make statistical comparisons. At first sight, the use of *in vitro* methods such as brush-border membrane vesicles, Ussing chambers or $CaCO_2$ cell layers are attractive because data collection is rapid. Thus the characteristics of several intestinal transporters have been defined in this way, the most notable being the discovery of the H^+-gradient energised di- and tripeptide transporter.[52,53] however, it should not be forgotten that the existence of this transporter was conclusively proven by the observation that patients

Table 4. 3 − Summary of water and electrolyte movement in the colon − comparison of perfusion methods

	Water (ml/min)	Water absorbed (ml/min)	Sodium (mmol/min)	Chloride (mmol/min)	Potassium (mmol/min)	Bicarbonate (mmol/min)
Colonic inflow						
Phillips *et al*[40]	1.06 (0.1 - 1.7)		0.14	0.07	0.0065	
Bowling *et al*[7]	2.01					
Total colon						
Levitan *et al*[38]		+1.70	+0.28	+0.39	-0.031	-0.18
Phillips *et al*[40]		+1.03	+0.14	+0.07	+0.003	NR
Right colon						
Levitan *et al*[38]		+0.16	+0.18	+0.26	-0.02	-0.15
Bowling *et al*[7]		+1.24	+0.3	+0.31	-0.0002	-0.04
Left colon						
Levitan *et al*[38]		+0.30	+0.05	+0.09	-0.008	-0.06
Bowling *et al*[7]		+0.86	+0.23	+0.21	-0.014	-0.05

with Cystinuria with a defect in the intestinal dibasic amino acid transporter were able to absorb arginine at normal rates when it was presented as an arginine-containing dipeptide.[24] These studies were, of course performed by jejunal and ileal perfusion. Despite the technical difficulties of human perfusion methods, they do yield information on the quantitative capacity of the intestine to absorb nutrients and absorb/secrete water and electrolytes. This can easily be applied to the clinical situation.

References

1. Sladen GE, Dawson AM. An evaluation of perfusion techniques in the study of water and electrolyte absorption in man: The problem of endogenous secretions An evaluation of perfusion techniques in the study of water and electrolyte absorption in man: the problem of endogenous secretions. *Gut* 1968; **9:** 530-535.

2. Sladen GE, Dawson AM. Further studies on the perfusion method for measuring intestinal absorption in man: The effects of a proximal occlusive balloon and a mixing segment Further studies on the perfusion method for measuring intestinal absorption in man: the effects of a proximal occlusive balloon and a mixing segment. *Gut* 1970; **11:** 947-954.

3. Phillips SF, Summerskill WHJ. Water and electrolyte transport during maintenance of isotonicity in human jejunum and ileum. *J Lab Clin Med* 1966; **70:** 686-698.

4. Modigliani R, Bernier JJ. Absorption of glucose, sodium, and water by the human jejunum studied by intestinal perfusion with a proximal occluding balloon and at variable flow rates. *Gut* 1971; **12:** 184-193.

5. Grimble GK. The physiology of digestion, absorption and metabolism in the human intestine. 'In:' Preedy V, R,, Watson R, R, eds. *Alcohol and the Gastrointestinal Tract.* Boca Raton: CRC Press., 1996.

6. Bowling TE, Raimundo AH, Grimble GK, *et al.* Reversal by short-chain fatty acids of colonic fluid secretion induced by enteral feeding. *Lancet* 1993; **342:** 1266-1268.

7. Bowling TE, Raimundo AH, Silk DBA. *In vivo* segmental colonic perfusion in humans: a new technique. *Eur J Gastroenterol Hepatol* 1993; **5:** 809-815.

8. Bowling TE, Raimundo AH, Grimble GK, *et al.* Colonic secretory effect in response to enteral feeding in humans. *Gut* 1994; **35:** 1734-1741.

9. Devroede GF, Phillips SF. Conservation of sodium, chloride and water by the human colon. *Gastroenterology* 1969; **56:** 101-109.

10. Purdum PP, III, Kirby DF. Short-bowel syndrome: A review of the role of nutrition support. *J Parent Ent Nutr* 1991; **15:** 93-101.

11. Schedl H. Poorly absorbed markers. *Gastroenterology* 1966; **51:** 1095

12. Maddrey WC, Serebro HA, Marcus H, *et al.* Recovery, reproducibility, and usefulness of polyethylene glycol, iodine-labelled rose bengal, sulphobromopthalein, and indocyanine green as non-absorbable markers. *Gut* 1967; **8:** 169-171.

13. Shaffer CB, Critchfield FH. The absorption and excretion of the solid polyethylene glycols (Carbowax compounds). *J Am Pharm Assoc Sci Ed* 1947; **36:** 152-157.

14. Schedl H. Use of polyethylene glycol and phenol red as unabsorbed indicators for intestinal absorption studies in man. *Gut* 1966; **7:** 159-163.

15. Shields R, Harris J, Davies MW. Suitability of polyethylene glycol as a dilution indicator in the human colon. *Gastroenterology* 1968; **54:** 331-333.

16. Miller DL, Schedl H. Total recovery studies of nonabsorbable indicators in the rat small intestine. *Gastroenterology* 1970; **58:** 40-46.

17. Wingate DL, Sandberg RJ, Phillips SF. A comparison of stable and C^{14}-labelled polyethylene glycol as volume indicators in the human jejunum. *Gut* 1972; 13: 812-815.

18. Davis GR, Santa Ana CA, Morawski SG, *et al.* Inhibition of water and electrolyte absorption by polyethylene glycol (PEG). *Gastroenterology* 1980; **79:** 35-39.

19. Grimble GK, Guilera Sarda M, Sesay HF, *et al.* The influence of whey hydrolysate peptide chain length on nitrogen and carbohydrate absorption in the perfused human jejunum. *Clin Nutr* 1994; **13(Suppl):** 46 (Abstract)

20. Sladen GE, Dawson AM. Inter-relationship between the absorption of glucose, sodium and water by the normal human jejunum. *Clin Sci Mol Med* 1969; **36:** 119-132.

21. Payne-James J, Grimble G, Cahill E, *et al.* Jejunal absorption of ornithine-oxoglutarate (OKGA) in man. *J Parent Ent Nutr* 1989; **13(Suppl):** 22S(Abstract).

22. Hellier MD, Holdsworth CD, Perrett D. Dibasic amino acid absorption in man. *Gastroenterology* 1973; **65:** 613-618.

23. Hegarty JE, Fairclough PD, Clark ML, *et al.* Jejunal water and electrolyte secretion induced by L-arginine in man. *Gut* 1981; **22:** 108-113.

24. Silk DBA, Perrett D, Clark ML. Jejeunal and ileal absorption of dibasic amino acids and an arginine containing dipeptide in cystinuria. *Gastroenterology* 1975; **68:** 1426-1432.

25. Grimble GK. The significance of peptides in clinical nutrition. 'In:' Olson R, E,, Bier D, M,, McCormick D, B, eds. *Annual Review of Nutrition, Volume 14.* Palo Alto: Annual Reviews Inc., 1994: 419-447.

26. Jones BJM, Brown BE, Loran JS, *et al.* Glucose absorption from starch hydrolysates in the human jejunum. *Gut* 1984; **24:** 1152-1160.

27. Jones BJM, Higgins BE, Silk DBA. Glucose absorption from maltotriose and glucose oligomers in the human jejunum. *Clin.Sci.* 1987; **72:** 409-414.

28. Grimble GK, Rees RG, Keohane PP, *et al.* The effect of peptide chain-length on absorption of egg-protein hydrolysates in the normal human jejunum. *Gastroenterology* 1987; **92:** 136-142.

29. Rees RG, Raimundo AH, Grimble GK, *et al.* Peptide based nitrogen source of enteral diets: studies with casein hydrolysates in man. *J Parent Ent Nutr* 1988; **12(Suppl):** 21S (Abstract).

30. Grimble GK, Rees RG, Raimundo AH, *et al.* Use of high performance liquid chromatography with pulsed amperometric detection (PAD-HPLC) to investigate an interaction between peptide and maltodextrin assimilation in the perfused human jejunum. *Clin Nutr* 1994; **13(Suppl):** 32 (Abstract).

31. Phillips SF. Absorption and secretion by the colon. *Gastroenterology* 1969; **56:** 966-971.

32. Kanaghis TM, Lubran M, Coghill NF. The composition of ileostomy fluid. *Gut* 1963; **4:** 322-338.

33. Kramer P, Kearney MM, Ingelfinger FJ. The effect of specific foods and water loading on the excreta of ileostomized human subjects. *Gastroenterology* 1962; **42:** 535-546.

34. Weinstein LD, Shoemaker CP, Hersh T, *et al.* Enhanced intestinal absorption after small bowel resection in man. *Arch Surg* 1969; **99:** 560-562.

35. Gallagher ND, Harrison DD, Skyring AP. Fluid and electrolyte disturbances in patients with long established ileostomies. *Gut* 1962; **3:** 219-223.

36. Levitan R, Goulston K. Water and electrolyte content of human ileostomy fluid after d-aldosterone administration. *Gastroenterology* 1967; **52:** 510-512.

37. Wrong O, Metcalfe-Gibson A, Morrison RB, *et al. In vivo* dialysis of feces as a method of stool analysis. 1. Technique and results in normal subjects. *Clin Sci Mol Med* 1965; **28:** 357

38. Levitan R, Fordtran JS, Burrows BA, *et al.* Water and salt absorption in the human colon. *J Clin Invest* 1962; **41:** 1754-1759.

39. Shields R. Absorption and secretion of electrolytes and water by the human colon, with particular reference to benign adenoma and papilloma. *Br J Surg* 1966; **53:** 893-897.

40. Phillips SF, Giller J. The contribution of the colon to electrolyte and water conservation in man. *J Lab Clin Med* 1973; **81:** 733-746.

41. Mekhijan HS, Phillips SF, Hofman AF. Colonic secretion of water and electrolytes induced by bile acids: perfusion studies in man. *J Clin Invest* 1971; **50:** 1569-1577.

42. Head LH, Heaton JW, Kivel RM. Absorption of water and electrolytes in Crohns disease of the colon. *Gastroenterology* 1969; **56:** 571-579.

43. Harris J, Shields R. Absorption and secretion of water and electrolytes by the intact human colon in diffuse untreated proctocolitis. *Gut* 1970; **11:** 27-33.

44. Devroede GF, Phillips SF. Studies of the perfusion technique for colonic absorption. *Gastroenterology* 1969; **56:** 92-100.

45. Devroede GF, Phillips SF. Failure of the human rectum to absorb electrolytes and water. *Gut* 1970; **1:** 438-442.

46. Devroede GF, Phillips SF, Code CF, *et al.* Regional differences in rates of insorption of sodium and water from the human large intestine. *Can J Physiol Pharmacol* 1971; **49:** 1023-1029.

47. Keohane PP, Attrill H, Jones BJM, *et al.* The roles of lactose and Clostridium difficile in the pathogenesis of enteral feeding associated diarrhoea. *Clin Nutr* 1983; **1:** 259-264.

48. Guenter PA, Settle RG, Perlmutter S, *et al.* Tube-feeding related diarrhea in acutely-ill patients. *J Parent Ent Nutr* 1991; **15:** 277-280.

49. Ruppin H, Bar-Meir S, Soergel KH, *et al.* Absorption of short chain fatty acids by the colon. *Gastroenterology* 1980; **78:** 1500-1507.

50. Binder HJ, Mehta P. Short-chain fatty acids stimulate active sodium chloride absorption *in vitro* in the rat distal colon. *Gastroenterology* 1989; **96:** 989-996.

51. Duncan HN, Cole SJ, Bowling TE, *et al.* Does the mode of feeding play a role in the pathogenesis of enteral-feeding related diarrhoea? *Proc Nutr Soc* 1997; **56:** 216A (Abstract).

52. Debongnie JC, Phillips SF. Capacity of the human colon to absorb fluid. *Gastroenterology* 1978; **74:** 698-703.

53. Fei Y, Kanal Y, Nussberger S, *et al.* Expression cloning of a mammalian proton-coupled oligopeptide transporter. *Nature* 1994; **368:** 563-566.

5

Assessing intestinal absorptive capacity and permeability *in vivo*

Ian S Menzies and Roger Crane

Summary

Methods available for assessing human intestinal absorption and permeability are considered in this chapter. These relate respectively to the efficiency of nutrient absorption and to barrier function, the former indicated by uptake of well-absorbed test probes that assess efficiency of diffusion and transport systems, and the latter by the permeation of larger, poorly absorbed probe molecules. The chemical and biochemical characteristics of available test substances, which determine the formulation of technical procedures, are discussed and recognised 'single-probe' procedures such as the D-xylose absorption test described. However, particular emphasis is placed on the advantages of more recently introduced non-invasive multi-probe sugar absorption methods that can be adapted for the simultaneous evaluation of intestinal permeability, absorptive capacity and, when required, disaccharidase activity. A well tried method for the simultaneous combined analysis of test sugars by thin-layer chromatography is also described: although quantitation by scanning densitometry gives the best results, visual assessment of the chromatograms by comparison of test with standard zones involves less labour and expenditure and can be sufficiently reliable to allow interpretation for clinical purposes.

Abbreviations

[51]Chromium-labelled ethylenediamine tetra-acetic acid	^{51}Cr-EDTA
polyethylene glycol	PEG
3-O-methyl-D-glucose	3mGluc
D-xylose	DXyl
L-rhamnose	Rham
mannitol	Man
lactulose	Lacl
lactose	Lac
sucrose	Suc
palatinose	Pal

Introduction

The uptake of nutrients involves an important aspect of intestinal permeability but, in its widest sense, intestinal permeability relates to three physiological requirements:

1. The uptake of nutrients and, in the therapeutic context, drugs. This is the outcome of efficient permeation or diffusion from the intestinal lumen usually refered to as 'absorption';

2. Secretion and diffusion of constituents into the intestinal lumen, related either to digestive or excretory functions;

3. Interposition of a protective barrier to reduce or prevent uptake of potentially harmful macromolecular constituents, achieved by a selective restriction of uptake, a further feature of mucosal permeability.

Alterations of intestinal permeability occur in a wide range of physiological, pathological and therapeutic situations, and techniques for the investigation of such changes can serve several purposes. The likelihood that hyperpermeability might enhance the uptake of antigenic or other potentially harmful macromolecules or micro-organisms has been mainly responsible for the current interest in the application of such techniques to research. In clinical contexts assessment of absorption is of obvious value when seeking an explanation for weight loss and other features of malnutrition, and investigation of intestinal permeability provides a useful indication of the integrity of the intestinal mucosa, for diagnostic screening or to monitor therapeutic progress in patients with villus atrophy due to gluten enteropathy, tropical malabsorption or inflammatory conditions such as Crohn's disease and gastroenteritis. The value of non-invasive tests as an alternative to repeated intubation with biopsy when assessing response to treatment was realised at quite an early stage,[1] especially after the introduction of more reliable differential tests of intestinal permeability,[2,3] which are described later in greater detail.

Methods for assessing absorption have been based upon the output of unabsorbed constituents in the faeces, for instance the estimation of faecal fat, widely adopted to investigate lipid absorption especially in pancreatic insufficiency.[4] Such procedures may be complicated by a loss of test substances due to bacterial action in the colon and the need for long collection periods to overcome day-to-day variations in bowel evacuation. Measurement of exsorption - the passage of constituents from blood to intestinal lumen - is employed for the clinical investigation of protein-losing enteropathy,[5-7] and has been used for assessing intestinal permeability in human and animal research.[8] Estimation of leucocyte influx for assessment of inflammatory bowel disease[9] is a further application of the same principle. Intestinal permeability has also been assessed by measurement of electrical resistance[10-12] and osmotic reflection.[13]

However, most methods for investigating absorption and permeability in humans[8,14-18] and laboratory animals[8,18-23] depend upon the uptake of selected test probes or their products from the intestine and are assessed by measuring recovery in urine or the rise in blood concentration following oral administration. When necessary greater anatomical specificity can be obtained, at the cost of further intervention, by delivering test solutions at defined levels in the intestine or by perfusing a selected intestinal segment by intubation (as described by Dr G.K. Grimble in the previous chapter). Transfer of selected probes across isolated portions of the intestinal epithelium *in vitro* has also been employed,[8,24-27] but deprivation of blood circulation may affect the integrity of epithelial cells.[28]

Over many years the search for sensitive test procedures with satisfactory reproducibility and discrimination has seen the introduction of many different test probes and variations of technique. As a result a large number of different procedures are currently in use, no consensus or standardisation having, so far, emerged. In this chapter, therefore,

critical reference is made to different methods, a selection of which are described in greater detail. With regard to tests of differential absorption and permeability the choice of probe combination and details of test procedure depend upon the aspects of intestinal function to be investigated and exact clinical or research situation, and should remain flexible. Formulation of test solutions and procedures should, however, take account of the properties of available probes and the impact of osmotic and other factors that may distort the outcome of such tests.

Methods

Choice of Probes

Probes should be known to cross the intestinal epithelium by a specific pathway of mediated or non-mediated diffusion so that test substances appropriate to the function or pathway to be investigated can be selected. Probes should resist metabolic degradation and be fully excreted by the kidney after reaching the circulation to ensure a reliable quantitative relationship between uptake from the intestine and concentration in the blood or recovery in the urine. Lack of toxicity, stability in test samples,

Table 5.1 – Physiological disposition of some intestinal test probes in the human[13,29,32,34-39]

| Probe | MW | Recovery in urine | | | | | Renal clearance | Degradation | |
| | | Following I.V. injection | | Following ingestion | | | (Inulin = 100 ml/min) | Metabolic | Bacterial |
		0–5 h	0–24 h	0–5h	0–10h	0–24h			
PEG-400	194-502	24-67%	26-68%	17%	19%	19%	–	Nil	Nil
[51]Cr-EDTA	359	85%	95%	0.44%	0.73%	1.16%	100 ml/min	Nil	Nil
FITC-dextran	3000	85%	98%	0.04%	–	–	100 ml/min	Nil	+
Lactulose	342	80%	90%	0.39%	0.54%	0.55%	100 ml/min	Nil	+
Melibiose	342	80%	90%	0.39%	0.54%	0.55%	100 ml/min	Nil	+
Mannitol	182	80%	90%	30%	38%	–	100 ml/min	Nil	+
L-rhamnose	164	62%	72%	11.7%	13%	14%	71 ml/min	minimal	+
D-xylose	150	43%	49%	31%	34%	35%	73 ml/min	50% loss	+
L-xylose	150	59%	72%	42%	50%	51%	91 ml/min	minimal	+
D-arabinose	150	51%	59%	22%	26%	27%	73 ml/min	minimal	+
L-arabinose	150	51%	58%	21.5%	24%	25%	78 ml/min	minimal	+
3-O-methyl-D-glucose	194	53%	80%	52%	74%	80%	59 ml/min	Nil	minimal

reasonable cost and availability of practical and reliable methods for quantitative analysis are also important, and it is necessary to know if and when a particular probe may normally be present in the diet or body fluids in order to avoid such circumstances during a test.

Information about mode of intestinal absorption, recovery in urine following intravenous and oral administration, renal clearance and susceptibility to systemic metabolism in the human, and degradation by bacteria, is given in Table 5.1. Additional details not included in Table 5.1 are mentioned below.

Probes with affinity for specific intestinal transport systems

D-xylose

Absorption of D-xylose in the human is mainly from the jejunum,[29] and is more efficient than that of mannitol, rhamnose and other pentoses so that concentrations in blood following ingestion are easier to measure. Involvment of a carrier-mediated pathway distinct from the active Na-dependant transport system available to D-glucose, D-galactose and 3-O-methyl-D-glucose is suggested by the observation that D-xylose absorption was not affected in two siblings with markedly reduced absorption of 3-O-methyl-D-glucose due to glucose-galactose malabsorption.[30] D-xylose is partly metabolised after reaching the circulation, about 50% of an intravenous dose being recovered in the urine.[29,31,32] Suitable oral test doses for adult subjects are 5.0 g or 0.5 g when concentrations in blood or urine, respectively, are to be estimated.

3-O-methyl-D-glucose

A synthetic monosaccharide which is efficiently absorbed from the human small intestine by an active Na-linked transport system shared with D-glucose and D-galactose.[29] 3-O-methyl-D-glucose resists metabolism in the human and is fully excreted in the urine after intravenous administration. Behaviour in other species may differ: for instance in calves 3-O-methyl-D-glucose did not appear in the urine following either intravenous or oral administration but persisted in the circulation for several days, re-absorption from the renal tubule evidently being complete as it is for D-glucose.[33] Suitable oral test doses are 2.5 g or 0.2 g when blood or urine concentrations, respectively, are to be estimated in adult human subjects.

Probes absorbed by non-mediated permeation (simple diffusion)

Molecular radius 0.4 nm

(permeating through high-incidence small aqueous mucosal pores)

L-rhamnose (Rham; 6-deoxy-L-mannose; a 'methylpentose'). McCance and Madders,[31] found the rate of rhamnose, arabinose and xylose uptake from the human intestine to be in the ratio 1/2.33/3.6 respectively, the comparatively slow rate for rhamnose suggesting a low or absent affinity for mediated intestinal transport.[31,15] 1.0 g is a suitable oral test dose for adult human subjects.

D-mannitol (D-mannose hexitol). Like rhamnose the uptake of mannitol from the human intestine is relatively slow suggesting lack of affinity for biochemically mediated mucosal transport.[34,35] Distribution after absorption appears to be confined to the extracellular space, with no evidence of metabolic degradation: renal clearance is similar to that of inulin and recovery after intravenous administration almost complete.[34,35] Apart from excretion of a small but unpredictable amount (of dietary or endogenous origin) in normal human urine[34] – a problem that can be overcome by using a ^{14}C-labelled preparation if necessary[34,35] – mannitol, like L-rhamnose, appears to be a suitable probe for assessing permeation through the 'high incidence' aqueous channels available in the small intestinal mucosa for the non-mediated diffusion of small polar molecules.[15,36] 1.0 g is a suitable oral test dose for adult human subjects.

Molecular radius ≥0.5 nm

(Permeating through low-incidence large aqueous mucosal pores)

Lactulose (*β1-4 fructo-galactoside*). Like most oligosaccharides lactulose resists metabolism and is rapidly and almost completely excreted in human urine following intravenous administration.[36-39] Melibiose, *raffinose, *stachyose and *fluorescein-labelled dextran (molecular weights 342, 504, 666 and 3000 daltons and radii 0.5, 0.59, 0.62 and 1.25 nm, respectively) also resist the action of human intestinal disaccharidases and are suitable for assessing intestinal 'large pore' permeability, >0.5 nm radius.[37,39] *They can be used in the same way as lactulose (N.B. for interpretation of results allowance must be made for Graham's Law viz. diffusion is inversely proportional to √molecular weight).

Melibiose can be given in the same dosage as lactulose when investigating intestinal permeability in patients receiving treatment with the latter sugar (e.g. for hepatic encephalopathy): 5.0 g is a suitable oral test dose for adults.

Polysucrose (mean MW 1500 Daltons). A synthetic co-polymer of sucrose and epichlorohydrin which resists the action of intestinal sucrase, is an alternative macromolecular probe suggested recently for the measurement of intestinal permeability.[43]

Cellobiose (ß1-4 diglucoside), also introduced as a permeability probe,[3,40,41] has the disadvantage of being susceptible to hydrolysis by intestinal lactase.[42] Sucrose has been proposed for assessing gastric permeability,[44,45] but the quantity excreted in urine following ingestion is equally determined by the permeability and level of sucrase activity in the small intestine.[46,47]

[51]Cr-Ethylenediaminetetra-acetate. Introduced for assessing intestinal permeability by Bjarnason *et al* in 1983,[48-50] ^{51}Cr-EDTA is confined to the extracellular space after reaching the circulation and undergoes complete renal clearance.[51] Resistance to degradation by bacteria makes it suitable for the estimation of permeability in the colon as well as the small intestine.[52,53] Recovery of ^{51}Cr-EDTA in urine following oral administration to patients with an established ileostomy (i.e. excluding the colon) is quantitatively identical to that of lactulose,[35,54] but excretion of ^{51}Cr-EDTA in subjects with intact colonic transit becomes progressively greater than that of lactulose during the course of a 24h urine collection[35,53] due to contribution of ^{51}Cr-EDTA from the colon. ^{51}Cr-EDTA has a gamma emission half life of 27 days which necessitates regular purchase to replace the stock, retention of reference standards for each batch of tests, and also puts a time limit on the storage of samples before analysis. 50 µCi is a suitable oral test-dose for adult human subjects.[54]

Polyethylene glycol (PEG)

Ethylene glycol polymers of many different molecular sizes have been introduced to assess intestinal permeability: PEG-400,[55] PEG-600,[56] PEG-1000.[57,58] PEG-4000, originally used as a non-absorbable reference marker for intestinal perfusion procedures,[13] has also been employed as a permeability probe.[59] Interpretation of tests incorporating PEG-400 is confusing, not only because renal clearance of the smaller polymers may be incomplete, but also because

uptake from the normal intestine is very much greater, and response to intestinal pathology quite different, from that of other polar probes of similar molecular dimension.[15,36,60] ^{14}C-labelled ethylene-glycols are available for use.

Clinical assessment of intestinal absorption: general points

Formulation of Test Solutions

Two different osmotic effects require attention when formulating test solutions .

1. *Hyperosmolar stress.* Ingestion of solutions of osmolality greater than 1000 mosmol/kg, due to a high concentration of many different solutes, including sugars, may temporarily increase intestinal permeability to polar probes with a molecular radius of 0.5 nm and above (e.g. lactulose, ^{51}Cr-EDTA, etc.) without affecting the absorption of monosaccharides.[36-39] For instance, raising the osmolality of a test solution containing lactulose from 1200 to 2800 mosmol/kg can produce a 6-fold increase in the recovery of lactulose in the urine.[38] Patients with mucosal pathology, especially villus atrophy, are more susceptible to this effect[37,39] and some authors have purposely made test solutions hyperosmolar (1500 mosmol/kg) to increase the sensitivity of permeability tests when screening for villus atrophy.[2,3,37,39-41] Care should be taken to ensure that test solutions are standardised to be iso-osmolar or of a specified hyperosmolarity at the time of use.

2. *Osmotic effect of poorly absorbed solutes.* Inclusion of poorly absorbed solute reduces intestinal absorption of test probes, especially affecting the uptake of lactulose, L-rhamnose, mannitol and, to a lesser extent, D-xylose.[54,61] This is largely due to accumulation of fluid within the intestine producing dilution and hurry. A progressive reduction in the percentage of D-xylose excreted in the urine by normal human subjects as the dose is increased, 4-hour recovery falling from 31% to 22.8% and 18.2% as the oral dose is increased from 5 g, to 25 g and 50 g[62,63] is probably an example of this effect. Because test-sugars such as lactulose, L-rhamnose, mannitol and D-xylose themselves are capable of affecting their own absorption in this way, dosage should be kept at a minimum level compatible with analysis in urine (e.g. not more than 5 g of lactulose and D-xylose, and 1.0-2.0 g of L-rhamnose or mannitol are advisable per test).

Preservation of oral test solutions

Solutions containing test sugars should be kept deep frozen under conditions appropriate for food storage, and thawed overnight before use. Alternatively such solutions can be made up as a concentrated stock solution of bacteriocidal osmolality (>2000 mosmol/kg). Shortly before use an appropriate volume of the stock solution should be dispensed with a graduated syringe and diluted to standard volume with drinking water (N.B. lactose and raffinose, less soluble than other sugars, may precipitate from concentrated solutions). Such concentrated solutions prevent degradation of sugars by bacteria at room temperature, but are better kept refrigerated (but not deep frozen).

Conduct of tests

It is convenient to start the test after an overnight fast and the patient should take nothing except plain water by mouth for a minimum period of 4 hours before and 2 hours after commencing the test. It is necessary to ensure that the whole of the test solution is ingested without undue delay (i.e. within a period of 4 minutes) and the time recorded.

As uptake from the intestine is progressive and usually takes several hours to complete it is necessary to express the efficiency of absorption as the quantity of a test substance absorbed within a specified time. It is therefore important to ensure that urine collection is complete and of a prescribed duration. Doubts about the reliability of urine collection or efficiency of renal clearance may be resolved by calculating a 'clearance index' from estimates of creatinine in urine and plasma collected during course of the test and for this it is necessary to ensure that bladder emptying is undertaken immediately before the start of the test.

Sugars such as sucrose and lactose may have prolonged excretion and should be excluded from the diet for 16 hours before administration as well as throughout the period of urine collection. A 'baseline' urine sample collected before the start of each test can be analysed to confirm satisfactory elimination.

Preservation of plasma and urine samples

Most sugars in blood and urine samples are subject to rapid degradation by bacteria if kept at room temperature. Urine collections should be made into receptacles that contain an effective preservative such as thiomersal (BDH Chemicals, Ltd) which should be above a minimum concentration 10 mg/100 ml

in aliquots stored for analysis (= 0.1 ml of 10% w/v aqueous thiomersal per 100 ml urine).[64] Preserved thus urine samples can be safely stored for many months at room temperature, but plasma or blood samples, which would require a higher concentration of thiomersal, are better frozen for storage.[64]

D-xylose absorption tests

Intestinal absorption of D-xylose in the human was originally investigated by Helmer and Fouts in 1937,[65] and first employed for the detection of malabsorption by Fourman in 1948.[66] The 'D-xylose absorption test' has since become established for routine clinical investigation of intestinal absorption but a variety of test procedures have been suggested. Choice of oral test dose has varied considerably: for adults some authors employ 25 g,[67-70] but others use 15 g[71] or 5 g[72-75] on grounds that the larger dose may, by producing intestinal hurry and osmotic purgation, give an unreliable estimate of intestinal absorption.[73-75] Infants and children have been given either a fixed 5 g dose[76] or a variable dose related to body weight[77,78] or surface area.[79] Interpretation is based upon the behaviour of the blood xylose concentration/time (or 'absorption') curve, or timed excretion in the urine. As with other 'single probe' absorption and permeability tests the influence of extramucosal factors (i.e. those not directly related to the intestinal absorptive surface, see Table 5.2) presents a problem. Fordtran et al.[29] demonstrated that although absorption of D-xylose from the human jejunum is quite efficient, uptake from the ileum is minimal, and approximately 20% of the ingested dose normally enters the colon unabsorbed. Lack of any 'reserve capacity' for uptake by the normal small intestine increases ability of D-xylose to detect minor impairment of absorptive capacity.

The 5 gram D-xylose absorption test

(After Haeney *et al.* 1978.)[75]

Sammons *et al.*[73] comparing different doses of D-xylose found the response to 25 g to be insensitive but that a smaller oral dose (5.0 g) gave a more reliable indication of small bowel malabsorption, especially if the urine collection was split to allow comparison of the 2 hour with 5 hour recovery. Eleven years later the same group[75] concluded from a very detailed study that reproducibility was optimal, and discrimination between normal subjects and patients with malabsorption due to villus atrophy greatest, when xylose concentration, estimated in a blood sample taken 60 minutes after an oral dose of 5 g dissolved in 250 ml water, was corrected to constant body surface area.[75] This gave false positive and negative assessments in 2.2% and 4.8%, respectively.

Normal ranges

Blood or plasma: The normal 60 min blood D-xylose range, corrected to 1.73 m² body surface area, is 9.8-20.0 mg/100 ml.[75] This is not thought to be affected by impaired renal clearance, whether due to old age[62,75,80] or renal disease.

Urine: The mean ± SD recovery in urine (percentage of 5 g dose) is 19.0 ± 7.9% in 0 to 2 hours and 35.0 ± 9.2% in 0 to 5 hours for healthy subjects under 60 years age.

Clinical assessment of intestinal permeability

The focus of interest regarding 'barrier function' is on the permeation of large molecules across the intestinal surface. Uptake of oligosaccharides (e.g. lactulose, melibiose, raffinose) and ⁵¹Cr-EDTA, molecular radius 0.5 nm and above, which indicate this aspect of permeability, is usually less than 1.0% of the oral dose. Plasma concentrations achieved are very low and difficult to estimate so that most methods involve measurement of concentrations in urine which are between 10 and 100-fold higher. Test solutions can be delivered by intubation when it is necessary to study specific portions of the intestine.[52,81]

Mathematically expressed, permeability is the amount transferred in unit time across unit area of membrane under defined conditions of concentration gradient, temperature, etc. with respect to a specified probe. The difficulty of imposing sufficient control over factors in the intact intestine, let alone of making the necessary measurements, makes it impractical to express intestinal permeability *in vivo* in this way. Consequently intestinal 'permeability' has been expressed in terms of timed uptake of macro-molecular probes from the whole or part of the intestine, for instance the percentage of a 50 μCi oral dose of ⁵¹Cr-EDTA recovered in urine during 24 hours.[43,48-50,52,53] The advantages of simultaneous use of multiple probes is discussed later.

Measurement of large intestinal permeability

Uptake of sugar probes which are rapidly degraded by bacteria in the large intestine relates mainly to the stomach and small intestine. Colonic permeability can be assessed by measuring urinary recovery of a bacterial resistant probe such as ⁵¹Cr-EDTA following direct infusion into the colon.[52] Such a 'test-probe enema' should be iso-osmotic and retained for a carefully standardised period of time.

Alternatively colonic permeation may be calculated from the recovery of ⁵¹Cr-EDTA and lactulose in urine following combined oral administration.[53] Urine recovery of lactulose, rapidly degraded by bacteria on entering the colon, represents upper intestinal permeation whereas ⁵¹Cr-EDTA, which resists the action of colonic bacteria, represents total intestinal permeation. Subtraction of lactulose from ⁵¹Cr-EDTA, both expressed as percentages of the oral dose recovered in a 24 hour urine collection, can therefore be used as an indication of colonic permeability.

Differential Absorption: combined use of test sugars

This principle can be applied to the investigation of intestinal permeability, absorptive capacity and disaccharide hydrolysis.[14,16]

D-xylose and 3-O-methyl-D-glucose (intestinal absorption). The traditional D-xylose absorption test is influenced by variations in gastric emptying rate: in addition, blood concentrations will be influenced by body size, state of hydration and the presence of ascites or oedema, and recovery of D-xylose in urine will be influenced by the state of renal clearance and competence of urine collection. Although blood xylose concentration at 60 minutes was considered to be unaffected by poor renal clearance whether due to old age[62,80] or renal disease, correction for body size improved reliability.[75]

In view of the observations of Fordtran *et al.*[29] contrasting the sensitivity of D-xylose with the insensitivity of 3-O-methyl-D-glucose to changes in small intestinal absorptive capacity, Noone *et al.*[82] compared diagnostic discrimination between small children with and without malabsorption (due to acute rotaviral enteritis) obtained by blood D-xylose concentrations in samples taken 60 minutes after simultaneous oral administration of D-xyl 2.5 g and 3mGluc 1.25 g dissolved in 25 ml water:

1. when not corrected for body surface area,

2. when corrected for body surface area, and

3. when expressed as a D-xylose/3-O-methyl-D-glucose ratio.

The results of this study, presented in Figure 5.1, demonstrate a remarkable advantage obtained by using both sugars together: whereas discrimination by the 60 minute D-Xyl/3mGluc blood concentration ratios is complete, separation between the two groups obtained from D-xylose levels alone, even when corrected for body size, was far from satisfactory.

Lactulose and L-rhamnose (intestinal permeability). The same principle has also been applied to the assessment of intestinal permeability, in this case by comparing permeation of two polar probes with different molecular dimensions ingested simultaneously, e.g. lactulose and L-rhamnose, molecular radii 0.5 and 0.4 nm, respectively, and calculating a ratio of the percentages recovered in urine.[2,3] As variations due to 'non-mucosal factors' (see Table 5.2) are likely to affect the transfer of both probes to the same extent, calculation of a differential excretion ratio determined by the relative incidence of the large and small aqueous channels (pore profile) of the mucosa, will eliminate most of the irrelevant factors and provide a specific evaluation of permeability.[15]

Furthermore, combination of lactulose and L-rhamnose which show diametrically opposite responses to

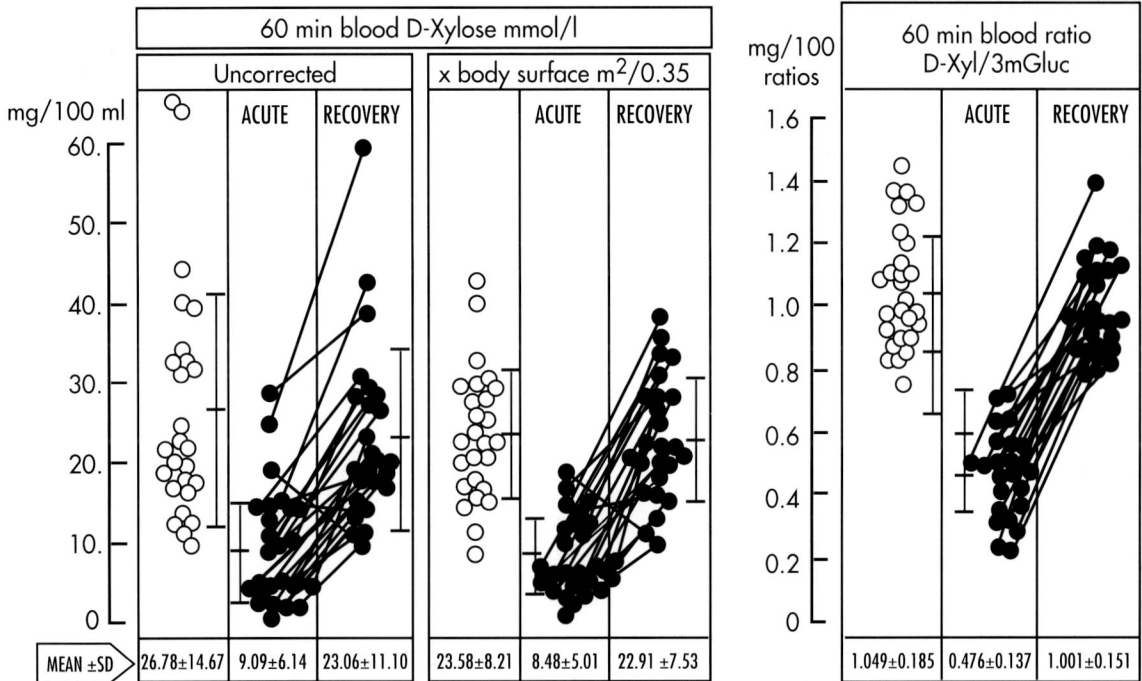

Figure 5.1 - Discrimination by plasma D-xylose compared with D-Xyl/3mGluc estimations in infants with malabsorption due to acute rotaviral enteritis.[82,83] Comparison of plasma D-Xyl (on left uncorrected and in center corrected to constant body surface area) with D-Xyl/3mGluc concentration ratio (on right, with no correction). 'Recovery' tests were performed after recovery, four weeks later. Unlike the plasma D-Xyl concentrations, D-Xyl/3mGluc concentration ratios gave complete discrimination.

Table 5.2 – Factors affecting the outcome of non-invasive absorption tests

Use of the principle of differential intestinal absoption to control variables.
Simultaneous administration of two test probes, A and B, which respond in an identical way to each variable except that selected for investigation, provides a non-invasive method for assessing specific aspects of intestinal function. Correctly devised A/B excretion ratio (of percentages recovered in the urine) provides a specific index of the selected function unaffected by the other variables.

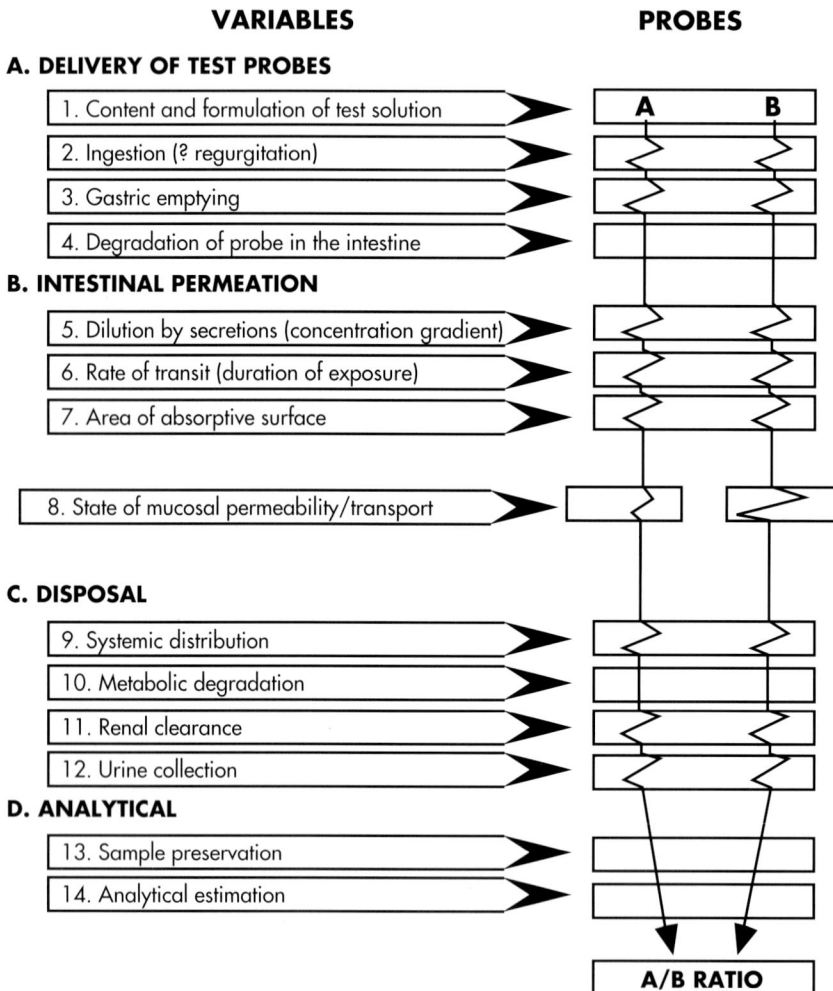

VARIABLES | PROBES

A. DELIVERY OF TEST PROBES
1. Content and formulation of test solution
2. Ingestion (? regurgitation)
3. Gastric emptying
4. Degradation of probe in the intestine

B. INTESTINAL PERMEATION
5. Dilution by secretions (concentration gradient)
6. Rate of transit (duration of exposure)
7. Area of absorptive surface

8. State of mucosal permeability/transport

C. DISPOSAL
9. Systemic distribution
10. Metabolic degradation
11. Renal clearance
12. Urine collection

D. ANALYTICAL
13. Sample preservation
14. Analytical estimation

A/B RATIO

intestinal pathology provides better discrimination than the use of either probe by itself[15, 84] (Figure 5.2). Probe combinations that are also employed include lactulose/mannitol,[85] cellobiose/rhamnose[41] and cellobiose/mannitol.[3,40] Combinations of ^{51}Cr-EDTA with either mannitol or rhamnose have also been proposed[35,86,87] but, unlike ^{51}Cr-EDTA, mannitol and rhamnose are degraded by bacteria in the colon. A satisfactory bacterial-resistant small-pore probe to combine with ^{51}Cr-EDTA for assessing large-intestinal pore profile has yet to be introduced. Use of the lactulose/rhamnose combination for measuring upper intestinal permeability[2,15,84,88-92] is described in greater detail below but, apart from the choice of probes and analytical procedure, all these dual-probe permeability tests can be conducted in the same way.

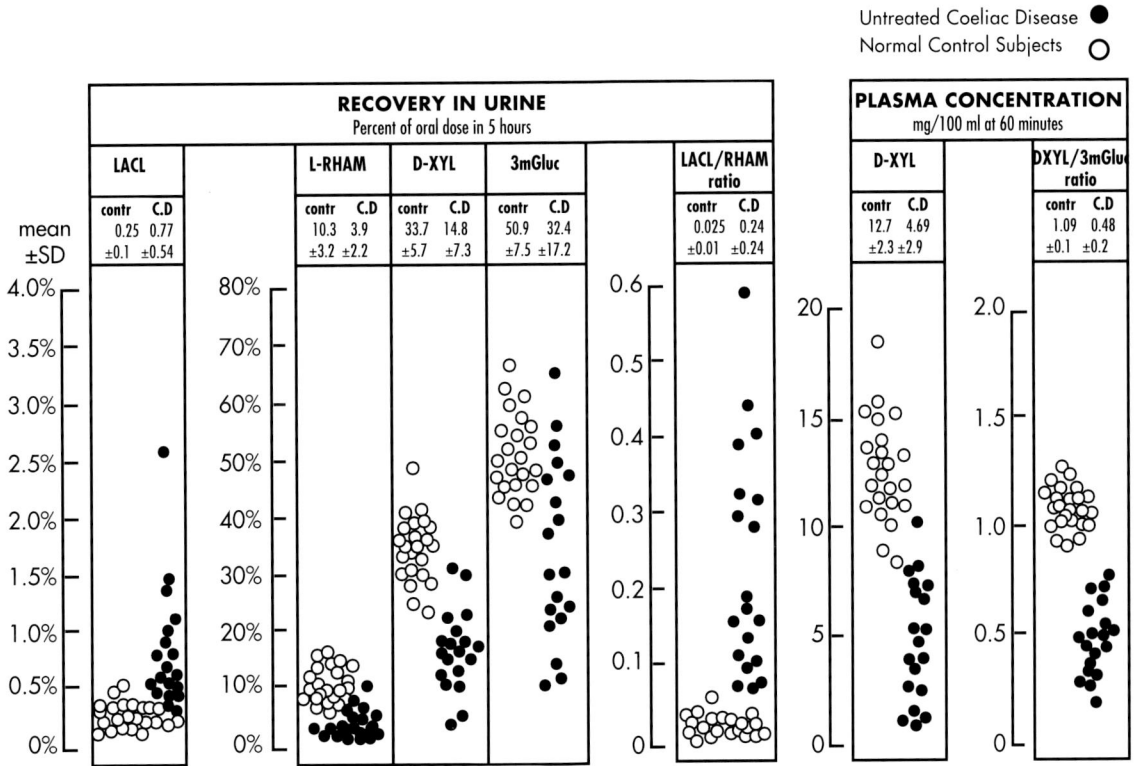

Untreated Coeliac Disease ●
Normal Control Subjects ○

Figure 5.2 – Response to the Lacl/Rham-DXyl/3mGluc four-sugar test in patients with untreated coeliac disease.
Oral Test Solution: Lacl, Rham, DXyl, 3mGluc: 5 g, 1 g, 5 g and 2.5 g, respectively, in 250ml.

● Patients with untreated coeliac disease.
○ Healthy control subjects.

The results demonstrate a considerable improvement in discrimination when Lacl/Rham (urine) and DXyl/3mGluc (plasma) ratios are calculated.

Differential four-sugar absorption/permeability test (After Cook & Menzies, 1986).[88]

The D-xylose/3-O-methyl-D-glucose and lactulose/L-rhamnose test procedures have been combined to assess intestinal absorptive capacity and permeability simultaneously.[88,89]

Test solution: lactulose 5.0 g (=7.5 ml 67% lactulose syrup), D-xylose 5.0 g, 3mGluc 2.5 g and L-rhamnose 1.0 g dissolved in 250 ml drinking water. For an alternative 'urine only' version of the test DXyl and 3mGluc in smaller amounts (0.5 and 0.2 g respectively) can be given with lactulose and L-rhamnose in 100 ml drinking water. Test solutions can be either kept deep frozen at full volume (as above), or made up as a concentrated syrup of bactericidal osmolarity (>2000 mosmol/litre) which

is stable at room temperature, the high dose in 25 ml (= 2,675 mosmol/l) and low dose in 10 ml (= 2,506 mosmol/l), to be diluted to 250 ml or 100 ml, respectively, shortly before the test.

Test procedure: After an overnight fast the subject voids urine, and then drinks the whole test solution within a period not longer than 4 minutes. All urine produced for exactly 5 hours is then collected into a 1-1.5 litre bottle containing thiomersal as preservative (>10 mg per 100 ml urine). The patient should finish the collection by voiding urine exactly (or as near as possible) at the end of 5 hours. Blood samples (5.0 ml each) should be taken into anticoagulant bottles at 30, 60, 90, and 120 minutes, separated and the plasma samples stored deep-frozen for analysis. The volume of the urine collection is recorded and a 20 ml aliquot kept for analysis.

Note. The patient is allowed to take food again 2 hours after commencing the test. For infants a single 60 minute 2.0 ml anticoagulated blood sample is sufficient if handled carefully. Haemolysed blood samples can be used for the analysis of sugars but not for creatinine.

Interpretation: (See box below)

Differential tests of intestinal disaccharide hydrolysis (After Maxton *et al.*).[46]

Urinary excretion ratios of intact hydrolysable/non-hydrolysable disaccharide following ingestion have been demonstrated to be inversely proportional to the efficiency intestinal hydrolysis.[37,46,47] This is the rationale for the non-invasive estimation of intestinal lactase, sucrase or isomaltase activity using lactose/lactulose, sucrose/lactulose or palatinose/lactulose ratio-tests respectively. These can be undertaken separately[84] or in combination[46,47] and are used to exclude disaccharidase deficiency in the clinical investigation of diarrhoea. Urine is collected for 10 hours following oral administration of lactulose (6.7 g), lactose, sucrose and, if necessary, palatinose (10 g each), dissolved in 300 ml drinking water. L-rhamnose 1.0 g is usually included to enable Lacl/Rham permeability to be monitored as well.

[46,47,84] Deficient intestinal hydrolysis is indicated by a rise in the hydrolysable/non-hydrolysable disaccharide urinary excretion ratio (of percentages excreted in 10 hours) above 0.3 and, when associated with a rise in lactulose/rhamnose ratio, the impairment of disaccharidase is likely to be secondary to intestinal disease.[46,47,84]

Note. Melibiose can be substituted for lactulose in the above tests if the latter sugar is being used therapeutically or the presence of lactose interferes with lactulose analysis. Excretion ranges for lactulose and melibiose are the same.

Miscellaneous factors affecting interpretation

1. *Drug effects*. Non-steroidal anti-inflammatory drugs increase intestinal permeability to ^{51}Cr-EDTA and lactulose:[87] there is evidence that this involves both the small and large intestine.[87,90,93] The small intestinal effect appears to be temporary, and lasts for less than 8 hours following ingestion of indomethacin.[93] The likelihood that irradiation, administration of cytotoxic drugs and antibiotics such as neomycin are capable of altering intestinal permeability and absorptive capacity[16] should also be considered when undertaking intestinal function tests.

Plasma DXyl and 3mGluc: Normal adult ranges, mg/100ml, following DXyl 5 g, 3mGluc 2.5 g dose for U.K.

Time	30 min	60 min	90 min	120 min
D-Xylose, Mean ± SD:	10.2 ± 3.10	12.72 ± 2.25	11.3 ± 2.22	9.24 ± 2.28
3mGluc, Mean ± SD:	10.27 ± 3.06	11.77 ± 2.02	9.91 ± 2.28	8.49 ± 1.98
D-Xyl/3mGluc, mg/100ml ratio:		1.089 ± 0.100		

Recovery in 5-hour urine (Mean ± S.D., see Figure 5.2 for scattergram).

Lactulose %/5hrs	L-rhamnose %/5hrs	D-xylose %/5hrs	3mGluc %/5hrs	Lacl/Rham ratio of %'s/5h
0.25 ± 0.1	10.3 ± 3.2	33.7 ± 5.7	50.9 ± 7.5	0.025 ± 0.01

Note. The normal ranges of urine lactulose and L-rhamnose recovery remain the same if D-xylose and 3mGluc are deleted from the test solution.

2. *Residence in tropical areas.* Caution is required when interpreting tests of intestinal permeability and absorption in residents of many tropical areas on account of tropical enteropathy.[94,95] This appears to be environmental, probably related to a high incidence of intestinal infestation with bacteria and other pathogenic microorganisms producing mucosal changes with increased permeability and reduced absorptive capacity.

3. *Age.* There is evidence of increased intestinal permeability to disaccharide in the pre-term neonate,[96] but otherwise differential sugar permeability remains unaltered even in advanced old age.[41] Urine D-Xylose recovery is reported to be significantly reduced in healthy infants below 6 months[97] and, on account of decreasing renal clearance, in subjects aged above 60 years.[62,80,98-101]

Application to animal studies

[51]Cr-EDTA and multiple-probe sugar tests have been adapted for assessing intestinal permeability in both rats[18-20] and dogs,[21-23] the principles and methods being similar to those employed for human investigation. These techniques are reported to be reliable and useful, but special problems concern the administration of test solutions and collection of urine samples, especially in the smaller laboratory animals, and also the use of test sugars which are susceptible to bacterial degradation. For rat experiments the dose of test sugars is scaled down (e.g. lactulose and mannitol, 100 mg and 40 mg, respectively)[19] and collection of urine can be undertaken through indwelling cannulae. Alternatively a 'metabolism cage' can be used, specially designed to collect urine and faeces separately.[19] For dog experiments sugar doses are similar to those used for humans (lactulose and D-xylose 5 g, 3mGluc and rhamnose 2.0 g for dogs over 20 Kg and half this for those under this weight), the solutions being given by mouth. Urine can be collected at the end of 5 hours by catherisation for dogs kept in a conventional cage, or into a vessel containing thiomersal in a metabolism cage.[102]

Analysis of test sugars

The great variety of procedures employed for quantitative sugar analysis bears witness to the problems presented. Estimation of xylose and other test monosaccharides, originally based upon reducing activity undertaken with[65,75] or without[66] prior removal of glucose by yeast fermentation, was later largely replaced by the specific reaction of pentoses with 4-bromoaniline described by Roe and Rice.[103] Mannitol has been estimated by oxidisation with periodic acid to formaldehyde which gives a purple colour with chromotropic acid,[104,3,40] but gas-liquid[105] and high pressure liquid[106,107] column chromatographic methods are now more widely used. Enzymatic methods are also available for the estimation of mannitol[108] and of disaccharides, the latter being based on measurement of monosaccharide products generated by incubation with ß-galactosidase – for instance fructose from lactulose and galactose from lactose[109] – and of glucose from cellobiose by incubation with β-glucosidase[40] (though glucose may also be generated from lactose). Alternatively, specific analysis of sugars can be facilitated by labelling with ^{3}H or [14]C. Chromatographic methods, however, not only have the advantage of greater specificity and sensitivity, but are capable of quantitating a combination of test sugars and are therefore particularly appropriate for differential sugar absorption tests.[105-107]

Quantitative estimation of sugars by thin-layer chromatography and scanning densitometry

(After Menzies, *et al.*).[110]

At the present time thin-layer chromatography with scanning densitometry[110] and high pressure liquid chromatography[107] are counted amongst the few reliable methods available for quantitating the combination of test sugars employed for the differential absorption/permeability tests described above. Details of an adaptation of thin-layer chromatography for the measurement of monosaccharides in plasma have been described previously.[110] The following account goes further, describing modifications such as 'multiple application with pre-run' for dealing with low disaccharide concentrations in urine.

Apparatus

SCANNING DENSITOMETER: Bio Rad Densitometer, model G57670 Molecular Analyst, from Bio Rad Systems, U.S.A. (other suitable instruments are also available).

CHROMATOGRAPHY TANK: Shandon SAA 21 44/DG 28 × 28 cm with cover and aluminium tray from Shandon Southern Products Ltd., 95-96 Chadwick Road, Runcorn, Cheshire.

MICROSYRINGE: R–GP type (5 μl) from Scientific Engineering (SGE) Ltd., Milton Keynes, Berks.

HOT-AIR OVEN: Type F with stainless steel interior, 24 × 20 × 20 inches with air circulating fan motor and door with glass panels, from Laboratories Thermal Equipment Ltd., Greenfield, Oldham, Lancashire.

ELECTRIC MOTOR (for rotating chromatograms during colour reaction): Type 82, 414/10 rev/min, from Crouzet, Thanet House, Brentford, Middlesex.

DIPPING CHAMBER. 'Roughcast' glass plates, 26.5 × 21.0 cm, 6 mm thick (two). Tygon heavy-wall sleeve tubing K 562-0005, 1/8 inch internal diameter (for spacer) from Gradko International Ltd., 77 Wales Street, Winchester, Hampshire SO23 7RH. The frame is not commercially available, for construction of chamber see Figure 5.4, inset 2a.

PYREX LOW-FORM BEAKERS. 200/250 ml capacity, to hold chromatograms during development, from Payne Products, 6 Iveley Road, London.

Materials and reagents

Thin-layer plates. Plastic-backed silica gel 60 (without fluorescent indicator, 0.25 mm layer) art. 5748 from E. Merck, Darmstadt, Germany. F1500 silica gel from Schleicher and Schuell, Dassel, Germany (but F1500 layers capable of providing a satisfactory separation of lactulose from lactose, as in Figure 5.3, are no longer available).

Standard sugar solutions (the pure sugars mentioned are available from Sigma Chemical Company).

monosaccharide *stock solution*:	L-rhamnose, D-xylose, 3-O-methyl-D-glucose 100 mg/100 ml
disaccharide *stock solution*:	melibiose, ★lactulose, ★lactose, sucrose 100 mg /100 ml
Internal *standard solutions*:	for monosaccharides: D-arabinose 40 mg/ 100 ml; for disaccharides: raffinose 50 mg/100 ml

★lactose and lactulose should not be used together if chromatographic separation is incomplete.

Note. All sugar solutions to be made up in distilled water with 20 mg/100 ml merthiolate as preservative,[64] and stored in the refrigerator (N.B. solutions must be brought to room temperature before using air-displacement pipettes).

DEPROTEINISATION/INTERNAL STANDARD REAGENT sulphosalicylic acid 5 g + arabinose 40 mg/ 100ml, aqueous.

DE-IONISING RESIN Zerolit DM-F (or equivalent), mixed cation/anion exchange resin is supplied in the H^+/OH^- phase and needs conversion to the $H^+/acetate^-$ phase to avoid sugar sequestration and the possibility of aldose/ketose conversion. 500 g of resin is stirred with 3 litres of 10% (v/v) acetic acid and washed with 3 litres distilled water followed by partial drying on an open tray at room temperature.

Note. The resin is hygroscopic, and damaged by complete desiccation.

SOLVENTS ethyl acetate, pyridine, glacial acetic acid, butan-1-ol, ethanol, methanol.

COLOUR REAGENT dissolve 4-aminobenzoic acid 1.4 g in methanol, add orthophosphoric acid (90 g/100 ml) 17.5 ml, mix and make up to 500 ml with further methanol.

obtainable for B.D.H. chemicals Limited.

Preparation of samples

This involves addition of internal standard and deproteinisation (for blood and plasma samples) followed by de-ionisation.

INTERNAL STANDARD. An internal standard correction is needed to reduce errors arising from imprecision of sample application, water content and molecular sieve properties of the desalting resin, and zone distortion. Sugars chosen as internal standards should separate well from those present in the sample and be of similar reactivity and molecular size to those requiring analysis.

URINE SAMPLES WITH SUGAR CONCENTRATIONS BETWEEN 10 AND 100 MG/100 ML: equal volumes (0.5 ml) of urine and internal standard solution (40 mg/100 ml arabinose for monosaccharide and 50 mg/100 ml raffinose or palatinose for disaccharide estimation) are mixed and then de-ionised. Dilution will be required for concentrations >100 mg/100 ml.

URINE SAMPLES WITH SUGAR CONCENTRATIONS BELOW 10 MG/100 ML: multiple applications are required to increase sensitivity.
For monosaccharides: two applications are usually sufficient, in which case 0.5 ml of urine sample is mixed

with 0.5 ml of half-strength internal standard (20 mg/100 ml arabinose) and de-ionised as above.

For disaccharides (often present at much lower concentration) multiple application with pre-run technique is required. For this 0.5 ml of urine sample is mixed with 0.5 ml of raffinose internal standard at a concentration appropriate to the number of applications required (= 50/n mg/100 ml, where n is the number of 5 µl applications proposed), and then de-ionised. The number of applications suitable for anticipated disaccharide concentrations of 10, 8, 4, 2 and 1 mg/100 ml are ×2, ×4, ×8, ×10 and ×20, respectively.

PLASMA, SERUM OR HAEMOLYSED WHOLE BLOOD SAMPLES: Equal volumes (0.5 ml) of sample and internal standard/deproteinising reagent (20 mg arabinose + 5 g sulphosalicylic acid/100 ml) are mixed and then centrifuged. The supernatant is transferred to a second tube for de-ionisation. Concentrations between 2 and 20 mg/100 ml are to be expected following an oral dose of 5 g DXyl + 2.5 g 3mGluc: two 5 µl applications required).

PREPARATION OF WORKING STANDARDS. Two series of four standards (12.5, 25, 50 and 100 mg/100 ml) are prepared from the 100 mg/100 ml stock sugar standard solutions, the first containing monosaccharides and the second, disaccharides. These are converted to 'working standards' by adding, as for the urine samples, an equal volume of internal standard, arabinose (40 mg/100 ml) for the monosaccharides and raffinose (50 mg/100 ml) for the disaccharides (de-ionisation not required).

QUALITY CONTROL (QC) SAMPLES. Urine and plasma obtained from a volunteer following exclusion of sugars from the diet for 16 hours should be used for preparing quality control samples. 20 mg/100 ml disaccharide and 40 mg/100 ml monosaccharide concentrations are suitable for urine and 10 mg/100 ml DXyl and 3mGluc concentrations for plasma. These should be prepared with each batch of test samples and de-ionised in the same way.

DE-IONISATION. Prepared resin is added (about 60% total volume) to deproteinised plasma or urine containing appropriate internal standard and shaken for 3.5 minutes. The supernatant is then ready for application.

Application technique

Application layout is illustrated in Figure 5.3: estimation of monosaccharides are performed on a half-plate (20 × 10 cm) to allow for a solvent rise of

8.5 cm from the origin, and of disaccharides on a full plate (20 × 20 cm) to allow for a 13.5 cm rise. The silica gel medium is scraped from 1.0 cm margins at the sides and a 0.5 cm margin along the top of each layer to allow handling without damage to the media, and a line of origin is marked in soft pencil 1 cm (for monosaccharide) or 6.5 cm (for disaccharide) above the lower border. To avoid zone distortion due to 'margin effects', which are difficult to control, the first and last application positions should be at least 2.5 cm from the lateral border (i.e. 1.5 cm from the edge of the silica media), and be allocated to less important samples (i.e. not to standards or quality controls). Application zones are marked out with a soft pencil, as shown in Figure 5.3, with care to avoid damaging the surface of the media. A template marked to indicate the position of 14 application areas (each 8 mm wide and separated by 3 mm intervals) along one edge is useful for marking out the chromatograms. 14 positions will allow 4 standard (12.5, 25, 50 and 100 mg/100 ml), one QC and 8 test sample applications per chromatogram, leaving one blank 'channel' for baseline assessment.

Applications of between 4 and 5 µl, suitable for both 'test', 'standard' and QC samples, are made manually with a microsyringe. The syringe is held slightly inclined to the surface of the silica gel layer with the bevel facing downwards: the needle is drawn gently along the origin while delivery is controlled to produce a uniform band-shaped zone not more than 5 mm wide within the appropriate application box. When further applications are required to increase sensitivity for monosaccharide estimations (especially of D-xylose and 3-O-methyl-D-glucose in plasma samples) the second application is superimposed after the first has dried completely (about 30 minutes required).

MULTIPLE APPLICATION AND PRE-RUN TECHNIQUE (to increase sensitivity when estimating urine disaccharide concentrations below 10 mg/100 ml). The appropriate number of 5 µl applications are made within longitudinal areas marked out in soft pencil on the lower 6.5 cm portion of a 20 × 20 cm layer, as shown in Figure 5.3. To avoid zone distortion adjacent applications are positioned sufficiently far apart to avoid any overlap, seven being the maximum number usually accomodated in each area. Should a larger application volume be required a further series can be superimposed when the first series has dried out completely (at least 30 minutes required). The sugars applied to each area are then 'brought up' to the effective '6.5 cm origin' by means of two consecutive upward developments, the first with a rise of 6.5 cm, and the second, following a 30 minute interval for drying and removal of the lower 4.5 cm portion of the application area, with a rise of 2 cm, using a water-rich solvent system in which the sugars move at the solvent front (see Figure 5.3).

Chromatographic development

The best results are obtained when the chromatogram is run as a cylinder inserted inside a standard-type 200-250 ml glass beaker, plastic backing facing outwards, as shown in Figure 5.4 (inset 1).[110] Radial symmetry ensures that exposure of the layer surface to solvent vapour is uniform, so that bowing of the solvent front with convergence and distortion of zones due to incomplete vapour saturation, seen with the traditional 'flat layer' technique, is avoided (Figure 5.4, inset 1), and development becomes more reproducible.

Solvent mixtures

A system: butanol, ethanol, acetic acid (glac.), water: 60, 30, 10, 10 by vol.

B systems: ethly acetate, butanol, pyridine, acetic acid (glac.), water: B_1: 75, 0 , 15, 10, 10; B_2: 70, 5, 15, 10, 10; and B_3: 65, 10, 15, 10, 10 by vol.

MONOSACCHARIDES: Rham, 3mGluc, DXyl and arabinose are adequately separated by two consecutive upward developments (rise 8.5 cm each) on Merck 60 plastic-backed silica gel layers (Dassel FRG) using the solvent sequence B_1, B_1 with 30 minute intervals minimum) between runs for drying. Urea, which inhibits the colour reaction, runs ahead of Rham in this system.

DISACCHARIDES: A satisfactory separation of Suc, Pal, Mel, and Raff is obtained on E. Merck silica gel 60 (0.25 mm art, 5748) plastic-backed layers following three consecutive upward developments (rise 13.5 cm each) using the solvent sequence A, B_3, B_3. This system does not separate lactose from lactulose on Merck 60 layers, as was previously possible using Schleicher and Schuell F1500 silica gel with a solvent sequence A, B_2, A (see Figure 5.3). Unfortunately the separation of lactose from lactulose, which has always been a problem, can no longer be achieved on the F1500 product at present available.

When pyridine, which inhibits the colour reaction, is included in the solvent drying should be continued overnight (or for at least 4 hours, minimum). After this layers may be safely stored in a protective poly-thene bag until the colour reaction can be performed.

Colour reaction

APPLICATION OF LOCATING REAGENT. Sufficient control of reagent distribution and concentration on the layer surface is not feasible by means of spraying techniques. A dipping technique standardises reagent uptake in accordance with layer absorbancy, but irregular distribution due to 'hesitation lines' and inadequate draining of reagent result when the traditional 'dipping tray' is used for thin-layer chromatograms.

DIPPING CHAMBER. A specially constructed dipping chamber can be used to overcome these problems. As shown in Figure 5.4 (inset 2) this consists of two rectangular glass plates mounted in a frame and held apart by a U-shaped spacer of thick-walled tygon tubing with a wire core to retain shape. Adjustable wing-nuts on the frame enable the plates to be compressed against the spacer, thus sealing the chamber for use. The faces of the chamber should be of 'rough cast' glass to prevent the plastic surface of a chromatogram from clinging during dipping, and the upper margins are rounded by honing to prevent damage to the layer surface when it is drained during withdrawal.

DIPPING PROCEDURE. Fill the chamber to within 0.5 cm of the top with 4-aminobenzoic acid/phosphoric acid reagent (see materials and reagents section) - approximately 250 ml required. The layer, held at one edge with a suitable clip, is lowered rapidly into the reagent, as shown in Figure 5.4 (inset 2a and 2b) and drawn slowly out against the smooth edge of the chamber to drain off excess reagent from the silica gel surface. Immersion should be as brief as possible to avoid zone trailing and loss of sugars. Return the reagent, which can be re-used if kept refrigerated, to the bottle without delay.

COLOUR REACTION. After drying for 5 to 10 minutes excess reagent is wiped from the posterior plastic surface of the layer and the colour reaction performed by heating in the hot-air oven at between 120 and 130°C for 10 minutes. Reproducibility is improved by rotating the layer, clipped to a light wooden frame in the oven as shown in Figure 5.4 (inset 3). The colours produced are relatively stable, but it is advisable to preserve the chromatogram by storing at -20°C in a polythene bag if densitometry is delayed. Exposure to light (especially short-wave ultraviolet) hastens background discolouration.

QUANTITATIVE THIN-LAYER CHROMATOGRAPHY

MONOSACCHARIDE APPLICATIONS

When more than a single 5 µl application is required additional aliquots should be superimposed, but only after the first has completely dried

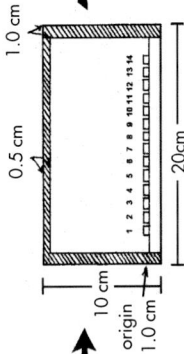

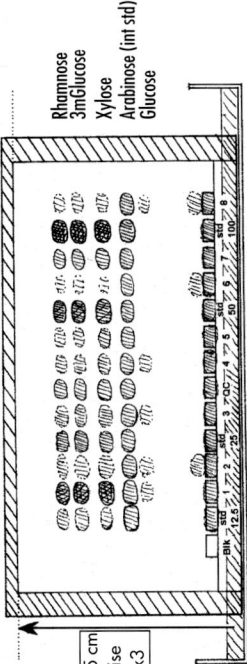

'MULTIPLE APPLICATIONS' FOR OLIGOSACCHARIDES

The purpose of the 'multiapplication and pre-run' technique is to increase sensitivity when estimating low oligosaccharide levels in the urine. Up to seven 5 µl applications of desalted urine can be made along a single 'sample area'. Further series can be superimposed if larger application volumes are required, but only *after the previous samples have had time to dry*. Adjacent applications should be spaced sufficiently far apart to avoid merging.

'PRE-RUN SOLVENT'

ethanol; 50 ml
butan-1-ol 10 ml
water 30 ml

Purpose to advance multiple sugar applications to the selected origin

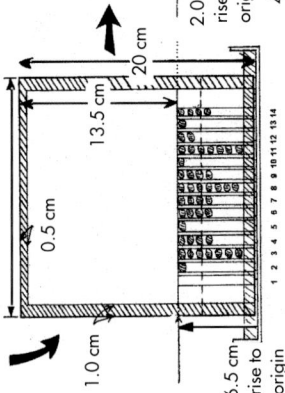

1. FIRST PRE-RUN
(6.5 cm rise to true origin)

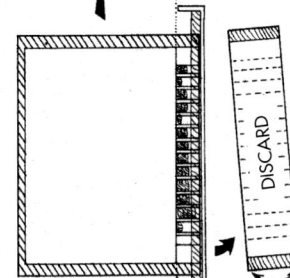

2. SECOND PRE-RUN
(2.0 cm rise to origin after cutting off lower 4.5 cm of chromatogram)

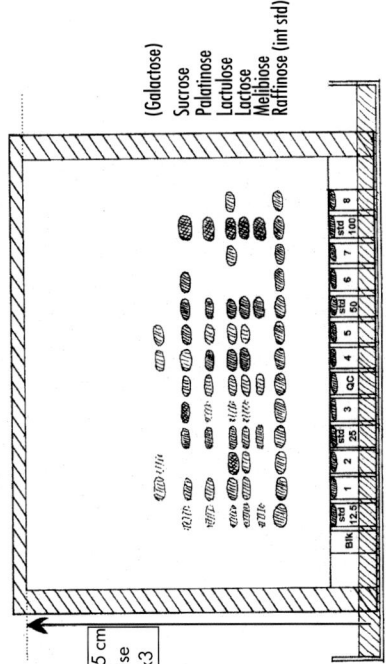

DISCARD

Rhamnose
3mGlucose
Xylose
Arabinose (int std)
Glucose

MULTIPLE DEVELOPMENT FOR MONOSACCHARIDES

Separation is achieved by two consecutive upward developments (rise 8.5 cm) on Merck 60 plastic-backed silica gel layers (Dassel FRG) using the following solvent mixture (i.e. B_1, B_1).

B_1 = ethyl acetate, pyridine, acetic acid (glac), water: 75, 15 10, 10 by vol.

(Galactose)
Sucrose
Palatinose
Lactulose
Lactose
Melibiose
Raffinose (int std)

MULTIPLE DEVELOPMENT FOR OLIGOSACCHARIDES

Separation is achieved by three consecutive upward developments (rise 13.5 cm) on plastic-backed silica gel layers (Merck 60 or Schleicher & Schuell F1500) using the following solvent mixtures (sequence A, B_3, B_3; or A, B_2, A, respectively).

A = butanol, ethanol, acetic acid (glac), water: 60, 30, 10, 10 by vol.
$B_{2,3}$ = ethyl acetate, butanol, pyridine, acetic acid, water; (2): 70,5,15,10 or (3): 65,10,15,10,10

Figure 5.3 – Quantitative thin-layer chromatography of test sugars. Sample preparation and solvent development for monosaccharides (above) and disaccharides (below).

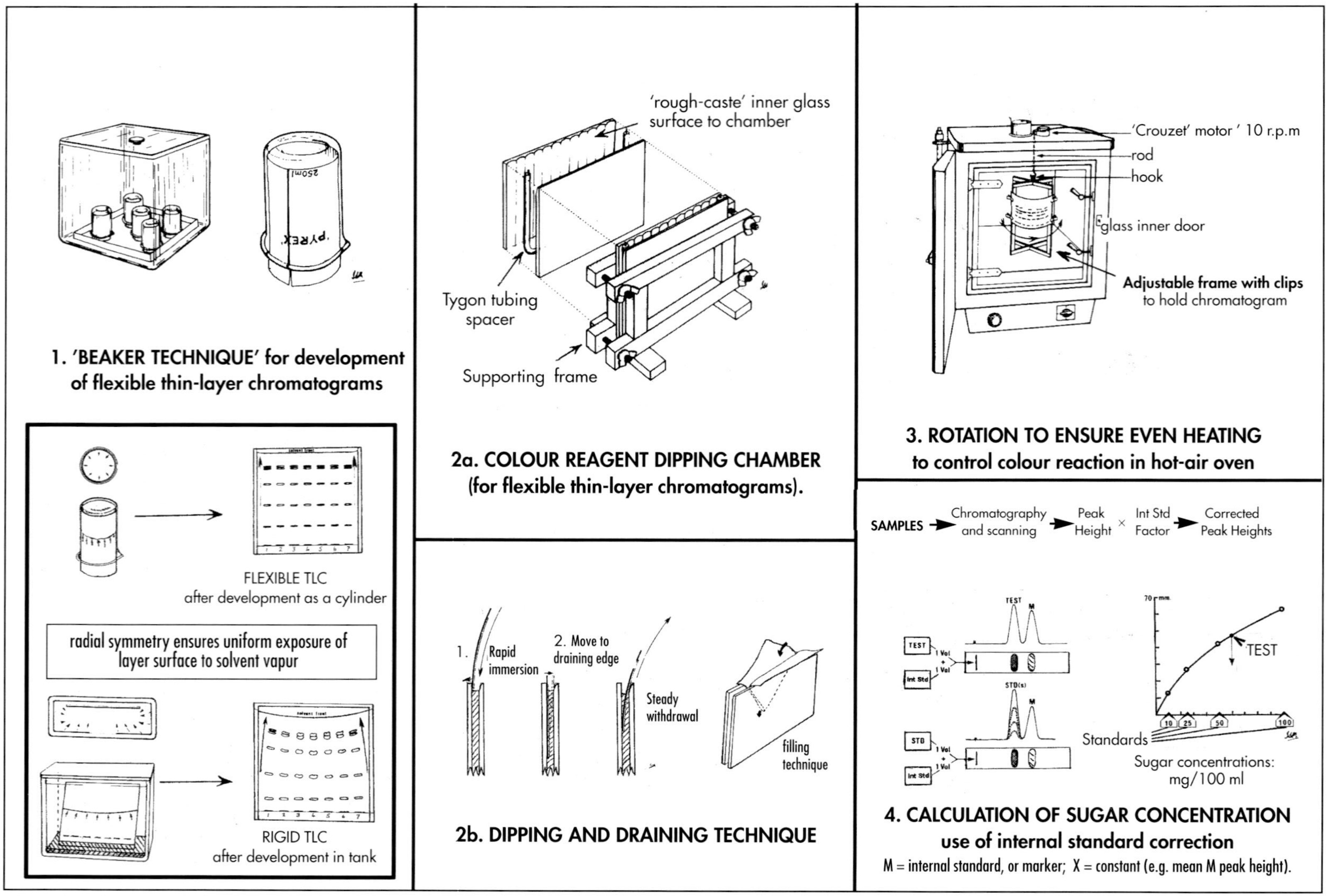
250ml
'PYREX'
1. 'BEAKER TECHNIQUE' for development of flexible thin-layer chromatograms
FLEXIBLE TLC
after development as a cylinder
radial symmetry ensures uniform exposure of layer surface to solvent vapur
RIGID TLC
after development in tank
'rough-caste' inner glass surface to chamber
Tygon tubing spacer
Supporting frame
2a. COLOUR REAGENT DIPPING CHAMBER (for flexible thin-layer chromatograms).
1. Rapid immersion
2. Move to draining edge
Steady withdrawal
filling technique
2b. DIPPING AND DRAINING TECHNIQUE
'Crouzet' motor ' 10 r.p.m
rod
hook
glass inner door
Adjustable frame with clips to hold chromatogram
3. ROTATION TO ENSURE EVEN HEATING to control colour reaction in hot-air oven
SAMPLES
Chromatography and scanning
Peak Height
×
Int Std Factor
Corrected Peak Heights
TEST
Int Std
1 Vol
+
1 Vol
TEST
M
STD(s)
STD
Int Std
70 mm.
TEST
Standards
10
25
50
100
Sugar concentrations: mg/100 ml
4. CALCULATION OF SUGAR CONCENTRATION use of internal standard correction
M = internal standard, or marker; X = constant (e.g. mean M peak height).

Figure 5.4 – Quantitative thin-layer chromatography of test sugars.
Refinements of technique introduced to improve precision and accuracy. [64,110]

Scanning densitometry.

Each chromatogram is subjected to scanning densitometry using a wide-band pass blue filter (400 to 530 nm). Baseline readings are taken from the blank pathway left for this purpose, and maximum (= peak) optic density readings are taken from the center of each sugar zone, using software that is available in several packages. Several suitable instruments, such as the Bio Rad Densitometer model G57670 Molecular Analyst, are available.

Calculations

SUGAR CONCENTRATION: After correction to constant internal standard value, optic density/concentration calibration curves are plotted using the sugar standard values (in accordance with the Kubelka-Munk law) and values for test sample concentrations are read off by interpolation as shown in Figure 5.4 (inset 4). A correction will be required for multiple applications ($\times 1/n$, where n = number of applications made) or dilution of concentrated samples ($\times$ n, where n = dilution factor).

SUGAR EXCRETION: mg excreted in urine = mg/100 ml in urine $\times$ urine volume in ml/100, percentage of oral dose recovered = mg excreted/mg administered $\times$ 100.

Performance

Provided all refinements of chromatographic technique are followed (inclusion of internal standards, multiple application and pre-run, 'cylinder' development in beakers, use of specialised dipping chamber, rotation as cylinder in hot-air oven during colour reaction, etc.),[110] the precision of the total procedure lies between 3.5 and 8.0% coefficient of variation for most sugars at concentrations above 10 mg/100 ml, but varies with sugar concentration and the experience of the analyst. Duplication of chromatograms with calculation of mean values will improve precision to between 2.5 and 6.0%. Suitable software programs will allow generation of calibration curves and calculation of concentrations to be automated.

Visual interpretation

An alternative method of quantitation by visual comparison of test with standard sugar zones on the same chromatogram can be undertaken without the incorporation of an internal standard, thus saving much labour and avoiding the expense of a scanner. Most of the errors associated with traditional methods of thin-layer chromatography arise from factors that are controlled by the technical refinements described[110] and, with practice, a precision between 8% and 15% coefficient of variation, adequate for most clinical purposes, can be achieved by this method.[111]

Acknowledgements

The multi-probe tests of differential absorption, permeability and disaccharide hydrolysis and the method of quantitative sugar analysis by thin-layer chromatography were developed in the Gastroenterology and Chemical Pathology Departments, St Thomas's Hospital Medical School and in the Clinical Biochemistry Department, King's College School of Medicine and Dentistry, London, UK.

References

1. Leading Article. Sugaring the Crosby Capsule. *Lancet* 1981; **1**: 593-594.

2. Menzies IS, Laker MF, Pounder R, Bull J, Heyer S, Wheeler PG, Creamer B. Abnormal intestinal permeability to sugars in villous atrophy. *Lancet* 1979; **2**: 1107-1109.

3. Cobden I, Dickinson RJ, Rothwell J, Axon ATR. Intestinal permeability assessed by excretion ratios of two molecules: results in coeliac disease. *BMJ* 1978; **2**: 1060.

4. Henry RJ. Fecal Lipids. In: *Clinical Chemistry, principles and technics.* Hoeber Medical Division: Harper and Row, New York, 1964; p873-883.

5. Van Tongeren JHM, Majoor CLH. Demonstration of protein losing gastroenteropathy. The disappearance rate of ^{51}Cr from plasma and the binding of ^{51}Cr to different serum proteins. *Clin Chim Acta* 1966; **14**: 31-41.

6. Tavill AS. Protein losing enteropathy. *J Clin Path* 1971; **24: Suppl (Roy. Coll. Path.):** 45-54.

7. Karbach U, Ewe K, Bodenstein H. α_1Antitrypsin, a reliable endogenous marker for intestinal protein loss and its application in patients with Crohn's disease. *Gut* 1983; **14**: 718-723.

8. Loehry CA, Kingham J, Baker J. Small intestinal permeability in animals and man. *Gut* 1973; **14**: 683-688.

9. Røseth AG, Fagerhol MK, Aadland E, Schjønsby H. Assessment of the neutrophil dominating protein calprotectin in feces. *Scand J Gastroenterol* 1992; **27**: 793-798.

10. Fromter E, Diamond J. Route of passive ion permeation in epithelia. *Nature New Biol* 1972; **235**: 9-13.

11. Claude P, Goodenough DA. Fracture faces of zonulae occludentes from "tight" and "leaky" epithelia. *J Cell Biol.* 1973; **58**: 390-400.

12. Turner MR. Electrical resistance of monolayers of cultured bovine epithelium in solutions of various resistivities. *J Physiol* (London) 1990; **425**: 63P.

13. Fortran JS, Rector FC, Ewton MF, Soter N, Kinney J. Permeability characteristics of the human small intestine. *J Clin Invest* 1965; **44**: 1935-1944.

14. Menzies IS. Medical importance of sugars in the alimentary tract. In: *Developments in sweeteners*. Grenby TH, Parker KJ & Lindley MG. eds. Applied Science Publishers Ltd., Lond & N.Y. 1983; 89-117.

15. Menzies IS. Transmucosal passage of inert molecules in health and disease. In: *Intestinal absorption and secretion*. Skadhauge E. & Heintze L., eds. Falk Symposium 36. Lancaster: MTP Press, 1984; 527-543.

16. Travis S, Menzies IS. Intestinal permeability: functional assessment and significance. Editorial review, *Clin Sci* 1992; **82**: 471-488.

17. Bijlsama PB, Peeters RA, Groot JA, Dekker PR, Taminiau JAJM, Meer R Van der. Differential *in vivo* and *in vitro* intestinal permeability to lactulose and mannitol in animals and human: a hypothesis. *Gastroenterology* 1995; **108**: 687-696.

18. Sandhu JS, Fraser DR. Assessment of intestinal permeability in the experimental rat with [³H]cellobiotol and [¹⁴C]mannitol. *Cli Sci* 1982; **63**: 311-316.

19. Cobden I, Rothwell J, Axon ATR. Intestinal permeability in rats infected by *Nippostrongylus brasiliensis. Gut* 1979; **20**: 716-721.

20. Davis NM, Wright MR, Jamali F. Anti-inflammatory drug-induced small intestinal permeability. The rat is a suitable model. *Pharmaceutical Res* 1994; **11**: 1652-1656.

21. Hall EJ, Batt RM. Enhanced intestinal permeability to ⁵¹Cr-labelled EDTA in dogs with small intestinal disease. *J Am Vet Med Assoc* 1990; **196**: 91-95.

22. Morris T, Sørensen S, Turkington J, Batt R. Diarrhoea and increased intestinal permeability in laboratory beagles associated with proximal small-intestinal bacterial overgrowth. *Lab Animals* 1994; **28**: 313-319.

23. Rutgers HC, Batt RM, Hall EJ, Sørensen SH, Proud FJ. Intestinal permeability testing in dogs with diet-responsive intestinal disease. *J Small Animal Practice* 1995; **36**: 295-301.

24. Wilson TH, Wiseman G. *J Physiol* 1954; **123**: 116-125

25. Miller D, Crane RK. *Biochim Biophys Acta* 1961; **52**: 293-298.

26. Peters TJ. Investigation of tissue organelles by a combination of analytical subcellular fractionation and enzymic microanalysis: a new approach to pathology. *J Clin Path* 1981; **34**: 1-12.

27. Storelli C, Vogel H, Semenza G. Reconstitution of a sucrase-mediated sugar transport system in lipid membranes *FEBS* Letters 1972; **24**: 287-292

28. Molitoris BA, Kinne R. Ischemia induces surface membrane dysfunction. *J Clin Invest* 1987; **80**: 647-654.

29. Fordtran JS, Clodi PH, Soergel KH, Inglefinger FJ. Sugar absorption tests with special reference to 3-O-methyl-D-glucose and D-xylose. *Annals Int Med* 1962; **57**: 883-891.

30. Menzies IS, Walker-Smith JA. Unpublished observations.

31. McCance RA, Madders K. The comparative rates of absorption of sugars from the human intestine. *Biochem J* 1930; **24**: 795-804.

32. Menzies IS, Laker MF, Heyer S, Bramley P, Pridham JB. Unpublished observations.

33. Hall G, Menzies IS. Unpublished observations.

34. Laker MF, Bull HJ, Menzies IS. Evaluation of mannitol for use as a probe marker of gastrointestinal permeability in man. *Eur J Clin Invest* 1982; **12**: 485-491.

35. Elia M, Behrens R, Northrop C, Wraight P, Neale G. Evaluation of mannitol, lactulose and ⁵¹Cr-EDTA as markers of intestinal permeability in man. *Clin Sci* 1987; **73**: 197-204.

36. Maxton DG, Bjarnason I, Reynolds AP, Catt SD, Peters TJ, Menzies IS. Lactulose, ⁵¹Cr-EDTA, L-rhamnose and PEG-400 as probe markers for assessment *in vivo* of human intestinal permeability. *Clin Sci* 1986; **71**: 71-80.

37. Menzies IS. Absorption of intact oligosaccharide in health and disease. *Biochem Soc Transac*, 1974; **2**: 1042-1047.

38. Laker MF, Menzies IS. Increase in human intestinal permeability following ingestion of hypertonic solutions. *J Physiol* 1977; **265**: 881-894.

39. Wheeler PG, Menzies IS, Creamer B. Effect of hyperosmolar stimuli and coeliac disease on the permeability of the human intestinal tract. *Clin Sci Mol Med* 1978; **54:** 495-501.

40. Strobel S, Brydon WG, Ferguson A. Cellobiose/mannitol sugar permeability test compliments biopsy histopathology in clinical investigation of the jejunum. *Gut* 1984; **25:** 1241-1246.

41. Sawiers WM, Andrews DJ, Low-Beer TS. The double sugar test of intestinal permeability in the elderly. *Age and Ageing* 1985; **14:** 312-315.

42. Dalqvist A. Method for assay of intestinal disaccharidases. *Anal Biochem* 1964; **7:** 18-25.

43. Oman H, Blomquist L, Henriksson AEK, Johanson SGO. Comparison of polysucrose 1500, ^{51}Cr-labelled EDTA and ^{14}C-mannitol as markers of intestinal permeability in man. *Scand J Gastroenterol* 1995; **30:** 1172-1177.

44. Meddings JB, Sutherland LR, Byles NI, Wallace JL. Sucrose: A novel marker for gastroduodenal disease. *Gastroenterology* 1993; **104:** 1619-1626.

45. Sutherland LR, Verhoef M, Wallace JL, Rosendaal G Van, Crutcher R, Meddings JB. A simple, non-invasive marker of gastric damage: sucrose permeability. *Lancet* 1994; **343:** 998-1000.

46. Maxton DG, Catt SD, Menzies IS. Combined assessment of intestinal disaccharidases in congenital asucrasia by differential urinary disaccharide excretion. *J Clin Path* 1990; **43:** 406-409.

47. Bjarnason I, Batt R, Catt S, Macpherson A, Maxton D, Menzies I. Evaluation of differential disaccharide excretion in urine for non-invasive investigation of altered intestinal disaccharidase activity caused by α-glucosidase inhibition, primary hypolactasia, and coeliac disease. *Gut* 1996; **39:** 374-381.

48. Bjarnason I, Peters TJ, Veall N. A persistent defect in intestinal permeability in coeliac disease demonstrated by a ^{51}Cr-labelled EDTA absorption test. *Lancet* 1983; **1:** 323-325

49. Bjarnason I, O'Morain C, Levi AJ, Peters TJ. Absorption of ^{51}Cr-EDTA in inflammatory bowel disease. *Gastroenterology* 1983; **85:** 318-322.

50. Aabakken L ^{51}Cr-EDTA absorption test, methodological aspects. *Scand J Gastroenterol* 1989; **24:** 351-358.

51. Chantler C, Garnett ES, Parsons V, Veall N. Glomerular filtration rate measurement in man by a single injection method using ^{51}Cr-EDTA. *Clin Sci* 1969; **37:** 169-180.

52. Jenkins RT, Ramage JR, Jones DB, Collins SM, Goodacre RL, Hunt RH. Small bowel and colonic permeability to ^{51}Cr-EDTA in patients with active inflammatory bowel disease. *Clin Invest Med* 1988; **11:** 151-155.

53. Jenkins AP, Nukajam WS, Menzies IS, Creamer B. Simultaneous administration of lactulose and ^{51}Cr-EDTA: a test to distinguish colonic from small-intestinal permeability change. *Scand J Gastroenterol* 1992; **27:** 769-773.

54. Jenkins AP, Menzies IS, Nukajam WS, Creamer B. The effect of ingested lactulose on absorption of L-rhamnose, D-xylose, and 3-O-methyl-D-glucose in subjects with ileostomies. *Scand J Gastroenterol* 1994; **29:** 820-825.

55. Chadwick VS, Phillips SF, Hoffman AF. Measurement of intestinal permeability using low molecular weight polyethylene glycols. *Gastroenterology* 1977; **73:** 241-251.

56. Olaison G, Leandersson P, Sjodahl R, Tagesson C. Intestinal permeability to PEG-600 in Crohn's disease. Peroperative determination in a defined segment of the small intestine. *Gut* 1988; **29:** 196-199.

57. Heuman R, Sjodahl R, Tagesson C. Passage of molecules through the wall of the gastrointestinal tract. Intestinal permeability to polyethyleneglycol in 1000 patients with Crohn's disease. *Acta Chir Scand* 1982; **148:** 281-284.

58. Falth-Magnusson K, Jansson G, Stenhammer L, Sundqvist T, Magnusson KE. Intestinal permeability assessed with different sized PEG's in children undergoing small intestinal biopsy for suspected coeliac disease. *Scand J Gastroenterol* 1989; **24:** 40-46.

59. Jackson PG, Lessof MH, Baker RW, Ferret J, MacDonald DM. Intestinal permeability in patients with eczema and food allergy. *Lancet* 1981; **1:** 1285-1286.

60. Iqbal TH, Lewis KO, Cooper BT. Diffusion of polyetheylene glycol-400 across lipid barriers *in vitro*. *Clin Sci* 1993; **85:** 111-115.

61. Menzies IS, Jenkins AP, Heduan E, Catt SD, Segal MB, Creamer B. The effect of poorly absorbed solute on intestinal absorption. *Scand J Gastroenterol* 1990; **25:** 1257-1264.

62. Guth PH. Physiological alterations in small bowel function with age. The absorption of D-xylose. *Am J Digest Dis* 1968; **13:** 565-571.

63. Rinaldo JA, Gluckman RF. Maximal absorption capacity for xylose in nontropical sprue. *Gastroenterology* 1964; **47:** 248-250.

64. Menzies IS. Quantitative estimation of sugars in blood and urine by paper chromatography using direct

densitometry. *J Chromatog* 1973; **81:** 109-127.

65. Helmer OM, Fouts PJ. Gastrointestinal studies VII, the excretion of xylose in pernicious anaemia. *J Clin Invest* 1937; **16:** 343-349.

66. Fourman LPR. The absorption of xylose in steatorrhoea. *Clin Sci* 1948; **6:** 289-294.

67. Benson JA, Culver PJ, Ragland S, Jones CM, Drummy GD, Bougas E. The D-xylose absorption test in malabsorption syndromes. *New Eng J Med* 1957; **256:** 335-339.

68. Fordtran JS, Soergel KH, Inglefinger FJ. Intestinal absorption of D-xylose in man. *New Eng J Med* 1962; **267:** 274-279.

69. Sladen GE, Kumar PJ. Is the xylose test still a worth-while investigation? *BMJ* 1973; **3:** 223-226.

70. Hindmarsh JT. Xylose absorption and its clinical significance. *Clin Biochem* 1976; **9:** 141-143.

71. Stevens FM, Watt DW, Bourke MA, McNicholl B, Fottrell PF, McCarthy CF. The 15g D-xylose absorption test: its application to the study of coeliac disease. *Clin Biochem* 1976; **9:** 141-143.

72. Santini R, Sheehy TW, Martinez-De-Jesus J. The xylose tolerance test with a five gram dose. *Gastroenterology* 1961; **40:** 772-774.

73. Sammons HG, Morgan DB, Frazer AC, Montgomery RD, Philip WM, Phillips MJ. Modification of the xylose absorption test as an index of intestinal function. *Gut* 1967; **8:** 348-353.

74. Kendall DF. Is the xylose test worthwhile? (Letter) *BMJ* 1973; **3:** 405.

75. Haeney MR, Culank LS, Montgomery RD, Sammons HG. Evaluation of xylose absorption as measured in blood and urine: a one-hour blood xylose screening test in malabsorption *Gastroenterology* 1978; **75:** 393-400.

76. Rolles CJ, Kendall MJ, Nutter S, Anderson CM. One-hour blood-xylose screening-test for coeliac disease in infants and young children. *Lancet* 1973; **2:** 1043-1045.

77. Jones WO, Di Sant Agnese PA. Laboratory aids in the diagnosis of malabsorption in pediatrics: II xylose absorption test. *J Pediatr* 1963; **62:** 50-56

78. Ducker DA, Hughes CA, Warren I, McNeish AS. Neonatal gut function measured by one hour blood D(+) xylose test: influence of gastrointestinal age and size. *Gut* 1980; **21:** 133-

79. Buts J-P, Morin CL, Roy CC, Weber A, Bonin A. One-hour blood xylose test: a reliable index of small bowel function. *J Pediatr* 1978; **90:** 729-733.

80. Montgomery RD, Haeney MR, Ross IN, Sammons HG, Barford AV, Balakrishnan S, Mayer PP, Culank LS, Field J, Gosling P., The ageing gut: a study of intestinal absorption in relation to nutrition in the elderly. *Quarterly J Med* 1978, **New Series XLVII:** 197-211.

81. Chadwick VS, Phillips SF, Hofmann AF. Measurements of intestinal permeability using low molecular weight polyethylene glycols (PEG 400). *Gastroenterology* 1977; **73:** 247-251.

82. Noone C, Beach RC, Bull J, Menzies IS. Differential absorption of D-xylose and 3-O-methyl-D-glucose in coeliac disease and acute gastroenteritis. *Gut* 1982; **23:** A921.

83. Noone C, Menzies IS. Unpublished observations.

84. Noone C, Menzies IS, Banatvala JE, Scopes JW. Intestinal permeability and lactose hydrolysis in human rotaviral gastroenteritis assessed simultaneously by non-invasive differential sugar permeation. *Eur J Clin Invest* 1986; **16:** 217-225.

85. Juby LD, Rothwell J, Axon ATR. Lactulose/mannitol test: An ideal screen for celiac disease. *Gastroenterology* 1989; **96:** 79-85.

86. Fotherby KJ, Wraight EP, Neale G. ^{51}Cr-EDTA/^{14}C-mannitol intestinal permeability test. Clinical use in screening for coeliac disease. *Scand J Gastroenterol* 1986; **23:** 171-177.

87. Bjarnason I, Felvilly B, Smethurst P, Menzies IS, Levi AJ. Importance of local versus systemic effects of non-steroidal anti-inflammatory drugs in increasing small intestinal permeability in man. *Gut* 1991; **32:** 275-277.

88. Cook GC, Menzies IS. Intestinal absorption and unmediated permeation of sugars in post infective tropical malabsorption. *Digestion* 1986; **33:** 109-116.

89. Griffiths CEM, Menzies IS, Barrison IG, Leonard JN, Fry L. Intestinal permeability in dermatitis herpetiformis. *J Invest Dermatol* 1988; **91:** 147-149.

90. Jenkins AP, Trew DR, Crump BJ, Nukajam WS, Foley JA, Menzies IS, Creamer B. Do non-steroidal anti-inflammatory drugs increase colonic permeability? *Gut* 1991; **32:** 66-69.

91. Lim SG, Menzies IS, Lee CA, Johnson MA, Pounder RE. Intestinal permeability and function in patients infected with human immunodeficiency virus. *Scand J Gastroenterol* 1993; **28:** 573-580.

92. Johnston JD, Harvey CJ, Menzies IS, Treacher DF. Gastrointestinal permeability and absorptive capacity in sepsis. *Crit Care Med* 1996; **24:** 1144-1149.

93. Menzies IS. Unpublished observations.

94. Ukabam SO, Homeida MMA, Cooper BT. Small intestinal permeability in normal Sudanese subjects: evidence of tropical enteropathy. *Trans R Soc Trop Med Hyg* 1986; **80:** 204-207.

95. Jenkins AP, Menzies IS, Nukajam WS *et al.* Geographical variation in intestinal permeability. *Gut* 1989; **30:** A1509-1510.

96. Beach RC, Menzies IS, Clayden GS, Scopes JW. Gastrointestinal permeability changes in the pre-term neonate. *Arch Dis Childh* 1982; **57:** 141-145.

97. Lanzowski P, Madenlioglu M, Wilson JF, Lahey ME. Oral D-xylose test in healthy infants and children. *New Eng J Med* 1963; **268:** 1441-1444.

98. Kendall MJ. The influence of age on the xylose absorption test. *Gut* 1970; **11:** 498-501.

99. Webster SGP, Leeming JT. Assessment of small bowel function in the elderly using a modified xylose tolerance test. *Gut* 1975; **16:** 109-113.

100. Mayerson MJ. The "xylose test" to assess gastrointestinal absorption in the elderly: a pharmacokinetic evaluation of the literature. *J Gerontol* 1982; **37:** 300-305.

101. Weiner R, Dietze F, Laue R. Age-dependent alterations of intestinal absorption. II. A clinical study using a modified D-xylose absorption test. *Arch Gerontol Geriat* 1984; **3:** 97-108.

102. Sørensen SH, Proud JH, Rutgers C, Markwell P, Adam A, Batt RM. A blood test for intestinal permeability and function: a new tool for the diagnosis of chronic intestinal disease in dogs. In press.

103. Roe JH, Rice EW. A photometric method for the determination of free pentoses in animal tissues. *J Biol Chem* 1948; **173:** 507-512.

104. Corcoran AC, Page IH. A method for the determination of mannitol in plasma and urine, *Biol Chem* 1947; **170:** 165-171.

105. Laker MN, Mount JN. Mannitol estimation in biological fluids by gas/liquid chromatography of tri-silyl derivatives. *Clin Chem* 1980; **26:** 441-443.

106. Kynaston JA, Fleming SC, Laker MF, Pearson DJ. Simultaneous quantification of mannitol, 3-O-methyl glucose, and lactulose in urine by HPLC with pulsed electrochemical detection, for use in studies of intestinal permeability. *Clin Chem* 1993; **39:** 453-456.

107. Srensen SH, Proud F, Adam A, Rutgers H, Batt R. A novel HPLC method for the simultaneous quantification of monosaccharides and disaccharides used in tests of intestinal function and permeability. *Clin Chim Acta* 1993; **221:** 115-125.

108. Lunn PG, Northrop CA, Northrop AJ. Automated enzymatic assays for the determination of intestinal permeability probes in urine. 2. Mannitol. *Clin Chim Acta* 1989; **183:** 163-170.

109. Northrop CA, Lunn PG, Behrens RH. Automated enzymatic assays for the determination of intestinal permeability probes in urine: lactulose and lactose. *Clin Chim Acta* 1990; **187:** 79-88.

110. Menzies IS, Mount JN, Wheeler MJ. Quantitative estimation of clinically important monosaccharides in plasma by rapid thin-layer chromatography. *Ann Clin Biochem* 1978; **15:** 65-76.

111. Menzies IS, Shine B, Crane R, unpublished observations.

6

Measurement of human intestinal secretion and absorption *in vitro*

Keith J Lindley and Rachel Menon

Summary

A variety of methods exist to measure intestinal secretion and absorption *in vitro*. This chapter focuses on two techniques: measurement of intestinal short circuit current, an invaluable tool with a well-established place in intestinal physiology; and measurement of colonic crypt absorptive function using laser scanning confocal microscopy. We describe the theory behind each method together with our personal experience of them.

Introduction

Many different and varied techniques may be used to measure the transport of water and solutes across the intestinal epithelium.[1] Choice of method depends upon the precise research question being asked and upon the availability of suitable subjects/tissues. It is important in this context that investigators realize the limitations of the method they are using and how the measurements relate to the 'normal' physiology of intestinal absorption and secretion *in vivo*.

The study of intestinal absorption and secretion in infants and children with rare gastrointestinal disease has been very fruitful in providing insights into the normal physiology of the gastrointestinal tract.[2] This chapter describes the use of measurements of short-circuit current and concentration of fluorescent impermeant solutes measured by confocal laser scanning microscopy to study intestinal absorption and secretion in human paediatric tissues *in vitro*.

Methods

Measurement of electrogenic ion secretion and absorption

Movement of charged particles across an epithelium generates a potential gradient across that epithelium. The absorption of glucose, galactose and some amino acids across the small intestine is coupled stochiometrically to the absorption of sodium by the sugar/amino acid transporter protein and this activity is therefore electrically overt. The reader will no doubt be familiar with the notion that it is the concentration gradient for sodium that drives the sugar/amino acid absorption. The presence of a low-resistance paracellular 'shunt' pathway between the individual enterocytes of the small intestine facilitates the passage of water and other ions across the intestinal barrier by solvent drag down the electro-chemical gradients set up by the various transporter proteins. Measurement of currents due to sodium-coupled solute absorption is therefore best viewed as an index of absorption. Secretion of ions down their electrochemical gradient across the apical enterocyte membrane is also an electrically overt process and will again provide an index of net secretion. Whilst such electrically overt movement of ions is a good index of net solute movement, the measurement of actual movement of each ion is dependent upon methods such as bidirectional radioisotopic fluxes. Potential differences across epithelia may also arise as a consequence of osmotic gradients (so-called electro-kinetic potentials) and diffusion gradients (diffusion potentials). These are discussed elsewhere.[3]

In the late 1940s, Hans Ussing validated the idea that an epithelium behaving as a simple ohmic resistance would have a transepithelial potential difference related directly to the current arising from ionic movement across the epithelium.[4] The apparatus described in this landmark paper included two celluloid half chambers which were tightly opposed with the tissue stretched across the aperture in the centre. These chambers to this day bear the author's name - Ussing chambers - although there have been many permutations of Ussing's basic design.

Ussing's short circuit current methodologies were extensively applied to the study of the small intestine of mammals during the 1950s and 60s[5-8] and when used to study intestinal transport *in vitro*, led to a series of advances in our understanding of normal intestinal transport physiology.[9-12]

The sheet of intestinal tissue stretched across the aperture between the half chambers is bathed on the mucosal and serosal sides by oxygenated (95% O_2/5% CO_2) Krebs-Ringer-bicarbonate solution which is traditionally circulated independently on each side of the tissue by a gas lift system. Potential sensing electrodes are opposed very close (usually within 1 mm) to either surface of the tissue (Fig. 6.1). We achieve this using salt-agar bridges (3% w/v agar in 1 M KCl) with one end opposed to the tissue and the other in a beaker containing 3 M KCl and a calomel electrode (Russell Electrodes, Fife, Scotland) connected to a potentiometer. The agar-salt (KCl) solution is syringed whilst boiling into lengths of 2 mm internal diameter PVC tubing (Portex), and when set the tubing is cut, leaving the agar protruding

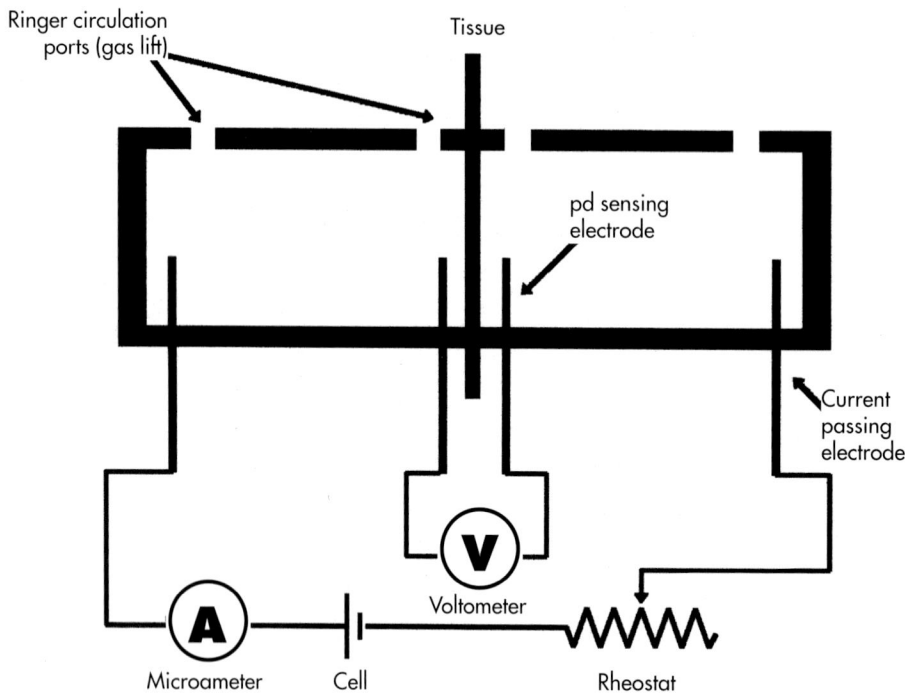

Figure 6.1 – Schematic representation of an Ussing chamber with simple short circuit current apparatus

slightly at each end of the tubing to facilitate good electrical contact. At the other end of each half chamber distant from the tissue (3 cm from the tissue plane in our apparatus) there are current passing electrodes. Again we find the salt-agar bridge arrangement with Ag/AgCl current passing electrodes dipped in 3MKCl most satisfactory (Clark Electromedical Ltd, Berks, UK).

Short circuit current (I_{sc}) is the external current necessary to abolish the transmural potential difference when the two sides of the tissue are bathed in identical ionic solutions, and may be considered a measurement of electrically overt secretion or absorption. Measurement of short circuit current is complicated if tissue resistance is low (as is the case with the small intestine) because the fluid resistance of the perfusion solution between the plane of the tissue and the tips of the potential sensing electrodes contributes significantly to the total resistance of the system. Hence during passage of a current across the mounted tissue, a potential difference is set up between the tips of the potential sensing electrodes and the tissue itself, and failure to take this into account will result in incomplete short circuiting of

the tissue. Fluid resistance between the potential sensing electrodes may contribute 50% or more of the total resistance of the circuit when working with human paediatric bowel mucosa (e.g. human paediatric jejunum (Crosby capsule biopsy)[13] 37 Ω cm²; human stripped rectosigmoid colon[14] 99 Ω cm²; typical fluid resistance 50 Ω cm²)). Fluid resistance will behave as a simple ohmic resistance and its contribution to measured potential difference will be a constant percentage of the current being passed to short circuit the tissue. It is therefore simple to correct for fluid resistance.

Measured tissue resistance is the sum of the contributions due to epithelial and subepithelial resistances.[15] Some authors prefer to take this into account when measuring short circuit current, arguing that without this consideration measured short circuit current will underestimate the current generated by the epithelial cell layer itself.[16] This approach is necessarily more complex and not in widespread use with no published normative data being available for human paediatric intestinal tissues; it is not described in this chapter. If one considers the mounted sheet of intestinal tissue as consisting of a number of compartments consisting of subepithelium, epithelium and any associated 'convective' compartments, then short circuiting the whole preparation to 0 mV will mean that the epithelial layer itself will necessarily have a potential drop across it and hence not be truly short circuited. This under short circuiting of the tissue results in an underestimate of net charge transfer across the epithelium. The reader is referred elsewhere for a more detailed discussion.[17]

We use one of three approaches to estimate short circuit current. When short circuit conditions are required for the purposes of the experimental protocol (e.g. bi-directional ^{22}Na ^{36}Cl flux measurements) this may be achieved either manually or automatically with a commercially available voltage clamp. Where one requires an estimate of short circuit current without requiring short circuit conditions, this may be achieved quite simply using a millivoltmeter and a battery as a current source together with a rheostat and microameter (Fig. 6.1) (see below).

Before mounting the tissues it is necessary to assemble the chambers and to circulate gassed (95% O_2, 5% CO_2) warmed Krebs-Ringer-bicarbonate solution to measure any asymmetrical potentials generated by the potential sensing electrodes themselves. These can be minimized by storing the electrodes in 3 M KCl with each pair connected to complete an electrical circuit. We normally accept an asymmetrical potential of up to 0.1 mV, and this is corrected for in due course. This procedure will also bring to light any junction potentials in the system which usually arise at the electrolyte/agar bridge interface, or as a result of cracks in the agar. Junction potentials need to be minimized by dealing with the cause and also taken into account as with the asymmetrical potential of the electrodes. The fluid resistance is measured by passing a current pulse of known amplitude and measuring the change in potential difference. The magnitude of this value will depend upon the composition and temperature of the electrolyte solution being circulated, the distance between the potential difference sensing electrodes, and the size of the aperture in the Ussing chambers.

Estimation of short circuit current under open circuit conditions

This simple method relies on the notion that the sheet of intestinal tissue behaves as a simple (variable) ohmic resistance. Thus the transepithelial potential difference is directly related (by Ohm's law) to the transepithelial current being generated by the net passage of ions across the epithelium. Hence if one measures open circuit potential difference and then passes a current pulse (commonly 100 µA) and measures the increase in potential difference enabling a calculation of tissue resistance, one can calculate short circuit current. In practice this may be performed with ease every 15 seconds or so enabling the response to secretagogues to be measured with ease.

An understanding of this approach may be obtained from the following argument in conjunction with Fig. 6.2. Assume that on setting up the chambers in the absence of tissue, the combined asymmetric potential of the calomel electrodes and any junction potentials at the tips of the agar bridges is measured as V_{ass}, and that passing a 100 µA pulse of current between the current passing electrodes increases this potential to V_{fc}. On mounting a tissue the measured potential across the tissues is V_t which rises to V_{tc} on passing a current of 100 µA across the tissue. By plotting the changes in measured potential as shown in Fig. 6.2, one can obtain two lines, the slopes of which (by Ohm's law) are a measure of fluid resistance (R_f) and tissue resistance (R_t), respectively. One may then use simple mathematics to predict intestinal short circuit current (I_{sc}) as follows:

Equation for a straight line is $y = a + bx$

Therefore

$$y_f = V_{ass} + (R_f \times I) \text{ and } y_t = V_t + (R_t \times I)$$

y_f will equal y_t when $I = I_{sc}$

Substituting for y under these conditions

$$V_t + (R_t \times I_{sc}) = V_{ass} + (R_f \times I_{sc})$$

Rearrange these

$$I_{sc} = \left[\frac{V_t - V_{ass}}{R_f - R_t} \right]$$

$$I_{sc} = \left[\frac{V_{fc} - V_{ass}}{0.1} \right] \text{ and } I_{sc} = \left[\frac{V_{fc} - V_{ass}}{0.1} \right]$$

In practice we have found it adequate to note the values V_{ass}, V_{fc}, V_t and V_{tc} at 15 second intervals and to enter the measured values into a spreadsheet which automatically calculates values for I_{sc} and R_t.

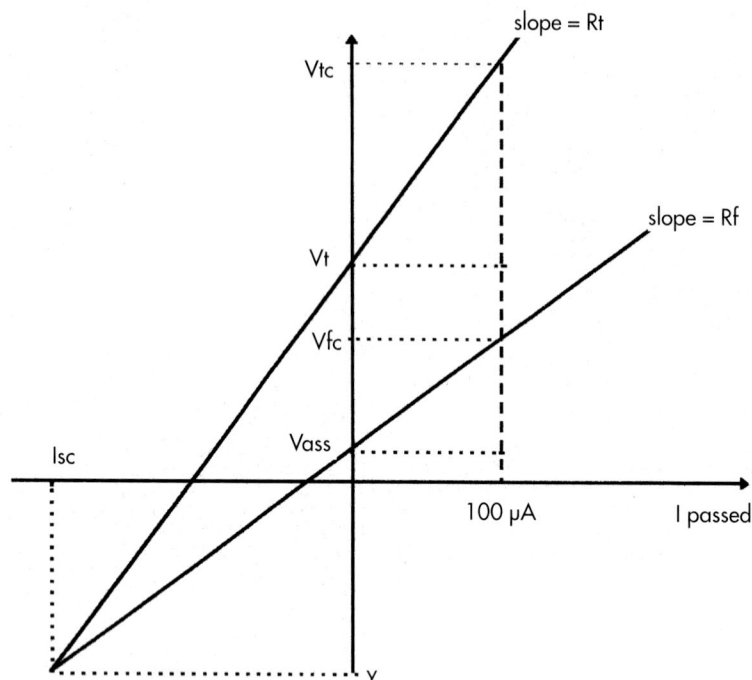

Figure 6.2 – Theoretical determination of short circuit (see text).

Measurement of short circuit current by manual short circuiting methods

This can be achieved using relatively simple apparatus, which has not changed in our laboratory for over 20 years. All that is required is a high impedance voltmeter (we have an Analogic AN 2570 digital voltmeter), a microameter (we have an Anders KM86 moving coil microameter) and a 9V battery attached to

a rheostat which is used to pass a variable current. To make the apparatus less cumbersome, all these elements are housed together in an easily moveable box. The manual short circuiting procedure is described by Field et al.[9] Fluid resistance has to be taken into account for each different short circuit current being passed. To calculate this a table is constructed before mounting the tissue and consists of values of current passed (I) in one column (in 5 µA increments) versus potential (I × R_{fluid}). After mounting the tissue, short circuit current is determined by successive approximations, the end point being the value of I which results in the same potential difference with the tissue in place as with the tissue absent

(where the two plots intercept in Fig. 6.2). This process is necessarily slow and cumbersome and is best suited to relatively steady-state experiments in which one is measuring radioisotopic fluxes (e.g. $^{22}Na/^{36}Cl$).

Automatic measurement of short circuit current using a voltage clamp

This is now the most common method in our laboratory and we use a commercially available voltage clamp (DVC 1000, World Precision Instruments, Herts, UK) of which a number are available (e.g. AD Instruments). Asymmetric potentials are offset with an equal and opposite potential using a dial on the front of the apparatus and fluid resistance accounted for by applying a current to the apparatus before the tissue is mounted and adjusting a rheostat on the front of the apparatus until the current pulse does not result in any change in potential between the pd sensing electrodes. Tissue is then simply mounted under open circuit conditions and the voltage clamp switched on to invoke short circuit current conditions. Tissue resistance may be measured by briefly returning to open circuit conditions every minute or so to measure transepithelial potential difference and applying Ohm's law, or by passing a current pulse under open circuit conditions.

The design of the Ussing chambers depends upon the source of human tissues used. Where surgically resected intestine is used there is generally ample tissue to stretch across a large aperture. We have found that the larger the surface area of the mounted tissue the more consistent are the results and we prefer under these circumstances to have a cross sectional area of 2 cm² or more. Our standard multipurpose chambers have a rectangular aperture with dimensions of 3 cm × 0.7 cm. Surgically resected tissue requires removal of external muscle layers before mounting. This is achieved by opening the intestine longitudinally along its mesenteric aspect, pinning the tissue mucosa downwards on dental wax, and removing the outer muscle layers under a dissecting microscope using microdissection scissors, leaving a mucosa/submucosa preparation for mounting in the chambers.

Mounting of Watson capsule biopsies of the small intestine or of endoscopic biopsies from either small or large intestine requires a highly modified chamber. We have developed a method which uses commercially available chambers (Snap Chamber CHM5 World Precision Instruments, Herts, UK) which were designed for use with tissue culture membranes ("Snapwells" Transwell, Costar, Bucks, UK). The polycarbonate membrane is removed from the Snapwell and can be replaced with a carefully machined circular piece of perspex in the centre of which has been drilled a hole 2 mm in diameter. The mucosal biopsy can be stuck carefully onto the perspex plate using a fast setting glue (Superglue). It is extremely important not to apply too much glue as this will narrow the aperture and change the passive electrical properties of the chambers. Equally, small junction potentials which have inadvertently not been corrected for will have a great impact on short circuit current when this is expressed as μA/cm².

Another drawback of such a small aperture is the effects of 'edge damage'. This is best regarded as the effects of low resistance pathways at the circumference of the preparation due either to mechanical damage of the epithelium by the edge of the chamber aperture or as a consequence of an imperfect seal. The consequences of this are both a fall in measured tissue resistance and, as a result of the low resistance pathway, true transepithelial potential difference will be underestimated. These effects are always proportionally larger with smaller aperture chambers and are a major drawback of Ussing chamber studies with endoscopic/Watson capsule biopsies.

The World Precision Instruments chambers dispense with the use of the long and unwieldy agar bridges normally used to connect potential difference sensing and current passing electrodes to the Ussing chamber, and have instead miniaturized Ag/AgCl electrodes which plug directly into the chamber via a luer fitting. The fitting still requires the space around the electrode to be filled with agar in KCl but on the whole this modification had made the apparatus much more robust.

Application to animal studies

Ussing chamber methods are widely used in a variety of other experimental systems, including animal intestine (both full thickness and mucosa/submucosa preparations stripped of the external serosal muscle layer), and cell lines grown in tissue culture. If the tissue allows, it is particularly beneficial to use rectangular Ussing chambers as a greater cross-sectional area of tissue is achieved than with spherical cross-sections. Typical aperture dimensions for rat small intestine would be 3 cm × 0.7 cm, giving a cross-section area of 2.1 cm². Methods for stripping the mucosa from its outer muscle layers will again vary depending on the source of the tissue. Rabbit ileum is best stripped under a dissecting microscope (see above), whereas rat ileum is more easily stripped by sliding the intestine as a tube over a moist, suitable sized rod (typically 4-5 mm in diameter), gently incising the antimesenteric border longitudinally with a blunt scalpel and then peeling the muscle layer off by gently rubbing with the thumb. The tube of intestine is then coverted into a sheet by cutting longitudinally adjacent to the mesenteric attachment.

Results and discussion

Basal electrical characteristics of human duodenal mucosal biopsies (4th part of duodenum adjacent to the Ligament of Trietze) from seven children (median age 2.7 years) with no histological abnormality evident in adjacent biopsies (biopsies taken using double port Watson capsule) were I_{sc} 18.4 ± 2.5 μcm⁻², Rt 43.5 ± 4.9 Ω cm², pd 0.8 ± 0.2 mV

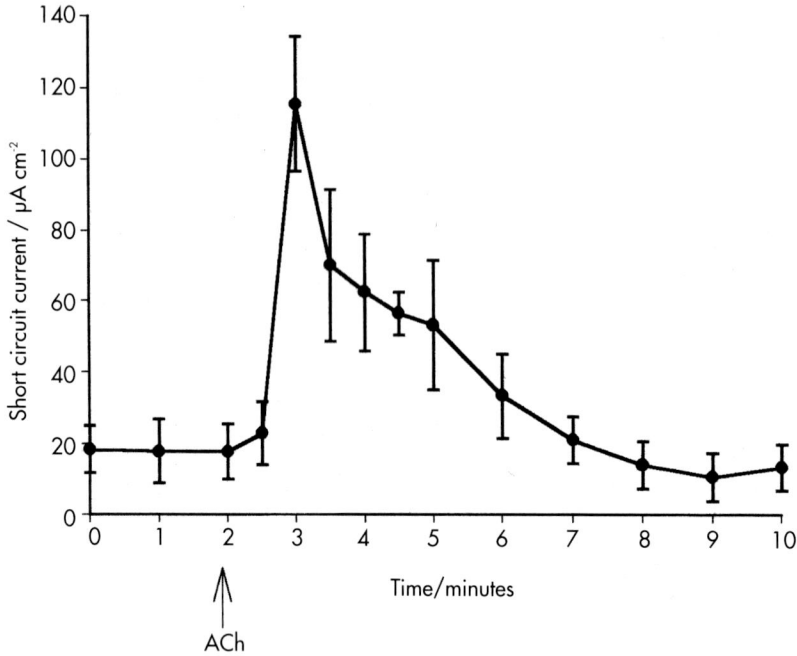

Figure 6.3 – Response of human paediatric Crosby - Watson capsule biopsies from the 4th part of the duodenum to serosally applied acetylcholine (ACh) (10^{-3}M) in Ussing chamber experiments. A 10 minute period was allowed after mounting to let the tissue stabilise before commencing the experiment. Data points are the mean of seven experiments with the 95th confidence interval for the mean given by the error bars.

(means ± sem). The secretory response to serosally applied acetylcholine (10^{-3} M) is shown in Fig. 6.3. There is little normative age-matched data with which to compare these results other than that provided by Taylor *et al.*[13]

Methods

Measurement of large intestinal crypt absorptive function in vitro

The colon is an organ of water and electrolyte salvage with a predominant role in the dehydration of lumenal contents. The driving force for the absorption of water is the active absorption of sodium resulting in high intramucosal concentrations of sodium and hence a transepithelial osmotic gradient to drive water absorption. The highest concentrations of sodium in the colonic mucosa are found in the pericryptal region with much lower concentrations near the lumenal surface epithelium. These findings have led to the (substantiated) proposal[18] that the lumenal surface epithelium is relatively 'leaky' with bi-directional passage of water and electrolyte (mucosa to serosa and serosa to mucosa) which, though providing a high capacity absorptive pathway, is unable to produce the high suction pressures necessary for the

formation of solid faeces because of the inability of this area to maintain high intramucosal sodium concentrations. By contrast, the crypt epithelium is very 'tight' and so it is possible to generate and maintain high concentrations of sodium as are found in the pericryptal space. The colonic crypt is therefore able to generate the high suction pressures necessary to dehydrate faeces and form solid stool.[19]

The process of fluid inflow into an absorbing colonic crypt can be shown by measuring the time dependent concentration of an impermeant dye within the crypt lumen. This *in vitro* approach using various derivatives of fluorescein was established and validated in various animal tissues by Naftalin and Pedley.[19,20] For example, in the rat descending colon the impermeant probe fluorescein isothiocyanate (FITC)-dextran (MW 10,000) placed on the lumenal side of a sheet of tissue flows into the crypt through the lumenal opening by convective flow and is then concentrated within the crypt lumen as a consequence of fluid absorption. Concentrations of FITC-dextran within the crypt are maximal at a depth of 60 μm and are 5 times that found at the crypt opening. From this is it possible by mathematical modelling to calculate the rate of fluid inflow into the crypt lumenal opening and also to demonstrate that 75% of the fluid entering the crypt is absorbed within the first 50 μm of the crypt.[20]

We have adapted these methods to study fluid absorption by human colonic crypts in isolated perfused biopsies taken using standard paediatric endoscopes (biopsy channel sizes 2-4 mm). The experiments described have all been performed using descending colon from children aged 6 months to 16 years.

Endoscopic biopsies are carefully removed from the biopsy forceps by gentle shaking in a universal container containing pre-warmed, gassed Tyrode's salt solution. The tissue is mounted mucosa side upwards (mucosa side downwards with an inverted microscope) using a dissecting microscope in a thermostatically controlled commercially available perifusion chamber (Clark Electromedical Instruments, Reading, UK; Series 20 chamber model RC-21B with heated platform PH-1). A minute amount of adhesive (Superglue), delivered by a capillary tube to the ends of the tissue only, secures the tissue in the chamber, which is then filled with Tyrode's solution and a glass coverslip is carefully applied over the top excluding any air. A watertight seal is achieved by pre-applying vacuum grease to the top coverslip. Heating elements, perfusion and suction tubing can then be attached to the chamber. The chamber is continually perfused with gassed (95% O_2, 5% CO_2) Tyrode's solution maintained at 37°C.

In our laboratory, the tissue is viewed by fluorescence microscopy with a Leica (Bedfordshire, UK) upright laser scanning confocal microscope using a ×10 (Numerical aperture 0.45 NPL Fluotar) objective oil immersion lens. Inverted microscopes are perhaps a little easier to use for *in vitro* work of this kind. Similar systems are available from a number of other manufacturers including Nikon and Biorad. The tissue is excited using a krypton/argon laser with low pass barrier filter set for ≤488 nm and the dichroic beam splitter in the lower position to transmit ≥510 nm. Emission light is collected at ≤515 nm (515 nm long pass barrier filter used). The detection pinhole is set for use with ×10 objective at 40 and offset the same for all experiments.

Once an image is located under bright field illumination, baseline fluid transport in the crypts is studied by changing the perfusate to Tyrode's solution containing 0.3 mM FITC-dextran. A confocal image is then obtained of a transverse optical section through the crypt lumen. From this FITC-dextran accumulation over time can be measured. Using the stepper motor attached to the focusing control of the microscope, optical sectioning at sequential steps down the crypt lumen can also be performed. This produces a concentration profile of FITC-dextran at different depths down the crypt lumen.

Concentration polarization of the FITC-dextran within the crypt lumen is measured as a ratio with the concentration at the crypt surface after subtraction of background fluorescence (mean fluorescence in areas without concentrated dye at the specified depth due to fluorescence detected outside of the plane of focus). The ratio $(I_x-I_{bkg})/(I_{co}-I_{bkg})$ in the crypt lumen is equivalent to the concentration at varying depths (x), where I_{co} and I_x are the mean fluorescence intensities in the crypt lumenal opening and at depth x, respectively, and I_{bkg} is the mean background fluorescence at each depth.[20] In practice these measurements are taken as the average of typically six crypts and fluorescence intensity is measured off line using a suitable software package. Until recently we have used a commercially available package (Sigmascan Pro-Jandel Scientific), but suitable public domain NIH Image programs (National Institutes of Health, USA) for both IBM and Macintosh computers are now available from the Internet (http://www.rsb.info.nih.gov/nih-image).

Application to animal studies

These methods are particularly suitable for use with sheets of animal-derived tissue and were initially developed using such tissues (bovine and ovine colonic tissues) obtained from abattoirs. The reader is referred to the original description of the methods for a fuller discussion.[20]

Results and discussion

The use of concentration polarization of impermeant fluorescent dyes to measure the concentrative capacity of colonic crypts *in vitro* has been well validated in a number of animal species.[19] We have applied this technology successfully to the study of human paediatric colonic mucosa (Fig. 6.4) documenting, as with the animal studies, a gradient of concentration along the colonic crypt and net concentration over time (Fig. 6.5), which can be impaired in the presence of a secretagogue. The methods are being used to study colonic function in healthy and diseased children.

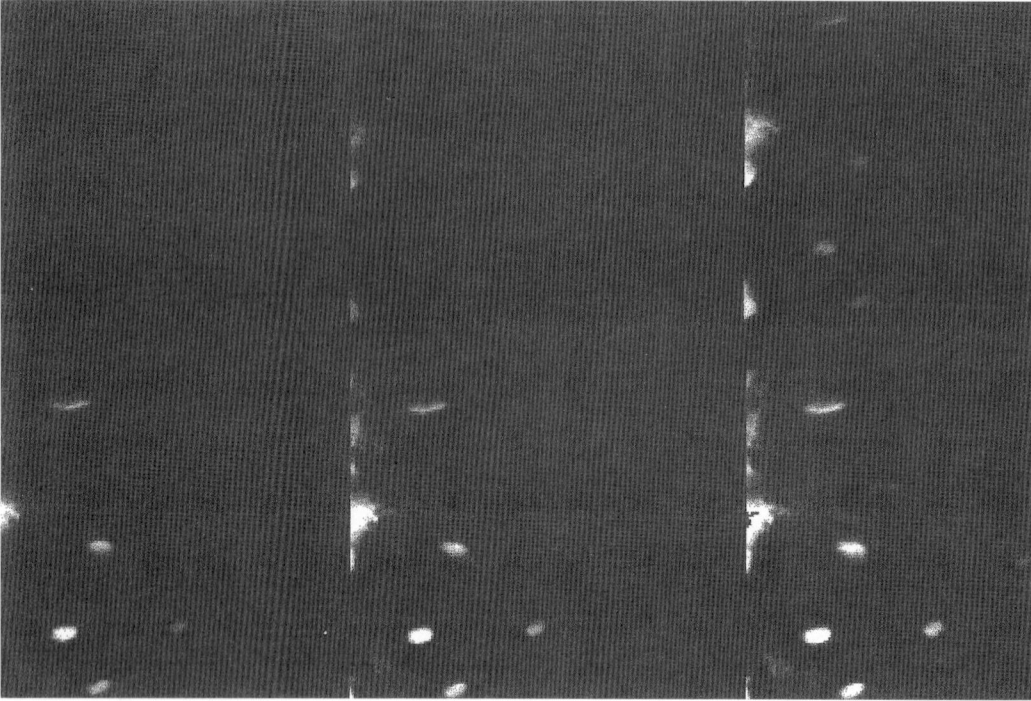

Figure 6.4 – Increasing concentration of FITC–dextran within crypt lumena of a paediatric colonic biopsy (2 mm biopsy forceps) with time at a depth of 30 μm. Images taken at 2 minute intervals.

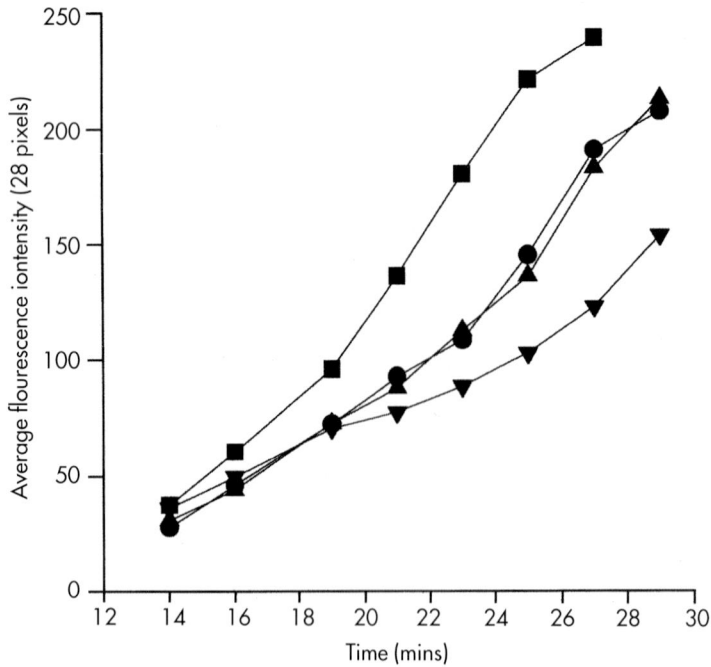

Figure 6.5 – Increasing fluorescence intensity of FITC–dextran over time in 4 adjacent crypt lumena at a depth of 30 μm below the surface mucosa. Human endoscopic biopsy from a 6 month old infant with a histologically normal colon.

Acknowledgements

We thank Peter Milla for his teaching and for providing the environment in which to carry out these studies. The financial support of the Dr Hadwen Trust for Humane Research has facilitated the development of the confocal microscopic methodology in human paediatric biopsies. KJL is supported by the Wellcome Trust.

References

1. Smyth DH. Methods of studying intestinal absorption. In: Smyth DH (Ed) *Biomembranes, Intestinal Absorption*, Vol 4A. Plenum Press, London, 1974, Ch 6.

2. Milla PJ. Paediatric gastroenterology: lessons of inborn errors. *Postgrad Med J* 1986; **62**: 101-105.

3. Levin RJ. Fundamental concepts of structure and function of the intestinal epithelium. In: Duthie HL, Wormsley KG (eds) *Scientific Basis of Gastroenterology*. Churchill Livingstone, Edinburgh, 1979, Ch 11.

4. Ussing HH, Zehran K. Active transport of sodium as the source of electric current in the short circuited isolated frog skin. *Acta Phys Scand* 1950; **23**: 110-128.

5. Curran PF, Soloman AK. Ion and water fluxes in the ileum of rats. *J Gen Physiol* 1957; **41**: 143-168.

6. Schultz SG, Zalusky R. Ion transport in the isolated rabbit ileum I: Short circuit current and sodium fluxes. *J Gen Physiol* 1964; **47**: 567-584.

7. Schultz SG, Zalusky R. Ion transport in the isolated rabbit ileum II: The interaction between active sodium and active sugar transport. *J Gen Physiol* 1964; **47**: 1043-1059.

8. Schultz SG, Zalusky R. Ion transport in the isolated rabbit ileum III: Chloride fluxes. *J Gen Physiol* 1964; **48**: 375-378.

9. Field M, Fromm D, McColl I. Ion transport in rabbit ileal mucosa I: Na and Cl fluxes and short circuit current. *Am J Physiol* 1971; **220**: 1388-1396.

10. Field M. Ion transport in rabbit ileal mucosa II: Effects of cyclic 3`,5`-AMP. *Am J Physiol* 1971; **221**: 992-997.

11. Field M, McColl I. Ion transport in rabbit ileal mucosa III: Effects of catecholamines. *Am J Physiol* 1973; **225**: 852-857.

12. Dietz J, Field M. Ion transport in rabbit ileal mucosa IV: Bicarbonate secretion. *Am J Physiol* 1973; **225**: 858-861.

13. Taylor CJ, Baxter PS, Hardcastle J, Hardcastle PT. Failure to induce secretion in jejunal biopsies from children with cystic fibrosis. *Gut* 1988; **29**: 957-962.

14. Hardy SP, Smith PM, Bayston R, Spitz L. Electrogenic colonic ion transport in Hirschprung's disease: reduced secretion to the neural secretagogues acetylcholine and iloprost. *Gut* 1993; **34**: 1405-1411.

15. Fromm M, Schulzke JD, Hegel U. Epithelial and subepithelial contributions to transmural electrical resistance of intact rat jejunum *in vitro*. *Pflugers Arch* 1985; **347**: 1-7.

16. Hemlin M, Jodal M, Lundgren O, Sjovall H, Stage L. The importance of the subepithelial resistance for the electrical properties of the rat jejunum *in vitro*. *Acta Physiol Scand* 1988; **134**: 79-88.

17. Hegel U, Fromm M. Electrical measurements in the large intestine. *Methods Enzymol* 1990; **192**: 459-484.

18. Naftalin RJ. The dehydrating function of the descending colon in relationship to crypt function. *Physiol Res* 1994; **43**: 65-73.

19. Pedley KC, Naftalin RJ. Evidence from fluorescence microscopy that rat, ovine and bovine colonic crypts are absorptive. *J Physiol* 1993; **460**: 525-547.

20. Naftalin RJ, Zammit PS, Pedley KC. Concentration polarisation of fluorescent dyes in rat descending colonic crypts: evidence of crypt fluid absorption. *J Physiol* 1995; **487**: 479-495.

7

Ambulatory oesophageal and gastric pH monitoring

HJ Stein and WKH Kauer

Summary

In recent years, ambulatory oesophageal pH monitoring has emerged as the gold standard for measuring oesophageal exposure to acid gastric juice in patients with symptoms suggesting gastro-oesophageal reflux disease. The overall percentage time with a pH below 4 on 24-hour oesophageal pH monitoring or a composite score (based on oesophageal exposure time with a pH below 4 during the upright und supine period and the number and duration of reflux episodes) allow an accurate diagnosis of the presence of gastro-oesophageal reflux disease even in the absence of oesophagitis. Interpretation of gastric pH recordings is more difficult than oesophageal recordings because the gastric pH environment is determined by a complex interplay of acid and mucous secretions, ingested food, swallowed saliva, regurgitated duodenal, pancreatic, biliary secretions, and the effectiveness of the mixing and evacuation of the chyme. Duodenogastric reflux and gastric acid secretion can, however, be assessed by gastric pH monitoring using a set of parameters describing the circadian gastric pH pattern based on the percentage time spent above or below several pH thresholds in the upright, supine, meal and postprandial periods, the number, height and duration of alkaline peaks, and the baseline pH. Ambulatory oesophageal and gastric pH monitoring thus allows integrated evaluation of gastro-oesophageal reflux, duodenogastric reflux and the gastric secretory state. This technology gives the physician and researcher the ability to evaluate foregut motor and secretory disorders in a physiological environment during a complete circadian cycle and thus provides a scientific basis for medical or surgical therapy of functional abnormalities of the foregut.

Introduction

Functional disorders are the most common reason for foregut symptoms. These disorders arise from disturbances of the motor or secretory function of the individual foregut compartments (i.e. oesophagus, stomach and duodenum) or are due to insufficiencies of the valves separating the compartments (i.e. the lower oesophageal sphincter and pylorus).[1] Symptoms are an unreliable indicator of the presence of a specific functional foregut disorder[2] and objective tests are required to determine the cause of a patient's symptoms. Because the individual compartments of the upper digestive tract are characterized by a typical pH environment, measurement of intraluminal pH offers the possibility to assess dysfunction of the co-ordinated interplay between the individual compartments.

Since Miller's original description of the use of an indwelling pH probe to evaluate 'acid-peptic diathesis', prolonged intraluminal pH monitoring has been shown to be an accurate method for detecting changes in the pH environment of the oesophagus and stomach.[3] With the development of miniaturized pH electrodes, portable digital data recorders and software to analyse pH records, ambulatory 24-hour pH monitoring of the oesophagus and stomach has become widely available and is commonly used as an office-based test.[1] The subtleties of performing the test, analysing the results and the application in both the clinical and research setting are discussed.

Methods

General

Oesophageal and gastric pH monitoring are usually performed after an overnight fast. All medications that affect acid secretion or the motility of the foregut should be stopped for a sufficiently long period before the study.

A variety of pH probes are available for prolonged intraluminal pH monotoring, i.e. glass electrodes, monocrystalline antimony electrodes, and ion sensitive field effect (ISFET) pH electrodes. We prefer bipolar glass probes with an internal reference electrode because of their accuracy, reliability and stability even at extreme pH values. Whichever electrode type is used, it is essential that the pH electrode is calibrated correctly at pH 1 and pH 7 in standard buffer solutions. Only recordings with an electrode drift of less than 0.2 pH units over a 24-hour period should be accepted.[4]

The pH probe is passed transnasally so that the tip of the electrode lies 5 cm above (for oesophageal pH monitoring) or 5 cm below (for gastric pH monitoring) the lower oesophageal sphincter (Fig. 7.1). Manometrically guided placement is the most accurate means of placing the probe in a reproducible position.[1] The pH electrode is then connected to a portable digital data recorder that stores pH readings every 4-6 seconds. Recording of intraluminal pH is performed over 24 hours on an outpatient basis, preferably while the subject is attending to normal

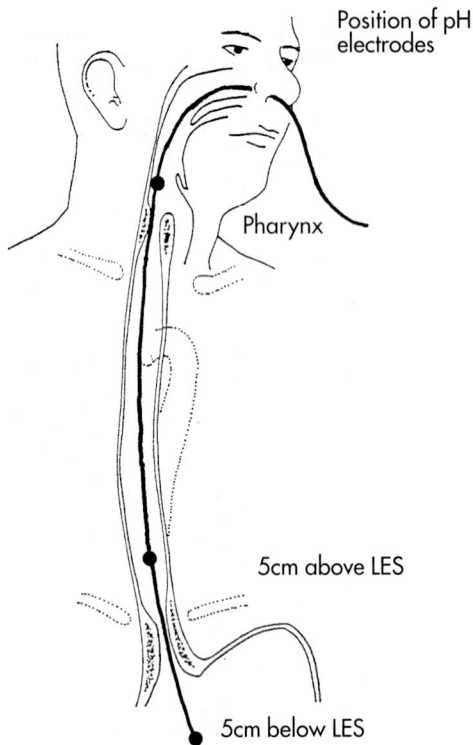

Figure 7.1 – Placement of pH probes for ambulatory oesophageal and gastric pH monitoring. LES = lower oesophageal sphincter.

daily activities. A 24-hour monitoring period is necessary so that measurements are made over one complete circadian cycle. This allows assessment of the effect of physiological activity such as eating or sleeping. The diet is standardized to exclude food and beverages with a pH of <5.0 or >7.0. Only water is allowed between meals. Patients are also instructed to keep a detailed diary of their symptoms during the study. After the 24-hour monitoring period the patient returns to the lab, the probe is removed and the data are loaded from the data-recorder onto a personal computer.

Ambulatory 24-hour oesophageal pH monitoring

Analysis of the oesophageal pH record can be fully automated using commercially available software. The oesophageal exposure to gastric contents as measured by 24-hour oesophageal pH monitoring is usually expressed as the cumulative time the pH is outside the normal range. In the normal situation oesophageal pH is above 4 for 98.5% of a 24-hour monitoring period.[5] Most centres therefore set a pH <4 as the threshold for acid reflux. With this threshold, there is a uniformity of normal values throughout the world.[4,5]

Single measurements of the time the pH is below 4, although concise, do not reflect how the exposure occurs, i.e. are there few but long reflux episodes or multiple episodes of short duration (Fig. 7.2)? Consequently, it is also necessary to measure the frequency and duration of each exposure below the threshold[6-8] by calculating the following parameters:

1. The % time with a pH <4 during the total monitoring period;

2. The % time with a pH <4 in the upright position;

3. The % time with a pH <4 in the supine position;

4. The total number of reflux episodes;

5. The number of reflux episodes lasting longer than 5 min;

6. The duration of the longest reflux episode.

Score values for each of these parameters can be calculated based on the standard deviation and mean of each of these parameters in 50 previously reported normal subjects.[5,9] When the score values for an individual patient are added, a composite score is obtained which reflects oesophageal acid exposure time and the mode of exposure over the 24-hour monitoring period. Extensive clinical studies and the results of a receiver operating characteristics analysis have shown that an overall acid exposure time above 4.5% of the monitoring period or a composite score above 15.6 are highly accurate in differentiating patients with and without increased oesophageal exposure to gastric juices (Table 7.1).[5]

Similar measurements can be made to assess elevations in pH above 7 as an indicator for alkaline intestino-oesophageal reflux.[10] Increased exposure in this pH range can, however, also be due to abnormal calibration of the pH recorder, the presence of a dental infection which increases salivary pH, or the presence of oesophageal obstruction, which results in static pools of saliva with an increase in pH secondary to bacterial overgrowth.[10,11]

In patients with symptoms of chronic cough, hoarseness or aspiration, the placement of an additional pH

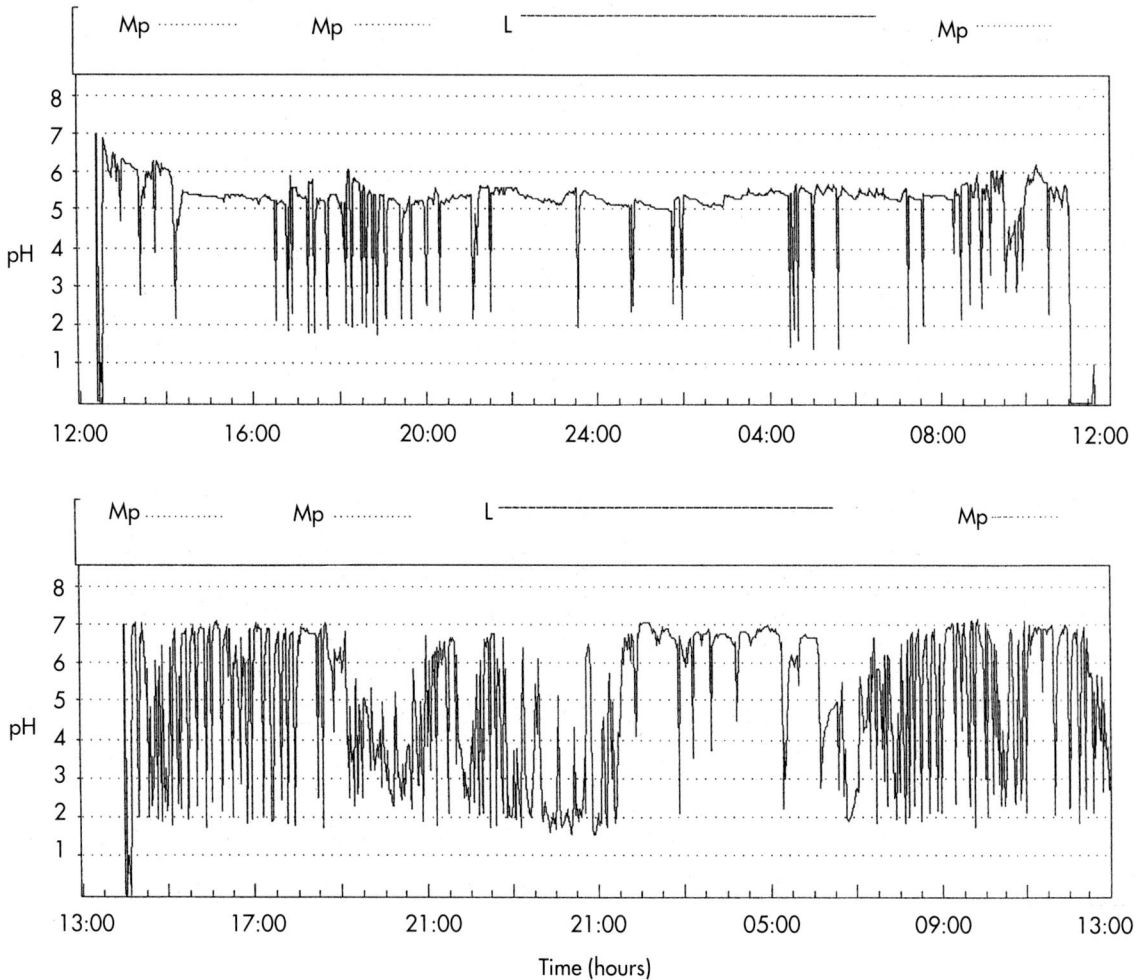

Figure 7.2 – 24-hour oesophageal pH record in a normal volunteer
(top) and a patients with gastro- oesophageal reflux disease (bottom).
M = meal period; p = postprandial period; L = supine period.

Table 7.1 – Sensitivity, specificity and accuracy of individual parameters of 24-hour oesophageal pH monitoring in the diagnosis of gastro-oesophageal reflux disease.

	Sensitivity (%)	Specificity (%)	Accuracy (%)
% Total time pH < 4	96	96	96
% Upright time pH < 4	92	88	88
% Supine time pH < 4	88	92	92
Number of reflux episodes	88	88	88
Episodes longer than 5 min	84	100	86
Duration of longest episode	84	100	86
Composite score	96	100	96

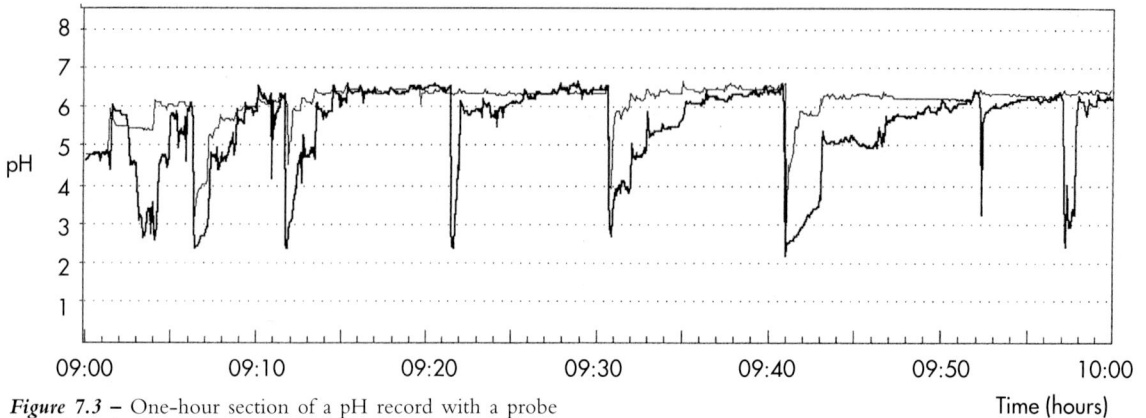

Figure 7.3 – One-hour section of a pH record with a probe located in the distal oesophagus (bold line) and pharynx (thin line) showing episodes with acid reflux reaching the pharynx.

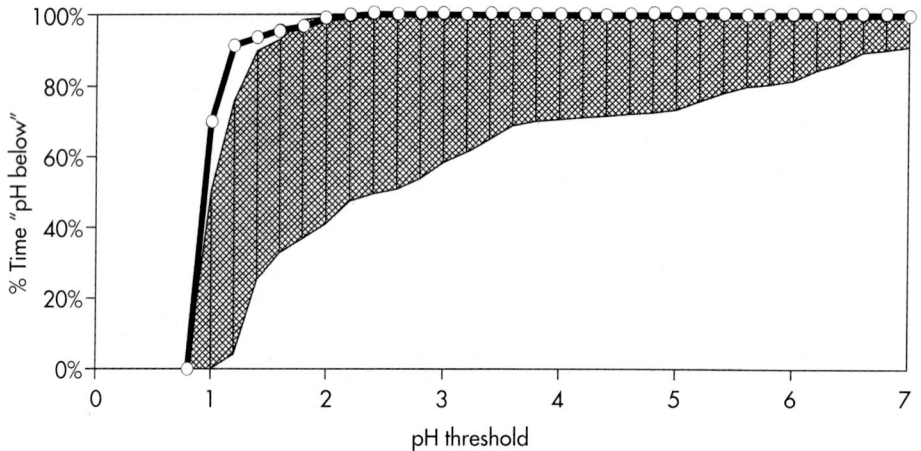

Figure 7.4 – Cumulative frequency of recorded gastric pH values during the supine period. The shaded area represents the 5th and 95th percentiles of 50 normal volunteers. The solid line shows a patient with acid hypersecretion and a marked 'left shift' beyond the normal range.

electrode in the pharynx can be helpful (Fig. 7.1). If reflux episodes reach the pharynx (Fig. 7.3) and a temporary relationship between these reflux episodes and the onset of the symptom can be documented, gastro-oesophageal reflux can be assumed to be the cause of the patient's respiratory complaint.[12]

Gastric pH monitoring and combined oesophageal/gastric pH monitoring

The interpretation of circadian gastric pH records is more difficult than the analysis of oesophageal pH recordings. This is because the gastric pH environment is determined by a complex interplay of acid and mucous secretion, ingested food, swallowed saliva, regurgitated duodenal, pancreatic, and biliary secretions, and the effectiveness of mixing and

evacuation of the chyme.[13]

For analysis the 24-hour gastric pH recording is divided into the upright period, the supine period, the prandial pH plateau, and the postprandial pH decline period.[14,15] For each of these periods the following parameters are calculated:

1. The pH frequency distribution;

2. The cumulative frequency distribution;

3. The frequency of pH changes;

4. The duration of pH exposure at each pH interval.

The gastric secretory state can be evaluated on the basis of the 24-hour gastric pH record by assessing the cumulative frequency distribution of luminal pH

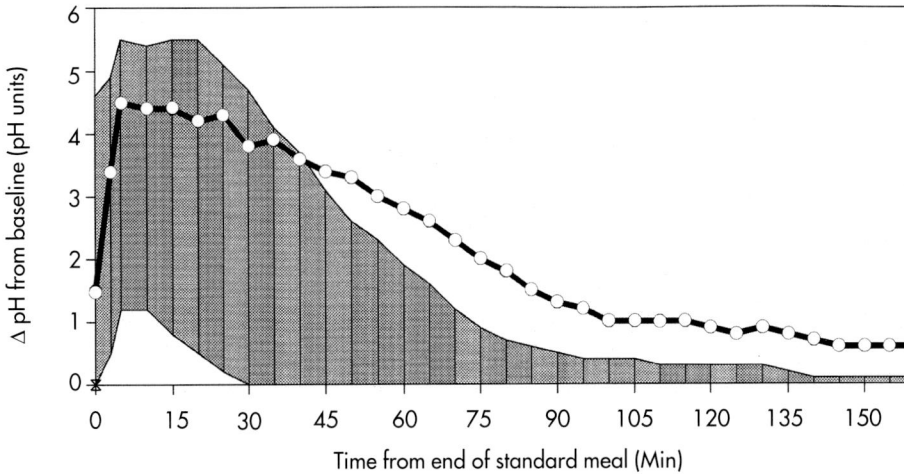

Figure 7.5 – Postprandial alkalinisation of the gastric luminal pH as measured by gastric pH monitoring. The shaded area represents the 5th and 95th percentiles of 50 normal volunteers. The solid line shows the values of a patient with prolonged postprandial alkalinisation.

values during the night. Gastric acid hypersecretion can be diagnosed by a 'left shift' on the frequency distribution graph (Fig. 7.4).

To estimate gastric emptying based on the gastric pH record, the postprandial intragastric pH profile must be assessed following a standard meal. The increase of the recorded luminal gastric pH values from the interdigestive baseline pH during the meal is plotted over the entire duration of the postprandial period, i.e. until the pH returns to its baseline value. A patient is considered to have prolonged postprandial alkalinisation if the postprandial pH record exceeds the normal range (Fig. 7.5).

Discriminant analysis has shown that a scoring system based on the above parameters can also differentiate the gastric pH profile of normal volunteers from patients with increased duodenogastric reflux. This scoring system is described in detail elsewhere[14] and is available with most commercial gastric pH analysis programs.

Combined ambulatory monitoring of gastric and oesophageal pH is suggested by some investigators to overcome the shortcomings of oesophageal pH monitoring to diagnose duodeno-gastro-oesophageal reflux.[16,17] This approach allows the correlation of episodes of oesophageal alkalization with gastric alkaline peaks, thus providing a strong indicator for a gastric or duodenal source of an alkaline oesophageal pH. In addition, combined monitoring may also help to identify episodes of duodeno-gastro-oesophageal reflux which do not alter the oesophageal pH beyond its normal range between 5 and 7, i.e. the so-called mixed reflux.[17]

Application to animal studies

Little data is available on ambulatory oesophageal or gastric pH monitoring in animals. We have used oesophageal pH monitoring in mini pigs to detect oesophageal exposure of acid reflux after excison of the lower oesophageal sphincter.[18] The test was performed exactly as in humans with the pH probe located 5 cm above the manometrically determined upper border of the lower oesophageal sphincter. The time with pH <4 and <5 was compared in the individual animals before and after the surgical procedure, i.e. the animals were used as their own controls.

Fuchs *et al.*[14] performed gastric pH monitoring in mongrel dogs. The dogs were sedated with ketamine and placed in the right lateral position. Two pH electrodes were attached to a nasogastric tube so that the tips were 5 cm apart. The distal portion of the nasogastric tube was advanced endoscopically into the duodenum to anchor the gastric pH electrodes 5 and 10 cm proximal to the pylorus. Their results indicate that the conversion of the continuous gastric pH plot to cumulative exposure at whole-number pH intervals accurately reflects induced changes in intraluminal gastric pH.

These studies show that oesophageal and gastric pH monitoring can be performed in animals without difficulty as long as the same precautions are observed as in humans. Since there are no normal values for any animal species these must either be established in a 'normal group' or each animal must be used as its own control, i.e. repeat measurements before and after the experiment-specific manipulations are required.

Results and discussion

Oesophageal and/or gastric pH monitoring offers the possibility to assess duodeno-gastro-oesophageal reflux and the gastric secretory state over an entire circadian cycle. It is now widely accepted that 24-hour oesophageal pH monitoring represents the gold standard for the detection of abnormal oesophageal acid exposure.[5,12] The use of 24-hour oesophageal pH monitoring to detect biliary intestino-oesophageal reflux by an alkaline exposure above pH 7 has been criticized due to methodological problems.[10,11] With the recent development of fibre-optic ambulatory 24-hour intraluminal bilirubin monitoring, the so-called BILITEC test, oesophageal pH monitoring has become obsolete as a test of biliary intestino-oesophageal reflux.[19]

Assessment of the gastric secretory state is an obvious application of 24-hour gastric pH monitoring. Initial studies have, however, shown that simple analysis of the mean or median pH or the time with a pH <1 is insufficient to identify gastric acid hypersecretion. Rather, a sophisticated analysis of the circadian record with exclusion of the meal and postprandial periods is necessary to avoid interference of meals and duo-denogastric reflux. In a recent study we showed that analysis of the frequency distribution of gastric pH values in steps of 0.1 pH units and calculation of the time the pH was <1.2 during the supine period allows discrimination of patients with acid hypersecretion from those with normal acid secretion.[15] With this approach gastric pH monitoring can be used to assess the effect of acid suppression therapy, predict patients at risk for recurrences of peptic ulcer after elimination of *Helicobacter pylori*, and identify patients that would benefit from proximal gastric vagotomy.

For a definite diagnosis of excessive duodenogastric reflux based on gastric pH records, a simple measurement of alkaline peaks has proved unreliable. This is because meals, liquids and the early morning reduction in acid secretion may also result in sudden changes of gastric pH mimicking alkaline reflux episodes. To overcome these problems Fuchs et al.[14] have developed a scoring system for duodenogastric reflux which uses a large number of computer-generated statistical measurements including the number and height of alkalinising peaks, the baseline pH, the pH of the meal plateau and the pattern of pH decline from the plateau. When tested against classical tests of duodenogastric reflux this scoring system has been found to be highly specific for the diagnosis of the abnormality.[20,21]

Evaluation of gastric emptying on the basis of the postprandial alkalinisation of the gastric pH record evolved from multiple probe gastric pH monitoring performed during scintigraphic gastric emptying studies.[22] These studies demonstrated a good correlation between the emptying of oatmeal and the duration of the postprandial plateau and decline phases of the pH in the gastric corpus. A prolonged postprandial decline time of the gastric pH may, however, also be due to excessive postprandial duodenogastric reflux or a decreased meal-induced stimulation of acid secretion. If these conditions are excluded a prolonged postprandial alkalinisation of the pH in the gastric corpus implies delayed gastric emptying.[15]

Taken together, ambulatory oesophageal and gastric pH monitoring allows integrated evaluation of gastro-oesophageal reflux, duodenogastric reflux and the gastric secretory state. This technology gives the physician and researcher the ability to evaluate foregut motor and secretory disorders in a physiological environment during a complete circadian cycle and provides a scientific basis for medical or surgical therapy of functional abnormalities of the foregut.[1]

References

1. Stein HJ, DeMeester TR, Hinder RA. Outpatient physiological testing and surgical management of foregut motor disorders. *Curr Probl Surg* 1992; **24:** 415-555.

2. Costantini M, Crookes PF, Bremner RM *et al.* Value of physiologic assessment of foregut symptoms in a surgical practice. *Surgery* 1993; **11:** 780-787.

3. Miller FA, DoVale J, Gunther T. Utilization of inlying pH-probe for evaluation of acid-peptic diathesis. *Arch Surg* 1964; **89:** 199-203.

4. Emde C, Garner A, Blum AL. Technical aspects of intraluminal pH-metry in man: current status and recommendations. *Gut* 1989; **28:** 1177-1188.

5. Jamieson JR, Stein HJ, DeMeester TR, Bonavina L, Hinder RA. Ambulatory 24-hour oesophageal pH monitoring: Normal values, optimal thresholds, specificity, sensitivity, and reproducibility. *Am J Gastroenterol* 1992; **87:** 1102-1111.

6. Johnson LF, DeMeester TR. Twenty-four hour pH monitoring of the distal oesophagus: A quantitative measure of gastrooesophageal reflux. *Am J Gastroenterol* 1974; **62:** 325-332.

7. DeMeester TR, Johnson LF, Joseph GJ *et al.* Patterns of gastrooesophageal reflux in health and disease. *Ann Surg* 1976; **184:** 459-470.

8. DeMeester TR, Wang CI, Wernly JA *et al.* Technique, indications, and clinical use of 24-hour oesophageal pH monitoring. *J Thorac Cardiovasc Surg* 1980; **79:** 656-670.

9. Johnson LF, DeMeester TR. Development of the 24-hour intraoesophageal pH monitoring composite scoring system. *J Clin Gastroenterol* 1986; **8:** 52-58.

10. Stein HJ, Feussner H, Kauer W, *et al.* 'Alkaline' gastrooesophageal reflux: Assessment by ambulatory oesophageal aspiration and pH monitoring. *Am J Surg* 1994; **167:** 163-168.

11. DeVault KR, Georgeson S, Castell DO. Salivary stimulation mimics oesophageal exposure to refluxed duodenal contents. *Am J Gastroent* 1993; **88:** 1040-1043.

12. Bremner RM, Bremner CG, DeMeester TR. Gastro-oesophageal reflux: the use of pH monitoring. *Curr Probl Surg* 1995; **32:** 429-568.

13. Fimmel CJ, Etienne A, Cilluffo T *et al.* Long-term ambulatory gastric pH monitoring: Validation of a new method and effect of H_2 antagonists. *Gastroenterology* 1985; **88:** 1842-1851.

14. Fuchs KH, DeMeester TR, Hinder RA, Computerized identification of pathologic duodenogastric reflux. *Ann Surg* 1991; **213:** 13-20.

15. Stein HJ, DeMeester TR, Peters J, *et al.* Indications, technique, and clinical use of ambulatory 24-hour gastric pH monitoring in a surgical practice. *Surgery* 1994; **116:** 758-767.

16. Mattioli S, Pilotti V, Felice V *et al.* Ambulatory 24-hr pH monitoring of oesophagus, fundus, and antrum. A new technique for simultaneous study of gastrooesophageal and duodenogastric reflux. *Dig Dis Sci* 1990; **35:** 929-938.

17. Attwood SEA, Ball CS, Barlow AP, *et al.* Role of intragastric and intra-oesophageal alkalinisation in the pathogenesis of complications in Barrett's columnar lined lower ooesophagus. *Gut* 1993; **34:** 11-15.

18. Stein HJ, Feussner H, Holste J, Experimentelle Ergebnisse mit einem partiell resorbierbaren Implantat zur Verhinderung des gastroösophagealen Refluxes. In: Hierholzer G (Ed) *Langenbecks Archiv für Chirurgie, Chirurgisches Forum '95 für experimentelle und klinische Forschung.* Springer Verlag, Berlin, 1995, pp 547-550.

19. Bechi P, Pucciano F, Baldini F *et al.* Long-term ambulatory enterogastric reflux monitoring: validation of a new fiber optic technique. *Dig Dis Sci* 1993; **38:** 1297-1306.

20. Stein HJ, Hinder RA, DeMeester TR, Clinical use of 24-hour gastric pH monitoring versus DISIDA scanning in the diagnosis of pathologic duodenogastric reflux. *Arch Surg* 1990; **125:** 966-971.

21. Stein HJ, Smyrk T, DeMeester TR, *et al.* Sensitivity and specificity of endoscopy and histology in the diagnosis of excessive duodenogastric reflux. *Surgery* 1992; **112:** 796-804.

22. Clark GWB, Jamieson JR, Hinder RA *et al.* The relationship of gastric pH and the emptying of solid, semisolid and liquid meals. *J Gastrointest Mot* 1993; **5:** 273-279.

8

Evaluation of cytokine profile in the gastrointestinal tract

James Y Wang and Dennis S Huang

Summary

Cytokines are regulatory proteins produced by a variety of cell type such as lymphocytes, monocytes/macrophages, epithelial cells and fibroblasts. Cytokines are composed of interleukins, monokines, chemokines, growth factors, interferons and colony stimulating factors. They are of central importance in the regulation of immunity and inflammation. The understanding of the mechanisms by which cytokines play important roles in mucosal immunity and inflammation as well as in some disease states will certainly contribute to the development of new therapies for, or the prevention of, infectious and inflammatory diseases of the gastrointestinal tract. This chapter describes techniques for assaying cytokine activities or measuring cytokine protein levels. The advantages and disadvantages for each technique are discussed.

Introduction

The evolution of multicellular organisms required the development of intercellular messengers, including cytokines and hormones, to co-ordinate cellular or physiological responses. Cytokines are low molecular weight regulatory proteins produced by virtually every nucleated cell type in the body, such as lymphocytes, monocytes/macrophages, epithelial cells and fibroblasts. They have pleiotropic regulatory effects on haematopoietic, immune and inflammatory cells and many other cell types. Cytokines are composed of interleukins (IL), monokines, chemokines, growth factors, interferons (IFN) and colony stimulating factors (CSF). An individual cytokine can stimulate the production of many others generating a network of interacting cytokines or cytokines interacting with each other or with other cell regulators such as hormones. In contrast to endocrine hormones that are generally produced by specialized glands or cells, are present in the circulation, and serve to maintain systemic homeostasis, cytokines usually act over short distances as autocrine or paracrine intercellular signals in local tissues and only occasionally circulate systemically to initiate systemic reactions. Despite these differences, cytokines and some polypeptide hormones form a large family of extracellular signalling molecules with fundamentally similar mechanisms of actions.

Cytokines are of central importance in the regulation of immunity, inflammation, tissue remodelling and embryonic development. An understanding of the cytokine network and its pathogenetic mechanisms in disease states has substantial clinical implications. As soluble mediators of immunity and inflammation, cytokines are being tested with increasing success in malignant diseases, chronic virus and parasitic infections, and some rare congenital immune deficiencies. In contrast, uncontrolled excessive production of cytokines may be associated with many pathological processes. Detection of cytokines in disease states promises to provide important diagnostic tools and cytokine inhibitors such as antagonists, binders or receptors to have therapeutic value when administered in therapeutic doses. In the past decade, therefore, cytokine research has become increasingly relevant to many different areas of biological sciences and medicine. The physiological role of cytokines in mucosal immunity and inflammation has also been increasingly recognized.[1,2]

Methods

Quantitative biological assays for individual cytokines

This chapter focuses on the detection of cytokines. Cytokine bioassays are based on various biological effects, and fall into six general categories with measurement of proliferation, cytotoxicity, intracellular changes, cell motility, and colony formation. Bioassays use primary cultures of cells or cytokine-dependent cell lines.

Proliferation assays are the first choice for many cytokines. Measurement techniques include enzyme-based colour changes as in the MTT (3-(4,5-dimethylthiazol-2-ys)-2,5-diphenyl tetrazolium bromide) assay,[3] in which yellow MTT is converted to a purple derivative by mitochondria, the colour change being proportional to the number of mitochondria and hence to cell number; and the tritiated thymidine incorporation assay in which the amount of new DNA synthesis and hence proliferative activity is estimated by the amount of radiolabelled thymidine incorporated into cellular DNA.

The most commonly used and reliable murine T cell assay systems which measure IL-1 biological activity are the subclone D10S of the murine T-helper cell line D10.64.1 and a subclone, NOB-1, of the murine thymoma cell line EL4.6.1.[4,5] They provide simple and sensitive IL-1 bioassays for most vertebrate species, including man. Another assay is the thymocyte assay, in which lectin-stimulated murine thymocytes proliferate in response to IL-1,[6] but is slow, unreliable and nonspecific. In any assay systems, use of an antibody specific to IL-1 is strongly recommended to confirm the specificity of the system. The protocol for the IL-1 bioassay is as follows. Take the D10.64.1 cells 2-3 days after feeding and wash three times in culture medium (CM; PRMI 1640 medium containing 10% fetal bovine serum, 2 mM glutamate, 7.5% (w/v) sodium bicarbonate, 100 units penicillin/ml and 100 µg/ml strepto- mycin/ml) by centrifuging the cells at 200 g for 10 min. Assess the viability of the cells by trypan blue exclusion assay and resuspend the cells to a final concentration of 1×10^6 cells/ml in CM. Distribute titration of an IL-1 standard, in triplicate, in 96-well microtitration plates. Start the titration of the standard at (100 pg/ml) IL-1 (10 U/ml) and make serial two-fold dilutions down to 0.10 pg/ml (0.01 U/ml) IL-1. Make appropriate dilutions of the samples to be measured for IL-1 activity at two-fold serial dilutions, in triplicate. The negative control is CM alone. The final volume of each well is 100 µl. Add 100 µl of the cell suspension to each well and incubate the plates for 24 hours at 37 °C in a humidi- fied 5% CO_2 incubator. Add 0.5 µCi of tritiated thymidine to each well and return the plates to the incubator for another 4 hours. Harvest the contents of each well on to filter mats, using a cell harvester, and determine the radioactivity by liquid scintillation counting. Plot a standard curve of counts per minutes (cpm) versus concentrations of IL-1.

The original assays for IL-2 used short-term lectin-induced T cell blasts, but they respond to other cytokines and some non-cytokine molecules. Currently, IL-2 is measured by its proliferative effect on IL-2-dependent cell lines such as MT-1, HT-2, and CTLL clones. The latter provides a reliable and easy method which responds to IL-2 from most mammalian species, including man.[7] As these cell lines also respond to other cytokines such as IL-4, IL- 6 and IL-12, the use of an antibody specific to IL-2 is strongly recommended to confirm the specificity of the system. The protocol for IL-2 bioassay is as for IL- 1 but CTLL-2 cells are used and these are resuspend- ed to a final concentration of 1×10^5 in CM. Titration of the standard is started at 100 U/ml IL-2 and serial two-fold dilutions are made down to 0.01 U/ml IL-2.

Bioassays for human IL-3 use AML 193 cells, MO-7

cells.[8] None of IL-3-dependent cell lines is specific. They often respond to G-CSF, M-CSF and GM-CSF. In any assay systems, an antibody specific to IL-3 is strongly recommended to confirm the specificity of the system. The protocol for IL-3 bioassay is as for IL-1 but MO-7 cells are used and these are resuspended to a final concentration of 5×10^5 cells/ml in CM. Titration of the standard is started at 400 U/ml IL-3 and serial two-fold dilutions are made down to 0.01 U/ml IL-3. The plates are ini- tially incubated for 36 hours at 37 °C in a humidified 5% CO_2 incubator.

The classical assay for human IL-4 is B-cell proliferation co-stimulated by anti-immunoglobulin, phorbol ester or *Staphylococcus aureus* Cowan strains 1.[9] Currently, some assays use the ability of IL-4 to induce proliferation in phytohaemagglutinin activated T lymphocytes or T cell lines such as CTLL-2, HT-2 and BCL-1. Assays measure the proliferative effect of human IL-4 on either B cell lines such as BLAM-4, HFB-1, and L4, or certain haemopoietic progenitor cell lines such as TF-1 or MO-7E.[9] None of these cell lines is very specific. They often respond to IL-2, IL-5 and IL-6, hence an antibody specific to IL-4 is strongly recommended to confirm the specificity of the system. The protocol for IL-4 bioassay is as for IL-1 but the MO-7 cells are used and are resuspended to a final concentration of 1×10^6 cells/ml in CM. Titration of the standard is started at 100 U/ml IL-4 and serial two-fold dilutions are made down to 0.01 U/µl IL-4. Add 50 µl of the cell suspension and 50 µl of phorbol ester (40 µg/ml) to each well and incubate the plates initially for 72 hours at 37 °C in a humidified 5% CO_2 incubator.

Human IL-5 is active on murine cells but with a greatly reduced specific activity; murine IL-5 is active on human cells. The commonest assay for IL-5 is the proliferation of murine BCL1 cells and TF-1.[10] These cell lines often respond to IL-2 or IL-4, hence an antibody specific to IL-5 is strongly recommended to confirm the specificity of the system. IL-5 can also be measured by stimulating the formation of eosinophil peroxidase.[10] The protocol for IL-5 bioassay is as for IL-1 but BCL-1 cells are used and resuspended to a final concentration of 2×10^5 cells/ml in CM. The titration of the standard is started at 200 U/ml IL-5 and serial two-fold dilutions are made down to 0.01 U/ml IL-5. The plates are initially incubated for 44 hours at 37 °C in a humidified 5% CO_2 incubator.

Human and murine IL-6 are equally active on murine

cells, whereas murine IL-6 is not active on human cells. Most bioassays for IL-6 depend upon the proliferative effect of this cytokine on IL-6-dependent hybridoma cell lines such as MH60, B9, and 7TD1. The IL-6-dependent murine hybrodoma cell line B9 provides a reliable and sensitive assay for measuring mammalian IL-6.[11] IL-4 also slightly stimulates the proliferation of these cell lines, hence an antibody specific to IL-6 is recommended to confirm the specificity of the system. The protocol for IL-6 bioassay is as for IL-1 but B9 cells are used and resuspended to a final concentration of 5×10^4 cells/ml in CM. Titration of the standard is started at 10 U/ml IL-6 and serial two-fold dilutions are made down to 0.01 U/ml IL-6. The plates are initially incubated for 72 hours at 37 °C in a humidified 5% CO_2 incubator.

Assay of human IL-7 can be achieved using a murine-dependent cell line, IxN/2b.[12] The IL-7 bioassay employs pre-B cell lines obtained from long-term Whitlock-Witte bone marrow cell cultures which are absolutely strictly dependent upon exogenous IL-7 for continuous growth and viability.[13] The protocol for IL-7 bioassay is as for IL-1 but clone 2b cells[14] are used and resuspended to a final concentration of 2×10^5 cells/ml in CM. Titration of the standard is started at 200 U/ml IL-7 and serial two-fold dilutions are made down to 0.001 U/ml IL-7. The plates are initially incubated for 44 hours at 37 °C in a humidified 5% CO_2 incubator and 2 µCi of tritiated thymidine is added to each well.

The classical assay for transforming growth factor (TGF)-β is based on its ability to reduce colony growth of fibroblasts in soft agar. Currently, TGF-β can be measured by decreased proliferation of the mink lung fibroblast MV3D9 cell line.[15] The decreased proliferation can be detected by reduced incorporation of labelled thymidine into DNA or by a decrease in the reduction of the MTT. To distinguish subtypes of TGF-β, antibodies specific to each subtype of TGF-β are recommended to confirm the specificity of the system. The protocol for TGF-β bioassay is as follows. Take the MV-3D9 cells 2-3 days after feeding and wash three times in CM by centrifuging the cells at 200 g for 10 min. Assess the viability of the cells by trypan blue exclusion assay and resuspend the cells to a final concentration of 2×10^5 cells/ml in CM. Add 50 µl of the cell suspension to each well of a microtiter plate and incubate for 3 hours. Distribute titration of an TGF-β standard, in triplicate, in 96-well microtitration plates. Start the titration of the standard at 350 U/ml TGF-β and

make serial two-fold dilutions down to 0.1 U/ml TGF-β. Make appropriate dilutions of the samples to be measured for TGF-β activity at two-fold serial dilutions, in triplicate. The negative control is CM alone. The final volume of each well is 100 µl. Transfer 50 µl from each well containing TGF-β standard or samples to the plate containing the cell. Incubate the plates for 96 hours at 37 °C in a humidified 5% CO_2 incubator. Add 10 µl of MTT to each well and return the plates to the incubator for another 2 hours. Add 25 µl of acid SDS (10% w/v SDS in 0.02M HCl) per well and mix carefully. Leave the plates in darkness at room temperature for 1 hours. Determine the absorbance at a wavelength of 620 nm using a microwell ELISA reader. Plot a standard curve of absorbance versus concentration of TGF-β.

Cytotoxicity assays use similar types of measurement to proliferation assays, although in the most common systems the target cells are normally not highly proliferative and hence tritiated thymidine is useless. In these situations simple vital stains such as crystal violet or amino blue-black give reliable results. Human tumour necrosis factor (TNF) is active on murine cells but with a slight reduction in specific activity. TNF shares many of the biological effects of IL-1 and may interfere with each other in bioassays. Bioassays for human TNF-α and -β use the cytotoxic action of these cytokines on murine fibroblasts such as L929 or L-M cells.[16] An antibody specific to TNF is strongly recommended to confirm the specificity of the system. The protocol for TNF bioassay is as follows. Take the L929 cells in log phase growth, trypsinize, wash three times and dilute to 2×10^5 cells/ml in CM. Aliquot 100 µl of cell suspension into each well of a microtiter plate and incubate for 24 hours at 37 °C, 5% CO_2 humidified incubator. Distribute titration of TNF standard and samples in duplicate in 200 µl in CM containing 2 µg/ml actinomycin D in a different microtiter plate. Start the titration of the standard at 100 U/ml and then make serial two-fold dilutions down to 0.10 U/ml. Make appropriate dilutions of the samples, in duplicate. For a positive control, add high TNF at 4000 U/ml. For a negative control, add CM alone. Incubate plates for 24 hours at 37 °C, in a 5% CO_2 humidified incubator. Suck out CM and blot plate dry by inverting on to adsorbent paper. Wash cells with 100 ml phoshate buffer solution (PBS; pH 7.2), and invert plate onto absorbent paper. Add 100 µl naphthol blue black (NBB stain; 0.05% NBB, 9% acetic acid in 0.1M sodium acetate). Leave plates to stain for 30 min. Fix cells for 15 min with 100 µl formalin fixative solution

(10% formalin, 9% acetic acid in 0.1M sodium acetate). Wash plates with tap-water and invert plates onto absorbent paper until dry. Add 150 µl of 50 mM NaOH to each well of the plate. Carefully agitate the plate until the dye is evenly dispensed throughout the wells, and determine the absorbance versus concentration of TNF.

Intracellular changes result in enhanced killing of ingested virus or bacteria. IFN–α and -β are usually assayed by their ability to reduce the viral killing of target cell types by inhibiting the replication of an infecting virus. Generally, cell lines of human origin (Hep2/C, WISH, A549) are best for the assay of human IFNs.[17] The challenge viruses commonly used in these assays are encephalomycarditis virus (ECMV), vesicular stomatitis virus, and Semliki forest virus. The cytopathic reduction effect is often used. It is rapid, economical and reliable. To distinguish the three types of IFN, antibody specific to each type of IFN is recommended to confirm the specificity of the system. The protocol for IFN bioassay is as follows. Culture the Hep2/C cells in CM. Add 100 µl of CM to all wells in the microtiter plate. Assign wells for cell and virus controls (usually lines 1 and 12). In line 2, rows B, C, and D are cell controls, and rows E, F, and G are virus controls. Add 100 µl of IFN sample at a known dilution to the wells, in triplicate. Make serial two-fold dilutions from rows A to H, using a multichannel micropipette. Trypsinize Hep2/C cells and resuspend cells to a concentration of 5×10^5 cells/µl. Add 100 µl of cell suspension to each well, including cell and virus controls, so that the final volume in each well is 200 µl. Incubate the plates for 16-24 hours at 37°C in a 5% CO_2 humidified incubator. Following overnight incubation, check the plates to see that a confluent monolayer of cells is present. Remove the CM in the wells by flicking out and blotting on a paper towel. Dilute the virus, ECMV, to around 10-30 PFU/cell in CM, or the dilution required to effect 100% cytopathic effect in the unprotected virus control. Add 200 µl of viral suspension to all wells except the cell controls. To the latter, add 200 µl of CM and return the plates to the incubator. After 36-48 hours incubation, examine the monolayer of the virus-control wells microscopically. Remove CM from all wells by flicking out. Add 100 µl of amino blue black (0.05% in 9% acetic acid with 0.1M sodium acetate) and stain for 15-30 min at room temperature. Remove the stain solution by flicking out. Fix the cell monolayer with 100 µl of formalin acetate fixative solution (10% formalin in 9% acetic acid with 0.1 M sodium acetate) and leave the plates at room temperature for at least 20 min. Flick off the fixative solution and wash the plates under running tap-water for 10 min. Dry the plates at room temperature. Add 100 µl of 0.38% NaOH to each well. Make sure that the contents of each well are uniformly distributed by tapping the sides of the plates. Read the absorbance at 620 nm with microwell ELISA reader for measurement of cell survival. Plot a standard curve of absorbance versus concentrations of IFN.

IL-8 can be measured by monitoring cell motility using either Boyden-chamber-type systems in which cells are allowed to migrate through filters of defined pore size, or out of drops of gelled agar. Directional movement can be assessed by monitoring polarization of individuals cells in a gradient of cytokine or by following bulk cell movements. Human IL-8 is an active chemotactic factor of rodent and rabbit neutrophils. Bioassays for IL-8 routinely use human peripheral blood neutrophils.[18] Cell migration can be determined by measuring the diameter of cell migration on a projected image of the well; digitizing tablets speed up porous filters and are commercially available.[19] Since other factors such as C5a des-arg, LTB4 and fMLP are also neutrophil chemoattractants, an antibody specific to IL-8 is strongly recommended to confirm the specificity of the system. No inhibitors of IL-8 have been reported. The protocol of IL-8 bioassay is as follows. Take 20 ml of freshly drawn venous blood and mix with 5 ml of 6% (w/v) dextran 70 in normal saline and 50 µl heparin (5000 U/ml). Leave the mixture to stand for 60 min at room temperature. Remove the upper leukocyte-rich layer and centrifuge at 200 g for 10 min. Resuspend the cell pellet in 10 ml 0.2% NaCl for 30 seconds, then quickly add 10 ml 1.6% NaCl. Filter through a lens tissue to remove cell debris, and centrifuge at 200 g for 10 min. Resuspend the pellet in 20 ml CM and centrifuge at 200 g for 10 min. Finally, resuspend the cell pellet to a concentration of 2×10^8 cells/ml in CM. Dissolve agarose 0.8% (w/v) in distilled water by gentle heating. Mix this agarose solution with an equal volume of warm 2× concentrated CM. To the diluted agarose/CM solution, add an equal volume of the cell suspension and mix thoroughly. Make sure the agarose/CM mixture is cool enough to ensure cell survival before pipetting 2 µl (containing 4×10^5 cells) into each well of cooled 96-well microtiter plates, sitting on ice. Allow agarose droplets to solidify and add appropriate dilutions of an IL-8 standard in 100 µl and as a negative control, include wells containing 100 µl of CM. Incubate the plates for 2 hours and determine the radial distance travelled by the cells from the agarose droplet for each sample by reading the plate, using a projecting microscope.

Classically, these factors are assayed by their ability to stimulate the formation of colonies of differentiated cells from bone marrow progenitor cells in soft agar. The type of colony produced depends upon the factor. IL-3 and GM-CSF stimulate the production of mixed colonies of different cell types. G-CSF, M-CSF and erythropoietin are lineage-restricted and produce granulocyte, monocyte and erythroid colonies, respectively. Human IL-3 and CSFs are fully active on murine cells. Colonies of more than 50 cells are counted and analysed after 7-14 days by eye using a binocular microscope.[20] The number of colonies usually relates to the specific activity or concentration of CSFs. Morphological analysis by staining dried and fixed gels allows proper identification of the colony type.[22] Alternative assays for CSFs measure the proliferative effect of these factors on cell lines derived from human leukaemia such as AML-193, TALL-101, MO-7E and TF-1 and murine lines such as NFS-60, WEHI 3BD+ and 32DC1.[21,22] Since none of these cell lines is specific for a given CSF, an antibody specific to each CSF is strongly recommended to confirm the specificity of the system. The protocol for IL-3, M-CSF, G-CSF and GM-CSF is as follows. Take the TF-1 cells 2-3 days after feeding and wash them three times in CM by centrifuging the cells at 200 g for 10 min. Assess the viability of the cells by trypan blue exclusion assay and resuspend the cells to a final concentration of 1×10^5 cells/ml in CM. Distribute titration of an appropriate standard (G-CSF, M-CSF or GM-CSF), in triplicate, in 96-well microtitration plates with 100 μl. Start the titration of the standard at 10 000 U/ml cytokine and make serial 10-fold dilutions down to 0.1 U/ml cytokine. Make appropriate dilutions of the samples to be measured for cytokine activity at 10-fold serial dilutions, in triplicate. The negative control is CM alone. The final volume of each well is 100 μl. Add 100 μl of the washed cell suspension to each well and incubate the plates for 48 hours at 37 °C in a humidified 5% CO_2 incubator. Add 0.5 μCi of tritiated thymidine to each well and return the plates to the incubator for another 4 hours. Harvest the contents of each well onto filter mats, using a cell harvester, and determine the radioactivity by liquid scintillation counting. Plot a standard curve of cpm versus cytokine concentration.

Immunoassays for cytokines

The lack of absolute specificity of cultured mammalian cells for the activities of individual cytokines and the often relatively poor reproducibility of cytokine bioassays have created the need for more specific and reproducible assays. This need has largely been filled by the development of immunoassays for cytokines. Such immunoassays are based on antibodies to each different cytokine, and are generally reasonably sensitive, reliable, rapid and easy to perform. Immunoassays for most cytokines have been published and many are now commercially available.

Three types of immunoassay have been developed: *radioimmunoassay (RIA), immunoradiometric assay (IRMA),* and *enzyme-linked immunoabsorbent assay (ELISA)*. All three require monoclonal or polyclonal antibodies. In general, most commercial cytokine immunoassays are either two-site ELISAs or IRMA and RIA with sensitivities of tens to several hundred pg/ml. The sensitivity of these assays largely depends on the specificity and affinities of cytokine antibodies. Careful selection of antibodies based on knowledge of the behaviour of particular cytokines should prevent the problem.

RIA requires the cytokine to be qualified as a pure, homogenous protein which can be radiolabelled to a high specific activity without untoward structural alterations. There are several ways in which cytokines may be radiolabelled with ^{125}I, but the choice of method largely depends on the robustness of the cytokine to the iodination conditions. For example, chloramine T will undoubtedly radiolabel cytokines to very high specific activities, but it is too denaturing and leads to loss of biological activity of cytokines. Other methods therefore are to be preferred including the iodogen (Sigma), Enzymobead (Bio-Rad) and Bolton-Hunter (Amersham) methods. The suitability of these for individual cytokines should be determined empirically. In general, most current radioimmunoassays for cytokines employ a competitive inhibition assay method. Briefly, this means that variable amounts of cytokine, as serial dilutions of a standard or samples, are incubated with a fixed amount of diluted polyclonal anti-cytokine antiserum, followed by a further incubation period with a fixed quantity of ^{125}I-labelled cytokine. Finally, antibody-cytokine complexes are removed from solution by the addition of a second antibody or other antibody-binding reagent (e.g. protein A). The amount of ^{125}I-cytokine bound therefore decreases as the concentration of unlabelled cytokine increases.[23,24]

The protocol for cytokine RIA is as follows. Coat an Eppendorf tube with 40 µl iodogen (1,3,4,6,-tetrachloro-3a, 6a-diphenyl-glycouril) at 1 mg/ml in trichloromethane by solvent evaporation. Add cytokines (IL-1β, IL-2, IL-3, IL-4, IL-5, IL-6, IL-8, IL-10, IL-12, TNF–α, TGF–β1, etc.), 5-10 µg in 30 µl of 0.25 M sodium phosphate buffer, pH 6.9, together with 10 µl (1 µCi) carrier-free [I^{125}]Na, to the iodogen-coated tube. Keep on ice for 10 min. Transfer the contents of the tube to a disposable 2 ml Sephadex G-25 column, previously equilibrated with bovine serum albumin (BSA; 2 mg/ml) in PBS. Wash the tube once with 40-50 µl PBS and add this to the Sephadex column. Elute the column with BSA-PBS and collect 10-20 200 µl fractions. Count these in a gamma-counter and determine the peak of radioactivity. Store radiolabelled [^{125}I]-cytokine at 4°C. It will be usable for up to 30 days. Add serial dilutions of cytokine standard (25 pg/ml to 25 ng/ml) or samples in 100 µl of assay diluent (BSA-PBS) to polystyrene tubes containing diluted rabbit polyclonal anti-cytokine (in 300 µl assay diluent/tube) and incubate for 24-48 hours at 4°C. The dilution of the rabbit polyclonal antibody giving maximum cpm of bound ^{125}I-cytokine (Bo) in the absence of unlabelled cytokine should be predetermined. Add ^{125}I-cytokine tracer (100 µCi/mg) in 100 µl assay diluent and incubate for a further 20 hours at 4°C. Separate free and bound cytokine by adding 1.5% sheep anti-rabbit IgG (0.5-1.0 ml) in 4% polyethylene glycol (16-20 kD). Mix and incubate for 1 hour at room temperature, then centrifuge at 1000 g for 30 min. Count the radioactivity (B) of the pellets in the assay tubes and express the results as a percentage of Bo (B/Bo × 100). Plot a standard curve of B/Bo × 100 versus cytokine concentration.

IRMA requires purified antibodies, but not pure cytokines. The concentration of cytokine in a sample is determined by the amount of ^{125}I-anti-cytokine IgG bound to cytokine that has been captured by a first, immobilized, anti-cytokine antibody. For optimal performance, it is necessary to use two cytokine-specific antibodies, each of which recognizes a different epitope or antigenic determinant on the cytokine molecule, particularly when the cytokine is monomeric. Steric separation of the epitopes recognized is essential for the development of highly sensitive assays. Ideally, the use of two complementary anti-cytokine monoclonal antibodies is the most effective combination for IRMAs, although polyclonal anti-cytokine IgG can also be effective.[25,26] The protocol for cytokine IRMA is as follows. Dilute purified capture monoclonal antibodies to the measured cytokines (IL-1β, IL-2, IL-3, IL-4, IL-5, IL-6, IL-8, IL-10, IL-12, TNF–α, TGF–β1, etc) to 200-400 µg/ml in PBS. Add 100 or so etched polystyrene balls (6.5 mm diameter; Northumbria Biologicals) to 14 ml of diluted antibody in a glass universal tube. Submerge the beads in the antibody solution overnight at 4°C, then aspirate the antibody solution and wash 4-5 times with 0.1% BSA-PBS. The beads may be stored under 0.1% BSA-PBS at 4°C for several weeks. Simultaneously fill a 100 or more Luckham LP4 tubes with 0.5% BSA-PBS to block any binding to plastic surfaces, and leave overnight at 4°C. Remove tube contents by aspiration just prior to setting up the assay. Prepare serial dilutions of cytokine standard, covering the range 2.5 pg/ml to 25 ng/ml in the assay diluent. The latter should be identical, if possible, to the medium of the samples to be tested. Add 200 µl of cytokine standard dilutions or samples to LP4 tubes. Blot the washed antibody-coated beads on paper towels until dry and add one bead per assay tube. The bead should be completely submerged and there should no bubbles. Incubate the assay tubes overnight at 4°C. On the following day, remove standard dilutions and samples by aspiration, and wash the beads extensively with 0.1% BSA-PBS or water before addition of 200 µl of [^{125}I]-anti-cytokine second antibody to the measured cytokines, diluted in 01% BSA-PBS at 10^6 cpm/ml, to all tubes. Leave the assay tubes for a further 4 hours at 4°C. Remove the unbound [^{125}I]-anti-cytokine second antibody by aspiration and wash the beads extensively with 0.1% BSA-PBS. Count the tubes containing beads in a gamma radiation counter. Plot a standard curve of cpm bound (minus negative control) versus cytokine concentration.

The major principles governing *ELISA* are the same as those for IRMA, except that the second anti-cytokine IgG is: (a) conjugated to an enzyme; (b) a third antibody-enzyme complex or variable combinations of biotinylated antibodies and streptavidin-enzyme complexes.[27,28] We have developed a protocol to measure human and murine cytokines in either body fluids (e.g. serum and intestinal fluid) or cell culture supernatant.[29-31] Briefly, the wells of 96-well microtiter plates are coated overnight at 4°C with 50 ml of mouse anti-human cytokine monoclonal antibody specific for the measured cytokines (IL-1β, IL-2, IL-3, IL-4, IL-5, IL-6, IL-8, IL-10, IL-12, TNF–α, TGF–β1, etc), diluted to 1-4 µg/ml in 0.05 M bicarbonate buffer (pH 9.6). Plates are washed once with PBS (0.01 M, pH 7.2-7.4) containing 0.05% (v/v) Tween-20 (PBST). Then 100 μl of standard or sample cytokines diluted in culture medium are added. Plates are incubated for 2 hours and washed three times. 50 μl of diluted goat anti-human cytokine polyclonal antibodies in PBS (1-4 μg/ml) is added into each well. Plates are incubated as above for 1.5 hours and washed four times with PBST. Then 50 μl of donkey anti-goat IgG-HRP (1:10 000) is added to each well. Plates are incubated as above for 1 hour, and washed five times with PBST and once with PBS. Finally, 100 μl of substrate buffer (ABTS in 0.1 M citrate buffer, pH 4.2 containing 0.03% (v/v) H_2O_2) is added to each well, and the colour is allowed to develop for 20-30 min at room temperature. Optical density is determined at 405 nm by a microwell ELISA reader and a standard curve of absorbance is plotted versus cytokine concentration.

Application to animal studies

This chapter has focused on experimental techniques used to detect cytokines in human systems and murine system. While the tissue dissection may differ between human and animal systems, the techniques for detection of cytokines can generally be applied to both.

Results and discussion

For analysis of assays by the *parallel line* approach, the unknown samples are titrated and then compared to the standard curve of known units. The parallel portions of these curves are then used to measure the displacement from the standard which is proportional to the biologically active cytokine content of the samples. These curves should be parallel if the molecule responsible for the activity in samples/ standards is the same.

One major advantage of bioassays is their sensitivity. Most can detect cytokines as low as 100 fg/ml. The detection of 1-20 pg cytokine/ml is achievable by bioassay. The results of bioassays directly reflect the biological activity of cytokines in the samples. The major disadvantages of bioassays are their poor reproducibility and specificity, as well as being time consuming and expensive. Specific neutralizing antibodies are often required to determine the

specificity of a bioassay and the cost will be substantial in a large-scale study. Furthermore, bioassays are not as reliable as most people think as the outcome of bioassays can be affected by a variety of factors such as cytokine inhibitors, binders or receptors, active proteins or lipids and hormones. Individual laboratory quality control and well-trained technical staff are key to consistent results. Large inter-coefficient and intra-coefficient variation often make the results obtained on different days incompatible.

For all types of immunoassays, correct calibration is vital. The standard used for calibration should contain the cytokine to be quantified in a known or predicted molecular form(s), which will be representative of the cytokine molecules present in samples. The diluent or matrix for immunoassays should be identical for the cytokine standard and for samples. Recognition of cytokines is often influenced by other molecules in the microenviroment (e.g. proteins and lipids).

Immunoassays for most cytokines have been published and many are commercially available (e.g. from R&D Systems, Genzyme, Endogen, Biosources International, Amgen, Amersham, Promaga and Sigma). In general, most cytokine immunoassays are either two-site ELISAs or radioimmunoassays and can detect cytokine levels down to 10-200 pg/ml. They are reliable, rapid, specific and reproducible. However, immunoassays may detect denatured biologically inactive cytokine molecules or fragments.

Immunoassays need to be very carefully validated to eliminate non-specific artifacts, particularly if they are used for assaying clinical samples. In some cases, the sensitivity of an immunoassay may also limit its application.

The choice of assay system depends on the type of sample studied. We recommend the following rules for the use of cytokine assays. Bioassays are applied for detecting cytokines in culture samples, as components in the culture medium are relatively well defined. Usually few interfering factors exist in the supernatant of the cell culture. To ensure the specificity of the bioassay, use specific neutralizing antibodies to measure cytokines. Immunoassays are applied for detecting cytokines in body fluids (e.g. serum and intestinal fluid), as components in body fluids cannot be well defined. If there is sufficient cytokine in the supernatant of cell culture, immunoassays can be applied. If possible, the optimal metthod for quantifying cytokine concentrations is to use a bioassay in combination with an immunoassay. Correlation of results between two systems should confirm the data obtained.

References

1. Kagnoff MF. Immunology of the intestinal tract. *Gastroenterology* 1993; **105:** 1275.

2. Beagley KW, Elson CO. Cells and cytokines in mucosal immunity and inflammation. *Gastoenterol Clinics N Am* 1992; **21:** 347.

3. Mosmann TR. Rapid calorimetric assay for cellular growth and survival: application to proliferation and cytotoxicity. *J Immunol Methods* 1983; **65:** 55.

4. Symmons TA, Diclcens EM, Di Giovine F *et al.* In: Clements MJ, Morris AG, Geraing AJH (Eds) *Lymphokins and Interferons: A Practical Approach*. IRL Press, Oxford, 1987, pp. 269.

5. Gearing AJH, Bird CR, Bristow A *et al.* A simple sensitive bioassay for interleukin-1 which is unresponsive to 10^3 U/ml of interleukin-2. *J Immunol Methods* 1987; **99:** 7.

6. Gery I, Gershon RK, Waksmann BH. Potentiation of the T-lymphocyte response to mitogens. I. The responding cells. *J Exp Med* 1972; **136:** 128.

7. Gillis S, Ferm MM, Ou W *et al.* T cell growth factor: parameters of production and a quantitative microassay for activity. *J Immunol* 1978; **120:** 2027.

8. Gascan H, Moreau JF, Jaques Y. Response of murine IL-3-sensitive cell lines to cytokines of human and murine origin. *Lymphokine Res* 1989; **8:** 79.

9. Callard RE, Shields JG, Smith SH. In: Clements MJ, Morris AG, Geraing AJH (Eds) *Lymphokins and Interferons: A Practical Approach*. IRL Press, Oxford, 1987, pp. 354.

10. O'Garra A, Sanderson CJ. In: Clements MJ, Morris AG, Geraing AJH (Eds) *Lymphokins and Interferons: A Practical Approach*. IRL Press, Oxford, 1987, pp. 323.

11. Helle M, Boeje L, Aarden LA. Functional discrimination between interleukin 6 and interleukin 1. *Eur J Immunol* 1988; **18:** 1535.

12. Park LS, Friend DJ, Schmierer AE *et al.* Murine interleukin 7 (IL-7) receptor: Characterization on an IL-7-dependent cell line. *J Exp Med* 1990; **171:** 1073.

13. Namen AE, Schmierer AE, Marh CJ *et al.* B cell precursor growth-promoting activity. Purification and characterization of a growth factor active on lympho-cyte precursors. *J Exp Med* 1988; **167:** 988.

14. Renauld J, Goethals A, Houssiau F *et al.* Cloning and expression of a cDNA for the human homolog of mouse T cell and mast cell growth factor p40. *Cytokine* 1990; **2:** 9.

15. Like B, Massague J. The antiproliferative effect of type beta transforming growth factor occurs at a level distal from receptors for growth-activating factors. *J Biol Chem* 1986; **261:** 13426.

16. Merger A, Leung H, Wooley J. Assays for tumor necrosis factor and related cytokines. *J Immunol Methods* 1989; **116:** 1.

17. Merger A. In: Clements MJ, Morris AG, Geraing AJH (Eds) *Lymphokins and Interferons: A Practical Approach*. IRL Press, Oxford, 1987, pp. 129.

18. Gibson UEM, Kramer SM. Enzyme-linked bio-immunoassay for IFN-gamma by HLA-DR induction. *J Immunol Methods* 1989; **125:** 105.

19. Binnold LP. Measurement of chemotaxis of polymor-phonuclear leukocytes *in vitro*. The problems of the control of gradients of chemotactic factors, of the control of cells and of the separation of chemotaxis from chemokinesis. *J Immunol Methods* 1988; **108:** 1.

20. Metclaf D. *The Hemopoietic Colony Stimulating Factors*. Elsevier, Amsterdam, 1984, pp. 1.

21. Morgan C, Pollard JW, Stanley ER. Isolation and characterization of a cloned growth factor dependent macrophage cell line, BAC1.2F5. *J Cell Physiol* 1987; **130:** 420.

22. Nakoinz I, Lee M, Weaver JF *et al.* In: *7th International Congress of Immunology*. Ges. Fur Immunologie, Gustav Fischer, Stuttgart, 1989, Abstr 40-23.

23. Reay P. Use of N-bromosuccinimide for the iodination of proteins for radioimmunoassay. *Ann Clin Biochem* 1982; **19:** 129.

24. Poole S, Bristow AF, Selkirk S. Development and application of radioimmunoassays for interleukin-1 alpha and interleukin-1 beta. *J Immunol Methods* 1989; **116:** 259.

25. Merger A. In: Clements MJ, Morris AG, Geraing AJH (Eds) *Lymphokins and Interferons: A Practical Approach*. IRL Press, Oxford, 1987, pp. 105.

26. Ey PL, Prowse SJ, Jenkin CR. Isolation of pure IgG1, IgG2a and IgG2b immunoglobulins from mouse serum using protein A-sepharose. *Immunochemistry* 1978; **15:** 429.

27. Kemeny DM, Challacombe SJ (Eds) *ELISA and Other Solid Phase Immunoassays*. Wiley, Chichester, 1989, pp. 1.

28. Wang JY, Wicklund BH, Gustilo RB *et al.* Titanium, chromium and cobalt modulate osteotropic cytokine release by human monocytes/macrophages *in vitro*. *Biomaterials* 1996, **17:** 2233.

29. Wang JY, Tsukayama DT, Wicklund BH *et al.* Titanium, chromium and cobalt inhibit immuno-regulatory cytokine release by human peripheral blood mononuclear cells. *J Biomed Mater Res* 1996, **32:** 655.

30. Watson RR, Wang JY, Deghanpisheh K *et al*. T cell receptor Vβ complementarily-determining region 1 peptide moderates immune dysfunctions and cytokine dysregulation induced by murine retrovirus infection. *J Immunol* 1995; **155**: 2282.

31. Wang Y, Ardestani SK, Liang B *et al*. Administration of interferon-γ and monoclonal anti-interleukin-4 retards development of immune dysfunction and cytokine dysregulation during murine AIDS. *Immunology* 1994; **83**: 384.

9

Ion transport in the gastrointestinal tract

David I Soybel

Summary

A primary function of the alimentary tract is the intake and excretion of water and electrolytes. This chapter summarises current *in vivo* techniques used for investigating transepithelial potential differences (P.D.) and fluxes of electrolytes, H^+ and HCO_3^- ions across mucosal surfaces in different regions of the gastrointestinal tract in human subjects. It is important to note that such measurements can only be interpreted in the context of previously performed *in vitro* studies. Measurement of P.D. and disappearance/appearance rates of various ions can be understood only if the underlying transport mechanisms are identified, if the actions of hormones or other neuroendocrine influences have been characterised, and if the specificities of different transport inhibiting agents have been established.

Introduction

A primary function of the alimentary tract is the intake and excretion of water and electrolytes. The goals of this chapter are: 1) to provide a brief overview of fundamental properties that describe ion and water transport in epithelial cells of the alimentary tract and the different types of epithelial ion transport processes; 2) to discuss the relationship of these transport properties to electrical properties of mucosal surfaces, thereby leading to a discussion of *in vivo* electrophysiological measurements in the alimentary tract; 3) to discuss techniques for intubation of different regions of the alimentary tract and sampling of luminal contents to measure transepithelial movements of monovalent ions such as Na^+ and Cl^-; and 4) to discuss techniques for measuring H^+ and HCO_3^- secretion and disappearance *in vivo*, and limitations resulting from the need to measure pCO_2. The discussion will be limited to those techniques that are feasible for *in vivo* measurement in human subjects.

Theory

Fundamental concepts of ion and water transport

Flux Current, Permeability, Conductance, and Resistance

The first fundamental concept is that of ion flux.[1-3] This term describes the magnitude of the movement of a given number of particles (unchanged solutes or charged ions) across a flat membrane per unit area per unit time. It is a general term and does not imply whether the movement of the ion occurs via cellular pathways (i.e. across the apical and then basolateral cell membranes) or via the paracellular pathways, through intercellular junctions and spaces. The flux term does not imply anything about the forces that cause ions to move across the mucosa.

When particles carry charges (ions) from one side of the membrane to the other, the movement of charge is a "flux" and is, in some sense, an electrical current. Permeability reflects the properties of the membrane in its interaction with movements of a specified ion. Conductance (G_i), is the inverse of resistance (R_i), and reflects both the intrinsic permeability of the membrane to the ion and the free concentration gradient of the ion across the membrane.

Pores (Channels), Carriers, and Pumps.[1-4]

From purely functional studies, three classes of membrane transport processes have been recognised (Fig. 9.1): channels, carriers, and pumps.[1,2] It is important to distinguish transport mechanisms that generate electrical charge and those which do not. Channels are distinguished by their dependence on transmembrane ion concentration gradients and behaviour as electrical conductances. Pumps are distinguished by the requirement for ATP hydrolysis for maximal activity and frequently by transport of ions against transmembrane concentration gradients. Carriers are characterised by dependence on transmembrane ion concentration gradients, by the absence of characteristics of electrical conductance, and by the absence of a requirement for ATP hydrolysis.

Equilibrium

A third fundamental concept is that of equilibrium. For this discussion equilibrium may be defined as a set of conditions under which there is no greater tendency for ions to move in one direction or the other across the cell membrane. For example, consider a simple cell membrane which accumulates K^+ ions and extrudes Na^+ by the well-recognised Na^+/K^+ ATPase. The membrane contains selective channels which permit K^+ to exit the cell, down its concentration gradient. The movement of these positively charged ions leaves the inside of the cell negatively charged. If the transmembrane potential (V_m) were to be measured at a sufficiently negative value (approx. -80mV), then the electrical potential difference would balance the tendency for K^+ to exit

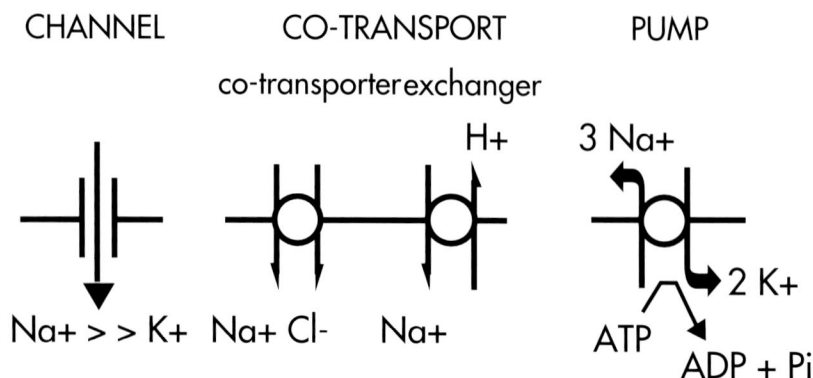

Figure 9.1 – Different classes of membrane ion transport processes.

the cell, and there would be no net transfer of K[+] across the membrane. The system would be at *electrochemical equilibrium* with respect to K[+]. A similar analysis can be used to describe equilibrium of passive diffusion of ions across an epithelial surface as a whole.[1-3]

In a second example, we consider the well recognised Na[+]/K[+] antiporter. Two questions are: 1) how to predict the directions in which Na[+] and H[+] have to move, if they are coupled; and 2) how to predict the conditions under which the tendency for Na[+] to cross the membrane be balanced by the tendency of H[+] to cross in the same direction. Such conditions would define the equilibrium state. To answer these latter questions, the easiest approach is to recall that any chemical reaction gives up or uses energy. If the concentration of [Na[+]] is less inside the cell than outside (10 mM vs. 100 mM) and [H[+]] is the same on the outside as on the inside (i.e. pH_i = pH_0 7.4), then Na[+] will enter and H[+] will exit the cell spontaneously. When the ratio of intracellular to extracellular Na[+] is equal to the ratio of intracellular to extracellular H[+], then the reaction cannot go forward or reverse spontaneously. This defines equilibrium when the exchanger will not produce net flux of either ion, into or out of the cell. These examples illustrate how simple ion fluxes may depend on concentration gradients, on potential differences, and on the presence of transport processes linked to other ionic species. The point is that measurements of P.D. and flux cannot be interpreted accurately without understanding how basic forces such as potential difference and concentration gradient influence the flux of ions across a membrane.

In vivo methods

Electrophysiological measurements

Measurements of transepithelial potential have been used for almost thirty years as an index of mucosal integrity.[2,5,6] In conjunction with manipulations of intraluminal conditions or exposure to bioactive substances in the lumen, such measurements have proven useful in exploring hypotheses about mechanisms of ion transport. In the *in vivo* setting, measurements of transepithelial potential difference are of limited usefulness for the following reasons: First, transepithelial recordings treat the mucosa as a flat sheet and homogeneous collection of epithelial cells, when in fact, the mucosa may have many glandular structures and is composed of several cell types. It is a constant concern that experimental manipulations alter the surface area, thus altering apparent transport rates without really affecting cell function. Also, manipulations of luminal conditions may influence transport activity in only a subset of mucosal cells, but transepithelial P.D. measurements will not separate effects on the cells of interest from others in the mucosa. In addition, it is necessary, and difficult, to prove that transport of one ion is independent of others. A third consideration is that when probes such as amiloride are used to define mechanisms of membrane transport, their specific mode of action should be carefully defined. For example, at relatively low concentrations (<5x 10[-4] M), the investigational drug amiloride (Sigma Chemical, St. Louis, MO) and its analogues are specific blockers of epithelial Na[+] channels. At higher doses (1 mM) the drug also inhibits Na[+]/K[+] transport in a variety of tissues.[6]

Further, it may not always be true that a drug present in the luminal solution acts only on one transport process located in the luminal cell membrane. Finally, without additional measurements of transepithelial resistance and short-circuit current, it is often impossible to know whether a change in P.D. is due to changes in tissue resistance, changes in permeability of cellular or paracellular pathways, or true changes in active or facilitated transport.[1,2] For all these reasons, interpretation of transepithelial P.D. measurements is difficult and it must be used, cautiously, as an overall parameter that assesses mucosal integrity and function.

In the stomach and intestines, measurement of transepithelial P.D. requires two electrodes. Premeasurement conditions must be established and strictly followed (npo after midnight, suction and sampling of gastric contents, etc.). A reference electrode consists of 0.9N normal saline (0. 15 M NaCl) in a 18 gauge, standard intravenous catheter, the tip of which is inserted under the skin of the forearm and the hub of which is connected, via calomel half-cell, to an electrometer instrument and recording instrument. A single lumen 16 Fr polyvinyl (LeVeen) tube, acting as recording electrode, and a 16 Fr (Salem) sump tube are positioned next to each other in the gastric lumen, with the tip of the tube placed proximal to the aspiration ports of the sump.

For many years, the recording electrode contained various salts dissolved in agar gel and was connected by means of calomel half cells to the recording device.[7] Read and Fordtran[8] described the use of a "flowing junction" electrode, which consists of isotonic saline or molar KCl flowing through the tip of the tube at a slow rate (0.005 ml/min for KCl, 0.05 ml/min for NaCl), but fast enough to prevent separations of charge that can arise at the junction of the agar and luminal solution (Fig. 9.2). The flowing junction is not available commercially, but easy to construct.[9] The magnitude of such junction potentials depends on gastric acidity and the "flowing junction" does not completely eliminate interference by junction potentials. Nevertheless, it is possible to take these into account, in order to obtain an accurate estimate of the true transepithelial P.D.[8]

As an example of the way in which meaningful measurements can be obtained, despite the uncertainties and difficulties in interpretation, Orlando and colleagues[10] reported the measurement of colonic and esophageal P.D. in control individuals and patients with cystic fibrosis (CF). Infusion of amiloride, a known inhibitor of Na^+ channels at the concentration of 10^{-4} M, into the lumen resulted in a greater magnitude of colonic mucosal depolarisation in CF patients, but no alterations in oesophageal mucosa. Because previous studies had shown that colonic P.D. depends substantially on electrogenic Cl^- secretion, and esophageal mucosal P.D. is not so dependent, these findings were consistent with the loss of a voltage-generating pathway for Cl^- in CF. This example illustrates the importance of obtaining extensive information from complementary *in vitro* studies, before attempting to obtain meaningful measurements of transepithelial P.D. in the *in vivo* setting.

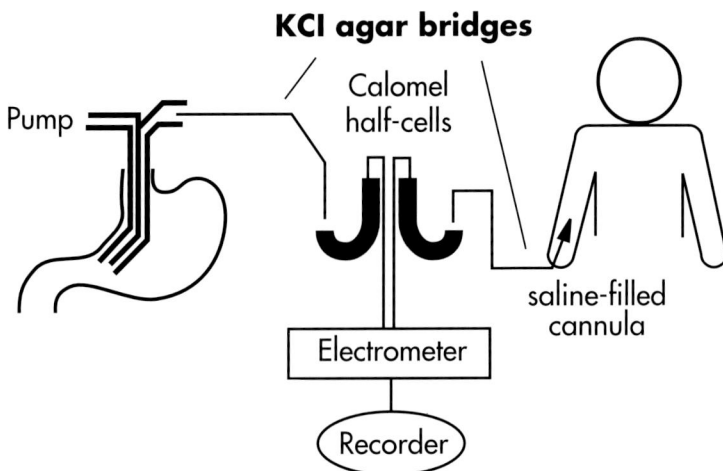

KCl agar bridges

Pump

Calomel
half-cells

saline-filled
cannula

Electrometer

Recorder

Figure 9.2 – Configuration of gastric P.D. measurements. A flowing intragastric electrode is connected, via a KCl bridge, to a calomel half cell. The reference electrode is placed subcutaneously and is filled with isotonic saline. (After Read NW, Fordtran JS. *Gastroenterology* 1979; **76**: 933.)

Gastrointestinal intubation and measurements of ion fluxes

The ability to perform P.D. measurements in other regions of the gastrointestinal tract has depended on access through intubation or access to exteriorized segments after surgical procedures such as ileostomy or colostomy. To measure gastric fluid secretion, a relatively simple sump tube (18 Fr) apparatus can be used if the pylorus is competent. If the pylorus has been resected or is not competent, a distal occluding balloon (Davol/Bard, Cranston, RI, USA) may be utilised to prevent contamination of gastric luminal contents by refluxing duodenal or intestinal fluid. In addition, investigators have reported the feasibility of passing long tubes (Davol/Bard, Cranston, RI, USA) transorally or transanally, in order to reach otherwise inaccessible regions such as the jejunum, ileum and proximal colon.[10] Fluoroscopy is used to verify the position of the tube. In addition, for measurements of colonic mucosal properties, a twenty four hour mechanical cleansing is required, a manoeuvre that can alter colonic flora and, potentially, other transport properties. For this, a standard preparation such as two bottles of commercially available 10% magnesium citrate solutions or polyethylene glycol 3350 (NuLytely balanced salt preparation, Braintree Laboratories, Inc., Braintree, Mass., USA).

To measure intestinal ion flux *in vivo*, a double or triple-lumen perfusion apparatus is used.[10-12] Sometimes a proximal occluding balloon is used to prevent contamination from more proximal luminal contents. The triple lumen apparatus utilises three ports, each opening to the gut lumen at different sites along the length of the tube. The more proximal port infuses the lumen with a "test" solution while the two distal ports are used to sample the contents of the lumen downstream. The test solution is iso-osmotic with respect to the plasma and usually contains plasma-like concentrations of Na^+, K^+, Cl^-, HCO_3^- and a known concentration (2 g/L) of a non-transportable, high molecular weight marker such as polyethylene glycol (PEG, mean 3350 molecular weight). To assure the integrity of the results, it is important, first and foremost, to establish a steady state of perfusion of the test solution. This requires about forty to sixty minutes of perfusion of the gut segment, utilising stable flow rates of 10-15 ml/min. An additional detail, emphasised by a number of investigators, is that sampling from the middle and distal ports should be staggered, so that the aspiration of the middle port begins 10 to 15 minutes

before aspiration at the distal port. The rate of aspiration at the distal ports should be small relative to the rate of perfusion (1 to 1.5 ml/min at each site). Collections are performed at regular intervals over periods of one hour or more, under control conditions and during any investigation manoeuvre.

Measurements of electrolytes concentrations in the aspirates are usually performed using commercially available automated analysers that are used in clinical chemistry laboratories. Analytic, radio-isotope or calorimetric methods may be used to assay PEG concentration.[12] The rate of ion movement, "delta S"(dS) is calculated from the following relationships

$$V2 = V1M1 / M2$$

$$V3 = V2M2 / M3$$

$$dH_2O = V2 - V3$$

$$dS = V2S2 - V3S3$$

where Vl is perfusion rate through Port 1, V2 is the flow rate at the middle port and V3 is the flow rate at the distal port. Ml, M2, and M3 are the concentrations of the marker at the proximal, middle and distal ports, respectively. Finally, S1 and S2 are the concentrations of the electrolyte or substrate of interest at the middle or distal ports, respectively.

Because access to and control of conditions in the lumen and the blood side is difficult, the technique of intubation and measurement of fluxes during controlled perfusion is a mainstay for evaluating ion transport across a mucosal surface under *in vivo* conditions. It is important to remember that changes in luminal concentrations of any ion can alter electrical, chemical or osmotic gradients that determine the rates of its movement across the epithelium. Changes in osmolality of the luminal perfusate can especially cause unappreciated changes in bulk flow of electrolytes and other solutes across an epithelium particularly in the highly permeable and electrically "leaky" mucosa of the small intestine.[1,2] In addition it must be remembered that electrolyte or solute transport rates reflect the surface area of the segment under study, not its length. Starvation, surgical resection and changes in the neurohumoral milieu can and do lead to atrophy or proliferation of the mucosa, thus altering the surface area of the intestinal segment. Any such changes in mucosal surface area must be anticipated and accounted for. Finally, it must be recalled that perfusion-based measurements can describe ion fluxes, i.e., rates of transport into or out of the lumen. They do not directly identify mechanisms or routes (cellular vs. paracellular) of transport. As discussed above in regard to P.D. measurements, inferences about mechanism require studies utilising conditions and transporter inhibitors which have undergone detailed characterisation in the *in vitro* setting.

Measurements of H^+ and HCO_3^- flux

Special problems are encountered in the determination of H^+ and HCO_3^- fluxes. Gastrointestinal intubation and aspiration techniques are utilised for measurement of H^+ and HCO_3^- movements and are most relevant in the stomach and duodenum. For such studies, H^+ concentrations are assessed by measurements of pH of the luminal contents, converting $[H^+]$ from the relationship $[H^+] = 10^{7pH \, (lumen)}$. It must be remembered that, unless distally occluding balloons are used and the aspiration tube is correctly positioned, 5 to 10% of gastric contents will escape at the duodenum.[13] Concentrations measured in gastric contents are in the millimolar range, but are less than 1 micromolar in the intestine and colon. In addition, the presence of organic buffers (especially bile salts, mucus, or food) directly affects the change in pH that is caused by movement of a given amount of H^+ into or out of the lumen. Moreover, pH measurements are directly influenced by ambient levels of CO_2 and HCO_3^- through the Henderson-Hasselbach relationship:

$$pH = pK - \log_{10} \{[HCO_3^- / (0.03 \times pCO_2)]\}.$$

More accurate, but more cumbersome, methodologies utilise a strategy of intragastric titration of luminal contents.[13-15] In this setting, a homogenised meal or indicator dye is infused into the stomach and its pH measured at regular intervals. By titrating the pH to a standard level with 0. 1 N NaOH the quantity of H^+ released to the lumen can be measured. The intragastric titration technique is, theoretically, more rigorous. However, it is also subject to more variability, due to difficulties in controlling the buffering capacity of the infused meal or dye.

These considerations have an even greater impact on measurement of luminal bicarbonate concentrations $[HCO_3^-]$, which cannot be measured directly. In one technique, measurements of HCO_3^- concentration in gastric aspirates are obtained from measurements of pH and estimates or direct measurements of ambient CO_2.[16]

It is also possible to measure luminal HCO_3^- secretion by performing intragastric titrations.[17] This method is also a more rigorous approach pen-permitting measurements of steady-state secretion of HCO_3^-, even when acid is present. A theoretical, two-compartment model of gastric secretion is used to analyse contributions of H^+ and HCO_3^- secretions to luminal pH levels and C)_2 accumulation / partial pressure. When CO_2 levels are physiologic (40 mmHg) a change in pH of 0.3 units reflects a doubling or halving of HCO_3^-. For both methods, it is very important to standardise conditions of aspiration and transport of samples, to minimise the presence of any contaminating organic matter in the aspirate, and to account for pCO_2 levels in luminal aspirates.

Applications in animal studies

With the qualifications noted above, the techniques described above are highly suitable for use in experimental animals. One variation of the intubation/perfusion technique, not feasible in humans for safety reasons, is the use of double isotopes to evaluate mucosal ion transport. In this variation, two radioisotopes of the same ionic species are used (e.g. ^{45}Ca and ^{47}Ca). Amounts of one isotope – given orally or via intubation – and the other – given intravenously – can be recovered and measured in the stool, in relationship to recovery of a non-transported marker. Changes in the amount of intravenously administered isotope would thus reflect secretion while changes in the amount of the orally administered isotope would reflect a net of absorption and secretion.[12]

Results and discussion

The techniques described above are relatively simple to perform and feasible for outpatients as well as inpatients. The fundamental measurements of transepithelial potential difference and rates of appearance/disappearance of different ionic species can provide an accurate picture of the overall balance of ion transport in the gut as a whole or in individual regions of the gut. Overall rates of H^+ and HCO_3^- secretion have been characterised in the stomach and duodenum under standardised conditions in healthy individuals and in patients with acid peptic disease or complications resulting from therapy for such diseases. In the intestines, it has been possible to evaluate fluid and electrolyte balance in healthy individual as well as patients with ion transport defects such as cystic fibrosis.

In this review, it has been emphasised that such measurements can only be interpreted in the context of previously performed *in vitro* studies. Care must be taken in establishing standardised conditions for making measurements of P.D. or luminal ion flux. The investigator must control for the potential influences of fasting, time of day, month or season. Along these lines, it should be emphasised that each laboratory should establish its own normative values in healthy individuals, under standardised conditions. The investigator must be aware of potential sources of inaccuracy in measurement, such as poor control of correlated variables (i.e. ambient CO_2 in the measurement of pH) or alterations in surface area of the mucosal surface. Above all, the measurement of P.D. and disappearance/appearance rates of various ions can be understood only if the underlying transport mechanisms are identified, if the actions of hormones or other neuroendocrine influences have been characterised, and if the specificities of different transport inhibiting agents have been established.

References

1. Schultz, SG Basic Principles of Membrane Transport. Cambridge: Cambridge University Press, 1980.

2. Soybel, DI. Applications of electrophysiologic techniques in studies of ion transport by gut mucosa. *J. Surg Res* 1994; **57**: 510.

3. Hille, B. Ionic Channels of Excitable Membranes. Sunderland, MA: Sinauer Assoc., Inc. 1984

4. Sachs, G, Chang, H H, Rabon E, Schackman R, Lewin, M and Sacchomani, G. A non electrogenic H+ pump in plasma membranes of Hog stomach. *J Biol Chem* 1976; **251**: 7690.

5. Davenport, HW, Wamer, HA, Code, CF. Functional significance of gastric mucosal barrier to sodium. *Gastroenterology* 1964; **47**: 142.

6. Soybel, D.I., Modlin, IM Overview of gastric mucosal injury and inflammation. In: *Gastritis*. Kozol, R-A. Boca Raton: CRC Press, 1992; p 1.

7. Benos, DJ. Amiloride: a molecular probe of sodium transport in tissues and cells. *Am J Physiol* 1982; **242**: C 13 1.

8. Read, NW, Fordtran, JS. The role of intraluminal junction potentials in the generation of the gastric potential difference in man. *Gastroenterology* 1979; **76**: 932.

9. Andersson S, Grossman MI. Profile of pH, pressure and potential difference at gastro-duodenal junction in man. *Gastroenterology* 1965; **49**: 364.

10. Orlando, RC, Powell, DW, Croom RD, Berschneider, HM Boucher, RC, Knowlees, RM Colonic and esophageal transepithelial potential difference in cystic fibrosis. *Gastroenterology* 1989; **96**: 1041.

11. Davis, GR, Santa Ana, CA, Morawski, SG, Fordtran, JS. Permeability characteristics of human jejunum, proximal colon and distal colon. *Gastroenterology* 1982; **83**: 844.

12. Cooper, R Levitan, R, Fordtran, JS, Ingelfinger, FJ. A method for studying absorption of water and solute from the human small intestine. *Gastroenterology* 1966; **50**: 1.

13. Acra, SA, Ghishan, FK. Methods of investigating intestinal transport. *J Parent Ent Nut* 1991; **15**: 93S.

14. Feldman, M. Comparison of acid secretion rates measured by gastric aspiration and by *in vivo* intra-gastric titration in healthy human subjects. *Gastroenterology* 1979; **76**: 954.

15. Fordtran, JS, Walsh, JH. Gastric acid secretion rate and buffer content of the stomach after eating. *J Clin Invest* 1973; **52**: 645.

16. Hogan, DL, Turken, D, Stern, AI, Isenberg, JI. Comparison of the serial dilution indicator and intra-gastric titration methods for measurement of meal-stimulated gastric acid secretion in man. *Dig Dis Sci* 1983; **28**: 1001.

17. Forsell, H., Stenquist, B., Olbe, L. Vagal stimulation of human gastric bicarbonate secretion. *Gastroenterology* 1985; **89**: 581.

10

Motility measurements

Sean P Devane

Summary

This chapter describes techniques for the investigation of gastrointestinal motor function at the levels of transit of luminal contents, of muscle actions responsible for this transit, of electrical activity underlying the control of and the effecting of these muscle actions, and of the endocrine and paracrine factors influencing these processes. The techniques include invasive and non-invasive methods, with the latter being particularly suitable for application to children and infants. All the techniques can be applied to animals, within constraints of size.

Introduction

The motility function of the gastrointestinal tract is the process responsible for the ordered movement of luminal contents from mouth to anus. It is crucially important for the proper functioning of the tract's various regions. Disturbances of this motility function account for the biggest sub-group of chronic ailments affecting the gastrointestinal tract in human beings. They result in vomiting, diarrhoea, constipation, abdominal pain, and the combination of these that is called 'irritable bowel syndrome'.

The ordered movement of luminal contents is effected by contractions of the gastrointestinal smooth muscle cells. These contractions are coordinated by the control mechanisms of the enteric nervous system and of the paracrine and endocrine milieu of the gastrointestinal tract wall. Measurement of the motility function of the gastrointestinal tract can be considered, therefore, under three headings. These are:-

1. *Transit measurement:*

The measurement of the actual movement of luminal contents through the tract.

2. *Luminal pressure recording:*

The recording of the effector system whose action and co-ordination leads to the transit of luminal contents.

3. *Control mechanisms assessment:*

Investigations of the processes (at the level of the smooth muscle cells, the enteric nervous system and the paracrine and endocrine environment of the gastrointestinal tract wall), that control the effector system, leading to movement of the luminal contents.

Tests of the anatomical integrity and anatomical position of the gastrointestinal tract are relevant to the assessment of the motility function, but are outside the scope of this chapter. For example, the position of the gastro-oesophageal junction relative to the diaphragm is important for the avoidance of gastro-oesophageal reflux, and can be assessed by a contrast X-ray study. Tests of the pathophysiological effects of motility abnormalities are useful clinically, but are also outside the scope of this chapter. For example, continuous intra-oesophageal pH monitoring provides a quantitative assessment of reflux of gastric acid into the oesophagus due to abnormal function of the gastro-oesophageal junction area.

Methods – transit measurement

The first studies of gastrointestinal motor activity were undertaken in the late 19th and early 20th century using fluoroscopic methods.[1] Contrast radiology, in the form of swallows, meals, follow through investigations and enemas, can still provide information about gut transit, and the fluoroscopic equipment needed is readily available in many hospitals. Major abnormalities of transit can be detected by delay in the passage of the contrast medium. However, these tests assess the transit of a non-physiological meal (contrast medium) and require radiation. As a result, alternative methods have been developed in an attempt to measure the passage of real or physiological foods.

Whole gut transit

Whole gut transit can be measured by the addition of a non-absorbable colouring to ingested food and watching for a change in colour in the stools. Carmine red is the traditional agent used. The dose for an adult human being is 3-4 g taken orally. The first appearance of the dye in the stools defines the transit time for the "head" of the meal (the first appearance of part of the meal), and usually occurs 24 – 48 hours after ingestion. Charcoal can be used as an alternative to carmine red.

Whole gut transit can be also be assessed by using radio-opaque markers,[2] but this method suffers from the disadvantage of requiring the use of radiation. 20-50 markers can be ingested mixed with food (e.g. with yoghurt), and their passage followed either by taking an abdominal X-ray, or alternatively by X-raying the stools (to avoid irradiation to the subject). The majority of the markers should have been expelled by 48 hours, so a single X-ray at this time is sufficient to detect slow transit. A convenient source of "home made" markers is radio-opaque tubing as used in cardiac catheterisation laboratories, which can be cut into 1-2 mm long fragments.

Mouth-to-caecum transit time

Mouth-to-caecum transit time can be measured by adding a non-absorbable carbohydrate (e.g. lactulose) to a test meal. The usual dose is 2 g/kg up to a maximum of 50 g. It can be mixed with water and taken as a drink, but the results obtained in this way are less reproducible than when it is mixed with a meal. The arrival of the "head" of the meal at the caecum is marked by the production of hydrogen by fermentation of lactulose by colonic bacteria resident there. Hydrogen diffuses readily through the blood stream and is exhaled within minutes of production. Breath hydrogen can be measured using an electro-chemical detector (e.g. Breath Hydrogen Monitor, GMI Ltd, Renfrew, Scotland). Breath samples can be collected using a Haldane-Priestley tube (a 2 metre long segment of garden hose will do) in co-operative subjects. The subject produces a long exhalation into the tube, then holds the breath in expiration while the operator extracts an aliquot (20 ml) of air via a needle, tap and syringe from the proximal part of the tube. A mask and an appropriate valve system (e.g. Hans Rudolf Inc., Kansas City, MO, USA) with a reservoir bag to collect exhaled air can be used to obtain mixed expiratory air in non-co-operative subjects. Mixed expiratory air is less sensitive to rises in hydrogen production than end-expiratory air. Multiple small aliquots from successive exhaled breaths obtained using a syringe and a fine bore plastic tube placed in the nasopharynx is an alternative in non-co-operative subjects,[3] but requires a monitoring device to assist with the timing of the sampling to coincide with expiration. Samples of air should be collected at 10 minute intervals until a rise in breath hydrogen to greater than 10 parts per million (ppm) is detected. The samples can be kept in sealed vacuum bottles such as those used for blood sampling with the Vacutainer system until analysis if this is not immediate. Usually, the head of a meal reaches the caecum at 45-120 minutes after ingestion. The normal range is wide. This measurement should be undertaken in an initially fasted state to ensure low base line breath hydrogen levels. Bacterial overgrowth in the small intestine, a feature of some gastrointestinal disorders, produces an early peak in breath hydrogen concentration and invalidates this method.

Abdominal scintigraphy

A gamma camera can be used to follow the movement of a radioactively labelled meal through the abdomen. The label must be an emitter of gamma rays and not be absorbed by the gastrointestinal tract. Technetium[99] labelled sulphur colloid can be used to label a mashed potato meal.[4] Other test meals used include technetium labelled chicken liver, and iodine labelled bran. Care must be taken in designing the test meal in relation to the information required. For example, if the transit of a solid meal is to be measured, the label must be a component of the solid phase and not in solution in a liquid phase that may separate from the solid phase in the stomach. Transit can be inferred by measuring the change in gamma ray counts within defined areas of interest in the abdomen. Gamma cameras are normally equipped with the analysis software to allow definition of these areas of interest and to quantify the changes in counts within them. The decline in count from the left upper quadrant reflects gastric emptying. The rise in count in the right lower quadrant reflects caecal filling.

Differential transit by marker studies

Radio-opaque markers can be used to follow luminal contents using repeated X-rays. This is an extension of the whole gut transit method using radio-opaque markers detailed above. It is most useful for measuring colonic transit and for differentiating whether delay in colonic transit is occurring in the proximal or distal colon. Markers made from cardiac catheterisation tubing can be used as described above, or shaped radio-opaque solid markers can be purchased commercially. X-rays at 24, 48 and 72 hours will show progress through the bowel. Radiation exposure can be reduced by using differently shaped markers taken on successive days. On 3 successive days, rings, cubes and stars are swallowed and a single X-ray is then taken on the 4th day. The progress of markers from the first, second and third days can be deduced. All of the first markers, most of the second markers, and perhaps some of the final markers should have been expelled.

Gastric emptying by dye dilution

The first studies of gastric emptying were conducted on subjects intubated with a nasogastric or orogastric tube. Gastric emptying can be assessed most simply by measuring the residual volume that can be aspirated after a given period of time. Marker dilution methods allow the determination of a profile of emptying from a single meal. Phenol red[5] and polyethylene glycol[6] can be used. At intervals after the instillation of a test meal (the sampling frequency is usually once every 10 minutes for a 40-60 minute period), a known quantity and concentration of marker is introduced, mixed with intragastric contents, and a defined small volume of intragastric contents is then aspirated. If the concentration of the marker present in the aspirate is measured, the residual volume can be calculated. This marker dilution method has been refined to improve its accuracy.[7,8] The use of two markers in the initial meal, only one of which is added at intervals during the test, provides even greater accuracy in allowing for gastric fluid secretion.[9] These methods require intubation, and are only suitable for liquid meals.

Measurement of gastric emptying using abdominal ultrasound

In co-operative subjects, absolute gastric volume can be calculated from dimensions measured while the ultrasound probe is moved in discrete and measured steps along a raster across the abdomen.[10,11] The cross-sectional area of the antrum in the plane of the superior mesenteric artery has been used as an index of gastric volume in infants.[12] Also in infants, a gastric filling index calculated from orthogonal parasaggital and transverse diameters of the antrum has been used.[13] A similar method has been used for the estimation of the changes in volume of the fetal stomach in utero.[14]

The most widely used of these methods is the measurement of a single parasaggital cross-sectional area in the plane of the superior mesenteric artery in a subject lying in the right lateral position.[15] Measurements are taken at 15 minute intervals using a 5 MHz sector scanner. Most ultrasound machines now incorporate the software to calculate the area of a defined region of interest. Care must be taken in imaging to ensure that the image is not taken during the passage of an antral contraction wave. In infants, a standard meal of 22 ml/kg of milk has been adopted by many investigators.

Measurement of gastric emptying by electrical impedance tomography

The availability of cheap and powerful desktop computers in recent years has allowed the development of electrical impedance tomography (previously called applied potential tomography), an enhancement of the technique of epigastric impedance.[16] Impedance measurements are obtained in turn from each pair of an array of electrodes placed in a ring around the abdomen in the plane of the stomach (in practice, 16 or 32 electrodes are used). Computerised tomographic algorithms are then used to obtain a two dimensional representation of the resistivity within the area of the stomach. The resistivity changes calculated in the area of the gastric lumen can be summated to give a measure of changes in gastric volume. This method allows the measurement of the emptying of substances with a relatively high (e.g. glucose solutions) or low (e.g. beef consommé) resistivity.[17] It is non-invasive, the equipment required is cheap compared to the cost of a gamma camera, and it does not require the use of radiation. The method of electrical impedance tomography has been validated in a direct comparison with radio-isotopic scintigraphy. Reproducibility in adults is moderately good but is improved by suppression of gastric acid secretion by administration of a single dose of cimetidine prior to the study.[16] Signal generation and detection equipment is available commercially (IBEES, Sheffield, UK).

Other methods of measuring gastric emptying

Non-invasive measurement of gastric emptying of a liquid meal by magnetic resonance imaging has been validated,[18] but the expense of the equipment makes it unlikely to be used widely.

Methods – luminal pressure recordings

In recent years, manometric recordings of intestinal motor activity using either constantly perfused multilumen catheters or electronic strain-gauge pressure transducers have become possible in the investigation of patients with severe chronic gastrointestinal symptoms. Parameters of the normal pattern of small intestinal motor activity have been published for adults[19] and for children.[20,21] In the fasting state, this pattern of activity shows 4 phases (Phase I, a phase of quietude, Phase II, a period of increasing activity, Phase III, a short period of continuous regular contractions, and Phase IV, a short period of declining activity[22]), occurring in sequence over 60-90 minutes and called the migrating motor complex. Phase changes occur proximally before being propagated to the more distal parts of the gut. In the fed state, this pattern is replaced by frequent irregular contractions responsible for mixing and lasting for 90-180 minutes). The abnormal patterns found in patients with chronic idiopathic intestinal pseudo-obstruction have been described,[23,24] as have the patterns found in patients with irritable bowel disease.[25,26]

Electronic strain gauge pressure transducers are becoming more common but are still very expensive. Systems are available from Synetics among others. Electronic transducers can be obtained with three or more pressure channels and with the pressure channels separated by distances from 2 to 5 cms. An appropriate catheter must be chosen for the size of the gastrointestinal tract under investigation.

Constantly perfused catheters are cheaper and can be home-made to suit. The raw materials needed are as follows:-

1. Multiple-lumen PVC catheters (obtainable from Dural Plastics, Dural, New South Wales, among others): these are available as triple lumen tubes with diameters from 2.5 mm (internal channel diameters 0.9 mm) down.

2. A glue to bond two triple lumen tubes together to make a 6 lumen tube; a solvent for PVC will produce bonding when applied to two catheters held in contact with one another.

3. A razor or scalpel blade to cut side holes in the lumens and a silicon glue to seal the lumen distal to the hole made. The distance between the side holes can be 2-5 cm, depending on the size of the subject.

4. Butterfly catheters, or small intravenous infusion catheters of the type commonly used in paediatric wards: these are inserted into the top of the triple lumen tube to provide a "Medusa's Head" to attach to the pressure transducers.

5. Pressure transducers: these are placed in line between the perfusion pumps and the multi-lumen catheters. They are available from many sources now supplying intensive care units.

6. A constant rate low compliance pump capable of perfusing the number of channels being used (e.g.

Harvard Infusion Pumps, Boston, MA, USA). A pump of the Arndofer design, incorporating a high resistance capillary coil provides maximum isolation of the transducer from the pump elements.

Once the catheter is ready and available, it can be passed into the required part of the gastrointestinal tract, usually under fluoroscopic control. Perfused side hole systems and electronic transducers are suitable for narrow parts of the gastrointestinal tract with predominantly liquid contents, and are therefore suitable for the oesphagus and the antroduodenal area. However, a balloon system (see below) is required for gastric body pressure measurements.

The output of the pressure transducers can be recorded on a chart recorder, but may also be recorded electronically if fed to an analogue to digital (A-D) convertor in a computer. As the highest frequency in the normal gastrointestinal tract is approximately 12 cycles per minute, the sampling frequency of an A-D convertor must be at least 24 samples per minute. If such a low sampling frequency is to be used, higher interference frequencies from respiration and cardiac activity must be filtered beforehand.

When using a constantly perfused system, care must be taken not to overload the gastrointestinal tract of a small animal or child with fluid. Measurements should be undertaken over at least a 3 hour period in the antroduodenal area because of the fluctuation in activity due to the migrating motor complex. The most constant feature of the fasting activity is the Phase III period, and the recordings can be analysed to produce the following parameters:

- The average time between successive Phase III periods
- The average duration of Phase III
- The maximum frequency of the contractions in Phase III
- The average amplitude of the contractions in Phase III

The fed activity pattern can be induced by infusing a glucose solution through the most proximal channel.

Special adaptations of luminal pressure recordings

Rectum

Because the rectum has a complex arrangement of muscles, multiple closely spaced recording sites are required. A balloon placed at the end of the catheter allows the measurement of the effect of rectal distension. Such balloons can be manufactured by using silicon sheeting with a silicon glue.

Stomach

Measurement of pressure in the fundus and body of the stomach, where receptive relaxation occurs after eating, is done best by using a constant volume balloon connected to a pressure transducer. The balloon can be filled with air or with water.

Oesophagus

Measurement of luminal pressure in the body of the oesophagus is similar to that described above for any small volume tubular part of the gastrointestinal tract. Repeated swallowing waves may be initiated by administering small volumes of fluid into the mouth of the subject. Alternatively, reflex swallowing in young human infants can be induced by blowing at the face (the Santmyer reflex). At least 20 swallows should be measured and the results integrated. The amplitude and rate of propagation of the swallowing waves can be measured.

The function of the gastro-oesphageal junction area is a special case. Its efficacy is the combined product of the anatomical arrangement of the gastro-oesophageal junction area and the pressure of the lower oesophageal sphincter. The pressure generated and the length of oesophagus over which that pressure is active can be measured with a single point pressure measuring device using the pull-through technique. This requires a constantly perfused side hole manometry catheter (or an electronic strain gauge transducer) which can be pulled through the lower oesophageal sphincter area while pressure is recorded. This method is necessary because the position of the gastro-oesophageal junction varies with swallowing and with position. The pull-through may be slow with frequent stops (the station pull-though) or fast without stopping. Passage through the diaphragm can be noted from the change of phase of the respiratory signal. The maximum pressure recorded is the maximum pressure achieved by the lower oesophageal sphincter area. The effective sphincter pressure can be calculated as the difference between gastric end-expiratory pressure and sphincter end-expiratory pressure. In adults, this pressure should be 10-40 mmHg, and should act over 2 to 4 cm. It is radially asymmetrical however.

Whether pull-through systems are accurate is a question of controversy. An alternative method regarded as more reliable is the use of a Dent sleeve,[27] a 6 cm long perfused slit sensitive to pressure through its length. A similar system is the Kraglund tube (Cook Europe). Recently a miniaturised Dent sleeve has been manufactured and used successfully in premature human infants.[28] The Dent sleeve has the advantage that it records the maximum pressure applied over the length of the sleeve area, and is not influenced by fore and aft movement of the sphincter.

Methods – control mechanisms

Implanted electrodes in animals allowed prolonged studies to be conducted of the electrical activity of the gastrointestinal tract, and it was this method in 1969 that led to the discovery of the migrating myoelectric complex before that of its motor correlate.[29] The techniques available for the measurement of control mechanisms in gastrointestinal motility are still very primitive in comparison to their undoubted complexity. Methods are available for detecting the electrical control activity of the stomach, and blood sampling can be used to measure changes in gastrointestinally active endocrine substances. Assessment of the enteric nervous system, and of paracrine substances in the gastrointestinal wall are experimental.

Electrogastrography

Electrogastrography is available for detecting the electrical control activity of the stomach. The smooth muscle cells of the gastrointestinal tract, with the exception of those in the oesophagus, have an intrinsic rhythmic fluctuation in their electrical control activity. The fluctuation of this electrical control activity in adjacent smooth muscle cells is entrained and as the stomach muscle cells are predominantly aligned in one direction the electrical vectors are additive and surface electrodes can detect the rhythmic fluctuation.

Definitive demonstration of the gastrointestinal electrical control activity can be obtained from surgically implanted electrodes placed on the serosal surface of the gastrointestinal tract, and such electrodes have provided useful information in cases requiring laparotomy.[30] Multiple electrodes can be implanted, allowing the localisation of areas of smooth muscle responsible for ectopic frequencies or rhythms.[31] Platinum or steel electrodes may be used, and removed transcutaneously when no longer required. This has not achieved a widespread clinically useful role at the present time.

Mucosal electrodes mounted on intestinal infusion tubes introduced through the mouth were used prior to the development of non-invasive methods,[32] and these are still required to detect small intestinal electrical control activity. Agar bridge Ag/AgCl electrodes, Ag/AgCl spike electrodes, platinum spike electrodes or metallic clip electrodes[33] have been used.

Recordings may be monopolar or bipolar. Mucosal recordings suffer from unstable contact between the electrodes and the inner surface of the gastrointestinal tract wall, though the use of improved fixation techniques such as platinum ring electrodes held in place by an external magnet[34] has attempted to address this problem. The invasive nature of intubation techniques restricts the usefulness of mucosal recordings.

Recordings of gastric electrical control activity obtained from surface electrodes have been shown to correlate well with mucosal recordings,[35,36] though internal and external recordings do not always agree [37] and internal electrogastrographic recordings have been found to be more sensitive for the detection of loss of coupling.[38]

Pairs of Ag/AgCl electrodes are placed over the antrum in the direction of the axis of the stomach. The signal is passed through isolation pre-amplifiers to amplifiers and a chart recorder, or alternatively to an A-D convertor for recording digitally. Low pass filtering at a frequency of approximately 15 cycles per minute will remove cardiac electrical activity. The resultant signal can be subjected to discrete Fast Fourier transformation. This method is based on the false premise of statistical stationarity of the signal but is an acceptable approximation. The advent of powerful desktop computers and the introduction of the technique of running spectral analysis[39] has allowed objective analysis of the recorded signals, complementing the use of visual analysis techniques. It is necessary to pass an analogue signal through a low-pass filter with a cutoff frequency of less than half the sampling frequency if an error, known as aliasing, is to be avoided.

As sampling truncates the signal measured at onset and completion, errors can be introduced into the frequency spectrum due to these discontinuities. This error is called leakage, and can be compensated for by tapering the sampled amplitudes with a data window such as a Bartlett window (a triangular function) or a Hanning window (a shifted cosine function). An alternative to Fast Fourier transformation is autoregressive modelling, which has advantages in frequency peak detection but loses power information.

Occasionally the 12 cycles per minute electrical control activity of the small intestine appears in the electrogastrography signal but this is not reliably detected as the electrical vector of the small intestine is randomly distributed.

Endocrine influences

The paracrine and endocrine control mechanisms governing the motor activity of the gastrointestinal tract are still poorly understood. However, many hormones including motilin, cholecystokinin, secretin, pancreatic polypeptide, enteroglucogon, peptide YY, gastric inhibitory peptide and many more are known to be involved. Many studies have measured the concentrations of these hormones at different times during the fasting migrating motor complex cycle and in the post-prandial state and this work has also been done during the development of the gastrointestinal tract in preterm infants. Further consideration of this is outside the scope of this chapter.

Results & discussion

As an illustration of the application of one of the techniques outlined above, the investigation of electrical control activity in a group of children with chronic idiopathic intestinal pseudo-obstruction (CIIP) will be outlined. CIIP is a condition in which gastrointestinal transit is severely abnormal, without evidence of a structural obstruction or partial obstruction.

Eleven children (0.1-16 years, median 11 years) with proven chronic idiopathic intestinal pseudo-obstruction were investigated. All had severe symptoms of intestinal psuedo-obstruction, including episodic vomiting, abdominal distension and intolerance of food. None of the patients had evidence of a central nervous system or an autonomic nervous system disorder. The diagnosis was supported in all 11 patients by contrast radiography, which showed severe delay in the passage of contrast through the small intestine.

Table 10.1 – Dominant electrical control activity frequency and histological categorisation of the 11 patients with chronic idiopathic intestinal pseduo-obstruction

Patient dominant frequency (cycles per minute)		Histology
Patient 1	6.4	Neuropathy
Patient 2	8.3	Neuropathy
Patient 3	9.4	Neuropathy
Patient 4	2.8	Neuropathy
Patient 5	None	Myopathy
Patient 6	None	Myopathy
Patient 7	None	Myopathy
Patient 8	None	Inconclusive examination
Patient 9	None	Insufficient material for full evaluation
Patient 10	2.2	No histology available
Patient 11	3.7	No histology available

Antroduodenal manometry was undertaken in all cases, and abnormalities of the pattern of small intestine contraction was shown. In 8 of the 11 patients, full thickness intestinal biopsies were available for histological examination. Electrical control activity was measured using the non-invasive technique of surface electrogastrography. The dominant frequency of the electrical control activity was determined by running spectral analysis of a one hour digital recording of surface electrical activity. The result of the spectral analysis is presented in Table 10.1. In conclusion, abnormalities were present in 8/11 patients. Persistent tachygastria (electrical control activity frequency > 5 cycles per minute) was found in 3 patients, all with a proven neuropathy. A continuously irregular frequency was found in 5 patients, 3 with a proven myopathy and 2 with undefined pathology. A normal electrical control activity frequency was present in 3 patients, 1 with a proven neuropathy and 2 with undefined pathology.

Application to animal studies

The techniques above are all applicable to animal studies, bearing in mind the size constraints. For those working with small animals, the techniques that have been used in the investigations of neonatal and infant gastrointestinal motor activity, are particularly relevant.

When choosing an animal model for human gastrointestinal motor function, care must be taken that the appropriate system is chosen. Ruminant animals have a different anatomical gastrointestinal tract construction, with an additional storage and mixing area (the rumen). The cyclical nature of gastrointestinal motor activity expressed as the migrating motor complex is a universal feature of all mammalian species. The duration of a complete cycle tends to be shorter with smaller species size. The cyclical pattern is present only in the fasting state in non-ruminant animals, but is present in the fasting and the fed state in ruminant animals. Curiously, pigs who are not fed *ad libitum* show a non-ruminant pattern rather than a ruminant pattern.[19] Rats and rabbits do not show a vomiting reflex, while the ferret has been used as a model of upper gastrointestinal dysfunction in studies of the pathophysiology of vomiting.

References

1. Cannon WB, Lieb CW. The receptive relaxation of the stomach. *Am J Physiol* 1911; **29**: 267-273.

2. Hinton JM, Lennard-Jones JE, Young AC. A new method of studying gut transit times using radio-opaque markers. *Gut* 1969; **10**: 842-847.

3. Perman JA, Barr RG, Watkins JB. Sucrose malabsorption in children: noninvasive diagnosis by interval breath hydrogen determination. *J Pediatr* 1978; **93**: 17-22.

4. Read NW, Al-Janabi MN, Holgate AM, Barber DC, Edwards CA. Simultaneous measurement of gastric emptying, small bowel residence, and colonic filling of a solid meal by the use of a gamma camera. *Gut* 1986; **27**: 300-308.

5. George JD. New clinical method for measuring the rate of gastric emptying; the double sampling test meal. *Gut* 1968; **9**: 237-242.

6. Cavell B. Gastric emptying in preterm infants. *Acta Paed Scand* 1979; **68**: 725-730.

7. Hunt JN. A modification to the method of George for studying gastric emptying. *Gut* 1974; **15**: 812-813.

8. Hurwitz A. Measuring gastric volumes by dye dilution. *Gut* 1981; **22**: 85-93.

9. Beeket.s EJ, Rehrer NJ, Brouns F, TenHoor F, Saris WIIM. Determination of total gastric volume, gastric secretion, and residual meal using the double sampling technique of George. *Gut* 1988; **29**: 1725-1729.

10. Bateman DN, Whittingham TA. Measurement of gastric emptying by real-time ultrasonography. *Gut* 1982; **23**: 524-527.

11. Holt CS, Stickler GB. A study of 44 children with the syndrome of recurrent cyclic vomiting. *Pediatrics.* 1960; **25:** 775-780.

12. Newell SJ, Chapman S, Durbin GM, Morgan MEI, Booth IW. Ultrasonic measurement of gastric antral transit: a novel method for measuring gastric emptying in the premature infant, In: *Proceedings of the British Paediatric Association.* London: British Paediatric Association 1991: p 58.

13. Lambrecht L, Robberecht E, Deschynkel K, Afschrift M. Ultrasonic evaluation of gastric clearing in young infants. *Pediatr Radiol* 1988; **18:** 314-318.

14. Devane SP, Soothill PW, Candy DCA. Temporal changes in gastric volume in the human fetus – a manifestation of intrauterine gastrointestinal motor activity. *J Pediatr Gastroenterol Nutr* 1991; **13:** 319.

15. Newell SJ, Chapman S, Booth IW. Ultrasonic assessment of gastric emptying in the preterm infant. *Arch Dis Child* 1993; **69:** 32-36

16. Brown BH, Barber DC, Seagar AD. Applied potential tomography: possible clinical applications. *Clin Phys and Physiol Meas* 1985; **6:** 109-121.

17. Mangnall YF. Baxter AJ, Avill R, *et al.* Applied potential tomography: a new non-invasive technique for assessing gastric function. *Clin Phys and Physiol Meas* 1987; **8 (Suppl A):** 119-129.

18. Schwizer W, Macke H, Fried M. Measurement of gastric emptying by magnetic resonance imaging in humans. *Gastroenterology.* 1992; **103:** 369-376.

19. Phillips SF. Normal gastrointestinal motility - small bowel. In: Kumar D, Gustavsson S, eds. *An illustrated guide to gastrointestinal motility.* Chichester: John Wiley. 1988; 187-206.

20. Devane SP, Coombs R, Smith VV, et al. Persistent gastrointestinal symptoms after correction of malrotation. *Arch Dis Child* 1992; **67:** 218 221.

21. Fenton T. Antroduodenal motor function in children. University of London: Doctoral Thesis MD- 1988.

22. Code CF, Marlett JA. The interdigestive myoelectric complex of the stomach and small bowel of dogs. *J Physiol.* 1975; **246:** 289-309.

23. Stanghellini V, Camilleri M, Malagelada J-R. Chronic idiopathic intestinal pseudo-obstruction: clinical and intestinal manometric findings. *Gut* 1987; **28:** 5-12.

24. Hyman PE, McDiarmid SV, Napolitano J, Abrams CL, Tomomasa T. Antroduodenal motility in children with chronic intestinal pseudo-obstruction. *J Pediatr* 1988; **112:** 899-905.

25. Kellow JE, Gill RC, Wingate DL Proximal gut motor activity in irritable bowel syndrome. Patients at home and at work. *Gastroenterology.* 1987; **92:** 1463.

26. Kellow JE, Phillips SF. Altered small bowel motility in irritable bowel syndrome is correlated with symptoms. *Gastroenterology.* 1987; **92:** 1885-1893.

27. Dent J. A new technique for continuous sphincter pressure measurement. *Gastroenterology* 1976; **71:** 263-267.

28. Omari TI, Miki K, Fraser R, *et al.* Esophageal body and lower esophageal sphincter function in healthy preterm infants. *Gastroenterology* 1995; **109:** 1757-1764.

29. Szurszewski JH. A migrating electric complex of the canine small intestine. *Am J Physiol* 1969; **217:** 1757-1763.

30. Blank EL, Karaus M, Glicklis M, Sarna SK, Werlin SL. Gastrointestinal myoelectric activity in an infant with congenital idiopathic motility disorder. *Dig Dis Sci* 1989; **34:** 1124-1131.

31. Cucchiara S, Janssens J, Vantrappen G, Geboes K, Ceccatelli P. Gastric electrical dysrhythmias tachygastria and tachyarrhythmia in a girl with chronic intractable vomiting. *J Pediatr* 1986; **108:** 264-267.

32. Christensen J, Schedl HP, Clifton JA. The small intestinal basic electrical rhythm slow wave frequency gradiant in normal man and in patients with a variant of diseases. *Gastroenterology* 1966; **50:** 309-315.

33. Pope CE II, Ask P, Tibbling L. Evaluation of intraluminal EMG electrodes for the esophagus and gastrointestinal tract. *Med Biol Eng Comput* 1984; **22:** 461-464.

34. Abell TL, Malagelada J-R. Glucagon-evoked gastric dysrhythmias in humans shown by an improved electrogastrographic technique. *Gastroenterology* 1985; **88:** 1932-1940.

35. Geldof H, Van der Schee EJ, Grashuis JL. Accuracy and reliability of electrogastrography. *Gastroenterology* 1986; **90:** 1425 abstract.

36. Hamilton JW, Bellahsene BE, Reichelderfer M, Webster JG, Bass P. Human electrogastrograms: comparison of surface and mucosal recordings. *Dig Dis Sci* 1986; **31:** 33-39.

37. Smout AJ PM, van der Schee EJ, Grashuis JL. What is measured in electrogastrography? *Dig Dis Sci* 1980; **25:** 179-187.

38. Familoni BO, Bowes KL, Kingma YJ, Cote KR. Can transcutaneous recordings recordings detect gastric electrical abnormalities? *Gut* 1991, **32:** 141-146.

39. Van der Schee EJ, Grashuis JL. Running spectrum analysis as an aid in the representation and interpretation of electrgastrographic signals. *Med Biol Eng Comput* 1987; **25:** 57-62.

11

Helicobacter pylori: Methods of detection and study

Shigemi Nakajima, Ana Maria Segura and Robert M Genta

Summary

Helicobacter pylori infection is the most important cause of chronic active gastritis, a condition which exists in several distinct patterns (e.g. antral predominant or multifocal atrophic gastritis) and may remain clinically silent or progress to diseases such as peptic ulcer, gastric adenocarcinoma or primary gastric B cell lymphoma.[1] Treatment of *H. pylori* infection can lead to disappearance of active gastritis, virtual elimination of peptic ulcer recurrence and regression of a significant percentage of primary gastric lymphoma of the mucosa-associated lymphoid tissue type.[2,3] Treatment is also believed to represent the first important step in the prevention of many gastric carcinomas.[4] Therefore, accurate diagnosis of *H. pylori* is of paramount importance. Invasive and non-invasive tests are available to the clinician and amongst the former, the histopathological examination of biopsy specimens is considered the gold standard, but new accurate, rapid urease tests are becoming increasingly accepted; bacterial culture and more sophisticated methods of bacterial detection, such as the polymerase chain reaction and *in situ* hybridization remain mostly confined to research settings. Of the non-invasive tests, serology and the urea breath test are the most widely available, although many office-based kits for the detection of antibodies in whole blood specimens, saliva and urine are rapidly emerging. This chapter reviews the use of these tests in different clinical settings.

Introduction

Since Warren and Marshall reported unidentified curved bacilli on gastric epithelium in active chronic gastritis in 1983, *H. pylori* has been investigated energetically all over the world, and is now regarded as the most important cause of chonic active gastritis and peptic ulcers.[5] Furthermore, there is now compelling evidence that *H. pylori* infection is associated with primary gastric B cell lymphomas of the mucosa-associated lymphoid tissue (MALT) type[2,3] and on the basis of epidemiological evidence the World Health Organization has declared this organism a type-1 carcinogen.[6]

As the clinical implications of *H. pylori* infection become increasingly apparent, the indications for treatment are steadily expanding. Gastric and duodenal ulcers and MALT lymphoma are universally considered indications for *H. pylori* treatment[7] and debate now focuses on whether to treat patients with non-ulcer dyspepsia and those at risk for gastric

cancer.[5] Since at least three billion people are currently infected with *H. pylori* and the antibiotic regimens for its cure are expensive and often complicated, the decision to treat must be founded on solid diagnostic criteria. In other words, the clinician must be confident that the patient has the infection and that he will be cured with available treatment.

A vast array of tests is now available for the diagnosis of *H. pylori* infection (Table 11.1).[8] Below we consider separately invasive tests (i.e. those that require gastric tissue obtained through an endoscopic procedure) and non-invasive tests (i.e. laboratory tests that can be performed without endoscopy). The distinction, although somewhat artificial, is practically useful. We shall then discuss the use of these tests in light of context-sensitive diagnostic strategies.

Methods

Invasive tests

Histopathological examination of gastric biopsy specimens

Curved or spiral bacilli can be detected in histological preparations of gastric biopsy specimens stained with a variety of methods.[9] For several years after the first description of *H. pylori*, pathologists – unaccustomed and uncomfortable with microbiological diagnoses based on histopathological observations – prudently called these bacilli CLO (Campylobacter-like organisms). It is now accepted that such bacilli are virtually always *H. pylori* (very rarely *H. heilmanni*). *H. pylori* can be detected in routinely stained haematoxylin and eosin-stained (H&E) biopsy specimens. However, variations in quality of the stain, the paucity of bacteria in some specimens, and the need for exceptional diligence on the part of observers make H&E a sub-optimal choice for the specific task of detecting *H. pylori*. Special stains include Warthin-Starry and Steiner silver stains, Giemsa, Diff-Quick®, Gimenez stain and Acridine orange, which has the disadvantage of requiring a microscope for fluorescent observation.[10-12] A triple stain (a combination of modified Steiner staining, H&E and Alcian blue at pH 2.5), known as the Genta stain, allows simultaneous visualization of the features of gastritis, including intestinal metaplasia, and the bacteria, which characteristically stain mid-brown with two dark polar dots (Fig. 11.1).[13] The application of this stain requires an experienced and dedicated technical staff, but its specificity and ease of use have

Table 11.1 — Methods for detection of *Helicobacter pylori* infection

---

Invasive tests (need endoscopic examination, or gastric juice collection)

1. **HISTOPATHOLOGICAL EXAMINATION IN BIOPSY SPECIMENS**

   Chemical (Non-immunohistochemical staining)
   a. non-silver staining
      haematoxylin and eosin
      Giemsa
      Diff-Quick®
      Gimenez
      acridine orange
      other (Gram, methylene blue, cresyl fast violet)

   b. Silver staining
      Warthin-Starry
      Steiner
      Genta, or modified Genta
      other (e.g. combined Warthin-Starry staining with haematoxylin and eosin)
   Immunohistochemistry staining
   In situ hybridization

2. **SMEAR, BRUSH AND TOUCH SAMPLE EXAMINATION**

   Cytological examination
      Gram staining

3. **BACTERIAL CULTURE**

4. **POLYMERASE CHAIN REACTION (PCR)**

5. **RAPID UREASE TEST**

6. **OTHER TESTS**

   Ammonia detection in gastric juice
   Endoscopic urease detection

Non-invasive tests

1. **SEROLOGICAL EXAMINNATION FOR IMMUNOGLOBULINS**

   Laboratory-based assays (ELISA)
   Simplified 'in-office' immunoenzymatic tests

2. **UREA BREATH TEST**

   Non-radioactive isotope (^{13}C) methods
   Radioactive isotope (^{14}C) methods

3. **OTHER TESTS**

   $^{15}NH_4^+$ excretion test in urine
   PCR in saliva, dental plaque of faeces
   Immunoglobulin detection in saliva or urine

contributed to its rapid acceptance amongst histopathologists. Modified versions of the Genta stain have recently become available.[14,15] Since local laboratory conditions and financial constraints often determine the choice of a stain more than the individual histopathologist's preference, no universal recommendation can be made as to which technique should be used. However, the 1994 Houston International Gastritis Workshop, a working party of gastric pathologists engaged in the revision and updating of the Sydney System for the classification of gastritis, issued the following guidelines: "In addition to H&E, many laboratories routinely undertake a special stain for *H. pylori*. This practice encourages proper assessment and may be more cost-effective than subsequent requests for an extra stain. The choice of stain, for example modified Giemsa, Warthin-Starry or the new Genta stain, is a matter of local perference, but the use of a special stain is strongly recommended, particularly when the H&E fails to reveal organisms in a biopsy specimen with chronic active inflammation. Thus, while many positive cases can be recognized in a good H&E stain, careful examination of a special stain is deemed essential before declaring an inflamed biopsy specimen histologically negative for *H. pylori*.[16]

Immunohistochemical staining and *in situ* hybridization

Several anti-*H. pylori* antibodies are now commercially available for the immunohistochemical detection of *H. pylori* in paraffin-embedded biopsy specimens. To obtain good and consistent staining, enzyme digestion with trypsin is recommended. This method is expensive and requires considerable technical and histopathological expertise. However, its sensitivity and specificity are high,[17,18] and some laboratories use it for routine clinical diagnosis. Immunohistochemistry may be particularly useful for the detection of the coccoid forms of *H. pylori*, believed by some to appear in some patients after failed attempts to treat the infection with antibiotics. *In situ* hybridization (ISH) may be used for the detection of *H. pylori* in paraffin-embedded sections. Some researchers believe that ISH may turn out to be the most specific and sensitive method for the visual detection of *H. pylori* in biopsy specimens, since it can detect not only small numbers of organisms but also the coccoid form. However, the high cost and the technical difficulty of this procedure may prevent the gathering of sufficient data to refute this optimistic view.

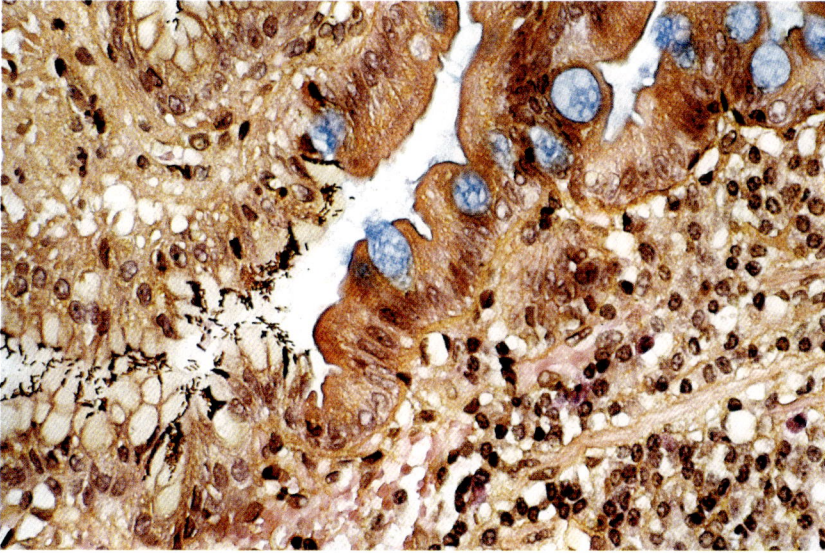

Figure 11.1 – The triple stain[13] allows the simultaneous visualization of the gastric morphology (e.g. type and intensity of the inflammatory infiltrate, presence of intestinal metaplasia) and *H. pylori*. In this photomicrograph innumerable organisms are seen in a gastric pit (left), away from areas of intestinal metaplasia (characterized by the Alcian blue-stained goblet cells). The lamina propria contains a marked mixed inflammatory infiltrate.

Smear, brush and touch preparations

Smears of gastric mucus and exfoliated epithelial cells may be prepared by techniques similar to those used to obtain specimens for cytological examination. Such smears are usually stained with Gram staining and can allow the detection of bacteria within minutes of the endoscopic procedure.[19,20] Although some laboratories perform this procedure routinely, these tests have been largely supplanted by the introduction of the rapid urease test (see below).

Bacterial culture

The fortuitous conditions that led to the isolation of *H. pylori* have becomne part of the folklore surrounding the initial phases of its discovery. According to a popular version of the story, a batch of culture dishes was forgotten in the incubator for several days because of the Easter holidays instead of being discarded after a 3-day incubation as usual. The longer incubation allowed the fastidious and slower growing 'cruved bacilli' to grow. [21] *H. pylori* is best cultured in a microaerophillic and humid atmosphere, usually 5% O_2, 10-15% CO_2, 80-85% N_2, 70-100% humidity, and a temperature between 33°C and 40°C, ideally 37°C. Incubators containing 10-15% CO_2 or anaerobic jars can also be used to culture *H. pylori*. Culture media require fresh horse and/or sheep blood, as well as antibiotics such as vancomycin, trimethoprim and amphotericin B to suppress contaminants. Skirrow's medium has a high isolation rate and is commonly used,[22] but some other good commercial media have recently become available. The incubation time may vary from 3 to 14 days; most laboratories routinely use 6 days. *H. pylori* may be identified by examining unstained smears with a phase-contrast microscope or by staining them with the Gram stain; biochemical identification may be performed based on positivity for urease, catalase and oxidase. Since many clinical facilities are not equipped to perform the time-consuming procedures necessary to culture *H. pylori*, several methods for transportation have been devised.[23,24] *H. pylori* is easily destroyed in dry or aerobic condition and cannot be stored like other anaerobic bacteria. Special techniques are necessary, the most widely used consisting of freezing the fresh biopsy specimens in storage media containing 20% glycerol with skimmed milk, Brucella broth or cysteine-Albini medium, preferably at -70°C but most commonly at -20°C.[24]

Although culturing specimens is generally the most reliable method to identify a bacterium species, in the case of *H. pylori* several factors prevent this technique from being the detection method of choice. First, as stated above, the cultures are technically more complicated than those usually performed by a clinical microbiology laboratory. Secondly, *H. pylori* may have a patchy distribution on the gastric mucosa, and there may be areas without bacteria even in infected stomachs. Culturing mucosal specimens from such areas would result in false negative results and there is an approximately 30% chance of this occurring in a laboratory not specifically devoted to the study of

H. pylori. Since there are now other simpler and more reliable methods to identify *H. pylori*, cultures are likely to be limited to research settings, where studies on bacterial toxins, the bacterial genome, and antibiotic resistance are performed.

Polymerase chain reaction

Polymerase chain reaction (PCR) is a technique that allows the amplification of a DNA template into multiple copies through sequential rounds of DNA replication by DNA polymerase. This permits the detection of a DNA fragment that can be resolved and visualized in agarose gels. For the detection of *H. pylori* DNA the urease gene is commonly used.[25] Reverse transcription (RT)-PCR has also been applied to the detection of *H. pylori* RNA, in which 16S rRNA is the common target.[26] To perform the procedure, specimens are taken from fresh biopsy tissues, gastric juice, saliva, dental plaque and faeces. A particularly useful technique that allows PCR in sections obtained from paraffin-embedded forma-lin-fixed biopsy specimens has been developed.[27] The initial step is the extraction of the bacterial DNA or RNA, but this is not always necessary since boiling has been shown to be sufficient to amplify the target nucleotide.[26,28,29] When performed in the appropriate conditions, with no contamination and appropriate primers, this technique has an extremely high sensitivity and a near perfect specificity. However, its high sensitivity may be a source of uncertainty when evaluating the results, since DNA or RNA from dead bacteria may also be detected, as well as rare bacteria or their products that may contaminate the work area or the tissues studied. Of particular concern is the contamination caused by inadequately disinfected endoscopes.[30] Another source of false positive results may be inadequate primers, since the specificity of this test hinges on the specificity of the primers.

The practical usefulness of PCR for the detection of *H. pylori* infection has been difficult to define because this technique is so much more sensitive than the considered 'gold standard', i.e. histopathological detection. Cases are frequent in which no bacteria can be identified by histopathological examination, yet the PCR yields a positive result. While the presence of coccoid forms of *H. pylori* and inevitable sampling errors may elucidate some of these discrepancies, many remain unexplained. In such cases the decision to accept the PCR results is an arbitrary one and only follow-up of the patient may provide retrospective information. False negative results are rare and are almost invariably due to technical problems. PCR is very expensive and requires a highly sophisticated molecular biology laboratory and the availability of appropriate primers. Important questions related to the transmission of *H. pylori* have been addressed using PCR,[31-33] but PCR must be considered a research tool with no documented clinical applicability.

Rapid urease tests

These assays exploit the high urease content of *H. pylori*.[34,35] To perform the test a fragment of gastric mucosa is placed into a broth (originally called Cristensen's broth) or in agar containing various concentrations of urea. The urease produced by *H. pylori* hydrolyzes the urea releasing ammonia, which raises the pH of the broth or agar. An appropriate indicator (e.g. phenol red) changes colour as the pH increases. In the first commercially poduced rapid urease test, the CLO test, the yellow gel capsule into which the specimen is placed turns red within minutes to hours, depending on the quantity of bacteria present. Several rapid urease tests are commercially available. Their specificity and sensitivity, compared to the histopathological examination, are extremely high, in most cases approaching 100%.[36,37]

Non-invasive tests

Serology

A correlation between the presence of organisms in the gastric mucosa, chronic active gastritis and serum anti-*H. pylori* antibodies was first documented using crude antigen preparations in complement fixation, bacterial agglutination tests, immunoblotting techniques and enzyme-linked immunosorbant assays (ELISA).[38,39] In later studies whole cell antigen preparations and cell lysates were used and significant correlations were reported between the presence of anti-*H. pylori* antibody in serum and the occurrence of gastroduodenal ulcers. Such relatively crude preparations contained antigens that cross-reacted wtih antibodies directed against other bacteria (e.g. *Campylobacter jejuni, C. fetus* and *Escherichia coli*) and new techniques were developed to minimize the problem of cross-reactivity. An effective method is the removal of cross-reactive antibodies from sera by adsorption with *C. jejuni*.[40] The pre-absorption of sera, when tested in an ELISA, showed that the sensitivity and specificity of the assay could be increased to 100% and 94%, respectively.[41] Another method uses cell-associated protein antigen prepared by extracting the 600,000 kDa protein fraction that has urease activity using gel filtration, and has shown 100% specificity and 99% sensitivity with light molecular weight cell-associated proteins (HM-CAP) ELISA.[42]

The selection of *H. pylori* strain(s) as sources of antigen is critical to the specificity and sensitivity of a test and it is of paramount importance to evaluate specific tests in the population to be studied before selection of a test for use in specific settings. Another interesting fact is that the measurement of serum IgG antibodies has been consistently shown to provide better sensitivity and specificty than the measurement of either IgM or IgA anti-*H. pylori* antibodies.[43-45]

Simplified 'in-office' immunoenzymatic tests

Several in-office kits have been developed for the detection of IgG anti-*H. pylori* antibodies. Most consist of disposable kits that provide a yes/no answer within a few minutes of placing a drop of serum on a well pre-absorbed with antigen and an immunoenzymatic detection system. Preliminary testing of some of the kits available in the US has shown an excellent level of accuracy.

Antibodies (mostly of the IgG class) against *H. pylori* have been detected in the saliva and urine of infected patients, and many attempts have been made to develop diagnostic tests using these body fluids.[46-48] Specificity and sensitivity, however, are poor and no such tests are available as yet.

Urea breath tests

The urea breath tests represent one of the most important and innovative methods to detect *H. pylori*.[42,49,50] The tests rely on the ability of *H. pylori* to produce large quantities of urease. Thus, the ingestion of a solution containing urea will be rapidly followed, in an infected subject, by the production of NH_3 and CO_2. The latter rapidly appears in the subject's breath. If the ingested urea is labelled with a detectable isotope, then the exhaled CO_2 will also be labelled and, therefore, measurable by an appropriate detection method. The two most commonly used breath tests employ urea labelled with either the radioactive isotope ^{14}C or with the non-radioactive isotope ^{13}C. When the former is used, the general method consists of the ingestion of a solution or a capsule containing quantities between 0.5 and 10 μCi

of the isotope-labelled urea.[51] When ^{13}C-labelled urea is used, test subjects are given a solution of 125 mg 99.9% labelled urea followed by a meal aimed at increasing the permanence of the labelled urea in the stomach. After various periods of time, the subject inflates a balloon, which is immediately sealed and sent to a laboratory for the detection of the isotope-labelled CO_2. Both tests are now standarized and approved by regulatory agencies in Europe and North America. The urea breath tests are extremely sensitive and specific and, in contrast to serological tests, detect current active infection and not evidence of a past infection. As their widespread use will probably reduce their cost, they are likely to become the test of choice in a variety of clinical situations.[52] Furthermore, as these tests are non-invasive and the only nuisance to the patient may be the quality of the meal administered to delay gastric emptying, these tests are ideal for children, pregnant women and patients who cannot undergo an endoscopic procedure.[53,54]

Application to animal studies

A fruitful strategy in the study of human disease is to introduce the disease, or one very similar to it, into an animal that can be conveniently maintained in the laboratory. Ideally, animal models of infectious diseases are created by infecting a mammal with an agent from an infected human, e.g. infection of guinea pigs with *Mycobacterium tuberculosis*. When the organism has a narrow host-specificity and either does not infect or does not cause disease in animals, a similar agent must be used, e.g. woodchucks hepatitis B virus to obtain an infection similar to human hepatitis B.

Numerous unsuccessful attempts were made to establish *H. pylori* infection in a variety of laboratory animals, including mice (both conventional and germ-free), rats, guinea pigs, ferrets and rabbits.[55] Next, several newly identified species of *Helicobacter* were found to cause gastritis in their hosts, e.g. *H. mustelae* in ferrits and *H. felis* and *H. heilmannii* in cats and dogs. Manipulations of these naturally occurring infections allowed the development of a number of models with specific characteristics that made them extremely useful for the study of individual aspects of the wide spectrum of *H. pylori*. A particularly successful model used gnotobiotic mice infected with *H. felis* who acquire chronic active gastritis reminiscent of human *H. pylori* chronic active gastritis.[56] More importantly, while examining the stomachs of sacrificed mice with long-standing infections, several mice were observed to have developed MALT lymphomas,[57] and the search for a model of gastritis resulted in the serendipitous discovery of a model of *H. pylori*-associated (or perhaps induced) primary gastric lymphoma.

Non-human primates could provide particularly useful models because they can be infected with *H. pylori* from infected patients. However, financial and humane considerations pose considerable restraints on their widespread usage.

A new promising model is Mongolian gerbils (Merionis ungulatus) infected with human strains of *H. pylori* which not only acquire a severe chronic active gastritis very similar to the human counterpart, but also develop prominent lymphoid infiltrates that may result in MALT lymphomas.[58]

The usefulness of these models resides in their potential for the study of the basic mechanisms of infection. An area in which the availability of suitable animal models is crucial is the development of vaccines,[59] the testing of new drug regimens and the study of *H. pylori*-associated carcinogenesis.

Results and discussion

The choice of a diagnostic test is strictly related to its intended use. If a study is to determine the prevalence of *H. pylori* in a population of 2000 school children, a laboratory-based sero-enzymatic assay able to detect anti-*H. pylori* IgG antibodies (e.g. an ELISA system) will be the method of choice. In this situation, the effect of the 10% or so false negatives carried by such tests may be considered negligible. A perfectly healthy individual may read an article on *H. pylori* and ask his general practitioner to test his infection status. In this case the practitioner my be perfectly justified to perform one of the less accurate, but quick and inexpensive, office-based whole-blood immunoenzymatic tests. On the other hand, a gastroenterologist seeing a patient referred for ulcer-type pain will probably want to perform an endoscopic examination and obtain several gastric biopsy specimens to evaluate not only the presence of *H. pylori*, but also the type and distribution of gastritis. Having found a duodenal ulcer and having decided to treat the infection, the gastroenterologist will also want to know whether the patient is cured. Thus, 4-6 weeks after the end of an antibiotic course, the patient may be asked to come back for a follow-up endoscopy (with more biopsy sampling) or, if available, a urea breath test to confirm the success of the therapy.[60]

These clinical vignettes underscore that universal guidelines on the use of tests to detect *H. pylori* cannot and perhaps should not be provided. Below, however, we will outline a sensible approach shared by most clinical researchers devoted to the investigation of *H. pylori* and its diseases. It must be emphasized that these guidelines may not be applicable to all healthcare settings and may need to be adapted as more is learned about this infection.

All patients with long-standing dyspepsia, ulcer-like symptoms, severe upper gastrointestinal manifestations (vomiting, bleeding) or unexplained weight loss should undergo an oesophago-gastro-duodenoscopy. During this procedure appropriate biopsy samples should be obtained from all lesions. If no gastric lesions are detected, at the very least one biopsy specimen from the antrum and one from the cropus should be obtained.[61] If a rapid urease test is available, an additional specimen may be obtained to perform this test. If *H. pylori* is detected and the decision to treat it is made, confirmation of cure is optional in the absence of gastric lesions (i.e. if the patient is deemed to have non-ulcer dyspepsia). However, if a gastric or duodenal ulcer or a MALT lymphoma are detected, confirmation of cure is mandatory and can be done with a urea breath test. If this is not available, re-endoscopy with biopsies is recommended. Serology alone (unaccompanied by endoscopic examination) should not be used for the initial diagnosis of *H. pylori* infection, and must not be used to assess the results of treatment, since the decrease in antibody levels is slow and unpredictable.[62]

In asymptomatic patients who request determination of their *H. pylori* status, or in subjects who may be at risk for gastric cancer (e.g. patients from a high-risk area or relatives of a gastric cancer patient), an office-based immunoenzymatic or serological test may be adequate.[63] If such individuals are treated, confirmation of cure is generally not considered essential.

All the other tests described above (cytological preparations, immunohistochemical staining of biopsy specimens, PCR and bacterial culture) are usefully employed in research settings and experimental protocols. However, at present they do not have a useful place in the clinical investigation of *H. pylori* infection.

Acknowledgement

This work was supported by a grant from the Department of Veterans Affairs, Washington, DC, USA.

References

1. Genta RM, Graham DY. *Helicobacter pylori*: the new bug on the (paraffin) block. *Virchows Arch* 1994; **425**: 339-347.

2. Isaacson PG. Gastrointestinal lymphoma. *Hum Pathol* 1994; **25**: 1020-1029.

3. Wotherspoon AC, Doglioni C, Diss TC *et al.* Regression of primary low-grade B-cell gastric lymphoma of mucosa-associated lymphoid tissue type after eradication of *Helicobacter pylori*. *Lancet* 1993; **342**: 575-577.

4. Parsonnet J, Friedman GD, Vandersteen DP *et al.* *Helicobacter pylori* infection and the risk of gastric carcinoma. *N Engl J Med* 1991; **325**: 1127-1131.

5. Graham DY. Benefits from elimination of *Helicobacter pylori* infection include major reduction in the incidence of peptic ulcer disease, gastric cancer, and primary gastric lymphoma. *Prev Med* 1994; **23**: 712-716.

6. IARC Working Group on the Evaluation of Carcinogenic Risks to Humans. Schistomsomes, liver flukes and *Helicobacter pylori*. In: *IARC Monographs on the Evaluation of Carcinogenic Risks to Humans* 1994; **61**: 1-241.

7. Soll AH. Consensus conference. Medical treatment of peptic ulcer disease. Practice guidelines. Practice Parameters Committee of the American College of Gastroenterology. *JAMA* 1996; **275**: 622-629.

8. Cutler AF, Havstad S, Ma CK, Blaser MJ, Perez-Perez GI, Schubert TT. Accuracy of invasive and noninvasive tests to diagnose *Helicobacter pylori* infection. *Gastroenterology* 1995; **109**: 136-141.

9. Genta RM. Helicobacter pylori infection in gastric pathology. In: Weinstein RS, Graham AR (eds) *Advances in Pathology and Laboratory Medicine*. Mosby Yearbook, St Louis, 1994, pp. 443-465.

10. Guglielmetti P, Figura N, Rossolini A *et al.* The usefulness of the acridine-orange stain in identifying *Helicobacter pylori* in gastric biopsies. *Microbiologica* 1991; **14**: 131-134.

11. Loffeld RJ, Stobberingh E, Arends JW. A review of diagnostic techniques for *Helicobacter pylori* infection. *Dig Dis* 1993; **11**: 173-180.

12. Zaitoun AM. Use of Ramanowsky type (Diff-3) stain for detecting *Helicobacter pylori* in smears and tissue sections. *J Clin Pathol* 1992; **45**: 448-449.

13. Genta RM, Robason GO, Graham DY. Simultaneous visualization of *Helicobacter pylori* and gastric morphology: a new strain. *Hum Pathol* 1994; **25**: 221-226.

14. Hayama M, Shimizu T, Akamatsu Y, Ota H, Katsuyama T. Histological diagnosis of Helicobacter infection. *Prog Med* 1995; **15**: 783-790.

15. Iwaki H, Takahashi K, Ohtanaka K *et al.* Comparison of a new staining (Genta stain) and other stainings for the detection of *Helicobacter pylori* and development of a modified Genta stain. *Pathol Clin Med* 1995; **13**: 1171-1174.

16. Dixon MF, Genta RM, Yardley JH, Correa P *et al.* Classification and grading of gastritis: The Updated Sydney System. *Am J Surg Pathol* 1996; **20**: 1161-1181.

17. Loffeld RJ, Stobberingh E, Flendrig JA, Arends JW. *Helicobacter pylori* in gastric biopsy specimens. Comparison of culture, modified Giemsa stain, and immunohistochemistry. A retrospective study. *J Pathol* 1991; **165**: 69-73.

18. Cartun RW, Kryzmowski GA, Pedersen CA, Morin SG, Van Kruiningen HJ, Berman MM. Immunocytochemical identification of *Helicobacter pylori* in formalin-fixed gastric biopsies. *Mod Pathol* 1991; **4**: 498-502.

19. Cardillo MR, Agnelli M. Brush cytology in the endoscopic diagnosis of benign gastric ulcers. A useful adjunct to biopsy? *Arch Anat Cytol Pathol* 1990; **38**: 86-91.

20. Debongnie JC, Mairesse J, Donnay M, Dekoninck X. Touch cytology. A quick, simple, sensitive screening test in the diagnosis of infections of the gastrointestinal mucosa. *Arch Pathol Lab Med* 1994; **118**: 1115-1118.

21. Goodwin CS. *Helicobacter pylori*: 10th anniversary of its culture in April 1982. *Gut* 1993; **34**: 293-294.

22. Tee W, Fairley S, Smallwood R, Dwyer B. Comparative evaluation of three selective media and a nonselective medium for the culture of *Helicobacter pylori* from gastric biopsies. *J Clin Microbiol* 1991; **29**: 2587-2589.

23. Veenendaal RA, Lichtendahl-Bernards AT, Pena AS *et al.* Effect of transport medium and transportation time on culture of *Helicobacter pylori* from gastric biopsy specimens. *J Clin Pathol* 1993; **46**: 561-563.

24. Han SW, Flamm R, Hachem CY *et al.* Transport and storage of *Helicobacter pylori* from gastric mucosal biopsies and clinical isolates. *Eur J Clin Microbiol Infect Dis* 1995; **14**: 349-352.

25. Westblom TU, Phadnis S, Yang P, Czinn SJ. Diagnosis of *Helicobacter pylori* infection by means of a polymerase chain reaction assay for gastric juice aspirates. *Clin Infect Dis* 1993; **16**: 367-371.

26. Engstrand L, Nguyen AM, Graham DY, el-Zaatari FA. Reverse transcription and polymerase chain reaction

amplification of rRNA for detection of Helicobacter species. *J Clin Microbiol* 1992; **30**: 2295-2301.

27. Ho SA, Hoyle JA, Lewis FA *et al*. Direct polymerase chain reaction test for detection of *Helicobacter pylori* in humans and animals. *J Clin Microbiol* 1991; **29**: 2543-2549.

28. Bickley J, Owen RJ, Fraser AG, Pounder RE. Evaluation of the polymerase chain reaction for detecting the urease C gene of *Helicobacter pylori* in gastric biopsy samples and dental plaques. *J Med Microbiol* 1993; **39**: 338-344.

29. Wang JT, Lin JT, Sheu JC, Yang JC, Chen DS, Wang TH. Detection of *Helicobacter pylori* in gastric biopsy tissue by polymerase chain reaction. *Eur J Clin Microbiol Infect Dis* 1993; **12**: 367-371.

30. Roosendaal R, Kuipers EJ, van den Brule AJ *et al*. Importance of the fiberoptic endoscope cleaning procedure for detection of *Helicobacter pylori* in gastric biopsy specimens by PCR. *J Clin Microbiol* 1994; **32**: 1123-1126.

31. Costas M, Owen RJ, Bickley J, Morgan DR. Molecular techniques for studying the epidemiology of infection by *Helicobacter pylori*. *Scand J Gastroenterol* 1991; **181(Suppl)**: 20-32.

32. Klein PD, Graham DY, Gaillour A, Opekun AR, Smith EO. Water source as risk factor for *Helicobacter pylori* infection in Peruvian children. Gastrointestinal Physiology Working Group. *Lancet* 1991; **337**: 1503-1506.

33. van Zwet AA, Thijs TC, Kooistra-Smid AM, Schirm J, Snijder JA. Use of PCR with feces for detection of *Helicobacter pylori* infections in patients. *J Clin Microbiol* 1994; **32**: 1345-1348.

34. Lee N, Lee TT, Fang KM. Assessment of four rapid urease test systems for detection of *Helicobacter pylori* in gastric biopsy specimens. *Diagn Microbiol Infect Dis* 19??; **18**: 69-74.

35. Fraser AG, Ali MR, McCullough S, Yeates NJ, Haystead A. Diagnostic tests for *Helicobacter pylori* - can they help select patients for endoscopy? *N Z Med J* 1996; **109**: 95-98.

36. Marshall BJ, Warren JR, Francis GJ *et al*. Rapid urease test in the management of *Campylobacter pyloridis*-associated gastritis. *Am J Gastroenterol* 1987; **82**: 200-210.

37. Ng TM, Fock KM, Ho J *et al*. Clotest (rapid urease test) in the diagnosis of *Helicobacter pylori* infection. *Singapore Med J* 1992; **33**: 568-569.

38. Newell DG, Johnston BJ, Ali MH, Reed PI. An enzyme-linked immunosorbent assay for the serodiagnosis of *Campylobacter pylori*-associated gastritis. *Scand J Gastroenterol* 1988; **142(Suppl)**: 53-57.

39. von Wulffen H, Grote HJ, Gatermann S, Loning T, Berger B, Buhl C. Immunoblot analysis of immune response to *Campylobacter pylori* and its clinical associations. *J Clin Pathol* 1988; **41**: 653-659.

40. Maeland JA, Bevanger L, Enge J. Serological testing for campylobacteriosis with sera forwarded for Salmonella and Yersinia serology. *APMIS* 1993; **101**: 647-650.

41. Perez-Perez GI, Dworkin BM, Chodos JE, Blaser MJ. *Campylobacter pylori* antibodies in humans. *Ann Intern Med* 1988; **109**: 11-17.

42. Evans DJ, Jr, Evans DG, Graham DY, Klein PD. A sensitive and specific serologic test for detection of *Campylobacter pylori* infection. *Gastroenterology* 1989; **96**: 1004-1008.

43. Best LM, Veldhuyzen van Zanten SJ, Sherman PM, Bezanson GS. Serological detection of *Helicobacter pylori* antibodies in children and their parents. *J Clin Microbiol* 1994; **32**: 1193-1196.

44. Kosunen TU, Seppala K, Sarna S, Sipponen P. Diagnostic value of decreasing IgG, IgA and IgM antibody titres after eradication of *Helicobacter pylori* (see comments). *Lancet* 1992; **339**: 893-895.

45. Talley NJ, Kost L, Haddad A, Zinsmeister AR. Comparison of commercial serological tests for detection of *Helicobacter pylori* antibodies. *J Clin Microbiol* 1992; **30**: 3146-3150.

46. Luzza F, Maletta M, Imeneo M *et al*. Salivary-specific immunoglobulin G in the diagnosis of *Helicobacter pylori* infection in dyspeptic patients. *Am J Gastroenterol* 1995; **90**: 1820-1823.

47. Luzza F, Imeneo M, Maletta M *et al*. Isotypic analysis of specific antibody response in serum, saliva, gastric and rectal homogenates of *Helicobacter pylori*-infected patients. *FEMS Immunol Med Microbiol* 1995; **10**: 285-288.

48. Wienholt MG, Erbling MC, Bennetts RW, Galen EA, Cimler BM. Detection of antibodies to *Helicobacter pylori* using oral fluid specimens. *Ann NY Acad Sci* 1993; **694**: 340-342.

49. Graham DY, Klein PD, Evans DG *et al*. Simple noninvasive method to test efficacy of drugs in the eradication of *Helicobacter pylori* infection: the example of combined bismuth subsalicyclate and nitrofurantoin. *Am J Gastroenterol* 1991; **86**: 1158-1162.

50. Marshall BJ, Surveyor I. Carbon-14 urea breath test for the diagnosis of *Campylobacter pylori*-associated gastritis. *J Nucl Med* 1988; **29**: 11-16.

51. Raju GS, Smith MJ, Morton D, Bardhan KD. Mini-dose (1 µCi) ^{14}C-urea breath test for the detection of *Helicobacter pylori*. *Am J Gastroenterol* 1994; **89**: 1027-1031.

52. Peura DA, Pambianco DJ, Dye KR *et al.* Microdose ^{14}C-urea breath test offers diagnosis of *Helicobacter pylori* in 10 minutes. *Am J Gastroenterol* 1996; **91**: 233-238.

53. Yamashiro Y, Oguchi S, Otsuka Y, Nagata S, Shioya T, Shimizu T. *Helicobacter pylori* colonization in children with peptic ulcer disease. III. Diagnostic value of the ^{13}C-urea breath test to detect gastric *H. pylori* colonization. *Acta Paediatr Jpn* 1995; **37**: 12-16.

54. Slomianski A, Schubert T, Cutler AR. [^{13}C]urea breath test to confirm eradication of *Helicobacter pylori*. *Am J Gastroenterol* 1995; **90**: 224-226.

55. Fox JG. *In vivo* models of *Helicobacter pylori* infections. In: Hurt RH, Tytgat G (Eds). *Helicobacter Pylori: Basic Mechanisms of Clinical Cure*. Kluwer, Dordrecht, 1994, pp. 3-27.

56. Lee A, Fox JG, Otto G, Murphy J. A small animal model of human *Helicobacter pylori* active chronic gastritis. *Gastroenterology* 1990; **99**: 1315-1323.

57. Enno A, O'Rourke JL, Howlett CR, Jack A, Dixon MF, Lee A. MALToma-like lesions in the murine gastric mucosa after long-term infection with *Helicobacter felis*. A mouse model of *Helicobacter pylori*-induced gastric lymphoma. *Am J Pathol* 1995; **147**: 217-222.

58. Yokota K, Kurebayashi Y, Takayama *et al.* Colonization of *Helicobacter pylori* in the gastric mucosa of Mongolian gerbils. *Microbiol Immunol* 1991; **35**: 475-480.

59. Lee A. Animal models and vaccine development (review). *Balliere's Clinics in Gastroenterology* 1995; **9**: 615-632.

60. Atherton JC, Spiller RC. The urea breath test for *Helicobacter pylori*. *Gut* 1994; **35**: 723-725.

61. Genta RM, Graham DY. Comparison of biopsy sites for the histopathologic diagnosis of *Helicobacter pylori*: a topographic study of *H. pylori* density and distribution. *Gastrointest Endosc* 1994; **40**: 342-345.

62. Cutler AF, Prasad VM. Long-term follow-up of *Helicobacter pylori* serology after successful eradication. *Am J Gastroenterol* 1996; **91**: 85-88.

63. Blecker U, Lanciers S, Hauser B, Mehta DI, Vandenplas Y. Serology as a valid screening test for *Helicobacter pylori* infection in asymptomatic subjects. *Arch Pathol Lab Med* 1995; **119**: 30-32.

12

Doppler sonography

Carlo Martinoli and Lorenzo E Derchi

Summary

Doppler sonography has made possible the noninvasive investigation of the hemodynamics of the gastrointestinal circulation in normal and pathological conditions. Information on the presence, direction and characteristics of blood flow can be reliably obtained in splanchnic vessels. Spectral evaluation of Doppler tracings can provide insight into the vascular impedance of downstream circulation and allows accurate calculation of peak velocity, mean velocity and flow volume in large arteries and veins. Quantitative data can be successfully used to estimate hemodynamic changes occurring during physiological stimulations and in a variety of bowel diseases. Increased splanchnic blood flow, as reflected in duplex Doppler (DDUS) analysis of mesenteric vessels, and mural hypervascularity seen with colour Doppler (CDUS), can be recognized in patients with acute inflammatory bowel disease. Although the relationship of hypervascularity to the level of disease awaits further evaluation, detection of both spectral changes in supplying vessels and mural hypervascularity may improve diagnostic specificity in evaluating patients with focal bowel wall thickening.

Introduction

Before the 1980s, knowledge of the mechanisms involved in splanchnic hemodynamics came mainly from experimental investigations in animals; direct evaluation of the blood flow supplying the gastrointestinal tract in humans was limited by the invasive nature and complexity of available techniques.[1] Measurements in humans made use of surgically implanted electromagnetic flowmeters,[2,3] dye dilution techniques[4-6] or catheters.[7] The development and refinement of Doppler technology has allowed the noninvasive evaluation of splanchnic hemodynamics. Ultrasound (US) waves transmitted through the intact skin are harmless, painless and do not affect blood flow. Different Doppler techniques can be used. Duplex Doppler (DDUS) systems allow measurement of flow velocity and, by simultaneously measuring the cross-sectional area of the vessel, provide quantitative information about blood flow volume.[8,9] Colour (CDUS) and power (PDUS) Doppler systems can depict flow in vessels and demonstrate tissue hyperperfusion associated with inflammation and tumours.[10,11] In other words, the first one is a functional technique which provides clinically useful

insight into pathophysiology; the second has much in common with angiography but without the need for contrast media and the ionizing radiation hazard. Several reports have demonstrated the reliability of these Doppler methods in evaluating gastrointestinal hemodynamics in normal subjects and patients with a variety of diseases, even though some inherent limitations of reproducibility and sensitivity and possible sources of error have been pointed out.[12,13] The accuracy of Doppler studies heavily depends on a good understanding of the basic principles of Doppler and hemodynamics, together with a good knowledge of the examination technique.

This chapter reviews quantitative duplex Doppler data analysis applied to the study of splanchnic hemodynamics as well as the correct methodology to investigate the mural flow in the bowel loops with colour Doppler equipment. The current range of clinical applications of Doppler techniques to the study of the gastrointestinal tract is briefly described.

Methods

Conventional DDUS and CDUS scanners equipped with low-frequency (3.5-5 MHz) transabdominal transducers can evaluate blood flow in splanchnic vessels.[14,15] DDUS devices combine a grey-scale (B-mode) imager and a pulsed Doppler unit with real-time spectral analysis. The grey-scale mode image allows visualization of the vessel of interest. Thus the vessel can be identified, the sample volume of the pulsed Doppler beam can be correctly placed into its lumen and Doppler spectra reporting velocity-related frequency shifts versus time waveforms are obtained. The insonation angle between the incident Doppler beam and the longitudinal axis of the vessel is visually checked and is the basis for the computer-derived calculation of duplex blood flow parameters based on Doppler frequency shift (ΔF).[8] It allows the system to compute the blood flow velocity (cm/s) in accordance with the Doppler equation:

$$V = \Delta Fc / 2F_o cos\theta$$

where F_o is the incident Doppler frequency, θ is the Doppler angle, and c the US velocity in soft tissue Fs. The major disadvantage of duplex scanning is that flow is not evaluated simultaneously throughout the whole US image but rather is sampled at a particular location selected by the examiner. Consequently, focal regions of abnormal flow can be overlooked.

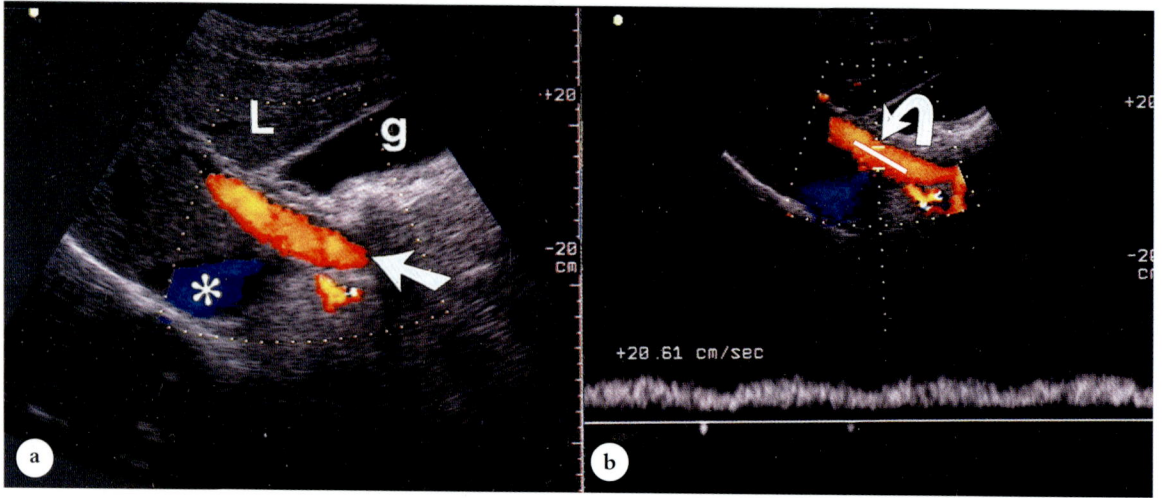

Figure 12.1 – Representative (a) colour and (b) duplex Doppler images of the normal portal vein. In (a) the hepatopetal portal flow (arrow), directed towards the transducer, is shown in red. Inferior to this, flow within the inferior vena cava (★) is in the opposite direction and is represented in blue. L = liver; g = gallbladder. In (b) subsequent spectral Doppler analysis of the portal vein is obtained by placing the sample volume (curved arrow) into the portal lumen and adjusting the angle bar correction for velocity measurements along the longitudinal axis of the vessel. The spectrum obtained is representative of velocity versus time waveforms and shows the portal flow to be continuous with only slight phasic changes.

CDUS equipment combines grey-scale imaging with two-dimensional mapping of flow information in real-time.[8] Flow is depicted throughout the field of view by superimposing different colours on the two-dimensional grey-scale image. Conventionally, red indicates motion towards the transducer and blue away from it. Colour hues parallel the values of Doppler shifts detected by the instrument and are usually representative of the mean velocity. CDUS systems can identify intraparenchymal vessels too small to be imaged with grey-scale US and are better at detecting the presence or absence of flow in peripheral vessels compared with DDUS. Nevertheless, the shades of red and blue are not precise indicators of velocity variation and, especially in the evaluation of splanchnic vessels, degradation of the image quality often occurs as a result of colour artifacts induced by the presence of intestinal gas.[16] Recently, power Doppler technology has been introduced as a new colour system that displays the total integrated Doppler shifts to calculate the amplitude of the Doppler signal, which is proportional to the number of moving red blood cells.[17] A major benefit of this method of flow mapping over mean-frequency shift colour Doppler is its higher sensitivity to slowly flowing blood. However, in the power Doppler mode, without comparison of the phase of the incident and reflected beam, no indication of the direction and velocity of the flowing blood is given.

Optimal results are usually obtained by the complementary use of CDUS and DDUS, the former as a real-time two-dimensional display and the latter as a temporal display required for quantitation studies (Fig. 12.1a, b). According to the method used, the Doppler results range from the highly qualitative to the precisely quantitative. Both techniques allow assessment of the presence and direction of flow, and identify distinct characteristics of flow (laminar vs. turbulent; plug vs. parabolic profile), or focal differences in velocity within the vessel (high velocity jets in stenoses).[12] Quantitative blood flow parameters, including peak velocity, mean velocity, flow volume, flow impedance and pulsatility can only be obtained from the DDUS spectrum.[12] A step-by-step guide to the complex and time-consuming methodology used in Doppler blood flow measurement is shown in Table 12.1.

Accurate measurements of blood flow velocity are only possible if the angle of the incident Doppler beam with respect to the vessel axis is carefully assessed on the screen and kept less than 60°.[14] This requires visualization of the vessel for a minimum length of 3-4 cm.[13] Inaccurate measurement of the angle of insonation can be an important source of error in the calculation of flow velocity. This possible error increases exponentially with increasing angle and becomes unacceptable when the angle is >60°.

Table 12.1 – Step-by-step guide for flow measurement in DDUS

To obtain adequate spectral Doppler tracings

1. Identify the vessel of interest with US or CDUS;
2. Place the transducer on the skin to image the vessel longitudinally with an angle <60°;
3. Put the sample volume in the vessel site selected for measurement;
4. Adjust the sample volume to encompass the entire diameter of the vessel;
5. Set carefully the angle bar correction along the direction of flow;
6. Use the most clear-cut tracings for flow measurements.

To calculate the maximum (peak systolic) velocity

7. Follow steps 1–3, 5–6;
8. Select the cursor for velocity calculation provided by the software menu of the scanner and position it at the maximum ΔF reported in the Doppler spectrum.

To calculate the mean velocity

9. Follow steps 1–6;
10. Trace (manually or automatically) the superior edge of the spectrum along a cardiac cycle with the cursor provided by the software menu. The mean velocity is computed from the outer and inner envelope of velocities.

To calculate the flow volume

11. Follow steps 1–6 and 10;
12. Set calipers for calculation of cross-sectional area across the vessel diameter. The flow volume is computed by the software menu of the scanner.

To calculate the resistive index

13. Follow steps 1–3 and 6;
14. Select the calipers provided by the software menu for calculation of resistive index and, in a single cardiac cycle, set one at the systolic peak and the other at the maximum ΔF in end diastole.

To calculate the pulsatility index

15. Follow steps 1–3 and 6;
16. Trace (manually or automatically) the superior edge of the spectrum with a cursor provided by the software menu for calculation of pulsatility index to compute the time average of the maximum ΔFs over one cardiac cycle;
17. In the same cardiac cycle, set the calipers at the systolic peak and at the maximum ΔF in end diastole.

For example, in the case of an angle of 45°, an error in angle measurement of 5° induces a final error of 9% in the calculation of velocity; at 70°, the same difference results in a 25% error.[12] On the other hand, at angles less than 20°, these errors are reduced and the calculation of flow velocity is quite accurate.

In clinical practice, optimal selection of the insonation angle is not always possible in the abdominal circulation because of anatomical variations and interference by intestinal gas which may obscure the vascular segment most appropriate for measurement.[18] Anatomical difficulties can be overcome by changing the patient position and/or adjusting the probe to obtain a suitable angle.

The calculation of the mean velocity (mean of the outer and inner envelope of the Doppler spectrum) requires, besides selecting an appropriate angle, the accurate insonation of the vessel using a sample volume whose size nearly corresponds to the vessel diameter.[12,19] In this way, the mean velocity can be determined directly on Doppler spectral analysis without making assumptions regarding the spatial flow profile in the vessel. In fact, an incomplete insonation of the vessel or too high levels of band-pass filters results in an overestimation of blood flow velocity due to the partial loss of peripheral slow components of flow from the sample volume.[12,14] As an alternative to this method, the mean velocity is calculated as the maximal velocity value multiplied by a correction factor of 0.57 for parabolic flow obtained from an experimental circulation model.[20,21]

To calculate the flow volume (Q), the mean velocity (V_m) is multiplied by the cross-sectional area (A) of the vessel,[12] using the equation:

$$Q = V_m A$$

The cross-sectional area is obtained from the transverse image of the vessel visualized on grey-scale US after defining its major and minor axes. The accuracy of diameter measurements is critical since the area depends on the product of diameters and, therefore, any given percentage of error in estimating diameters will result in an exponential error in estimating flow volume: for example, a 1 mm uncertainty in the measurement of the diameter of a 10 mm vessel may cause a flow error of about 20%.[12] It has, however, been demonstrated that the diameter obtained by repeated measurements can decrease the final error of the flow volume calculation to as low as 10%.[22] The aspect ratio of a vessel represents an additional challenging problem in the measurement of the cross-sectional area. In fact, most vessels, and especially compressible veins, are not circular in section. By assuming an elliptical vessel to be circular, one can introduce an important error. For example, for an elliptical vessel with a major diameter 50% longer than the minor one, a 50% error can result.[19] However, the machine's computer software can alternately calculate the area using the geometric formula of a circle ($\pi D^2/4$) or an ellipse ($\pi D_1 D_2/4$).[23]

In summary, some bias is difficult to control and may influence the calculation of angle-derived measurements based on Doppler spectral analysis and many sources of error and variability may result especially when calculation of flow volume rate is attempted. In spite of all the efforts to standardize these measurements, the Doppler technique has still to be considered a subjective method for flow quantitation.[13] Currently, the results of duplex Doppler methodology from different institutions and equipment are not universally acceptable and it is possible that the velocity values expressed by Doppler measurements do not correspond to the actual flow in a vessel.[13] Intra- and inter-observer variability applied to the study of portal venous flow range between 8% and 18% and no guidelines are available as to how many measurements should be averaged in velocity calculations.[18,24] As a general rule, intra-observer variability does not seem to affect the determination of rapid and large hemodynamic changes within a short period of time, but produces low precision in monitoring chronic changes.[18] In addition, a recent paper has demonstrated poor inter-observer agreement, at least in part due to the different levels of experience of operators.[25] This implies that follow-up examinations should be carried out using the same equipment and with the same transducer, and that measurements taken in different institutions are not comparable. Before accepting Doppler as a method for measuring changes in flow characteristics, investigators must assess its variability within their patient populations using a controlled technique to avoid possible bias.[18] In clinical studies, these problems are magnified in non-cooperative patients in whom meticulous measurements are not always possible. A lack of cooperation, particularly in maintaining suspended respiration and remaining motionless for at least 10 seconds, must be regarded as exclusion criteria for quantitative Doppler studies.[13]

In addition to quantitative estimates of blood flow derived from the calculation of blood flow velocity, semiquantitative indices have proven increasingly helpful in defining many physiological and pathological changes of splanchnic flows. Hemodynamically, these indices describe the shape of the Doppler waveform and reflect the impedance of the vascular bed downstream.[8] Practically, this means that changes within peripheral arteries that supply a given organ, but are too small to be imaged directly, can influence flow characteristics upstream. This is of great significance for the application of Doppler techniques to the study of the gastrointestinal tract in which the distal vascular bed of the mesentery and bowel loops is almost inaccessible to direct US scanning. Although numerous indices have been proposed in the literature, the pulsatility and resistive indices are most commonly referred to as indicators of vascular impedance. The pulsatility index, described by Gosling et al,[26] is obtained by the following ratio:

(peak-systolic velocity) - (end-diastolic velocity) / (time average of the maximum ΔFs over a cardiac cycle).

As this is a ratio it does not matter whether velocities or kiloHertz shifts are used. The resistive index, described by Pourcelot,[27] is equal to:

(peak-systolic velocity) - (end-diastolic velocity) / (peak-systolic velocity)

Although the pulsatility index has the advantage of being relatively insensitive to heart rate, the resistive index is easier to calculate without the need to determine the mean velocity.[12] Pulsatility and resistive indexes should be calculated for each of at least three cardiac cycles and an average value taken.

The investigation of the circulatory dynamics in the human intestine is essentially based on the evaluation of spectral waveforms from a) the coeliac axis (CA), the superior (SMA) and inferior (IMA) mesenteric arteries and b) the superior mesenteric (SMV) and portal (PV) veins. Patients are prepared for Doppler studies with overnight fasting. The CA and SMA can be easily identified just ventral to the aorta.[28,29] Intervening gas and obesity can prevent their visualization. To avoid flow turbulence at the vessel origin, Doppler recordings are generally taken from a straight segment 1-2 cm distal to the origin of these arteries but proximal to the first side branches, where the most favourable vessel-beam angle is found.[30,31] Likewise SMA, recent US studies have shown that the initial segment of the IMA can be reliably detected in the great majority (up to 92%) of patients.[32,33] To eliminate low frequencies related to vessel wall movement in the study, the sampling gate can be adjusted to encompass as much of the lumen of the vessel as possible without touching the vessel wall and a high band-pass filter of 200 Hz can be selected.[32]

Recent US studies have shown that the initial segment of the IMA can be reliably detected in the great majority (up to 92%) of patients.[32,33] The IMA must be sought by scanning the aorta in cross section, starting from the renal arteries and ending at the aortic bifurcation. The vessel originates at the left anterior aspect of the aorta. Dopper flow examination of the PV is generally performed by slightly oblique right paramedian scanning in order to visualize the mesenteric-portal axis.[34] In order to avoid any fluctuation in flow velocity, velocity measurements must be obtained while patients are holding their breath in expiration for at least 4-6 seconds long, a condition which may be easily standardized and in which the portal venous flow appears to be more constant.[14]

Improvements in the sensitivity of CDUS equipment have made possible the visualization of small distal vessels within the bowel wall and the adjacent mesentery using both transabdominal and endorectal high-resolution transducers.[10,35,36] Analysis of mural

vascularity requires US evidence of focal bowel wall thickening and accurate scanning technique, including graded compression and optimized sensitivity of the CDUS system with maximal power and gain, maximal gate, low pulse repetition frequency and lowest band-pass filters.[16] The colour box must be kept as small as possible to minimize the effects of flash artifacts from vascular pulsatility and bowel peristalsis and to maximize temporal resolution. Similarly, breath-hold imaging reduces flash artifacts from respiratory motion. In order not to misinterpret flash artifacts as true flow, mural blood flow should be recognized only if it is consistently reproducible in the same location with continuous observation and after DDUS analysis.[16] Despite a higher sensitivity to tissue motion and consequent possible artifacts, detection of intramural gastrointestinal vascularity can be substantially improved with the use of PDUS technology.[37]

The recent introduction of endocavitary transducers connected to fibre-optic endoscopes has allowed new perspectives to be seen in DDUS and CDUS evaluation of peri-oesophageal vessels.[38-40] The endoscopic transducer is directed laterally with respect to the fibroscope axis and the resultant US image is longitudinal to the major axis of the oesophagus. Information on direction, velocity of flow and the presence of turbulences in the azygos system, downstream of the confluence of all the hepatofugal collaterals, can be obtained in most cases.[40]

Application to animal studies

Doppler US has been introduced as a noninvasive means to measure transcutaneously blood flow velocity in vessels. Animal studies have been performed to validate the accuracy of spectral measurements compared with those obtained with invasive techniques, e.g. electromagnetic flowmetry[15,21,41] and cineangiography.[20] Significant correlations were observed between pulsed Doppler and these invasive techniques in measurements of flow velocity from both the SMA[15] and PV[20] over a wide range of values in dogs. The application of Doppler studies to experimental animals is quite similar to the techniques described above for humans. According to the body mass of the animal examined, a different transducer shape and US beam frequency can be selected. As a general rule, small animals are better imaged using

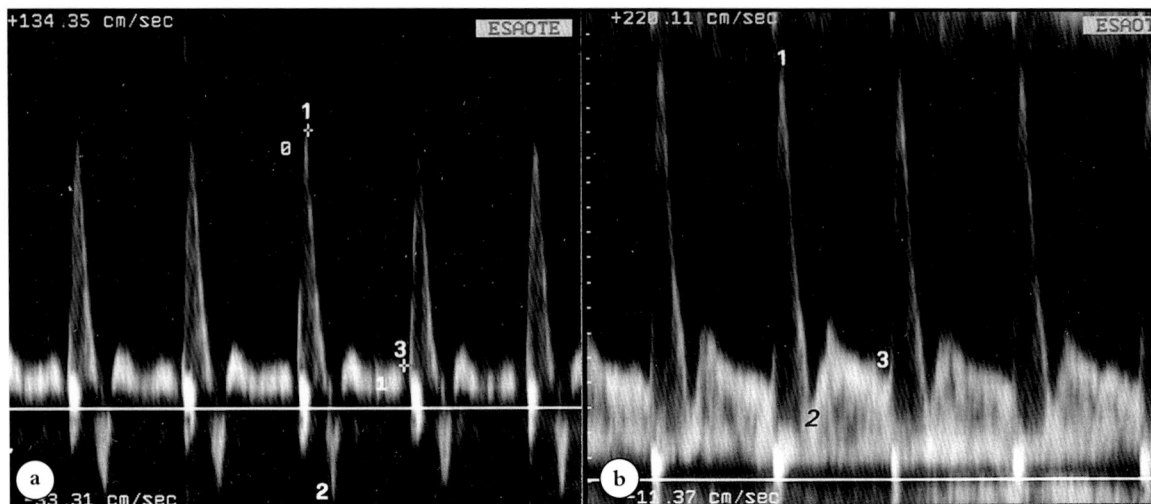

Figure 12.2 – Typical waveforms obtained from the superior mesenteric artery in healthy subject (a) at rest and (b) 30 minutes after a meal. Note the increases in both peak-systolic velocity (1) and end-diastolic velocity (3), and loss of reverse flow (2) after feeding.

smaller probes and higher frequencies than for humans. Small-parts transducers with high US frequency (up to 20 MHz) are now commercially available and can be readily adapted for experimental uses in small animals.

Due to the intrinsic noninvasive nature of Doppler techniques and because anaesthesia is not required, most physiological studies over the last decade have been conducted in humans. However, new interest may focus on animal studies when Doppler techniques are used to provide insight into the pathophysiological processes in simulated conditions such as ischaemia and other pathological conditions inducing vessel stenosis and occlusion, as well as in testing the effect of drugs.

Results and discussion

The ability of Doppler US to measure noninvasively blood flow changes has provided insight into the mechanisms regulating human splanchnic blood flow under different physiological conditions and in response to disease. As regards physiological studies, DDUS has been shown to measure blood flow alterations in the SMA and PV after a meal in conscious subjects.[14,42-46] Doppler techniques have shown that there is at least a three-fold increase in blood flow volume in the SMA in response to feeding compared with fasting values.[28] In fasting subjects, the normal Doppler flow pattern of the SMA is characterized by a high systolic flow, followed by a short reverse flow in the early diastole and forward flow in end diastole (Fig. 12.2a).[43] After a meal, flow is increased mostly by the selective elevation of the diastolic component as a result of arteriolar vasodilatation of the intestinal vascular bed (Fig. 12.2b).[14,42-46] This phenomenon can be also demonstrated after administration of glucagon.[44] According to different meal types, the increase in flow appears to be maximal 20-30 min after the test meal and persists for at least 90 min.[44] After a meal, a significant increase in flow volume (30-125%),[14,42] can be observed in the PV. In healthy subjects, this seems to be essentially due to the increased inflow from the mesenteric arterial bed.[28] As assessed by DDUS, the arterial response to a test meal is reduced or absent in patients with intestinal angina.[28,47] In patients with liver cirrhosis, blood flow is basally increased in the SMA as a result of the hyperdynamic flow state of the disease,[15] and the PV flow response after meal is less marked than in normal subjects as a probable consequence of congestion and a lack of compliance of splanchnic venous vessels.[14,48] Doppler US has been used to analyse the modulatory effects of drugs, such as glucagon, secretin, octreotide, β-blockers and other vasoactive substances on splanchnic circulation in different experimental settings.[42,49-52] Additionally, as far as the intestinal hemodynamics are concerned, DDUS has proved a simple method for evaluating splanchnic flow changes during physical exercise.

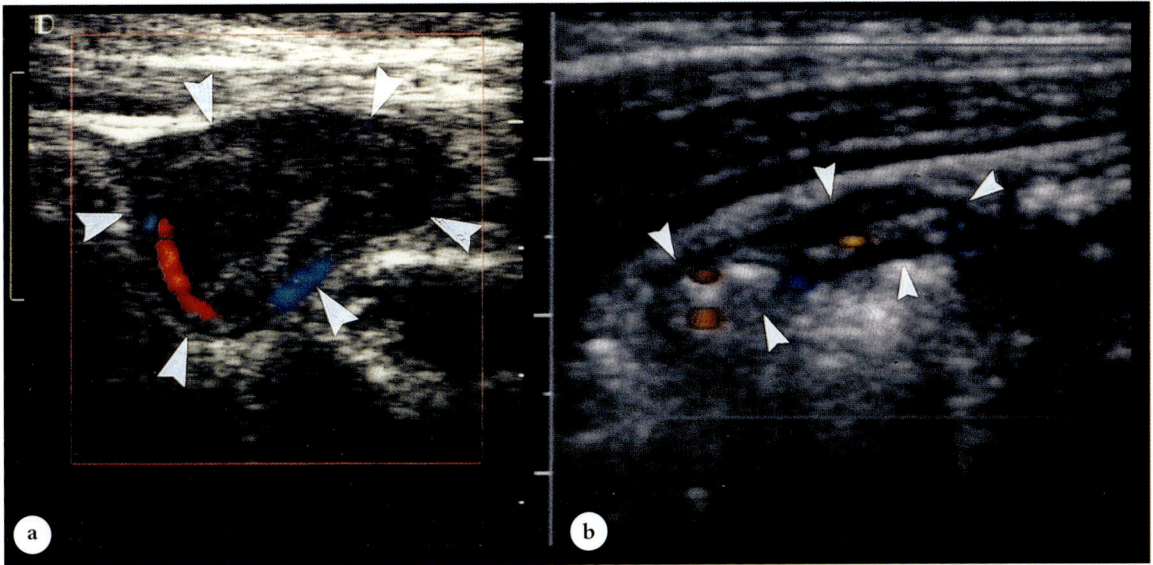

Figure 12.3 – Colour Doppler images of inflammatory bowel diseases. Intramural colour signals of flow are demonstrated in an involved bowel loop (arrowheads) of a 45-year-old patient with active Crohn's disease (a) and in an inflamed nonperforating appendix (arrowheads) of an 8-year-old boy (b).

On the basis of presence or absence of blood flow, the patency of splanchnic vessels can be reliably assessed with CDUS and DDUS. CDUS has improved the sensitivity of spectral analysis in detecting either nonocclusive PV thrombosis or PV branch occlusion.[53-55] In chronic PV thrombosis, cavernous transformation can be accurately demonstrated with CDUS and PDUS by showing numerous periportal tortuous vessels with continuous venous flow.[56] US and Doppler studies of mesenteric vessels can give useful information in the study of bowel obstruction. In midgut malrotation, the SMA lies anteriorly or on the right of the SMV.[57] In duodenal or afferent loop obstruction, the superior mesenteric vessels are displaced anteriorly by the obstructed duodenal loop which crosses the midline interposed between them and the aorta.[58] In bowel strangulation following volvulus and intestinal infarction, Doppler analysis can detect no flow or flow with very low or absent diastolic component in the SMA, consistent with a high resistance vascular bed.[59] Unfortunately, these pathological conditions present with air-filled obstructed loops in the mesogastrium and US and Doppler exploration of mesenteric vessels can be reliably performed in a minority of cases only. In contrast, in patients with chronic intestinal ischaemia, Doppler studies can play a role in identifying flow-reducing mesenteric arterial stenoses. A peak-systolic velocity >275 cm/s was described as the cut-off value to predict a diameter-reducing SMA stenosis of 70% or more.[60,61] In neonates predisposed to necrotizing enterocolitis, significant changes in blood flow velocity in the SMA and estimated flow volume have been described.[62]

In acute inflammation, the increased blood perfusion to the inflamed bowel and surrounding tissues can manifest itself in several ways. There may be evidence of increased mural vascularity, decreased arterial resistence, increased arterial and venous velocities or loss of venous phasic pattern.[10] The pathophysiology of inflammation is relatively uniform and the vascular response is independent of aetiology and the affected intestinal segment. In Crohn's disease, CDUS can show increased bowel-wall and mesenteric blood flow (Fig. 12.3a).[10,16,30,35,63-67] The flow volume in the SMA is elevated when Crohn's disease is active and correlates well with the disease activity assessed by the Crohn's disease activity index.[30] Other inflammatory bowel conditions, such as acute bacterial infections, acute diverticolitis, ulcerative and pseudo-membranous colitis and cytomegalovirus infections, as well as intestinal tumours, can cause increased mural blood flow.[16,37] In the acute abdomen, DDUS and CDUS may prove useful in differentiating ischaemic from inflammatory lesions in patients with focal bowel wall thickening.[37] Likewise, in paediatric intussusception the presence or absence of blood flow in the intussusceptum as shown by CDUS seems to be a promising predictor of the success of pneumatic or surgical reduction.[68,69] Absence of flow indicates that necrotic changes have occurred in the intussusceptum, and that vigorous reduction should be not attempted.[68,69] Acute appendicitis is usually accompanied by a low resistance hypervascular pattern within the appendix and mesoappendix on CDUS (Fig. 12.3b).[70-72] In necrosis and perforation, the vascularity decreases and few or no Doppler signals are found, especially at the appendiceal tip which is usually the site of perforation.[63,72] Because perforation leads to inflammation of the peritoneum, peri-appendiceal hyperemia can be demonstrated in the adjacent right lower quadrant bowel loops, bladder wall and soft tissues.[63,72]

Evaluation of tumour neoangiogenesis with Doppler techniques has recently been performed in gastrointestinal tumours using transabdominal probes and for rectal wall masses using endorectal US.[16,36,73] Preliminary experience indicates that endorectal CDUS may offer information in discriminating hypervascular recurrent or residual tumours from hypovascular surgical scarring.[73]

References

1. Granger DN, Kvietys PR. Recent advances in measurement of gastrointestinal blood flow. *Gastroenterology* 1985; **88**: 1073-1076.

2. Schenk WG, Dedichen H. Electronic measurement of blood flow. *Am J Surg* 1967; **114**: 111-118.

3. Schenk WG, McDonald KE, Camp FA, Pollock L. The measurement of regional blood flow. *J Thorac Cardiovasc Surg* 1963; **46**: 50-56.

4. Caesar J, Shaldon S, Chiandussi L *et al.* The use of indocyanin green in the measurement of hepatic blood flow and as a test of hepatic function. *Clin Sci* 1961; **21**: 43-57.

5. Huet PM, Lavoie P, Viallet A. Simultaneous estimation of hepatic and portal blood flows by an indicator dilution technique. *J Lab Clin Med* 1973; **83**: 836-846.

6. Bosch J, Groszmann RJ. Measurement of the azygos venous blood flow by a continuous thermodilution technique. An index of blood flow through gastroesophageal collaterals in cirrhosis. *Hepatology* 1984; **4**: 424-429.

7. Okuda K, Suzuki K, Husha H *et al.* Percutaneous transhepatic catheterization of the portal vein for the study of portal hemodynamics and shunts. *Gastroenterology* 1977; **73**: 279-284.

8. Taylor KJW, Holland S. Doppler US. Part I. Basic principles, instrumentation and pitfalls. *Radiology* 1990; **174**: 297-307.

9. Scoutt LM, Zawin ML, Taylor KJW. Doppler US. Part II. Clinical applications. *Radiology* 1990; **174**: 309-319.

10. Stavros AT, Rapp CL, Thickman D. Sonography of inflammatory conditions. *Ultrasound Q* 1995; **13**: 1-26.

11. Newman JS, Adler RS, Bude RO, Rubin JM. Detection of soft-tissue hyperemia: value of power Doppler sonography. *Am J Radiol* 1994; **163**: 385-389.

12. Burns PN, Jaffe CC. Quantitative flow measurements with Doppler ultrasound: techniques, accuracy and limitations. *Radiol Clin North Am* 1985; **23**: 641-657.

13. Bolondi L, Gaiani S, Barbara L. Accuracy and reproducibility of portal flow measurement by Doppler US. *J Hepatol* 1991; **13**: 269-273.

14. Gaiani S, Bolondi L, Li Bassi S, Santi V, Zironi G, Barbara L. Effect of meal on portal hemodynamics in healthy humans and in patients with chronic liver disease. *Hepatology* 1989; **9**: 815-819.

15. Sato S, Ohnishi K, Sugita S, Okuda K. Splenic artery and superior mesenteric artery blood flow: nonsurgical Doppler US measurement in healthy subjects and patients with chronic liver disease. *Radiology* 1987; **164**: 347-352.

16. Jeffrey RB Jr, Sommer FG, Debatin JF. Color Doppler sonography of focal gastrointestinal lesions: initial clinical experience. *J Ultrasound Med* 1994; **13**: 473-478.

17. Rubin JM, Bude RO, Carson PL, Bree RL, Adler RS. Power Doppler: a potentially useful alternative to mean-frequency based color Doppler sonography. *Radiology* 1994; **190**: 853-856.

18. Sabbà C, Weltin GG, Cicchetti DV *et al.* Observer variability in echo-Doppler measurements of portal flow in cirrhotic patients and normal volunteers. *Gastroenterology* 1990; **98**: 1603-1611.

19. Gill RW. Pulsed Doppler with B-mode imaging for quantitating blood flow measurement. *Ultrasound Med Biol* 1979; **5**: 223-235.

20. Ohnishi K, Saito M, Koen H, Nakayama T, Nomura F, Okuda K. Pulsed Doppler flow as a criterion of portal venous velocity: comparison with cineangiographic measurements. *Radiology* 1985; **154**: 495-498.

21. Moriyasu F, Nishida O, Ban N *et al.* Clinical application of an ultrasonic duplex system in the quantitative measurement of portal blood flow. *J Clin Ultrasound* 1986; **14**: 579-588.

22. Eik-Nes SH, Marsal K, Kristoffersen K. Methodology and basic problems related to blood flow studies in the human fetus. *Ultrasound Med Biol* 1984; **10**: 329-337.

23. Sabbà C, Ferraioli G, Buonamico P *et al.* Echo-Doppler evaluation of acute flow changes in portal hypertensive patients: flow velocity as a reliable parameter. *J Hepatol* 1992; **15:** 356-360.

24. De Vries PJ, Van Hattum J, Hoekstra JBL, De Hooge P. Duplex Doppler measurements of portal venous flow in normal subjects: inter- and intraobserver variability. *J Hepatol* 1991; **13:** 358-363.

25. Sabbà C, Merkel C, Zoli M *et al.* Interobserver and interequipment variability of echo-Doppler examination of the portal vein: effect of a cooperative training program. *Hepatology* 1995; **21:** 428-433.

26. Gosling RG, King DH, Newman DL, Woodcock JP. Transcutaneous measurement of arterial blood velocity by ultrasound. In: *Ultrasonics for Industry Conference Papers*. IPC, Guildford, 1969, pp. 16-32.

27. Pourcelot L. Applications cliniques de l'examen Doppler transcutane. In: Peronneau P (Ed) *Velocimètre Ultrasonore Doppler*, Vol 34. Inserm, Paris 1974; pp. 780-785.

28. Jäger K, Bollinger A, Valli C, Ammann R. Measurement of mesenteric blood flow by duplex scanning. *J Vasc Surg* 1986; **3:** 462-469.

29. Taylor GA. Blood flow in the superior mesenteric artery: estimation with Doppler US. *Radiology* 1990; **174:** 15-16.

30. van Oostayen J, Wasser MNJM, van Hogezand RA, Griffioen G, de Roos A. Activity of Crohn disease assessed by measurement of superior mesenteric artery flow with Doppler US. *Radiology* 1994; **193:** 551-554.

31. Qamar MI, Read AE, Skidmore R, Evans JM, Wells PNT. Transcutaneous Doppler ultrasound measurement of superior mesenteric artery blood flow in man. *Gut* 1986; **27:** 100-105.

32. Denys AL, Lafortune M, Aubin B, Burke M, Breton G. Doppler sonography of the inferior mesenteric artery: a preliminary study. *J Ultrasound Med* 1995; **14:** 435-439.

33. Mirk P, Cotroneo AR, Palazzoni G, Bock E. Valutazione con eco-Doppler dell'arteria mesenterica inferiore. Studio di fattibilità e definizione dei caratteri morfologici e flussimetrici. *Radiol Med* 1994; **87:** 275-282.

34. Patriquin H, Lafortune M, Burns PN, Dauzat M. Duplex Doppler examination in portal hypertension: technique and anatomy. *AJR* 1987; **149:** 71-76.

35. Sturm W, Judmaier G, Propst A, Kathrein H. Color Doppler imaging for examination of bowel wall vessels in inflammatory bowel disease: preliminary results. *Eur J Ultrasound* 1994; **1:** 229-233.

36. Alexander AA, Liu JB, Palazzo JP *et al.* Endorectal color and duplex imaging of the normal rectal wall and rectal masses. *J Ultrasound Med* 1994; **13:** 509-515.

37. Clautice-Engle T, Jeffrey RB, Li KCP, Barth RA. Power Doppler imaging of focal lesions of the gastrointestinal tract: comparison with conventional color Doppler imaging. *J Ultrasound Med* 1996; **15:** 63-66.

38. Sukigara M, Komazaki T, Yamazaki T *et al.* Color flow mapping of the oesophageal varices and vessels in and around the oesophagus with real-time two-dimensional Doppler echography. *Clin Radiol* 1987; **38:** 487-489.

39. Kimura T, Moriyasu F, Kawasaki T *et al.* Changes in the azygos venous flow evaluated using transoesophageal Doppler ultrasound after vasopressin infusion in portal hypertension. *Hepatology* 1989; **10:** A 42.

40. Sukigara M, Shimoji K, Komazaki T, Omoto R. An assessment of the correlation between the azygos flow volume measured by transesophageal real-time two-dimensional Doppler echography and that measured by continuous thermodilution technique. *J Ultrasound Med* 1988; **7:** S189.

41. Dauzat M, Layarargues GP. Portal vein blood flow measurements using pulsed Doppler and electromagnetic flowmetry in dogs: a comparative study. *Gastroenterology* 1989; **96:** 913-919.

42. Okazaki K, Miyazaki M, Onishi S, Ito K. Effects of food intake and various extrinsic hormones on portal blood flow in patients with liver cirrhosis demonstrated by pulsed Doppler with the Octoson. *Scand J Gastroenterol* 1986; **21:** 1029-1036.

43. Moneta GL, Taylor DC, Helton WS, Mulholland MW, Strandness DE. Duplex ultrasound measurement of postprandial intestinal blood flow: effect of meal composition. *Gastroenterology* 1988; **95:** 1294-1301.

44. Lilly MP, Harward TRS, Flinn WR, Blackburn DR, Astleford PM, Yao JST. Duplex ultrasound measurement of changes in mesenteric flow velocity with pharmacologic and physiologic alteration of intestinal blood flow in man. *J Vasc Surg* 1989; **9:** 18-25.

45. Sabbà C, Ferraioli G, Genecin P *et al.* Evaluation of postprandial hyperemia in superior mesenteric artery and portal vein in healthy and cirrhotic humans: an operator-blind echo-Doppler study. *Hepatology* 1991; **13:** 714-718.

46. O'Brien S, Keogan M, Patchett S, McCormick PA, Afdhal N, Hegarty JE. Postprandial changes in portal haemodynamics in patients with cirrhosis. *Gut* 1992; **33:** 364-367.

47. Buchardt Hansen HJ, Engell HC, Ring-Larsen H, Ranek L. Splanchnic blood flow in patients with abdominal angina before and after arterial reconstruction. A proposal for a diagnostic test. *Ann Surg* 1977; **186:** 216-220.

48. Zwiebel WJ, Mountford RA, Halliwell MJ, Wells PNT. Splanchnic blood flow in patients with cirrhosis and portal hypertension: investigation with duplex Doppler US. *Radiology* 1995; **194:** 807-812.

49. Zoli M, Marchesini G, Brunori A, Cordiani MR, Pisi E. Portal venous flow in response to acute β blocker and vasodilatatory treatment in patients with liver cirrhosis. *Hepatology* 1986; **6:** 1248-1251.

50. Sabbà C, Ferraioli G, Buonamico P *et al.* A randomized study of propranolol on postprandial portal hyperemia in cirrhotic patients. *Gastroenterology* 1992; **102:** 1009-1016.

51. Bolondi L, Gaiani S, Li Bassi S, Zironi G, Casanova P, Barbara L. Effect of secretin on portal venous flow. *Gut* 1990; **31:** 1306-1310.

52. Li Bassi S, Sangermano A, Festi D, Orsini M, Roda E. Effect on splanchnic haemodynamics of acute administration of furosemide in liver cirrhosis. *Eur J Ultrasound* 1994; **1:** 235-240.

53. Ohnishi K, Saito M, Nakayama T *et al.* Portal venous hemodynamics in chronic liver disease: effects of posture change and exercise. *Radiology* 1985; **155:** 757-761.

54. Parvey HR, Eisenberg RL, Giyanani V, Krebs CA. Duplex sonography of the portal venous system: pitfalls and limitations. *Am J Radiol* 1989; **152:** 765-770.

55. Tanaka K, Numata K, Okazaki H *et al.* Diagnosis of portal vein thrombosis in patients with hepatocellular carcinoma: efficacy of color Doppler sonography compared with angiography. *Am J Radiol* 1993; **160:** 1279-1282.

56. Tessler FN, Gehring BJ, Gomes AS *et al.* Diagnosis of portal vein thrombosis: value of color Doppler imaging. *Am J Radiol* 1991; **157:** 293-297.

57. Zerin JM, DiPietro MA. Superior mesenteric vascular anatomy at US in patients with surgically proved malrotation of the midgut. *Radiology* 1992; **183:** 693-694.

58. Derchi LE, Bazzocchi M, Brovero PL. Sonographic diagnosis of obstructed afferent loop. *Gastrointest Radiol* 1992; **17:** 105-107.

59. Moneta GL, Yeager RA, Dalman R, Antonovic R, Hall LD, Porter JM. Duplex ultrasound criteria for diagnosis of splanchnic artery stenosis and occlusion. *J Vasc Surg* 1991; **14:** 511-518.

60. Neumyer MM, Healy DA, Thiele BL. Ultrasound assessment of mesenteric and renal ischemia. *Ultrasound Q* 1994; **12:** 89-103.

61. Roobottom CA, Dubbins PA. Significant disease of the celiac and superior mesenteric arteries in asymptomatic patients: predictive value of Doppler sonography. *Am J Radiol* 1993; **161:** 985-988.

62. Van Bel F, Van Zwieten PHT, Guit GL, Schipper J. Superior mesenteric artery blood flow velocity and estimated volume flow: duplex Doppler US study of preterm and term neonates. *Radiology* 1990; **174:** 165-169.

63. Lim JH, Ko YT, Lee DH, Lim JW, Kim TH. Sonography of inflammatory bowel disease: findings and value in differential diagnosis. *Am J Radiol* 1994; **163:** 343-347.

64. Lee SH, Lees WR. Color Doppler imaging in inflammatory bowel disease. *Gut* 1989; **30:** A 1480.

65. Bolondi L, Gaiani S, Brignola C *et al.* Changes in splanchnic hemodynamics in inflammatory bowel disease. Non invasive assessment by Doppler ultrasound flowmetry. *Scand J Gastroenterol* 1992; **27:** 501-507.

66. Quillin SP, Siegel MJ. Color Doppler US of children with acute lower abdominal pain. *Radiographics* 1993; **13:** 1281-1293.

67. Quillin SP, Siegel MJ. Gastrointestinal inflammation in children: color Doppler ultrasonography. *J Ultrasound Med* 1994; **13:** 751-756.

68. Lim HK, Bae SH, Lee KH, Seo GS, Yoon GS. Assessment of reducibility of ileocolic intussusception in children: usefulness of color Doppler sonography. *Radiology* 1994; **191:** 781-785.

69. Lagalla R, Caruso G, Novara V, Derchi LE, Cardinale AE. Color Doppler ultrasonography in pediatric intussusception. *J Ultrasound Med* 1994; **13:** 171-174.

70. Patriquin HB, Garcier JM, Lafortune M *et al.* Appendicitis in children and young adults: Doppler sonographic-pathologic correlation. *Am J Radiol* 1996; **166:** 629-633.

71. Quillin SP, Siegel MJ. Appendicitis in children: color Doppler sonography. *Radiology* 1992; **184:** 745-747.

72. Quillin SP, Siegel MJ. Diagnosis of appendiceal abscess in children with acute aappendicitis: value of color Doppler sonography. *Am J Radiol* 1995; **164:** 251-1254.

73. Sudakoff GS, Gasparaitis A, Michelassi F, Hurst R, Hoffmann K, Hackworth C. Endorectal color Doppler imaging of primary and recurrent rectal wall tumors: preliminary experience. *Am J Radiol* 1996; **166:** 55-61.

13

Techniques of endoscopic ultrasonography in investigating gastrointestinal pathologies and therapeutic options

---

Harry   Snady

Summary

Endoscopic ultrasonography (EUS) can provide highly accurate gastrointestinal tumour characterization and staging without surgery. However, this method is particularly operator dependent; to produce accurate and consistent results, it requires the understanding of endosonographic techniques and artifacts. EUS often establishes a diagnosis in malignant and, in certain patients, benign disease, accurately evaluates anastomoses for recurrent tumours, and characterizes submucosal masses. When histology is required, EUS plays a critical role in defining an abnormal area for deep biopsy from the gastrointestinal lumen. Precise preoperative EUS staging according to the TNM pathological staging system can be used to stratify treatment for oesophageal, gastric, rectal and pancreatobiliary tumours. EUS can be used to monitor treatment of downstaged tumours and is unsurpassed in determining resectability of gastrointestinal neoplasms. Using EUS for earlier diagnosis and precise staging will significantly improve the clinical outcome of patients with gastrointestinal disease as advances in surgical techniques and in combined chemoradiotherapy continue to be made and applied selectively.

Introduction

Attempts to combine ultrasonography (US) and endoscopy have developed to the point where endoscopic ultrasonography (EUS), also known as echoendoscopy, has become the most significant advance for imaging the gastrointestinal (GI) tract wall and contiguous organs in the past 20 years.[1-3] The detailed resolution seen on EUS images is unmatched by any other current method.[4] EUS is regarded by endoscopists as the most difficult procedure in gastroenterology.[5,6] In a survey of 21 centres representing over 12,000 EUS cases (Snady H, unpublished observations, 1993), all but one rated pancreatic EUS as at least as difficult as papillotomy with stent placement, the endoscopic procedure generally regarded as requiring the most training and skill. Thirteen of 21 centres rated EUS as more difficult. Artifacts that complicate image interpretation are to a great extent responsible for the difficulties in mastering EUS. Nevertheless, the unsurpassed accuracy of EUS, as compared to any other imaging technique, has been established repeatedly through retrospective, prospective, *in vitro* and *in vivo* studies.[7-14] Studies have been performed

on normal tissues as well as for non-operative GI tumour characterization and staging, documenting the high accuracy of TNM staging that is possible with EUS.[4] EUS can provide unique information, essential to diagnose malignancy, that is often otherwise obtainable only by surgical techniques.

The number and influence of animal studies have been limited. However, advances in the clinical application of EUS depend on refining image interpretations. The study of EUS in animals should improve interpretation of sonographic images through correlation of histology of disease to sonography.

In this chapter, optimal methods for performing EUS and factors such as ultrasound image artifacts, which contribute to accurate EUS interpretation, will be reviewed and discussed. The EUS technique can then be applied to understanding mechanisms inherent to GI tissue pathologies. The applicability of EUS to clinical problems will also be addressed.

Methods

Successful performance of EUS requires both specific equipment and special technique. In addition, a basic understanding of sonographic imaging is necessary. Finally, image interpretation requires a thorough knowledge of anatomical relationships of vessels and organs.[4,7,8,10,11,15-19]

Equipment

Mechanical and electrical methods of ultrasound scanning have been applied to intraluminal sonography. For the mechanical Olympus UM sector scan systems (Olympus Optical Co Ltd, Tokyo, Japan), a motor rotates a single piezoelectric transducer to produce a 360° circular scan that is perpendicular to the echoendoscope shaft. This circular sector facilitates orientation of the probe in the lumen of the GI tract and is the most widely used for scanning because rapid orientation allows faster, more efficient scanning. However, biopsies are not usually performed with this instrument. Because the needle is seen only as a single point where it pierces the perpendicular ultrasound image plane, the needle is difficult to direct. The linear array sector echoendoscopy system (Pentax/Hitachi, Pentax Precision Instruments Corp., Orangeburg, NY, USA) electronically switches an array of piezoelectric transducers to produce a linear scan image that is parallel to the endoscope shaft. Although the effective image provided is only a 105° wedge, making scanning more difficult, particularly in the oesophagus, this image orientation allows a biospy needle to be more easily directed and followed into the target because it is in line with the scanning plane.[20] Equipment has been developed to complement biopsy capabilities of the Olympus system.

A reflecting mirror converts the sector scan from perpendicular to parallel to the scope. Most echoendoscopes currently have a side or oblique angle of view with the exception of the echocolonoscope which is forward viewing. The echocolonoscope has an accessory channel with the optical components resulting in a 40° wedge cut from the full 360° EUS image. The echoendoscope can be passed into the distal duodenum, and the caecum can be reached with the echocolonoscope.

Small 2-3.7 mm diameter probes with a frequency of up to 50 MHz have been developed which can be passed through standard endoscopes. These probes are then placed against a target area. Because of significant attenuation of high frequency sound waves, depth of resolution of these probes is <1 cm. Their clinical utility is still being defined. Probes have been developed by numerous manufacturers including: Olympus Optical Co., Aloaka Co., Machida Co., Toshiba Medical Co., Fuji Photo Optical Co., Boston Scientific Corp. and Brual and Kjaeer Medical Systems.[10,21-28]

Technique

As with all endoscopic techniques, passing the instrument through the lumen is relatively easy. The difficulty arises in passing the scope to the target area, identifying and examining the target, and then interpreting the images and artifacts.

EUS is performed in a fasting patient. Pharyngeal anaesthesia and intravenous sedation are generally used, but are not required. Endoscopy with a standard endoscope is performed initially because the echoendoscope has limited capabilities as an endoscope. The rigid tip and the oblique viewing optics of the echoendoscope make examination of the mucosa and the lumen more difficult than with standard endoscopes, and similar to that with a large diameter side-viewing endoscope. Initial standard endoscopy allows for assessment of endoscopic anatomy and detection of areas such as strictures that may be at risk for a complication.

During EUS scanning, the transducer is guided through the GI lumen and placed directly adjacent to the area of interest. Bones, adipose tissue and air-filled structures, which limit the sound wave imaging clarity of extracorporeal sonography, are avoided. The close proximity of the ultrasonic source to the organs imaged permits the use of high frequency, high resolution sound waves that have too short a penetration depth to be used in transcutaneous sonography. Current EUS instruments use the higher sound wave frequencies of 7.5 and 12 MHz, as compared with 3.5 MHz for transcutaneous US and 5 MHz for blind rectal and oesophageal probes.

As with all sonography, the sound wave imaging plane can be oriented at any angle to bring the lesion into optimal focus simply by turning the probe. The operator is not limited to parallel sections, usually 1 cm apart, as with computed tomography (CT). When the echoendoscope is in the target area, intraluminal gas is aspirated to increase contact with the GI wall, thus maximizing available acoustic windows. The area to be imaged is brought into focus by filling a thin Latex rubber balloon (Olympus Optical Co. Ltd) surrounding the transducer at the tip of the echoendoscope with approximately 15 ml water. The water-filled balloon serves as a non-attenuating acoustic coupling medium between the transducer and the surface of the GI wall. If the target area is in the wall itself, water (up to 1000 ml) can be placed directly into the lumen for optimal acoustic coupling. The scanning plane is then manoeuvered, using scope controls and turning, pushing or pulling the scope shaft to orient the lesion into optimal position and focus. The technique will vary according to the indications and objectives of the examination.

EUS images of normal anatomy

EUS sonographic layers of the wall of the GI tract have been correlated to histopathological layers in several studies.[4] The standard five layer EUS image of the GI tract wall and its correlation to histological layers is shown in Fig. 13.1a.[16] However, additional histological layers can be seen when different factors change the sonographic resolution of the intestinal wall. When a pathological process changes sonographic interfaces, seven layers (Fig. 13.1b) can be seen (Snady H, unpublished observations). Up to nine layers have been observed when different frequencies are used.[27,28] Optimal imaging of the GI wall is essential to determine the wall layer(s) affected by disease. With the sonographic plane oriented as

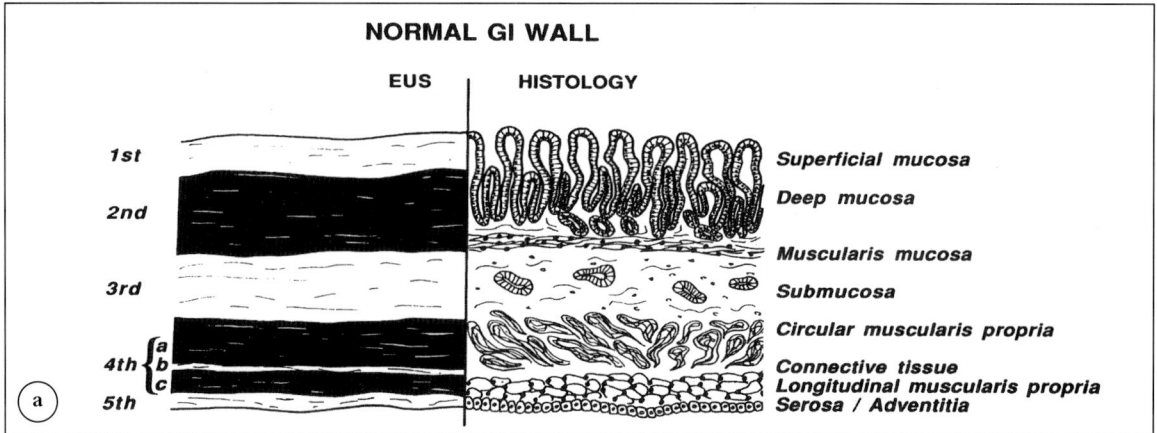

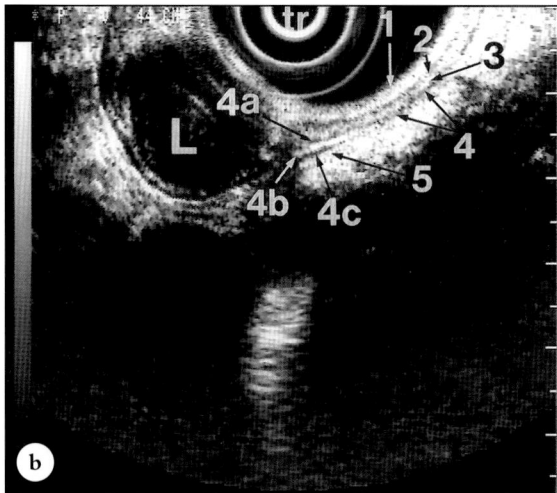

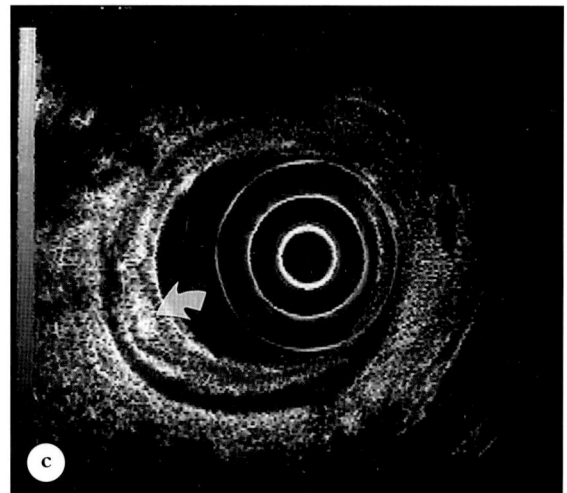

Figure 13.1 — (a) Correlation between the standard five EUS layers and histological layers of the normal intestinal wall. 1st = interface between fluid in the lumen and the superficial mucosa; 2nd = lamina propria and muscularis mucosa, or deep mucosa; 3rd = submucosa and interface between submucosa and muscularis propria; 4th = muscularis propria; circular (4a) and longitudinal (4c) are not usually seen as separate layers since the thin connective tissue layer (4b) is normally not seen; 5th = interface between serosa and surrounding adventitial tissue. Reproduced from Ref. 16, with permission. (b) EUS image showing five layers of the gastric wall that become seven layers near a leiomyoma (L) arising from the inner layer of the muscularis propria. 1, 3, 4b and 5 = 1st, 3rd, 5th and 7th layers are hyperechoic (white). 2, 4a and 4c = 2nd, 4th and 6th layers are hypoechoic (black). 4b = the connective tissue layer between the 4a = inner, circular layer and 4c = outer, longitudinal layer of the muscularis propira is generally not seen in the typical five layer image. Transducer (tr) is surrounded by a water-filled balloon. EUS magnification range scale = 6 cm. (c) Hyperechoic area (arrow) developing in deep mucosal, hypoechoic, 2nd layer of colonic wall after injection of normal saline into colonic wall with a 3-4 mm 23 gauge endoscopic injection needle (Varijet, Boston Scientific Corp., Watertown, MA, USA). EUS magnification range scale = 6 cm.

close as possible to perpendicular to the intestinal wall, optimal imaging and limitation of artifacts can be achieved. Substances injected into the GI wall can be located with EUS (Snady H, unpublished observations) to demonstrate which layers of the GI tract wall are altered (Fig. 13.1c).

EUS images of organs, large vessels and lymph nodes contiguous to the GI tract each have their own characteristic appearance from seven standard positions[7] used for orientation and finding anatomical landmarks. The normal anatomy of the oesophagus, stomach, pancreas, retroperitoneum and hepatobiliary tract have been described previously.[4,7,8,10,11,15-19]

Direct correlation of EUS images to anatomy, particularly for the pancreatobiliary system, have been difficult to perform. Consequently, precise correlation of various EUS findings to actual histopathology has been possible only through indirect methods, which rely on the analysis of pathology from operative or autopsy specimens. Although the pancreatobiliary system can be imaged in various animal models, the variations in anatomy from the human anatomy make EUS animal studies of limited value (H Snady, unpublished observations). Intraoperative EUS has also not been helpful; when the peritoneal cavity is opened, air distorts the EUS image (H Snady, unpublished observations). However, intraoperative EUS has been useful for analysis of lymph nodes.[29] An understanding of lymph nodes associated with each organ is crucial to understanding where to scan for spread of disease to regional lymph nodes.

Tumour staging

The role of EUS in determining patient outcome, both in terms of prognosis and quality of life, depends upon co-ordination of EUS with meaningful pathological staging and effective treatment. As more effective treatments for GI neoplasms involving combined chemotherapy/ radiotherapy plus surgery have evolved, increased response rates and improved survival have been reported.[4,14] Even when not curative, therapy may alter the course and life history of GI cancer. Studies show that accurate preoperative staging is essential in determining the timing and dosage of specific treatments for greatest efficacy and impact.[4]

For most cancer sites, the staging recommendations that are accepted and used worldwide are concerned only with anatomical extent of disease. An untreated primary cancer or tumour (T) progressively increases in depth of invasion, spreads to regional lymph nodes (N), and finally, as a result of continued extension of disease, metastasizes (M) to distant lymph nodes or organs. TNM classification and stage grouping is thus a method of designating the extent of a particular type of cancer as it is related to the natural course. Manuals[30,31] with recommendations for stage groupings of cancer at all anatomical sites have been published by The American Joint Committee of Cancer (AJCC) and The International Union Against

Cancer (UICC). These evolving recommendations of the TNM system, developed by Denoix,[32] are based on contributions from 400 expert participants over 40 years and replace other non-uniform staging methods.[33,34] The TNM tumour staging method has proven to be very accurate in determining prognosis. For GI tumours, EUS is the most accurate single technique to determine stage according to the TNM system.

Progress in predicting prognosis of a tumour will continue with further refinement of both the TNM system as well as the ability of EUS to predict the extent of tumour spread. Limitations of the TNM system for GI neoplastic disease have been reviewed.[35] Limitations of prediction of tumour stage with EUS are related to the overlap of current criteria used to differentiate the echo patterns and features of disease processes. Part of this overlap is inherent to the ultrasound pulses; however, part is a result of limited experience with the subtle distinctions required for the most refined EUS interpretation that is possible. As criteria continue to be developed, clarified and conjoined, image interpretation will continue to improve.[36-38] In addition, EUS will have a major role in defining abnormal areas as small as 5-10 mm for directed deep biopsies from the GI lumen through the GI tract wall.[20,39-41] Combining histology of a tissue sample with EUS imaging of the entire tumour will improve the process of differentiating neoplastic tissue from inflammation.

Sonographic principles and artifacts

The display of the interaction of sound waves with tissues on a monitor is the basis of clinical US. Understanding this interaction is the primary factor in using artifacts and in achieving optimal images. Accurate clinical US image interpretation depends on understanding the properties of sound waves, the mechanics of the equipment, the characteristics of the tissue or suspension media. as well as the proper technique.[3-6,42-46] Errors in EUS can occur at any phase of image generation and interpretation.[5,6,43-47] They can be divided into categories according to origin (Table 13.1). If maximum effort is not made to produce an optimal image, artifacts inherent to ultrasonography are magnified and even created, so that accurate interpretation is virtually impossible. Each of these features of EUS will be discussed to highlight aspects required to produce consistent, quality imaging.

Table 13.1 – Sources of EUS errors and artifacts.

1. Equipment

    a) Malfunction or improper operation

    b) Improper calibration

    c) Imaged object out of frequency's focal range

    d) Improper adjustment of electrical controls

2. Acoustic presentation of the image

    a) Assumptions made by the sonographic instrument
       to produce an image

    b) Physical properties of the sound beam

    c) Acoustic properties of the tissue

    d) Interaction of sound and tissue

3. Characteristics of the tissue or medium

4. EUS technique

    a) Improper operation of the transducer resulting in:

       1) non-perpendicular scanning

       2) object compression artifacts

       3) insufficient contact at appropriate anatomical
          acoustic window

       4) misinterpretation of anatomy

    b) Improper focal length adjustment altering acoustic
       presentation of the image

Properties of the sound beam

The term ultrasound refers to sound wave frequencies >20,000 Hz that are beyond human hearing. Ultrasound frequencies from 1 to 50 MHz have been investigated for clinical use. When performing US, factors that must be considered include: certain basic and necessary reductive assumptions that must be made to build an image-producing machine, the physical nature of the sound beam itself, and the acoustic properties of the objects being imaged.[43-46]

Absorption, reflection, refraction and scatter are behaviours of sound waves as they propagate through and interact with tissue. Through absorption the mechanical energy of the sound pulse is converted to heat. Reflection and refraction refer to the portion of sound that returns or emerges from a boundary or interface of a medium. Scattering occurs because of diffusion or redirection of sound in various angles when it encounters a particle suspension or a rough surface, resulting in sound energy not returning to the transducer and, therefore, loss of its detection by the transducer. Acoustic impedance (resistance) is the

product of wave velocity through the medium and density of the medium. All biological tissue and media have inherent acoustical properties and impedance. As sound travels through a medium, it looses energy through interactions of sound and tissue, and becomes attenuated. Higher frequency sound waves are subject to a greater degree of attenuation. Spatial resolution is also related to frequency. The higher the frequency, the better the spatial resolution. Although high frequency sound waves can penetrate deeper levels, images will be out of focus when attenuation overcomes the gain in spatial resolution.

Reflection is an important property of sound waves required for image formation in US. Sound reflection is maximized when a high amplitude beam strikes a soft tissue-gas or fluid-gas interface at a perpendicular angle. When the acoustic impedance of two adjacent tissues is different, sound striking the tissue interface is reflected, producing a sound wave echo which returns to the transducer. The reflected sound wave is translated to the screen, placing the interface at a specific point in the image that correlates with the distance from the transducer to the interface in the tissue. The greater the difference in tissue impedance, the stronger the amount of reflection. Reflection is also intensified with greater amplitude of the incident beam.

Imaging artifacts

Imaging artifacts are misrepresentations of the true nature of the structure or tissue being displayed on a monitor. Artifacts can cause misreading of EUS images because of optical illusions, errors of interpretation, and interobserver variability related to perception and/or incorrect or incomplete definitions and criteria of various terms and findings.[36-38,42-47]

Equipment artifacts

There are certain artifacts which relate to equipment malfunction. These occur when air, water or dust gain access to the oil-immersed-transducer housing, the transducer, or the electrical connections. These types of artifacts are generally easy to detect as they will be present on the screen even when the instrument is not being used for scanning.

Because of attenuation, the optimal focal range of an instrument will vary with frequency. For higher frequencies, the focal length is smaller and closer to the transducer; for lower frequencies, the focal length

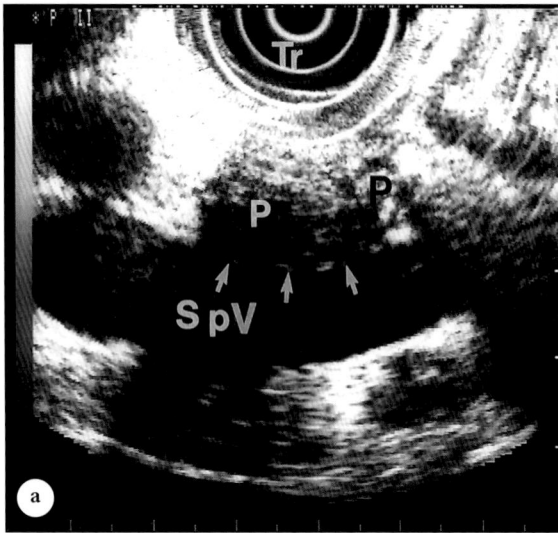

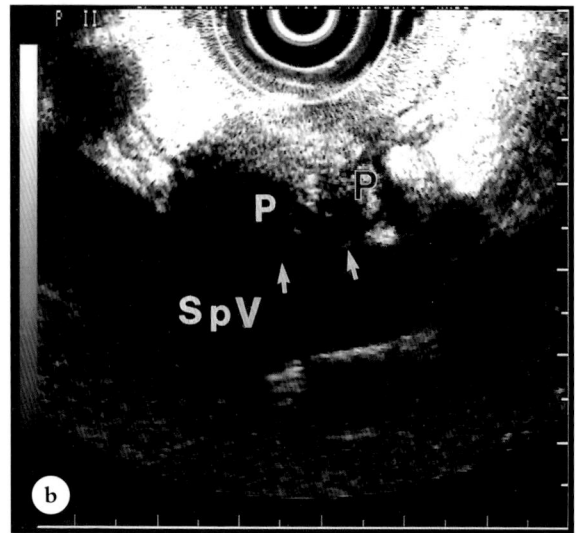

Figure 13.2 – (a) 7.5 MHz EUS image of pancreas (P) with the transducer (Tr) against the posterior wall of the stomach. Hyperechoic interface (arrows) between pancreas and splenic vein (SpV) is clearly seen. EUS magnification range scale = 6 cm. (b) 12 MHz EUS image of pancreas with transducer in exactly the same position as in (a). Hyperechoic interface between pancreas and splenic vein not clearly seen. EUS magnification range scale = 6 cm.

is further away from the transducer. The optimal focal range for 7.5 MHz is 1-4 cm and for 12 MHz, 2-20 mm. Objects that are not in the focal range of the sound beam cannot be consistently and accurately deciphered (Fig. 13.2a and b). Adjustment of image intensity with amplification (gain) or using adjustments in contrast, focal zone and depth can compensate for some of these factors in producing an accurate image. However, improper machine settings as well as improper adjustments of equipment controls during scanning can cause artifacts.

Acoustic artifacts

Artifacts of acoustic origin are pervasive throughout grey-scale imaging and are related to resolution, propagation and attenuation. This type of artifact can be grouped in terms of the effects they produce such as: added objects, missing objects, and incorrect object brightness, location, size or shape. These artifacts can be related to specific causes such as pulse length, pulse width, inteference, reflection, refraction, side lobes, grating lobes, attenuation, focusing, reverberation, resonance speed error and high pulse repetition frequency.[42-46] In ultrasound, acoustic artifacts arise as a consequence of reductive assumptions when the machine produces an image, physical characteristics of the sound beam, and tissue acoustic properties.

Artifacts occurring as the necessary consequence of reductive assumptions

The US instrument generates, records and processes complex signals using assumptions that are simple and consistent, but flawed in all but ideal situations. Artifacts result when significant violations of these assumptions occur. These assumed principles include: sound always travels in straight lines; only the properties of the imaged object directly determine the intensity of returning echoes; distance is directly proportional to the time it takes for an echo to make a round trip and return along the propagation path to the surface of the transducer.

Reverberation occurs as sound strikes a subjacent interface and is reflected many times between the interface and the transducer surface. When these multiple reflections are strong enough, they are detected by the receiver and given a spatial alignment that is a multiple of the depth of the original reflective interface. These artifactual echoes occur especially within soft tissue or fluid structures, and significantly alter the echo texture of the object. Reverberations can simulate disease, such as a pseudomass or thrombus in a vessel, when the additional 'non-real' reflectors are placed on the image. The water-filled balloon around the EUS transducer can also be a cause of reverberation artifacts.

Short-path reverberations cause comet tail or ring down artifacts, seen behind a small but intense reflector such as air, metal, plastic or calcified objects. They appear as a series of closely spaced echoes that trail off in intensity as distance from the object increases. The short path is probably produced by microbubbles or crystalline structures that set up reverberation chambers.

Multipath artifacts occur when the reflected sound beam maintains its intensity and coherence at flat and smooth interfaces. Acoustic noise is produced by back scattering of many secondary sound waves from surrounding tissue which reflect again off the smooth interface and return signals to the transducer surface. The result is the visible acoustic noise or dirty shadowing behind a reflecting surface such as a large, smooth calcification or gas pocket. However, the coherence of the reflected beam depends on the diffractive nature of the presenting surface. If the insonified surface is rough and/or has a small radius of curvature, the back-scattered beam will be diffuse, producing phase incoherence in the return beam. Since absorption, not reflection, of sound wave is the dominant process, phase cancellations and loss of signal occur, which cause clean shadowing.

Mirror image artifacts occur when sound takes a longer, more indirect path from the primary interface to a secondary interface before finally returning to the transducer surface. The processor assumes a straight line path and places a phantom lesion at a location deep to the primary reflector due to misregistration of some secondary reflectors. Mirror image artifacts are commonly found around the diaphragm, pleura and bowel. Similar phenomena are seen in colour Doppler.

Side lobe artifacts (from single element transducers) and grating lobe artifacts (from arrays) result from several low-intensity side lobe sound beams around the main ultrasound beam. These side beams can interact with reflectors and present sound back to the transducer face causing objects to be displayed incorrectly in a lateral position. The instrument, believing the integrity of a single main beam, assigns these side echoes a fictitious position within the path of the main beam. Side lobe signals are most significant at highly reflective interfaces and cause the true echo texture of the imaged object to be altered by low level echoes.

Focal zone banding artifacts occur because brighter shades on the grey scale are always assigned to higher amplitude echoes. However, a sound beam varies in amplitude along its propagation path, resulting in focal zones of increased intensity. Electronic focusing can therefore create focal zone bands of alternating high and low intensity in an organ that is actually homogeneous. A pseudohypoechoic mass can be created in an organ through such banding.

Flash artifact is seen with colour Doppler and has not played a significant role in EUS. It occurs when colour is suppressed where grey-scale echoes are present, but assigned to anechoic or hypoechoic areas.

Artifacts due to sound beam shape

Spatial resolution limitations can result in artifacts. Objects that are separated by a small distance can merge on the screen if the pulse length is not short enough to distinguish two closely spaced points. Axial resolution is superior to lateral resolution because pulse length is normally much less than pulse width. Axial resolution generally improves with higher frequencies. Lateral resolution can range up to 3 cm, whereas axial resolution is usually no more than 2-3 mm. Therefore, small objects may appear larger or thicker when reflectors are parallel to the beam compared to those that are encountered perpendicular to the beam. Measurements are best made in the axial direction as often as possible.

Image speckle, an interference pattern close to the transducer, causes a parenchymal echopattern, but also image degradation. This acoustic noise is produced by the constructive and destructive interference of rotating echoes from a scatter distribution. Speckle can be reduced by photographic averaging and deconvolution resulting in, improved images.

Slice thickness artifact, also termed section thickness, off-axis or beam-width artifact, results in the melding of the image of different tissues that may not belong together. A focused US pulse has a finite width in the direction perpendicular to the scan plane. The beam can therefore sonographically locate more than one tissue at the same location of a scan plane. The two simultaneously imaged tissues produce an image that has a combined echo texture.

Artifacts related to acoustic properties of the tissue or medium

Speed propagation artifact occurs because sound propagates through different body tissues or media at different velocities. Sound travels more slowly through soft tissue than fluid, and even more slowly through fat. As a result, sound that must traverse fatty tissue completes its round trip back to the transducer in a longer period of time. However, to produce an image, US equipment assumes an average tissue velocity of 1540 cm/s. Based on round-trip time an inaccurate depth assignment is made to reflectors posterior to tissue such as fat, fluid and cartilage which have acoustical velocities significantly different from the average.

Through-transmission artifacts occur when sound travels through a medium with low attenuation properties before reaching the imaged object. Scanning through fluid will cause objects to be more echogenic than usual. This is particularly relevant for EUS when cysts or peritoneal fluid are encountered around an area of disease.

Artifacts related to the interaction of sound and tissue

Refraction occurs when the sound beam at an oblique angle of incidence strikes a boundary between two media which conduct sound at different velocities. The transmitted part of the sound wave can be bent. The proportion of refraction and reflection that occurs depends on the angle of incidence. Complete bending of the beam can occur when the beam is parallel to the interface, obscuring the image of tissue posterior to the interface. Depending on the direction of the sound be am through the two adjacent media, sound waves will converge or diverge.

Posterior shadowing artifacts occur when sound wave penetration of a structure is very limited or absent. When impedance of two tissues differs to such a degree that a near complete reflection of the sound beam is produced, a dark shadow is noted where there are no echoes posterior to the interface. Shadowing also occurs at two apposed transitional zones in the same tissue. Refraction can also cause shadowing from the edge of a curved object, typically at the interface of calcium/soft tissue or gas/fluid.

Enhancement artifacts are due to contrasting acoustic impedance in adjacent structures. Posterior enhancement is a deceptive brightness behind a dark area. The higher amplitude of these echoes compared to those of equivalent adjacent tissue arises posterior to a contrastingly low attenuating area, such as a fluid structure. This sound transmission artifact can be used to distinguish cystic from solid structures. Edge enhancement is an infrequently seen artifact which can occur due to refraction at a curved edge.

Focal enhancement can occur in the focal region of the transducer.

Phase cancellation occurs when reflected wave segments are out of phase and cancel each other in summation. When a coherent sound wave crosses boundaries between media that conduct sound at different velocities, the adjacent waveforms become distorted and out of phase. The destructive interference produces an area of cancellation resulting in a black streak or absence of signal on the screen.

Attenuation is a loss of sound wave intensity as a consequence of the behaviours of sound as it interacts with matter. The greatest loss is due to absorption. The higher the frequency, the greater the absorption of sound energy. The degree of attenuation is related to wave frequency and the tissue type and shape. Hypoechoic regions, which could be misinterpreted as masses, can occur behind certain tissues that significantly attenuate the sound beam. Because of the high frequency used with EUS, attenuation artifacts must always be considered. Accuracy in imaging the deep parts of soft tissue structures can be limited by shadows produced when a sound beam does not traverse the structure.

Anisotrophy artifacts result from changes in tissue plane orientation relative to the main second beam axis due to the modulating shape of an imaged organ. Tissue echogenicity changes as sound waves are transmitted at different angles through the same structures due to alterations of sound wave behaviour at the tissue reflectors.

Perivascular colour artifact occurs when intravascular blood flow becomes turbulent resulting in vibrations within disturbed tissue surrounding the blood vessel. When the tissue is examined with colour Doppler, the motion of this vibration will be colour-encoded producing a sonographic equivalent of a soft tissue thrill.

Artifacts and errors related to characteristics of tissue

The composition of different tissues and organs determines their ultrasound image characteristics. Acoustic impedance of soft tissues can differ by as much as 22%. The presence and uniformity of distribution of different tissue components in a soft tissue structure alters its US image. Changes in tissue density and uniformity due to disease can also alter sound wave/tissue interactions. Inherent complexity of tissue properties will be the major consideration for *in vitro* studies. For *in vivo* and human studies, knowledge of anatomical relationships is also critical to proper EUS interpretation.

Artifacts and errors of EUS technique

Important sources of artifacts and errors that arise from improper instrument placement are non-perpendicular scanning, object compression, insufficient contact at the appropriate anatomical acoustic window, and misinterpretation of anatomy. When the incident sound wave encounters a reflector at an angle, the reflected wave will emerge at an equal angle. Part of the incident wave may not reflect, but may be transmitted into the next tissue or medium. The angle of scanning will affect the amplitude of reflected sonographic echoes and the corresponding degree of refraction. Transducer position can affect these properties of sound waves and can produce artifacts.

The most important source of EUS transducer positioning artifact is oblique or tangential scanning, which can result in the appearance of pseudotumours or indistinct margins between parenchyma and vessels through acoustic artifacts such as reverberation, shadowing and enhancement. However, the most common distortion of non-perpendicular scanning is the appearance of a widening or thickening of the layers of the intestinal wall. The best measurements are obtained with the transducer at right angles to the target so that the sound beam is perpendicular to any boundaries between two tissues or media. In performing EUS, one is always trying to optimize image clarity by balancing the highest frequency to obtain the best spatial resolution with a frequency that penetrates deep enough to view the target area. The higher the frequency, the less divergence occurs, and the easier it is to focus the narrowed beam.

The amount of water placed in the balloon surrounding the transducer affects the way the image is generated and can alter the size of the field of optimal focus. Changing the amount of water in the balloon can also be used to move the focal point. However, changing the angle of the echoendoscope and the amount of water in the balloon can easily compress structures so that distortion occurs. Superficial layers of the wall are more sensitive to this distortion than other parts of the intestinal tract or surrounding structures.

Repeat scanning for the same as well as different angles during introduction and withdrawal of the instrument while varying the focal length with the balloon will limit misinterpretation of an EUS image.

The effects of artifacts can be minimized by scanning from different angles, using the narrowest sound beam possible, focusing properly on the target area, avoiding scanning at edges of objects, recognizing secondary images, and adjusting equipment settings (usually the gain). Misinterpretation of anatomy often results from improper transducer location and/or orientation. Misinterpretation also results if surrounding anatomy and structures of the area being scanned are not considered. This is particularly true at the distal oesophagus where the diaphragm complicates interpretation, especially if a hiatal hernia is present.

Application to animal studies

Animal studies have not been as numerous as human studies. Since future improvements of the clinical application of EUS will depend on advances in image interpretation, useful information could potentially be gained through animal studies. Models could be developed to improve correlations of sonographic findings to histology. The investigation of various agents which enhance or change sound wave characteristics of tissues will assist in differentiating normal and pathological states.

In vitro studies

The study of GI tissue from surgical or autopsy material has resulted in many important findings. Correlation of the EUS wall structure to histology (Fig. 13.1) is the most significant.[48-53] Accuracy of these studies has depended on use of experimental systems that ensured maximum axial resolution and optimal focusing during sonographic imaging. Generally, specimens are mounted with needles into a container constructed to permit accurate spatial localization of the tissue and corresponding ultrasound image. Tissue are immersed in different media including water, deaerated water, saline, water soluble gels and fat emulsions. The acoustic coupling properties of these media have not been studied systematically. Fresh specimens as well as tissue fixed with different agents have been studied. Microdissection techniques are generally utilized.

Lymph nodes have also been studied with *in vitro* models.[29,54,55] In addition, contrast agents which can enhance grey scale and Doppler signals have been evaluated with various systems.[56-61] These agents include: fluorocarbons, galactose microspheres, oil–water and fat emulsions. They are used for tissue suspension media, for intraluminal media, and for intravenous injection to alter and enhance vessels and lymph node acoustic properties. Substances injected into the GI wall can be located with EUS (Fig. 13.1c). With *in vitro* and *in vivo* models this technique could be used to investigate disease or the effects of various substances on specific layers of the GI wall.

In vivo techniques

Swine, canine and sheep animal models have been used to study EUS (Snady H, unpublished observations).[20-22,42,62-65] Models studying gastric ulcers and portal hypertension have been reported.[63,64] Experimental systems have been used to test new probes.[21-26] Human intraoperative studies have also been performed (Snady H, unpublished observations). Recognizing anatomy correctly for proper image orientation is one of the most difficult aspects of EUS. Consequently, animal models are limited in their applicability to humans because animal anatomy is significantly different. This is particularly true for the pancreas. The normal pig pancreas appears as an inhomogenous structure with scattered hyperechoic, and round or linear foci within the parenchyma. The pancreatic duct is not visibile.[62] In contrast, the human pancreas is homogeneous with a visible duct. The pancreatic duct is visible in dogs, but limited surrounding fat and a separate ventral and dorsal pancreas make correlations to human disease difficult (Snady H, unpublished observations). Investigating and formulating an effective diagnostic system for early chronic pancreatitis has been limited by the difficulty of gaining direct one-to-one histological confirmation of EUS findings. The exquisite detail that EUS produces is likely eventually to make it the gold standard against which other methods are compared.[66]

Results and discussion

Pathology in GI organs can be imaged with EUS using anatomical landmarks for orientation. In patients without gastric surgery, all landmarks can be located in at least 90% of cases. However, scanning all organs completely would take more than an hour. Thus, in any given examination, certain unrelated structures or areas need not be recorded, if the focus is a specific anatomical site.

Table 13.2 – Accuracy (%) of GI tumour staging and resectability with EUS and CT.

		EUS	CT
Oesophagus	T stage	85	60
	N stage	80	55
	M stage	70	70
	Resectability	80	55
Gastric	T stage	80	40
	N stage	75	50
	M stage	75	75
	Resectability	80	70
Pancreas	T stage	90	50
	N stage	75	50
	M stage	65	65
	Resectability	80	40
Biliary system	T stage	85	45
	N stage	60	50
	M stage	85	85
	Resectability	80	50
Rectum	T stage	85	70
	N stage	80	55
	M stage	—	75

Values are median estimates in % from references in text.

Table 13.2 shows the median accuracy of TNM staging and assessment of resectability for EUS compared to CT scan for various major GI neoplasms.[4] Errors in T stage occur because EUS cannot always distinguish between neoplastic tissue and benign inflammation or fibrosis. Because high frequency sound waves have a penetration depth of only 2-4 cm from the probe, optimal focus of vessels or structures around a tumour larger than 5 cm may not always be achieved, and vessel or organ involvement may be missed.

Errors in N stage can occur for similar reasons.[4,29,52,55] A malignant node can appear to have benign characteristics because micrometastases have not yet caused parenchymal changes that can be seen sonographically. Criteria for lymph node boundaries and echogenicity appear to overlap less than those for size and shape (Table 13.3). Most metastatic lymph nodes are <10 mm. By relying almost exclusively on size to evaluate N stage, CT has been insensitive for neoplastic regional lymph nodes. In contrast, because most lymph nodes >10 mm are usually neoplastic, specificity is good when CT is positive. Unlike CT scan, size resolution is not a limitation for EUS. Lymph nodes >3 mm can be found easily. However,

Table 13.3 – Criteria to differentiate malignant and inflammatory lymph nodes.

	Malignant	Benign
Boundaries	Sharp	Indistinct
Echogenicity★	Echo-poor Homogeneous	Echo-rich Non-homogeneous
Shape	Round	Irregular
Size	>10 mm	< 5 mm

★Criteria are useful only for frequencies of 7.0 MHz or greater.

even though EUS is superior to other imaging methods in differentiating malignant from inflammatory benign lymph nodes, criteria (Table 13.3) overlap and still require improvement.

In a prospective series of 1000 patients where EUS was performed in an office setting, the major complication rate was 0.2% (Snady H, unpublished observations, 1996). Two perforations occurred in patients with oesophageal tumours, one related to preEUS dilation of the tumour. Transient laryngospasm occurred in a third patient. In a world-wide retrospective survey of 42,105 patients,[67] the major complication rate was also reported to be low (0.05%). Two-thirds of upper GI EUS complications occurred in patients with oesophageal strictures. In 10 of 13 perforations, oesophageal dilation had been performed immediately prior to EUS. Mortality within 30 days of EUS occurred in only 1 of 42,105 patients surveyed, and was related to one such perforation. Therefore, aggressive dilation of an oesophageal stricture at the time of EUS is not recommended.

EUS provides detailed images of the GI tract. Clinical applications continue to expand. Proper use of equipment and understanding sound wave properties will minimize errors of the method. Appreciation of how artifacts produce certain changes in tissues improves the operator's facility not only to distinguish the true image, but also to use the artifact to interpret pathology and make a diagnosis. Shadowing and enhancement artifacts are frequently useful in this regard. Section thickness and reverberation artifacts are generally more difficult to interpret and use constructively. The sonographer can be seriously misled by artifacts, which if properly recognized can be used to reveal and inform.

Improvements in correlations of sonographic findings to histology will continue to improve with further studies. Development of various agents to enhance or change sound wave characteristics of tissues and differentiate normal and pathological states will become valuable. Further human and animal studies will continue to establish and clarify parameters that will decrease interobserver variability.[36-38,47] The role of EUS in selection of appropriate treatment will depend upon alternatives available for amelioration of symptoms and improvement of quality of life, survival and outcome.[4,14] Utility of EUS will continue to increase with application of major advances in ultrasound technology.[68]

Acknowledgement

The author is grateful to Laurel Kiefer for editorial and graphic assistance.

References

1. Wild JJ, Reid JM. Diagnostic use of ultrasound. *Br J Phys Med* 1956; **19:** 248-257.

2. Lutz H, Rosch W. Transgastroscopic ultrasonography. *Endoscopy* 1976; **8:** 203-205.

3. Sasai T. Development of ultrasonic endoscope. In: Kawai K (Ed) *Endoscopic Ultrasonography in Gastroenterology* Igaku-Shoin Ltd, Tokyo, 1988, pp.18-34.

4. Snady H. The role of endoscopic ultrasonography in diagnosis, staging and outcomes of gastrointestinal disease. *Gastroenterologist* 1994; **10:** 91-110.

5. Snady H. Technical and interpretive pitfalls in initial experience with endoscopic ultrasonography for upper gastrointestinal disease. Lessons learned. *Gastroenterology* 1989; **96:** A480.

6. Rosch T. Endoscopic ultrasonography artifacts and problems of interpretation. *Gastrointest Endosc* 1996; **43:** S10-S12.

7. Tytgat GNJ, Tio TL (Eds). Endoscopic Ultrasonography: Proceedings of the 4th International Symposium on Endoscopic Ultrasonography. *Scand J Gastroenterol* 1986; **21(suppl 123):** 1-172.

8. Kawai K (Ed). *Endoscopic Ultrasonography in Gastroenterology* Igaku-Shoin, Tokyo, 1988.

9. Snady H. Endoscopic ultrasonography: an effective new tool for diagnosing gastrointestinal tumors. *Oncology* 1992; **6:** 63-74.

10. Rosch T, Classen M. *Gastroenterological Endosonography (Textbook and Atlas).* Thieme Medical Publishers, New York, 1992.

11. Lightdale C (Ed). Endoscopic ultrasonography. In: Sivak M Jr (Ed) *Gastrointest Endosc Clinics N Am* 1992; **2**: 557-749.

12. Rosch T (Ed). Endoscopic ultrasonography: State of the art - 1995. Part I. In: Sivak M Jr (Ed) *Gastrointest Endosc Clinics N Am* 1995; **5**: 475-698.

13. Rosch T (Ed) Endoscopic ultrasonography: State of the art - 1995. Part II. In: Sivak M Jr (Ed) *Gastrointest Endosc Clinics N Am* 1995; **5**: 699-898.

14. Gillard V, Mainguet P, Vicari F, Florent Ch (Eds). 3rd Endoscopic Ultrasonography Belgian Meeting. *Acta Endoscopia* 1995; **25**: 407-556.

15. Erickson R, Chang K. Normal anatomy, part I. In: *Training for Endosonography - An Interactive Learning Tool.* CD-ROM, Olympus America and Astra Merck Inc, 1996.

16. Caletti G, Gerrari A, Barbara L. Normal endosono-graphic anatomy of the esophagus and stomach. In: Lightdale C (Ed) Endoscopic ultrasonography. *Gastrointest Endosc Clinics N Am* 1992; **2**: 601-614.

17. Snady H. Endoscopic ultrasonography images of the normal retroperitoneum. In: Lightdale C (Ed) Endoscopic ultrasonography. *Gastrointest Endosc Clinics N Am* 1992; **2**: 637-655.

18. Dancygier H. Endosonographic evaluation of biliary tract disease. In: Lightdale C (Ed) Endoscopic ultrasonography. *Gastrointest Endosc Clinics N Am* 1992; **2**: 697-714.

19. Wiersema MJ, Hawes RJ. Normal colorectal anatomy and benign colon lesions. In: Lightdale C (Ed) Endoscopic ultrasonography. *Gastrointest Endosc Clinics N Am* 1992; **2**: 715-728.

20. Vilmann P. Endoscopic ultrasonography-guided fine-needle aspiration biopsy of lymph nodes. *Gastrointest Endosc* 1996; **43**: S24-S29.

21. Silverstain FE, Martin RW, Kimmey MB, Jiranek GC, Francklin DW, Proctor A. Experimental evaluation of an endoscopic ultrasound probe: *in vitro* and *in vivo* canine studies. *Gastroenterology* 1989; **96**: 1058-1062.

22. Taniguchi D, Martin R, Trowsers E, Silverstein F. Simultaneous M-mode echoesophagram and manometry in sheep esophagus. *Gastrointest Endosc* 1995; **41**: 582-586.

23. Gress F, Park K, Sangvi N, Kopecky K, Hawes R. A comparison study of high frequency ultrasound imaging of the canine GI tract at 20, 30 and 50 MHz frequencies. *Gastrointest Endosc* 1996; **43**: s54.

24. Takemoto T, Yanai H, Tada M *et al.* Application of ultrasonic probes prior to endoscopic resection of early gastric cancer. *Endoscopy* 1992; **24(suppl 1)**: 329-333.

25. Bartram CI. Anal sphincter disorders. *Gastrointest Endosc* 1996; **43**: S32-S34.

26. Yasdua K. Ultrasonic probes for pancreaticobiliary strictures. *Gastrointest Endosc* 1996; **43**: S35-S37.

27. Odegaard S, Kimmey M. Location of the muscularis mucosae on high frequency gastrointestinal ultrasound images. *Eur J Ultrasound* 1994; **1**: 39-50.

28. Wiersema M, Wiersema L. High-resolution 25 Megahertz ultrasonography of the gastrointestinal wall: histologic correlates. *Gastrointest Endosc* 1993; **39**: 499-504.

29. Tio TL, Tytgat GNJ. Endoscopic ultrasonography in analyzing per-intestinal lymph node abnormality. Preliminary results *in vivo* and *in vitro*. *Scand J Gastroenterol* 1986; **21(suppl 123)**: 158-163.

30. Behahrs O, Henson D, Hutter R (Eds). *Manual for Staging of Cancer,* 3rd edn. American Joint Committe on Cancer. JB Lippincott Co, Philadelphia, 1988.

31. Hermanek P, Sobin L (Eds). *International Union Against Cancer (UICC): TNM Classification of Malignant Tumors,* 4th edn. Springer-Verlag, Berlin, 1987.

32. Denoix PF. Six annees d'enquete permanente cancer. *Bull Inst Natl Hyg* 1944; **1**: 1-69.

33. Denoix PF. De l'importance d'une nomenclature unifiee dans l'etude du cancer. *Rev Med Franc* 1947; **36**: 1124-1128.

34. Hutter RV. At last - Worldwide agreement on the staging of cancer. *Arch Surg* 1987; **122**: 1235-1239.

35. Tio L. The TNM staging system. *Gastrointest Endosc* 1996; **43**: S19-24.

36. Snady H, Bruckner H, Siegel J, Cooperman A, Neff R, Kiefer L. Endoscopic ultrasonographic criteria of vascular invasion by potentially resectable pancreatic tumors. *Gastrointest Endosc* 1994; **40**: 326-333.

37. Palazzo L, Burtin P. Interobserver variation in tumor staging. In: Rosch T (Ed) Endoscopic ultrasonography: State of the art - 1995. Part I. In Sivak M Jr (Ed) *Gastrointest Endosc Clinics N Am* 1995; **5**: 559-568.

38. Roubein L. Inter-observer variability in endoscopic ultrasonography: a prospective study. *Acta Endoscopica* 1995; **25**: 549-550.

39. Caletti GC, Brocchi E, Ferrari A *et al.* Guillotine needle biopsy as a supplement to endosonography in the diagnosis of gastric submucosal tumors. *Endoscopy* 1991; **23**: 251-254.

40. Wiersema M, Hawes R, Tao L-C *et al.* Endoscopic ultrasonography as an adjunct to fine needle aspiration cytology of the upper and lower gastrointestinal tract. *Gastrointest Endosc* 1992; **38**: 35-39.

41. Snady H. Combined endoscopic ultrasound and guillotine needle biopsy in the diagnosis of submucosal tumors of the gastrointestinal tract (Abstract). *Am J Gastroenterol* 1993; **88**: 1599.

42. Kimmey M, Martin R. Fundamentals of endosonography. In: Lightdale C (Ed) Endoscopic ultrasonography. *Gastrointest Endosc Clinics N Am* 1992; **2**: 557-573.

43. Kremkau F, Taylor K. Artifacts in ultrasound imaging. *J Ultrasound Med* 1986; **5**: 227-237.

44. Scanlan KA. Sonographic artifacts and their origins. *Am J Radiol* 1991; **156**: 1267-1272.

45. Rubin J, Adler R, Bude R, Fowlkes J, Carson P. Clean and dirty shadowing at US: a reappraisal. *Radiology* 1991; **181**: 231-236.

46. Kliewer MA, Hertzberg BX, George PY, McDonald JW, Bowie JD, Carroll BA. Acoustic shadowing from uterine leiomyomas: sonographic-pathologic correlation. *Radiology* 1995; **196**: 99-102.

47. Catalano M. Normal structures on endoscopic ultrasonography: visualization measurement data and interobserver variation. In: Rosch T (Ed) Endoscopic ultrasonography: State of the art - 1995. Part I. In: Sivak M Jr (Ed) *Gastrointest Endosc Clin N Am* 1995; **5**: 474-486.

48. Kimmey MB, Martin RW, Haggitt RC, Wang Y, Franklin DW, Silverstein FE. Histologic correlates of gastrointestinal ultrasound images. *Gastroenterology* 1989; **96**: 433-441.

49. Aibe T, Fuji T, Okita K, Takemoto T. A fundamental study of the normal layer structure of the gastrointestinal wall visualized by endoscopic ultrasonography. *Scand J Gastroenterol* 1986; **21(suppl 123)**: 6-15.

50. Tio TL, Tytgat GNJ. Endoscopic ultrasonography of normal and pathologic upper gastrointestinal wall structure. *Scand J Gastroenterol* 1986; **21(suppl 123)**: 27-33.

51. Boscaini M, Montori A. Transrectal ultrasonography: Interpretation of normal intestinal wall structure for the preoperative staging of rectal cancer. *Scand J Gastroenterol* 1986; **21(suppl 123)**: 87-98.

52. Bolondi L, Caletti G, Casanova P, Villanacci V, Grigioni W, Labo G. Problems and variations in the interpretation of the ultrasound feature of the normal upper and lower GI tract wall. *Scand J Gastroenterol* 1986; **21(suppl 123)**: 16-26.

53. Silverstein F, Kimmey M, Martin R *et al*. Ultrasound and the intestinal wall: Experimental methods. *Scand J Gastroenterol* 1986; **21(suppl 123)**: 34-40.

54. Heinz A, Mildenberger P, Georg M, Garcia A, Junginger Th. *In vitro* studies of lymph node analysis. In: Rosch T (Ed) Endoscopic ultrasonography: State of the art - 1995. Part I. *Gastrointest Endosc Clin N Am* 1995; **5**: 577-586.

55. Aibe T, Ito T, Yoshida T *et al*. Endoscopic ultrasonography of lymph nodes surrounding the upper GI tract. *Scand J Gastroenterol* 1986; **21(suppl 123)**: 164-169.

56. Bhutani M, Hoffman B, Van Velse A, Hawes R. SHU508A (galactose microparticles) as contrast agent during endoscopic ultrasound. *Gastrointest Endosc* 1996; **43**: A416.

57. Andre M, Nelson T, Mattrey R. Physical and acoustical properties of perfluoroocytlbromide, an ultrasound contrast agent. *Invest Radiol* 1990; **25**: 983-987.

58. Mattrey R. The potential clinical impact of perflubron emulsion on general sonography. *Invest Radiol* 1991; **26**: S186-187.

59. Mattrey RF, Strich G, Shelton RE *et al*. Perfluorochemicals as US contrast agents for tumor imaging and hepatosplenography: preliminary clinical results. *Radiology* 1987; **163**: 339-343.

60. Fritzsch T, Hilmann J, Kampfe M, Muller N, Schobel C, Siegert J. SHU508, a transpulmonary echocontrast agent: initial experience. *Invest Radiol* 1990; **25**: S160-S161.

61. Gallez B, Demeure R, Debuyst R *et al*. Evaluation of nonionic nitroxyl lipids as potential organ specific contrast agents for magnetic resonance imaging. *Mag Res Imag* 1992; **10**: 445-455.

62. Bhutani MS, Hoffman BJ, Hawes RH. A swine model for endosonographic pancreatic imaging (Abstract). *Gastrointest Endosc* 1996; **43**: s53.

63. Maruoka A, Fujishima H, Misawa T, Chijiiwa Y, Nawata H. Evaluation of acetic acid-induced gastric ulcers in dogs by endoscopic ultrasonography. *Scand J Gastroenterol* 1993; **28**: 1055-1061.

64. Jutabha R, Jensen D, Machicado G, Hirabayashi K. Reliability of endoscopic ultrasound probe imaging of canine abdominal veins before and after sclerotherapy in a blinded study. *Gastrointest Endosc* 1996; **43**: A297.

65. Taniguchi D, Martin R, Trowers E, Silverstein F. Simultaneous M-mode echoesophagram and manometry in sheep esophagus. *Gastrointest Endosc* 1995; **41**: 582-586.

66. Lees WR. Endoscopic ultrasonography of chronic pancreatitis and pancreatic pseudocysts. *Scand J Gastroenterol* 1986; **21(suppl 123)**: 123-129.

67. Rosch T, Dittler HK, Fockens P, Yasuda K, Lightdate C. Major complications of endoscopic ultrasonography: results of a survey of 42 105 cases (Abstract). *Gastrointest Endosc* 1993; **39**: 370.

68. Wayt Gibbs W. Ultrasound's new phase. *Sci Am* 1996; **274**: 32-34.

14

Metabolic studies on isolated intestinal tissue

Barry J Campbell and Jonathan M Rhodes

Summary

Metabolic labelling using radioactive isotope incorporation is a valuable and rapid method for the assessment of mucosal protein or glycoprotein synthesis and of the metabolism of mucosal nutrients.

We describe two techniques with which whole epithelial biopsy specimens from patients attending routine endoscopy can be examined in an *in vitro* culture system that allows (i) the assessment of their ability to incorporate radiolabelled precursors (e.g. N-acetylglucosamine, sialic acid and sulphate) into mucosal glycoproteins, particularly but not exclusively mucins, and (ii) metabolism of nutrients to be examined (e.g butyrate and glutamine) by isolated intestinal mucosa.

Introduction

Intestinal mucus glycoprotein (mucin) synthesis

The method of isolated organ culture was originated by Trowell[1] and adapted by Trier *et al* for mucosal biopsies of the small intestine, colon and rectum, providing excellent cell morphology and function for at least 16 hours and sometimes as long as 24-48 hours.[2-4] Following incubation in the presence of radioactive precursors, labelled macromolecules (proteins and glycoproteins) released into the culture medium can be separated and characterized.

Metabolic incorporation of radioactive precursors into intestinal mucosal glycoproteins can be performed using either 'steady-state' labelling or 'pulse (pulse-chase)' labelling techniques. 'Steady-state' labelling is the better method to assess glycoprotein synthesis. Here, the isolated tissue is incubated for long periods (12-48 hours) in the presence of a high concentration of radioactive precursor in the culture medium, typically 0.5-5 µCi/ml for monosaccharide precursors and 50-100 µCi/ml for sulphate. This is sufficient to obtain high incorporation of radiolabel into all the tissue glycoconjugates and to allow their subsequent isolation and structural analysis. It is important to ensure that the growth media contain sufficient glucose and serum throughout the culture in order to maintain normal glycosylation and rates of maturation of the synthesized tissue glycoproteins.

In contrast, the 'pulse' method of labelling is performed for short periods, typically <1 hour. It is particularly useful for studying secretion. However, the time course for maturation of many glycoproteins is known to be hours and therefore it is of limited value in studying glycoconjugate synthesis as many may still be in precursor form, unless the pulse is followed by a prolonged 'chase'.

One of our main interests has been the role of mucus in the protection of intestinal mucosa. Secreted mucus is the major component of the glycoprotein synthesized by the intestinal mucosa. The intact mucus glycoprotein (mucin) molecules are very large (MW $1-20 \times 10^6$ Da), form gels and are heavily O-glycosylated (accounting for over 70% of their dry weight), and are often highly charged due to sialylation and/or sulphation (colonic mucins are particularly rich in acidic oligosaccharide side-chains with a high degree of sulphation). In mucus, approximately half of the carbohydrate component is N-acetyl-D-glucosamine, N-acetyl-D-galactosamine or sialic acid. These particular sugars are supplied to the glycoprotein molecule from the activated nucleotide sugar donors UDP-galactose, UDP-N-acetylglucosamine, UDP-N-acetylgalactosamine, GDP-fucose and CMP-sialic acid using glycosyltransferase for their attachment in the Golgi network. Subsequent addition of O-sulphate esters to mucin oligosaccharide chains occurs in the trans Golgi.

We have investigated the possibility that an underlying mucus abnormality might be present in conditions such as inflammatory bowel disease, peptic ulceration and intestinal cancer.[5] We have been particularly interested in the changes in oligosaccharide side-chain structure and sulphation that occur in these conditions.

This chapter describes a method for the metabolic labelling of isolated intestinal tissue in organ culture which is simple, easy to perform and which in our hands has provided a useful means for directly examining the synthesis and secretion of mucus glycoproteins (mucins) in both healthy and diseased colorectal mucosa.[6-11] The methods of tissue culture, metabolic radiolabelling and mucin purification described can also be applied to a wide range of other mucosal tissues where mucins are produced (e.g. lung).[12]

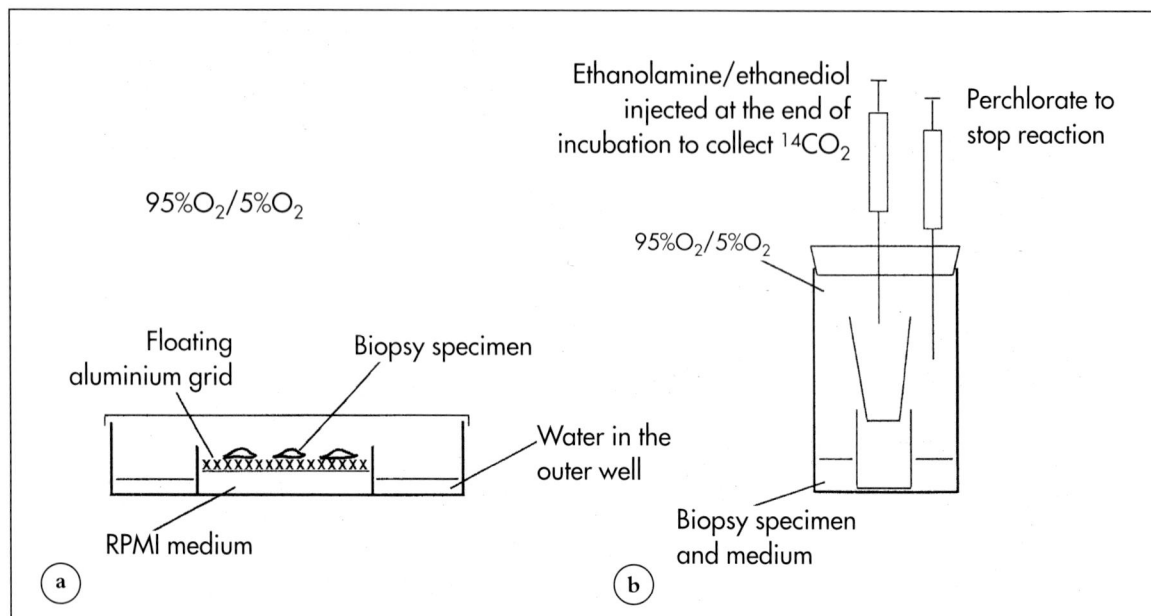

Figure 14.1 - a) Apparatus for short-term organ culture of whole intestinal biopsy specimens. **b**) Apparatus for measurement of metabolism by intestinal biopsy specimens (b is reproduced from reference 24 with permission). For detailed descriptions see respective methods section.

Methods

Culture of biopsy specimens of intestinal mucosa

1. Take control biopsies (approximately 10-15 mg wet weight) from a site at least 5 cm from any macroscopic abnormality. Colonic and ileal biopsies may be studied. They may be obtained either at endoscopy or by dissection of resected mucosa within 30 min of resection. For the latter, standard colonoscopic biopsy forceps can be used or alternatively a sterile surgical blade.

2. Collect endoscopic biopsies on lens tissue (Whatman Ltd, Maidstone, UK) soaked in Roswell Park Memorial Institute 1640 (RPMI) culture medium supplemented with 2 mM glutamine, 10% (v/v) fetal calf serum, 100 µg/ml gentamicin and 60 U/ml nystatin (Gibco Ltd, Edinburgh, Scotland). Transport to the laboratory within 10 min. Longer transportation times may be acceptable if transported in a suitable container pre-gassed with 95% O_2/5% CO_2.

3. Gently place up to three tissue biopsies, orientated with mucosal surface facing upward, on an aluminium wire grid (W David & Sons Ltd, Wellingborough, UK) in a Falcon® 60 mm × 15 mm organ culture dish with centre well (Becton Dickinson, Lincoln Park, NJ, USA). The aluminium mesh is floated on 1 ml of RPMI culture medium (supplemented with 2 mM glutamine, 10% (v/v) fetal calf serum, 100 mg/ml gentamicin and 60 U/ml nystatin) in the organ culture dish central well (Fig. 14.1a). Take care not to submerge the biopsies.

4. Add 2 ml of sterile deionized water to the outer well of the culture dish so as to obtain humidity saturation and prevent the biopsies drying out during incubation.

5. Place the culture dish in a water-jacketed Forma Scientific incubator (Jencons Ltd, Leighton Buzzard, UK) with protected circuitry to permit use of high % O_2. Maintain for 18 hours at 37°C in an atmosphere of 95% O_2 and 5% CO_2.

Mucus glycoprotein (mucin) synthesis assessed by [³H]-N-acetyl-D-glucosamine incorporation

New glycoprotein synthesis can be quantitatively measured through the addition of 0.5-2 µCi N-acetyl-D-[1-³H]-glucosamine (2-10 Ci/mmol, Amersham, Little Chalfont, UK) per ml medium, at the start of the culture period. Alternatively, D-[1-³H]glucosamine hydrochloride (1-5 Ci/mmol, Amersham) can be used.

It should be noted that incorporation of [³H]-N-acetylglucosamine or [³H]-glucosamine into mucus glycoproteins results in the labelling of the aminosugars N-acetylglucosamine, N-acetylgalactosamine and N-acetylneuraminic acid.[13]

Isolation of metabolically radiolabelled mucins

1. From each dish harvest the biopsies (stored macromolecules) and the culture medium (containing secreted macromolecules) separately.

2. Rinse the biopsies in ice cold 0.1 M Tris-HCl pH 8.0 containing 0.01% (w/v) thimerosal (as a broad-spectrum protease inhibitor) to remove adherent mucus. Pool the wash containing adherent mucus with the collected medium. Store at -40°C.

3. Place the biopsies in 5 ml ice-cold 0.1 M Tris-HCl pH 8.0 containing 0.01% (w/v) thimerosal and ultrasonicate with 8 × 15 second bursts (number 4 power setting), on ice, using an MSE ultrasonic disintegrator (MSE Instruments, Crawley, UK). The biopsies should then appear a ghostly white.

4. Centrifuge the samples at 105,000 g for 60 min at °4C. Collect the supernatant.

5. Retain 100 µl of the supernatant for either (i) protein estimation by a modified Lowry method standardized using bovine serum albumin, or (ii) DNA estimation by indirect fluorimetry (using bisbenzamide/Hoechst No.33258 DNA stain) for a size estimation of the biopsy.

6. To remove unincorporated radiolabelled substrate, desalt the biopsy supernatant and the medium separately by application of 2.5 ml aliquots to PD10 Sephadex GM25 gel columns (5 ×1.6 cm) (Pharmacia Ltd, Uppsala, Sweden) pre-equilibrated with deionized water.

7. Collect the excluded material, freeze at -80°C and lyophilize overnight in a freeze drier at -47°C and under a vacuum of 54 mBar.

8. Redissolve the lyophilized crude mucin in 0.1 M Tris-HCl pH 8.0, at a concentration of 5-10 mg/ml. Inject aliquots via a 200 µl sample loop onto a 10 mm x 30 cm Superose 6 HR10/30 gel filtration column. Elute at room temperature with 0.1 M Tris-HCl pH 8.0, at a rate of 15 ml/h, using a borosilicate glass pump fast protein liquid chromatography (FPLC) system (Pharmacia Ltd).

9. Collect 1 ml fractions for 2 hours and monitor continuously at an optical density (OD) of 280 nm. This procedure has been shown to yield mucus glycoprotein of high purity in the void volume fractions, free from contaminating non-mucus glycoprotein which are included.[14,15]

10. Remove a 100 µl aliquot of each fraction for total mucin quantification by enzyme-linked immunosorbent assay (ELISA) using an anti-mucin antibody (e.g. CAM17.1, a mouse monoclonal antibody with specificity for human colonic mucins (Euro DPC, Llanberis, UK)),[14,15] or by enzyme-linked lectin-binding assay (ELLA) with peroxidase-conjugated wheat germ agglutinin (WGA, Vector Lab. Ltd, Peterborough, UK).[15]

11. Retain the void volume fractions (7-10 ml) corresponding to the high molecular weight mucins. Remove 100 µl from each fraction for protein estimation by a modified Lowry method standardized using bovine serum albumin.

Measurement of radiolabelled metabolic products

1. Quantify the label incorporated into mucin by placing 100 µl of each Superose 6-purified mucin fraction into 20 ml polypropylene scintillation vials (May & Baker; Manchester, UK). Add 5 ml of Optiphase Safe scintillation fluid (Wallac, Milton Keynes, UK) to each sample and mix.

2. Count on a LKB Wallac 1219 RACKBETA liquid scintillation counter (Wallac) or equivalent.

3. Express results as disintegrations per min (dpm) ^{3}H incorporated into mucin/mg protein or /μg DNA in the biopsy ultrasonicate (or /mg total mucin protein). This gives an indication of the synthesis of mucin during the experiment. Although N-acetylglucosamine incorporation is only an indirect marker of mucus synthesis, it allows useful comparison between synthetic rates in different tissues.

Labelling of mucin O-sulphate esters using [^{35}S]-sulphate

To quantify mucin sulphation, add 50 μCi [^{35}S]-sulphate (250-1000 μCi/mmol) (NEN Products, Brussels, Belgium) and 2 μCi N-acetyl-D-[1-^{3}H]-glucosamine per ml medium, at the start of the culture period.

It should be noted that analysis of the ratio of dpm of ^{35}S to dpm of ^{3}H incorporated into the isolated pure mucin fractions gives an indication of the degree of sulphation. Analysis of the amount of ^{35}S or ^{3}H incorporated into isolated mucin/mg protein or /mg DNA in the biopsy ultrasonicate again gives an indication of the synthesis of mucin during the experiment.

Labelling of mucin sialic acids using [^{3}H]-N-acetyl-D-mannosamine

To quantify mucin sialylation, add 2 μCi N-acetyl-D-[6-^{3}H]-mannosamine (10 Ci/mmol) (NEN Products, Brussels, Belgium) and 2 μCi N-acetyl-D-[1-^{14}C]-galactosamine (800 mCi/mmol) (ICN Radiochemicals, Irvine, CA, USA) per ml medium, at the start of the culture period.

It should be noted that N-acetylmannosamine is a specific sialic acid precursor with no significant incorporation of radiolabel as N-acetylglucosamine and N-acetylgalactosamine.[13] N-acetylgalactosamine is useful as an index of the number of O-linked oligosaccharides (since N-acetylgalactosamine only occurs either as an initial O-linked carbohydrate or as a terminal residue in blood group A) and moreover results in no formation of labelled sialic acid.[13] Analysis of the ratio of dpm of ^{3}H to dpm of ^{14}C incorporated into the isolated pure mucin fractions gives an indication of the degree of sialylation. Analysis of the amount of ^{3}H or ^{14}C incorporated into isolated mucin/mg biopsy protein or /μg DNA in the

ultrasonicate, gives an indication of the synthesis of mucin during the experiment.

Application to animal studies

The techniques of metabolic labelling of whole biopsy specimens described in this chapter can easily be adapted for the metabolic study of isolated animal gastrointestinal tissues.

The study of macromolecular synthesis in mucosal explants was originally performed by Trier *et al* on tissue biopsies of both human and rabbit small intestine, colon and rectum.[2-4,16] In these studies, the viability of rabbit biopsies in short-term culture provided a convenient model for pilot studies of protein and glycoprotein synthesis and secretion assessed by incorporation at a steady rate of radiolabelled leucine and N-acetylglucosamine into proteins and glycoproteins. All regions of the rabbit gastrointestinal tract culture extremely well (including gastric fundus and antrum, small intestine, colon, rectum), whereas in humans the gastric fundus mucosa degenerates rapidly. However, culture of the small intestinal mucosae from the rat, mouse and hamster is more difficult.[17] The viability of biopsies in culture should be established over a 48 hour period, including cell morphology, protein and DNA (using ^{3}H-thymidine incorporation) synthetic activity, prior to studies examining factors which control normal epithelial function. Such studies using rabbit colon biopsies in short-term organ culture have been important in showing the increased uptake of [^{3}H]-N-acetylglucosamine into secretory glycoproteins of the colon in response to intracellular cyclic AMP and agents which elevate cAMP.[18]

Results and discussion

Control experiments have demonstrated that [^{3}H]-N-acetylglucosamine ([^{3}H]-GlcNAc) can be incorporated reproducibly into intestinal mucins. Initially there is a lag of 6-8 hours when the rate of mucin synthesis is low, followed by a period when the rate of mucin synthesis (total mucin in the biopsy and culture medium) is roughly linear for up to 26 hours. Radiolabelling of mucin in the biopsy specimen homogenate increases gradually to a peak at around 20-25 hours (Fig. 14.2).[8,10] Indeed by the end of the

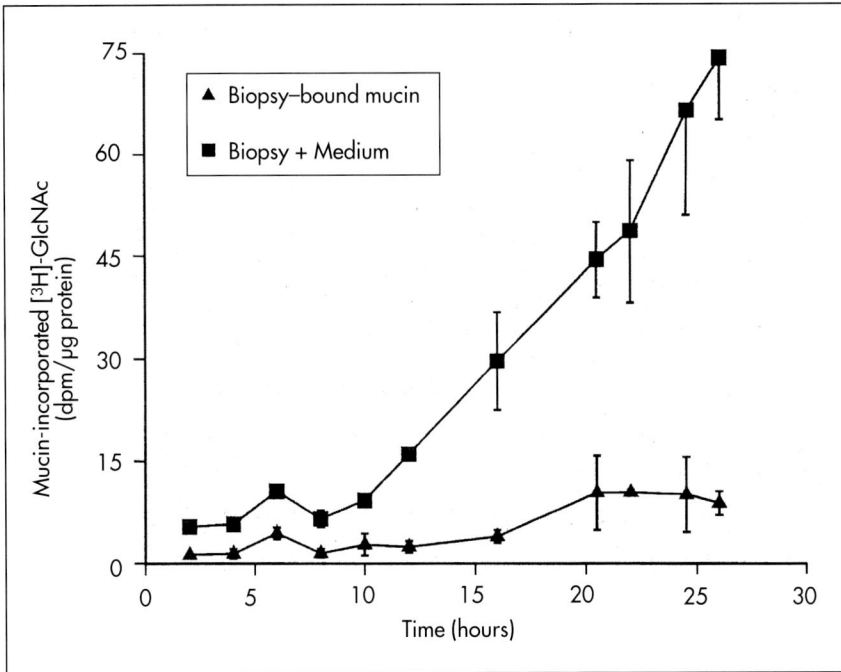

Figure 14.2 - Time course for incorporation of [³H]GlcNAc into mucin by colonic biopsy specimens (from a patient with cancer of the colon). ■ = biopsy specimen, ▲ = sum of biopsy specimen and culture medium. Note the time lag with little incorporation of [³H]N acetylglucosamine into mucin in the first 6-8 hours, followed by a period when the rate of incorporation is roughly linear. Reproduced from reference 10, reprinted with permission.

incubation more macromolecular radioactivity may be recoverable from the incubation medium than from the tissue.

We use radiolabelled N-acetylglucosamine rather than radiolabelled glucosamine as the former is more readily utilized in tissue from patients with inflammatory bowel disease.[19] The use of unlabelled precursor in a steady-state rather than pulse-chase labelling experiment is not recommended as this will decrease the specific activity of the label in the medium and consequently radiolabelled precursor incorporation into the mucin. Unlabelled glucose, already in the medium, provides both energy and a glycoconjugate precursor pool. It is also a rate-limiting step in the biosynthesis of radiolabelled glycoconjugates.

Abnormalities of mucin have been shown in ulcerative colitis using histochemical, biochemical and tissue culture techniques and an attractive hypothesis is that a primary abnormality of mucin synthesis predisposes subjects to an as yet undefined enviromental factor that induces the disease.[5] The mucins synthesized by the colorectal mucosa are normally rich in carbohydrate O-sulphate esters and sialic acids giving these molecules their characteristic high charge. Previous histochemical studies have identified goblet cell depletion and a reduction in staining for sulphated mucin associated with ulcerative colitis and colon cancer.[20] Increased sialylation of peripheral carbohydrate structures has been reported in mucins secreted by colorectal cancer cells.[21]

Using the method described above, we have compared mucin synthesis, sulphation and sialylation in a series of patients with inflammatory bowel disease with those with a histologically normal colon. In patients with ulcerative colitis we have demonstrated a highly significant reduction in the ability of the colorectal mucosa to incorporate radiolabelled-sulphate into mucin (Fig. 14.3)[6] and an increased incorporation of sialic acid precursor, N-acetylman-nosamine, compared to controls.[9] There is a well recognized increase in relative risk for colorectal cancer in patients with extensive ulcerative colitis,[22] so the functional significance of these changes may be of considerable interest,[23] since there is evidence of a correlation between (i) increased risk for colitis-associated colon cancer with reduced sulphation[24] and (ii) increased metastatic potential with increased sialylation.[25]

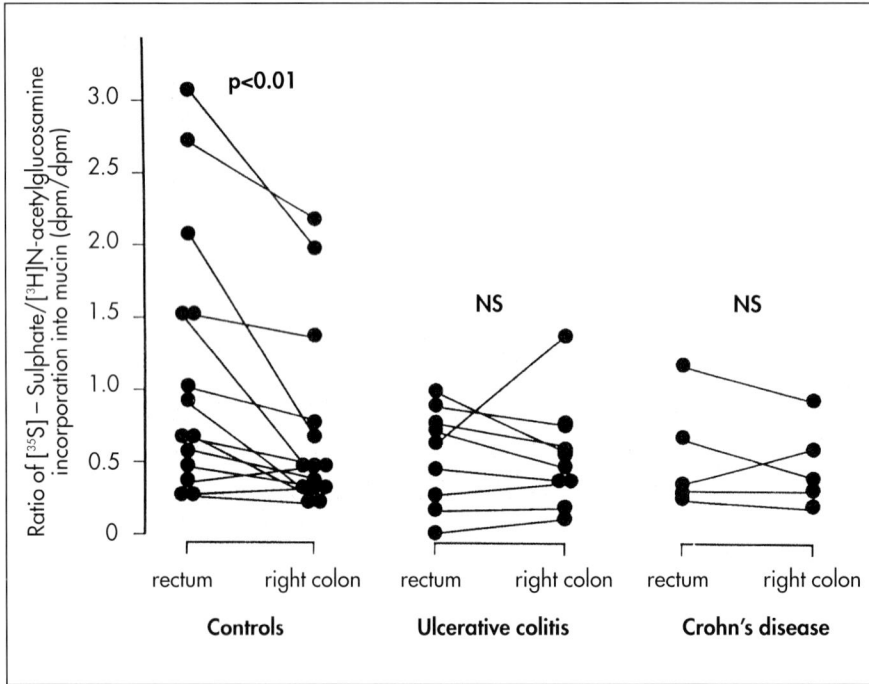

Figure 14.3 –
Ratio of [³⁵S]sulphate to N-[³H]acetylglucosamine incorporated into purified mucin by cultured biopsies in the rectum and their paired proximal colonic biopsies in control subjects, patients with ulcerative colitis and patients with Crohn's disease. Reproduced from reference 6 with permission.

In addition, we have successfully used the method described above to examine factors which alter mucus synthesis. Agents of therapeutic potential or of unclear therapeutic effect in intestinal disease can be assessed for their effect on mucosal synthesis. For example, exacerbations of ulcerative colitis can be treated successfully with sodium butyrate,[26] although its exact mode of action is unclear. Butyrate is an important source of colonocyte energy and deficiency in its metabolism has been implicated in the disease.[27-29] We have shown that sodium butyrate,[10] as well as other agents of therapeutic use such as the corticosteroids prednisolone and hydrocortisone,[11] strikingly enhance colonic mucin synthesis (as assessed by incorporation of radiolabelled N-acetyl-D-glucosamine) at concentrations that are therapeutically relevant. We have also demonstrated that although mucus synthesis is abnormal in ulcerative colitis it is unrelated to cigarette smoking,[8] a factor thought to influence inflammatory bowel disease activity; however, at nicotine levels likely to occur following smoking, nicotine does indeed enhance mucin synthesis and may very well be of some therapeutic benefit.[11] Dietary lectins have also been shown to alter colonic mucus synthesis using this technique.[7]

It is possible to extend the *in vitro* colonic biopsy culture system described above to examine mucolytic erosion of the mucus gel barrier by proteinases in the intestinal lumen. Here, radiolabelled amino acids (e.g. [U-¹⁴C]-L-threonine) can be incorporated into synthesized mucus glycoprotein and we have used this labelled mucin successfully as a substrate to analyse increases in mucolytic activity in intestinal disease.[30]

Introduction

Intestinal epithelial metabolism of butyrate and glutamine

The method described here to study intestinal mucosal metabolism is based on the technique of Veerkamp *et al*, originally devised to study fatty acid metabolism in skeletal muscle.[31] A previous adaptation of this original technique to the study of intestinal metabolism entailed preparation of a pure intestinal epithelial cell population.[27] However, because of uncertainties about possible damage to the cells during the isolation procedure, we have developed this technique for use on whole mucosal biopsies.

It is well established that both glucose and glutamine are important energy sources for many rapidly dividing cells, particularly of the intestine. However, in the colon, there is likely to be little or no glutamine available to the colonic lumen because it is so readily utilized by colonic flora[28] and peripheral blood concentrations are less than 0.5 mM.[32] Instead, the colonic epithelium obtains much of its energy from short-chain fatty acids, particularly butyrate, resulting from bacterial fermentation of dietary fibre in the lumen.[33] Butyrate is oxidized to provide energy through the citric acid cycle, resulting in the production of 4 molecules of CO_2 per molecule of butyrate.

There is evidence to suggest that a metabolic defect within intestinal epithelial cells could contribute to the pathogenesis of intestinal mucosal diseases, with this abnormality resulting in energy deficiency at the cellular level.[27,29] The occurrence of colitis in animals that are vitamin deficient[34] or are treated with inhibitors of fatty acid metabolism[35] supports the theory. Thus, we applied the metabolic labelling technique described above to assess the metabolism of luminal nutrients (such as glutamine and butyrate) by ileal and colonic biopsies from patients with idiopathic inflammatory bowel disease and controls.[36]

Methods

1. Take control biopsies (10-15 mg wet weight) from a site at least 5 cm from any macroscopic abnormality. Take adjacent biopsies to check histology. Perform assays in duplicate at least, at each site studied.

2. Place endoscopic biopsies onto lens tissue soaked in ice-cold pregassed modified Krebs-Henseleit buffer containing 11 mM glucose (118 mM NaCl, 4.7 mM KCl, 1.17 mM $MgSO_4$ 1.17 mM KH_2PO_4; add sodium bicarbonate to give pH 7.4 as per manufacturers instructions; Sigma, Poole, UK). Transport on ice to the laboratory within 10 min.

3. Divide each specimen into 10 pieces (approximately 1 mg) using a sterile surgical blade.

4. Place in a glass scintillation vial with 1 ml buffer to which has been added either 1 µCi [1-^{14}C] n-butyric acid (30-50 mCi/mmol, ICN Biomed Inc, Thame, UK) and 1 mM sodium butyrate, or 1 µCi L-[U-^{14}C]-glutamic acid (165-225 mCi/mmol, ICN Biomed Inc) and 1 mM L-glutamine.

5. Suspend an Eppendorf reaction vial above the culture medium using a 2 ml polyethylene sample cup (Elkay Products, Shrewsbury, MA, USA) and gas the vial with 95% CO_2/5% O_2 and close tightly with a rubber seal (Fig. 14.1b).

6. Culture vials for 2 hours at 37°C in a shaking water bath (Grant Instruments, Cambridge, UK) set at 120 oscillations per min.

7. Inject 0.25 ml 10% (v/v) perchloric acid in water, through the rubber seal, into the culture medium to stop the reaction.

8. Inject 0.5 ml of 6:3 ethane-1,2-diol:ethanolamine, through the rubber seal, into the Eppendorf reaction tube to absorb ^{14}C-labelled CO_2.

9. Store vials at 4°C for 90 min to allow equilibration.

10. Remove the reaction Eppendorf and place in 10 ml of scintillatiom fluid (4 g/l Omniflour in 2:1 toluene/methanol). Shake vigorously and count in a scintillation counter.

11. Express results as nmol substrate metabolized/hour/mg protein.

Application to animal studies

The above method has also been used to assess animal intestinal nutrient utilization. The technique was first established to study fatty acid metabolism in rat skeletal muscle.[31] Many studies since have also used isolated intestinal epithelial cells from rat jejunum, caecum and colon to study mucosal nutrient utilization.[37,38] Using these methods, it has been possible to demonstrate that starvation reduces the rate of metabolism of glutamine but not of ketone bodies in colonic epithelial cells of the rat.[38]

Results and discussion

Using the technique described above, we have assessed the metabolism of butyrate and glutamine by ileal and colonic biopsies from patients with idiopathic colitis and controls,[36] with a view to establishing whether the metabolism of the short-chain fatty acid butyrate is impaired in ulcerative colitis as previously suggested.[27,29]

Control experiments have shown acceptable reproducibility (overall coefficient of variation, 20-23%) with minimal contribution to butyrate metabolism from non-epithelial cells in the intestinal biopsies (4.5-8.5%). Further control experiments were performed to assess the effects of varying concentrations of butyrate. Metabolism was optimal at concentrations 1 mM but concentrations >5 mM were found to be relatively toxic. However, the rate of metabolism of 1 mM ^{14}C-labelled butyrate and glutamine to $^{14}CO_2$ by colonoscopic biopsies (10 mg wet weight) taken from a resected colon incubated in 1 ml of medium was linear for at least 3 hours (Fig. 14.4). In the case of butyrate (1 µmol total butyrate in 1 ml of medium), after 2 hours incubation about 200 nmol of CO_2 was produced for each mg of tissue protein. Given that the complete oxidation of 1 molecule of butyrate results in 4 molecules of CO_2, this represents the utilization of 50 nmol of butyrate per mg tissue protein.

This technique confirmed the high rate of butyrate metabolism by the normal colonic mucosa, indicating that such short-chain fatty acids rather than glutamine are the preferred energy source for colonocytes (Table 14.1). There was also regional variation of nutrient utilization throughout the colon. In contrast to the isolated colonocyte studies, we have illustrated with this technique that mucosal biopsy specimens from sufferers of quiescent ulcerative colitis possess a normal ability to oxidize butyrate compared with controls (Table 14.1), a fact now corroborated by two

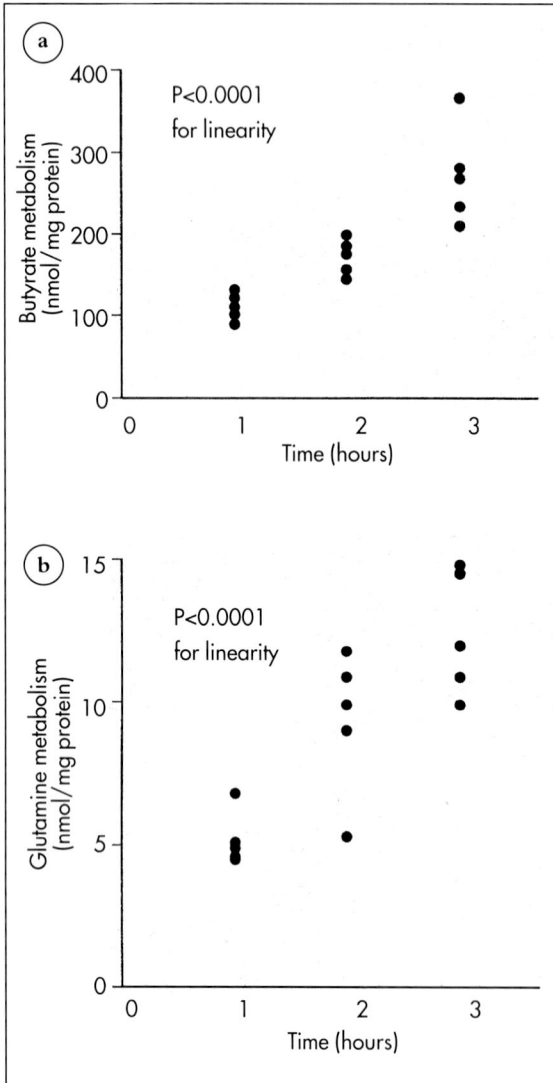

Figure 14.4 - Rate of metabolism of **a**) butyrate and **b**) glutamine by colonic biopsies. The rate of metabolism of sodium [1-^{14}C] butyrate or [U-^{14}C] glutamine to $^{14}CO_2$ by colonoscopic biopsies taken from a resected colon was found to be linear for at least 3 hours (p<0.0001 for linearity test using grouped regression analysis (Arcus Pro-Stat, Aughton, Lancs, UK)). Metabolism is measured as number of nmol $^{14}CO_2$ produced from sodium [1-^{14}C]-butyrate per mg biopsy protein. Adapted from reference 24, with permission.

Table 14.1 – Metabolism of glutamine and butyrate by mucosal biopsy specimens.

	Controls (n=12)	Ulcerative colitis (n=12)
Ascending colon, butyrate	62.6 (44.2)	92.5 (58.3)
Ascending colon, glutamine	4.9 (3.2)*	6.2 (7.7)
Ascending colon, butyrate/glutamine	14.3 (9.6)†	14.6 (9.3)
Descending colon, butyrate	51.5 (32.0)	93.3 (115.0)
Descending colon, glutamine	1.4 (0.7)*‡	7.8 (7.9)‡
Descending colon, butyrate/glutamine	20.6 (14.3)†	15.9 (15.6)

Mean figures for metabolism (nmol/mg biopsy protein/hour) of each nutrient are given with standard deviation in parentheses. Values with the same superscript are significantly different at p<0.05 (*,†) or p<0.01 (‡) using Mann Whitney U test.
Reproduced from reference 36 with permission.

recent studies.[39,40] In addition, an increased rate of glutamine utilization in the distal colonic mucosa was observed in ulcerative colitis biopsies compared to controls (Table 14.1). This probably relates to the increased rate of colonocyte proliferation seen in this condition. Control experiments suggest that inflammatory cells contribute little to the butyrate metabolism by the biopsy.[36]

An important additional effect is the need to avoid variation in bowel preparations prior to harvesting of the biopsy tissue. Starvation reduces the rate of glutamine metabolism[38] and as far as possible diet should be equivalent in the diseased and control patients.

Acknowledgements

Funding was obtained from the Medical Research Council, the National Association for Colitis & Crohn's Disease, the British Digestive Fund and the North West Regional Health Authority. Studies were approved by the Ethical Committee of the South Sefton Health Authority and the Royal Liverpool University Hospital Trust. The authors would also like to thank the Gastroenterology Unit, the Cancer Tissue Bank and the Departments of Surgery and Pathology (University of Liverpool and the Royal Liverpool University Hospital Trust) for their co-operation in obtaining tissue specimens.

References

1. Trowell OA. The culture of mature organs in a synthetic medium. *Exp Cell Res* 1959; **16:** 118-147.

2. Browning TH, Trier JS. Organ culture of mucosal biopsies of human small intestine. *J Clin Invest* 1969; **48:** 1423-1432.

3. Eastwood GL, Trier JS. Organ culture of human rectal mucosa. *Gastroenterology* 1973; **64:** 375-382.

4. McDermott RP, Donaldson RM, Trier JS. Glycoprotein synthesis and secretion by mucosal biopsies of rabbit colon and human rectum. *J Clin Invest* 1974; **54:** 545-554.

5. Rhodes JM. Colonic mucus and mucosal glycoproteins: the key to colitis and cancer? *Gut* 1989; **30:** 1660-1666.

6. Raouf AH, Tsai HH, Parker N, Hoffman J, Walker RJ, Rhodes JM. Sulphation of colonic and rectal mucin in inflammatory bowel disease: reduced sulphation of rectal mucus in ulcerative colitis. *Clin Sci* 1992; **83:** 623-626.

7. Ryder SD, Parker N, Eccleston D, Haqqani MT, Rhodes JM. Peanut lectin stimulates proliferation in colonic explants from patients with inflammatory bowel disease and colon polyps. *Gastroenterology* 1994; **106:** 117-124.

8. Ryder SD, Raouf AH, Parker N, Walker RJ, Rhodes JM. Abnormal mucosal glycoprotein synthesis in inflammatory bowel diseases is not related to cigarette smoking. *Digestion* 1995; **56:** 370-376.

9. Parker N, Tsai HH, Ryder SD, Raouf AH, Rhodes JM. Increased rate of sialylation of colonic mucin by cultured ulcerative colitis mucosal explants. *Digestion* 1995; **56:** 52-56.

10. Finnie IA, Dwarakanath AD, Taylor BA, Rhodes JM. Colonic mucin synthesis is increased by sodium butyrate. *Gut* 1995; **36:** 93-99.

11. Finnie IA, Campbell BJ, Taylor BA *et al.* Stimulation of colonic mucin synthesis by corticosteroids and nicotine. *Clin Sci* 1996; **91:** 359-364.

12. Cheng PW, Sherman JM, Boat TF, Bruce P. Quantification of radiolabelled mucous glycoproteins secreted by tracheal explants. *Ann Biochem* 1981; **117:** 301-306.

13. Diaz S, Varki A. Glycosylation: Metabolic radiolabelling of animal cell glycoconjugates. In: Colligan JE *et al* (Eds) *Current Protocols in Protein Science*, Vol 1. John Wiley & Sons, Inc, New York, 1995, pp.12.2.1-12.2.9.

14. Parker N, Finnie IA, Raouf AH *et al.* High performance gel filtration using monodisperse highly cross-linked agarose as a one-step system for mucin purification. *Biomed Chromatogr* 1993: **7:** 68-74.

15. Raouf AH, Parker N, Iddon D *et al.* Ion-exchange chromatography of purified colonic mucus glycoproteins in inflammatory bowel disease: absence of a selective subclass defect. *Gut* 1991; **32:** 1139-45.

16. Kagnoff MF, Donaldson RM, Trier JS. Organ culture of the rabbit small intestine: prolonged *in vitro* steady state protein synthesis and secretion and secretory IgA secretion. *Gastroenterology* 1972; **63:** 541-551.

17. Trier JS. Organ culture methods in the study of gastrointestinal-mucosal function and development. *N Engl J Med* 1976; **295:** 150-155.

18. Lamont JT, Ventola A. Stimulation of colonic glycoprotein synthesis by dibutyryl cyclic AMP and theophylline. *Gastroenterology* 1977; **72:** 82-86.

19. Burton AF, Anderson FH. Decreased incorporation of ^{14}C-glucosamine relative to ^{3}H-N-acetylglucosamine in the intestinal mucosa of patients with inflammatory bowel disease. *Am J Gastroenterol* 1983; **78:** 19-24.

20. Filipe MI. In: Whitehead R (Ed) *Gastrointestinal and Oesophageal Pathology*. Churchill-Livingstone Edinburgh, 1979, pp. 65-89.

21. Kim YS, Yuan M, Itzkowitz SH *et al.* Expression of Le Y and extended Le Y blood-group antigens in human malignant, premalignant and non-malignant colonic tissues. *Cancer Res* 1986; **46:** 5985-5992.

22. Gyde S, Prior P, Dew MJ. Mortality in ulcerative colitis. *Gastroenterology* 1982; **83:** 36-43.

23. Rhodes JM. A unifying hypothesis for inflammatory bowel disease and associated colon cancer: sticking the pieces together with sugar. *Lancet* 1996; **347:** 40-44.

24. Probert CSJ, Warren BF, Perry T, Mackay EH, Mayberry JF, Corfield AP. South Asian and European colitics show characteristics differences in colonic mucus glycoportens type and turnover. *Gut* 1995; **36:** 696-702.

25. Fogel M, Atterogt P, Schirrmacher V. Metastatic potential severely altered by changes in tumor cell adhesiveness and cell surface sialylation. *J Exp Med* 1983; **157:** 371-376.

26. Scheppach W, Sommer H, Kirchner T *et al.* Effect of butyrate enemas on the colonic mucosa in distal ulcerative colitis. *Gastroenterology* 1992; **103:** 51-56.

27. Roediger WEW. The colonic epithelium in ulcerative colitis: an energy deficient disease. *Lancet* 1980; **ii:** 712-715.

28. Chapman MAS, Grahn MF, Boyle MA, Hutton M, Rogers J, Williams NS. Butyrate oxidation is impaired in the colonic mucosa of sufferers of quiescent ulcerative colitis. *Gut* 1994; **35:** 73-76.

29. Chapman MAS, Grahn MF, Hutton M, Rogers J, Williams NS. Failure of colonic mucosa to oxidise butyrate in ulcerative colitis. *Gut* 1992; **33:** S40 (Abstract).

30. Dwarakanath AD, Campbell BJ, Tsai HH, Sunderland D, Hart CA, Rhodes JM. Faecal mucinase activity assessed in inflammatory bowel disease using ^{14}C-threonine labelled mucin substrate. *Gut* 1995; **37:** 58-62.

31. Veerkamp JH, Van Moerkerk HTB, Glatz JFC, Van Hinsbergh VWM. Incomplete palmitate oxidation in cell-free systems of rat and human muscles. *Biochem Biophys Acta* 1983; **753:** 399-410.

32. Deim K, Lentner C (Eds). *Documenta Geigy*, 7th edn. Geigy Pharmaceuticals, Macclesfield, 1970, pp. 574.

33. Roediger WEW. Role of anaerobic bacteria in the metabolic welfare of the colonic mucosa in man. *Gut* 1980; **21:** 793-798.

34. Wintrobe MM, Follis RH, Alcayaga R, Paulson M, Humphreys S. Panthothenic acid deficiency in swine. *Bull John Hopkins Hosp* 1943; **73:** 313-333.

35. Roediger WE, Nance S. Metabolic induction of experimental ulcerative colitis by inhibition of fatty acid oxidation. *Br J Exp Pathol* 1986; **67:** 773-782.

36. Finnie IA, Taylor BA, Rhodes JM. Ileal and colonic epithelial metabolism in quiescent ulcerative colitis: increased glutamine metabolism in distal colon but no defect in butyrate metabolism. *Gut* 1993; **34:** 1552-1558 and Letters to the Editor; *Gut* 1993; **34:** 1646 and 1152-1153.

37. Fleming SE, Fitch MD, DeVries S, Liu ML, Kight C. Nutrient utilisation by cells isolated from rat jejunum, caecum and colon. *J Nutr* 1991; **121:** 869-878.

38. Ardawi MSM, Newsholme EA. Fuel utilisation in colonocytes of the rat. *Biochem J* 1985; **231:** 713-719.

39. Clausen MR, Mortensen PB. Kinetic studies of colonocyte metabolism of short-chain fatty acids and glucose in patients with ulcerative colitis. *Gut* 1995; **37:** 685-689.

40. Allan ES, Winter S, Light AM, Allan A. Mucosal enzyme activity for butyrate oxidation; no defect in patients with ulcerative colitis. *Gut* 1996; **38:** 886-893.

15

Fibre optic confocal imaging (foci) for *in vivo* subsurface microscopy of the colon

Peter M Delaney, Glenn D Papworth and Roger G King

Summary

Fibre optic confocal imaging (FOCI) is a technique allowing visualisation of microscopic details of living tissue *in vivo*. The technology which enables FOCI has been miniaturised to produce an 'endomicroscope', a device having the dimensions of a conventional gastrointestinal endoscope. This creates the potential for 'optical biopsy' of gastrointestinal tissue, without the need for surgical biopsy and subsequent tissue processing.

Techniques were developed utilising FOCI to image components of the gastrointestinal tract *in vivo*, including the mucosa, enteric nervous system and microvasculature.

Endomicroscope images of the microvasculature of the rat colon *in vivo* revealed characteristic microvascular structure comparable with other *in vivo* confocal imaging studies. The myenteric plexus of rat colon imaged *in vivo* revealed ganglia, primary fibre tracts, secondary fibre bundles and neuronal cell bodies. Cells surrounding mucous crypts in samples of pig stomach *in vitro* were also imaged using FOCI, leading to ongoing *in vivo* investigations of the gastric mucosa in piglets using experimental confocal endomicroscope probes.

Work in progress to find the predominant areas of clinical usefulness and engineer devices specifically to these tasks may see the emergence of confocal endomicroscopy as an important clinical diagnostic technique in the future.

Introduction

Gastrointestinal biopsy makes a substantial contribution to our understanding of gastrointestinal diseases such as adenocarcinoma, Barrett's oesophagus, ulcerative colitis, Crohn's disease, oesophagitis, oesophageal, gastric or colonic neoplasms and gastritis.[1]

However, despite the wealth of information to be gained through microscopic examination of the various biopsies obtained from the gut, as with other tissues, biopsy procedures have certain limitations and drawbacks:

- the clinician must be selective in sampling a small area of tissue, and cannot guarantee sampling of the optimal region of tissue required for definitive assessment.

- the surgically invasive nature of biopsy procedures may be associated with risk of patient discomfort or even perforation.[2-4]

- processing of biopsies is laborious and time consuming, often incurring significant delays between the procedure and the assessment.[5] The post processing and delayed follow up are associated with significant costs,[6] which could potentially be reduced if diagnosis could be made at the time of the initial procedure.

- the biopsy represents a sample of the state of the host tissue at the time of the procedure. Therefore, the ability to perform dynamic observations of tissues or measure responses to exogenous stimuli at a microscopic level *in situ* is not offered by biopsy procedures.

A method for observing microscopic details of gastrointestinal tissue without the need for surgical excision is desirable. However, this has not been possible to date due to the inaccessibility of the area combined with the necessity for thin tissue sections, a requirement imposed by conventional microscope optics.

Limitations of conventional microscopy

With a conventional light microscope, the depth of field is very shallow, and diminishes with increasing magnification. When viewing thick translucent specimens, light returning from out-of-focus elements in the sample severely degrades the quality of the image. Thus fluorescence and reflectance images of samples suffer from reduced contrast.[7,8] This problem is overcome by slicing the tissue of interest to a thickness which is close to the depth of field at the desired magnification. Hence there is little purpose in attempting to miniaturise a conventional light microscope, or to utilise conventional microscopic techniques to image cellular or other microscopic details for diagnostic purposes *in vivo*.

Confocal microscopy

In recent years, the technique of confocal microscopy (first described by Minsky in 1957)[9] has become well established as a powerful research tool for the examination of living cells and tissues. A confocal microscope can isolate clear, high magnification views of individual focal planes at or beneath the surface of intact translucent specimens. It achieves this by optical sectioning, which is non-destructive and allows imaging in three dimensions. Confocal microscopy is thus well suited to *in vivo* microscopic imaging of living tissues otherwise impossible to image via conventional optical microscopy.

Several groups have used confocal microscopy to image a variety of tissues *in vivo*. Such tissues include skin,[10,11] teeth,[10,12] eye,[13-20] brain vasculature,[21-27] and epididymis, adrenal glands, liver, thyroid, muscle, nerve and connective tissue.[28]

Limitations of confocal microscopy

The bulky nature of conventional confocal microscopes, combined with movement artifacts (e.g. due to respiration) has hindered the progress of *in vivo* confocal microscopy, or the development of methods utilising the technology for non-invasive biopsy and histology of internal organs.

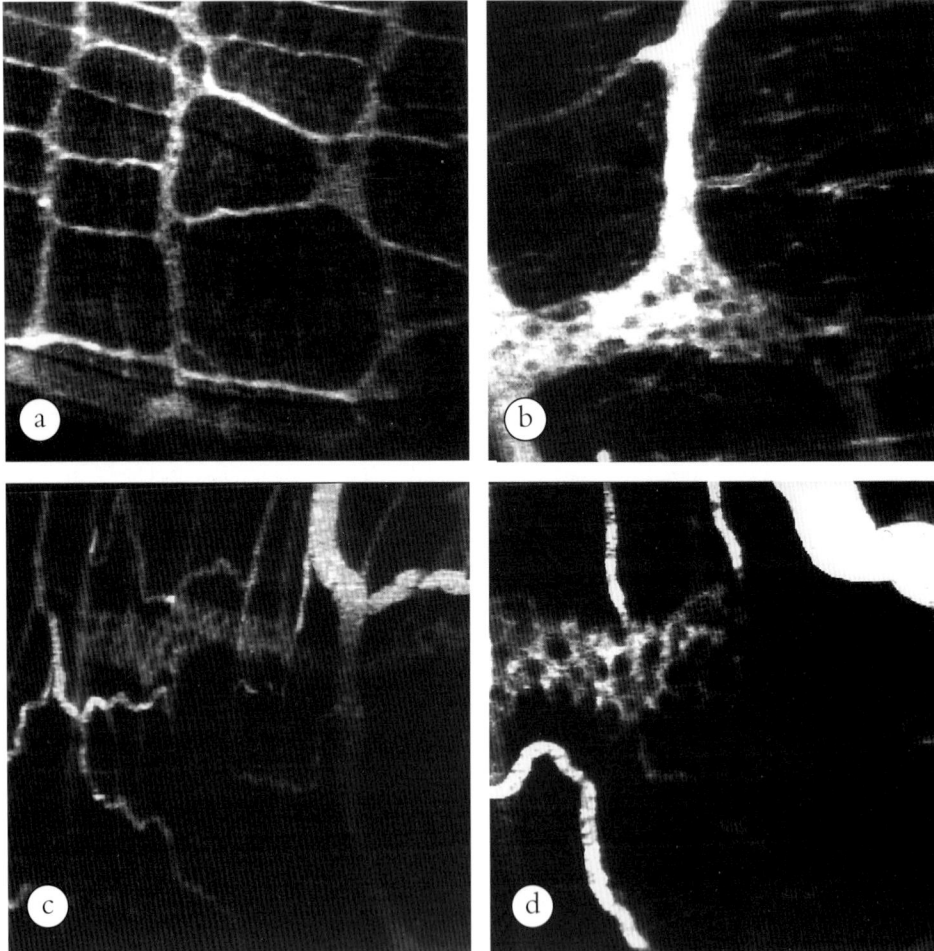

Figure 1 – Myenteric plexus of rat intact descending colon (serosal aspect) imaged *in vivo* following topical staining with 4-Di-2-ASP (10 μM). Visible in ***a*** are ganglia, primary fibre tracts, and secondary fibre bundles (field of view, FOV= 600 μm). At higher magnification ***b*** an individual ganglion and fibre tracts are seen, along with fine nerve fibres that are part of the tertiary nerve plexus. Within the ganglion, neuronal cell bodies are outlined as dark shapes (FOV= 300 μm). ***c, d*** show myenteric plexus of rat intact descending colon (serosal aspect) imaged *in vivo* following topical staining with 4-Di-2-ASP (10 μM) and i.v. 150kDa FITC-dextran (0.5 ml of 10 mg/ml). ***c*** shows the essentially planar nature of the myenteric plexus with few visible blood vessels running through this plane (FOV= 600 μm). At higher magnification ***(d)*** a myenteric plexus ganglion containing nerve cell bodies as dark shapes can be seen, but also visible are overlying vascular components with blood cells visible as dark shapes. Fine nerve fibres can also be seen in the background of the image (FOV= 300 μm).

Fibre optic confocal imaging (FOCI)

The fibre optic confocal imaging (FOCI) microscope[29] replaces a pinhole (used to deliver and/or collect light in the conventional confocal microscope) with an optical fibre, giving a reduction in bulk optics at the imaging end, and therefore a more compact and mobile instrument suited to *in vivo* work. Furthermore, the approach enables extreme miniaturisation,[30] and the development of tools akin to conventional endoscopes having confocal microscope capabilities.

The authors have developed several prototype confocal endomicroscope systems which have been trialed in animals with a view to eventually developing methodologies for diagnostic use in humans. A prototype endomicroscope with confocal microscope imaging capabilities in shown in Figure 15.2a.

Use of FOCI in the gastrointestinal tract

The potential to examine living cells in the gastrointestinal tract directly and without surgical excision presents obvious diagnostic potential. However, the existence of this technology in itself does not immediately enable new diagnostic procedures. The information offered by *in vivo* confocal microscopy or endomicroscopy is not yet directly comparable with conventional histological views in a diagnostic context.

To be useful for diagnosis, fibre optic confocal endomicroscopy of the gut would have to allow reproducible visualisation of specific parameters of tissues (such as cell morphology and categorisation, innervation, microvascular architecture or responsiveness) as they relate to particular pathologies. The optical capabilities of the technology are already well established, and therefore the future of "optical biopsy" procedures utilising fibre optic confocal endomicroscopy rests on the development and refinement of specific methodologies for vital tissue labelling and advances in miniaturisation. Using FOCI, we have previously imaged several tissues *in vivo*, including cellular and microvascular structure of hairless mouse skin,[31] microvasculature of rat gingiva and skin,[32] microvasculature of rat colon,[33] and rat colonic mucosal structure.[34]

For the remainder, we describe the main issues relating to putative clinical diagnostic applications, vital staining techniques and results of *in vivo* fibre optic confocal imaging of particular components of tissues of the gastrointestinal tract accessible by endoscopy.

We present images of the enteric nervous system, mucosal glandular microarchitecture and microvasculature of the rat colon obtained using FOCI *in vivo*. We also review comparisons of *in vivo* fibre optic confocal microscopy of mucosal glandular micro-architecture in the rat colon with that of rat and human colonic biopsies. Finally we discuss possible diagnostic significance and comment on the current status of miniaturisation of prototype endomicroscopes and associated trials in piglets *in vivo*.

Imaging of the enteric nervous system

In conditions associated with degeneration of the enteric nervous system (e.g. Hirschsprung's disease), a method of non-destructively examining the microarchitecture of this expansive structure would be a useful diagnostic tool. In order to be useful in experimental and clinical studies for *in vivo* imaging of the enteric nervous system and other autonomic nerves, a fluorescent vital dye must be: non-toxic and without pharmacological effects on the tissue; preferably water soluble; non-fading; visible without further manipulation of the tissue; and specific for nervous tissue.[34] The vital fluorescent dye 4-(4-(diethylamino)styryl)-N-methylpyridinium iodide (4-Di-2-ASP, Molecular Probes Inc, Eugene, Oregon, USA) has been shown in prior work to fulfill all these requirements. This dye is well suited to microscopic imaging of the enteric nervous system *in vivo*. Although its mechanism of staining action is not completely clear, it is thought to preferentially stain nerves.[36]

It has been suggested,[37] that a rapid and reliable technique that does not require sectioning would be useful for examining the enteric nervous system for evidence of certain pathologies of the gut. Many of the existing methods used for vitally staining the intact enteric nervous system have proved unsuitable because they involve fixation or are time consuming or expensive procedures,[35] e.g., staining for acetylcholine esterase or silver impregnation. Immunohistochemical staining of nerve elements is sensitive and selective, but is also slow and expensive. The successful use of 4-Di-2-ASP for examining unfixed whole mount bowel specimens from patients with Hirschsprung's disease (characterised by aganglionosis of the diseased segment of gut), using epifluorescent illumination has been reported.[37] However, this method required a biopsy to be taken, the tissue pinned out and the mucosa, submucosa and circular muscle removed under a dissecting microscope to expose the myenteric plexus for visualisation under a conventional epifluorescence microscope. This was necessary due to the depth of the plexus within the gut wall, since the myenteric plexus lies between the outer longitudinal and inner circular muscle layers of the muscularis externa. Difficulties inherent in the use of stereo or electron microscopes to observe plexus structure following stripping off of muscle layers of whole mount samples have also been reported.[38] Other workers have used topically applied fluorescent dyes and have confocally imaged *in vitro* mounts of gut mucosa to study various aspects of colonic crypt function, including fluid absorption,[39] and quantitation of cell cycle biomarkers.[40] Regional differences in autofluorescence have been examined confocally in human colonic mucosa samples.[41]

Here we present methods and results for FOCI of enteric nerves of the rat colon *in vivo*.

Methods

All experiments were approved by the relevant Institutional Animal Ethics Committee. In urethane anaesthetised male Sprague-Dawley rats (200-300 g), a midline abdominal incision was made and a 10 mm region of the descending colon was exposed and stabilised by positioning it across gauze, keeping it continually soaked with warmed saline. An adjustable micropositioner ring was used for stabilisation of the surrounding tissue, without applying any pressure directly to the colon itself. The animal was then transferred to a specialised heated platform attached to the confocal microscope stage, and 4-Di-2-ASP was topically applied (10 µM, 3 minutes staining, 1 minute saline wash) to the tissue surface prior to application of a 15 mm diameter circular coverslip to the stabilised tissue surface.

The concentration of 4-Di-2-ASP applied and the period of staining was the result of extensive trials of different staining conditions with visual evaluation of image quality for each condition.

Confocal imaging was performed using the Optiscan F900e fibre optic laser scanning confocal microscope system equipped with an argon ion laser (Optiscan Imaging Ltd., Melbourne, Victoria, Australia). Single channel fluorescence imaging was performed using an excitation wavelength of 488 nm (blue), with detection >514 nm (green). The confocal system was fitted to an Olympus BH-2 light microscope equipped with Olympus objectives (×10, 0.4NA or ×20, 0.7NA). In the colon, imaging was performed through the intact serosal surface.

Results

Various components of the enteric nervous system of the rat colon were identifiable using this *in vivo* subsurface imaging technique. The image quality and degree of magnification achieved are such that morphological characteristics of ganglia and the connecting nerve fibre tracts in the myenteric plexus are quite distinctly visible (Fig. 15.1a).

At higher magnification, individual nerve ganglia and fibre tracts could be visualised, along with fine nerve fibres that form part of the tertiary nerve plexus (Fig.15.1b). Neuronal cell bodies were outlined as dark shapes within ganglia.

Microvascular imaging

Observation of microvascular dynamics *in vivo* is generally not possible due to the limitations of conventional microscope optics discussed previously. This means only the most superficial, semi-isolated vessels can be visualised without surgically exposing deeper regions of the tissue. This has proved to be the limiting factor in many such experiments, for example, in the study of the microvasculature of the endometrium of the rat uterus.[42] Other *in vivo* preparations used to investigate various aspects of microvascular function have also required delicate and complex physical isolation of a single tissue plane containing a chosen vessel to ensure no reduction in contrast due to underlying vessels; for example the hamster cheek pouch,[43,44] the rat cremaster muscle,[45] and various mesenteric preparations.[46, 47]

The collapse of the vasculature on excision likewise limits microvascular observations of biopsied tissue to ultrastructural changes in vessel wall morphology using high power light or electron microscopy (e.g.[48]).

Microvascular imaging experiments utilising bulk optical confocal microscopy, such as those performed in the intact rat brain cortex *in vivo*[21, 22] and the living rat kidney,[25] are limited by the experimental complexity associated with the inflexibility of the

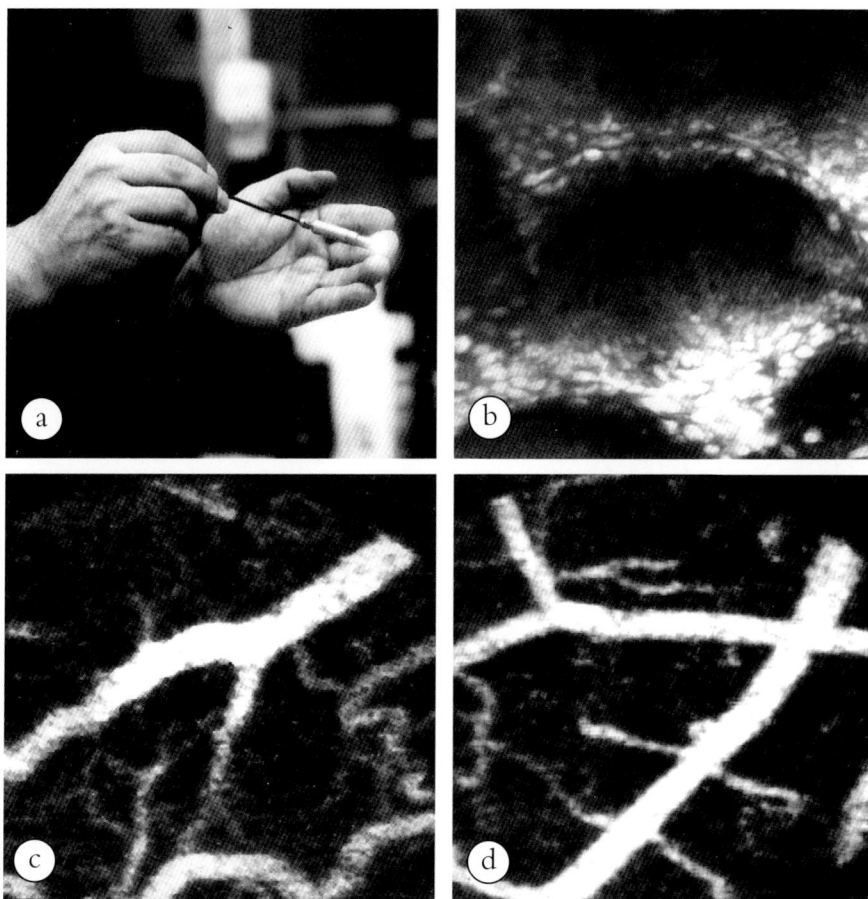

Figure 2. *– **a** shows a current prototype confocal endomicroscope possessing an imaging end with tip diameter of 10 mm. **b** shows cells surrounding mucous crypts in an in vitro sample of pig stomach topically stained with acridine orange (1% solution, 1 minute staining time) FOV=300 μm. **c,d** show confocal endomicroscope images of microvasculature (imaged from the serosal surface) of the intact rat colon in vivo following i.v. FITC-dextran (0.5 ml, 10 mg/ml). Characteristic microvascular architecture was readily observed comparable with other in vivo microvascular confocal imaging studies. FOV=250 μm.*

instrumentation. Previously we have used FOCI to image subsurface microvascular structure *in vivo* in rat gingiva and skin,[32] and rat colon.[33] Here we present a methodology for the use of a common high molecular weight fluorescent tracer molecule, fluorescein isothyocyanate conjugated dextran (FITC-dextran) to obtain images of the rat colon microvasculature *in vivo*.

Methods

All experiments were approved by the relevant Institutional Animal Ethics Committee. In urethane anaesthetised male Sprague-Dawley rats (200-300 g), a midline abdominal incision was made adequate for insertion of the 10 mm diameter confocal endomicroscope. A jugular vein cannula was inserted for intravascular dye administration. The concentration of the dye (FITC-dextran, MW 150kDa, Sigma, St Louis, MO, USA) was determined following extensive trials of different staining conditions with visual evaluation of image quality for each condition. FITC-dextran was administered via a cannulated jugular vein (0.5 ml, 10 mg/ml in saline) when required. Confocal imaging was performed using a 10 mm prototype confocal endomicroscope attachment fitted to the Optiscan F900e system setup (described above for neuronal plexus imaging). The imaging end of this attachment can be seen in Fig. 15.2a.

Results

Confocal endomicroscopy allowed clear visualisation of characteristic microvascular architecture of the muscle layers of the rat descending colon (Fig. 15.2 c, d). Arterioles and venules were readily observed with image quality comparable with the previously cited *in vivo* microvascular confocal imaging studies.[32,33] More importantly, however, is the simplicity with which the images were obtained under manual manipulation of the flexible probe across any region of the tissue of interest.

Simultaneous nerve/microvascular imaging

Given the neuronal and microvascular imaging reported above, it is conceivable that concurrent observation of these two tissue components would yield more informative images.

In one set of experiments FITC-dextran was administered intravascularly in combination with topically applied 4-Di-2-ASP in animal preparations as per the individual descriptions above.

This dual label imaging enabled simultaneous visualisation of the same nerve components of the myenteric plexus as were visible with single label imaging, as well as showing the spatial relationship of the myenteric plexus with components of the microvasculature (see Fig.15.1 c, d).

Mucosal imaging

Previously during the early development of fibre optic confocal imaging we demonstrated simple staining protocols utilising the application of sodium fluorescein crystals to the gastric mucosa. This revealed the overall crypt pattern and structure. Comparable images were obtained in human and rat gastric biopsy samples and the rat gastric mucosa *in vivo*.[34]

More recently, staining protocols involving topical application of the fluorescent nuceic acid stain acridine orange (Sigma, St Louis, MO, USA) are enabling prototype endomicroscope imaging trials in anaesthetised piglets. Results thus far reveal glandular microarchitecture in samples of pig stomach imaged *in vitro* (see Fig. 15.2b), which are comparable to those obtained using the confocal endomicroscope

in vivo (unpublished data). Superior subcellular detail was obtained than in the earlier biopsy imaging (which was performed at lower magnification). However, it is unlikely that acridine orange would be safe for clinical application in humans. Hence while such trials indicate the imaging capability of the technology, further development of staining protocols would be required to fully exploit this optical performance in imaging subcellular details of gastric mucous crypts for diagnostic purposes.

Discussion

Very little confocal microscopy of the colon has been performed in living animals.

That which has been performed *in vivo* (e.g. in the mouse colonic mucosa[49]), like the *in vitro* imaging of the colon described herein utilised confocal microscopy as a tool for measuring parameters of colonic crypt function.

Results presented here represent the successful extension of the epifluorescence microscopy of whole mounts by Hanani[35] to subsurface confocal visualisation of nerve and blood vessel morphology in the rat colon *in vivo*. The fact that these images were taken from the serosal side of the intact colon (and thus through the serosa and intact muscle layer) illustrates well the subsurface 'optical sectioning' capabilities of FOCI. This gives the technique potential for imaging the architecture of the myenteric plexus in normal or diseased segments of gut *in vivo*.

The *in vitro* FOCI of pig gastric samples described in this study has led to current *in vivo* investigations of the gastric mucosa in piglets using experimental confocal endomicroscope probes. It is the results of these true endoscopic experiments which are directly driving the refinement of both the confocal endomicroscope technology and the associated methodologies required to realise the potential for investigation of gastrointestinal mucosa in humans.

Thus we have described the establishment of an imaging technique useful as a means of observing and morphologically characterising living neuronal and vascular and glandular microarchitectural elements *in vivo*. Further investigation may show this technique to be useful as a tool in the study of neurodegenerative disorders, vascular pathology or inflammatory conditions in animal models, and potentially in humans.

In the future, confocal endomicroscopy may provide an alternative to many gastrointestinal biopsy procedures. In other cases, it may allow microscopic pre-examination of a larger area of tissue than can be excised, therefore assisting the selection of a biopsy site. However, rapid progress is being made both in the development of specific vital staining techniques and in the miniaturisation and refinement of the confocal endomicroscope technology. Research grade high resolution rigid endomicroscopes and flexible confocal endomicroscopes of less than 10 mm diameter are now becoming available. Work in progress to identify the predominant areas of clinical usefulness and engineer devices specifically to these tasks may see the emergence of confocal endomicroscopy as a clinical diagnostic technique in the foreseeable future.

References

1. Rotterdam H. Contributions of gastrointestinal biopsy to an understanding of gastrointestinal disease. *Am J Gastroenterol* 1983; **78:** 140-148.

2. Foliente RL, Chang AC, Youssef AL, Ford LJ, Condon SC, Chen YK. Endoscopic cecal perforation: mechanisms of injury. *Am J Gastroenterol* 1996; **91:** 105-708.

3. Jiménez-perez FJ, Echarri A, Jimenez E, Borda F. Colonic hemorrhage after standard biopsy (letter). *Am J Gastroenterol* 1994; **89:** 1123-1124.

4. Tytgat GN, Endoscopic transmission of *Helicobacter pylori*. *Aliment Pharmacol Therapeut* 1995; **9(suppl.2):** 105-110.

5. Tytgat GN, Ignacio JG Technicalities of endoscopic biopsy. *Endoscopy* 1995; **27:** 683-688.

6. Rubio CA, Slezak P, Befrits R. The costs of colonoscopy in patients with ulcerative pan-colitis in Sweden. *Endoscopy* 1994; **26:** 228-230.

7. White JG, Amos WB, Fordham M. An evaluation of confocal versus conventional imaging of biological structures by fluorescence light microscopy. *J Cell Biol* 1987; **105:** 41-48.

8. Brakenhoff GJ, Van Der Voort HTM, Van Spronsen EA, Nanning N. Three-dimensional imaging in fluorescence by confocal scanning microscopy. *J Microscopy* 1989; **153:** 155-159.

9. Minsky M (1957) U.S. Patent No. 3,013,467.

10. New KC, Petroll WM, Boyde A, Martin L, Corcuff P, Leveque JL, Lemp MA, Cavanagh HD, Jester JV. *in vivo* imaging of human teeth and skin using real-time confocal microscopy. *Scanning* 1991; **13:** 369-372.

11. Rajadhaksha M, Grossman M, Esterowitz D, Webb RH, Anderson RR. *In vivo* confocal scanning laser microscopy of human skin: melanin provides strong contrast. *J Invest Derm* 1995; **104:** 946-952.

12. Waston TF, Petroll WM, Cavanagh HD, Jester JV. *In vivo* confocal microscopy in dental research: an initial appraisal. *J Dent* 1992; **20:** 352-358.

13. Auran JD, Koester CJ, Rapaport R, Florakis GJ. Wide field scanning slit *in vivo* confocal microscopy of flattening-induced corneal bands and ridges. *Scanning* 1994, **16:** 182-186.

14. Beuerman RW, Laird JA, Kaufman SC, Kaufman HE. Quantification of real-time confocal images of the human cornea. *J Neurosci Meth* 1994, **54:** 197-203.

15. Chew SJ, Beuerman RW, Kaufman HE, McDonald MB. *In vivo* confocal microscopy of corneal wound healing after excimer laser photorefractive keratectomy. *CLAO Journal* 1995; **21:** 273-280.

16. Corbett MC, Prydal JI, Verma S, Oliver KM, Pande M, Marshall J. An *in vivo* investigation of the structures responsible for corneal haze after photorefractive keratectomy and their effect on visual function. *Ophthalmology* 1996; **103:** 1366-1380.

17. Jester JV, Petroll WM, Barry PA, Cavanagh HD. Expression of alpha-smooth muscle (alpha-sm) actin during stromal wound healing. *Invest Ophthalmol Visual Sci* 1995; **35:** 809-819.

18. Jester JV, Maurer JK, Petroll WM, Wilkie DA, Parker RD, Cavanagh HD. Application of *in vivo* confocal microscopy to the understanding of surfactant-induced ocular irritation. *Toxicol Path* 1996; **24:** 412-428.

19. Petroll WM, Cavanagh HD, Jester JV. Three-dimensional imaging of corneal cells using *in vivo* confocal microscopy. *J Microscopy* 1993; **170:** 213-219.

20. Wiegand W, Thaer AA, Kroll P, Geyer OC, Garcia AJ. Optical sectioning of the cornea with a new confocal *in vivo* slit-scanning videomicroscope. *Ophthalmology* 1995; **102:** 568-575.

21. Villringer A, Dringl U, Gebhardt R, Haberl RL, Einhaupl KM. Non-invasive optical sectioning of the living rat brain. In *MICRO* 1990; pp. 353-356. IOP Publishing Ltd., London.

22. Villringer A, Drinagl U, Them A, Schurer L, Krombach F, Einhaupl KM. Imaging of leukocytes within the rat brain cortex *in vivo*. *Microvasc Res* 1991; **42:** 305-315.

23. Lindauer U, Dreier J, Angstwurm K, Rubin I Villringer A, Einhaupl KM, Dringl U Role of nitric oxide synthase inhibition in leukocyte-endothelium interaction in the rat pial microvasculaure. *J Cereb Blood Flow Metabol* 1996; **16:** 1143-1152.

24. Lorenzl S, Koedel U, Dirnagl U, Ruckdeschel G, Pfister HW. Imaging of leukocyte-endothelium interaction using *in vivo* confocal laser scanning microscopy during the early phase of experimental pneumococcal meningitis. *J Inf Dis* 1993; **168**: 927-933.

25. Andrews PM, Petroll WM, Cavanagh HD, Jester JV Tandem scanning confocal microscopy (TSCM) of normal and ischemic living kidneys. *Am J Anat* 1991; **191**: 95-102.

26. Andrews PM The histopathology of kidney uriniferous tubules as revealed by noninvasive confocal vita microscopy. *Scanning* 1994; **16**: 174-181.

27. Pulver M, Petroll WM, Andrews PM. Noninvasive microscopic evaluation of the intact living nephrotic kidney. *Lab Invest* 1993; **68**: 592-596.

28. Jester JV, Andrews PM, Petroll WM, Lemp MA, Cavanagh HD. *In vivo*, real-time confocal imaging. *J Electron Microsc Tech* 1991; **18**: 50-60.

29. Delaney PM, Harris MR, King RG. Fibre optic laser scanning confocal microscope suitable for fluorescence imaging. *Appl Optics* 1994; **33**: 573-577.

30. Harris MR. Scanning confocal microscope including a single fibre for transmitting light to and receiving light from an object. U.S. Patent 5, 1992, **120**: 953

31. Bussau LJ, Delaney PM, Papwoth GD, Barkla DH, King RG. Fibre optic confocal imaging of hairless mouse skin: comparison with conventional histology. *Proceedings of the Australian Physiological and Pharmacological Society* 1995; **26**: 233P.

32. Papworth GD, Delaney PM, Bussau LJ, King RG. *In vivo* subsurface microvascular imaging using fibre optic confocal microscopy (FOCI). *Proceedings of the Australian Physiological and Pharmacological Society* 1995; **26**: 200P.

33. Delaney PM, Harris MR, King RG Novel microscopy using fibre optic confocal imaging and its suitability for subsurface blood vessel imaging *in vivo*. *Clin Exp Pharmacol Physiol* 1993; **20**: 197-198.

34. Delaney PM, King RG, Lambert JR, Harris MR. Fibre optic confocal imaging (FOCI) for subsurface microscopy of the colon *in vivo*. *J Anat* 1994b; **184**: 157-160.

35. Hanani M. Visualization of enteric and gallbladder ganglia with a vital fluorescent dye. *J Auton Nerv Syst* 1992; **38**: 77-84.

36. Molecular Probes Inc., Personal Communication (1995)

37. Hanani M, Udassin R, Ariel I, Freund H. A simple and rapid method for staining the enteric ganglia: Application for Hirschsprung's disease. *J Ped Surg* 1993; **28**: 939-941.

38. Miura H, Ohi R, Tseng SW, Takashi T. The structure of the transitional and aganglionic zones of Auerbach's plexus in patients with Hirschsprung's disease: a computer-assisted three-dimensional reconstruction study. *J Ped Surg* 1996; **31**: 420-426.

39. Naftalin RJ, Zammit PS, Pedley KC. Concentration polarization of fluorescent dyes in rat descending colonic crypts: evidence of crypt fluid absorption. *J Physiol* 1995; **487**: 479-495.

40. Konishi H, Steinbach G, Hittelman WN, Fujita K, Lee JJ, Glober GA, Levin B, Andreeff M, Goodacre AM, Terry NH. Cell kinetic analysis of intact rat colonic crypts by confocal microscopy and immunofluorescence. *Gastroenterology* 1996; **111**: 1493-1500.

41. Fiarman GS, Nathanson MH, West AB, Decke;baum LI, Kelly L, Kapadia CR. Differences in laser-induced autofluorescence between adentaomatous and hyperplastic polyps and normal colonic mucosa by confocal microscopy. *Dig Dis Sci* 1995; **40**: 1261-1268.

42. Rogars PAW and Macpherson AM. *In-vivo* microscopy of the rat endometrial subepithelial capillary plexus during the oestrus cycle and after ovariectomy. *J Reprod Fert* 1990; **90**: 137-145.

43. Fulton GP, Jackson RG. Cinephotomicroscopy of normal blood circulation in the cheek pouch of the hamster. *Science* 1947; **105**: 361-362.

44. Duling BR. The preparation and use of the hamster cheek pouch for studies of the microcirculation. *Microvascular Research* 1973; **5**: 423-429.

45. Baezs. An open cremaster muscle preparation for the study of blood vessels by *in vivo* microscopy. *Microvascular Research* 1973; **5**: 384-394.

46. Zweifach BW Direct observations of mesenteric circulation in experimental animals. *Anatomical Record* 1954; **120**: 277-291.

47. Gore RW. Mesenteric preparations for quantitative microcirculatory studies. *Microvascular Research* 1973; **5**: 368-375.

48. Langer K, Seidler C, Partsch H. Ultrastructural study of the dermal microvascular in patients undergoing retrogade intravenous pressure infusions. *Dermatology* 1996; **192**: 103-109.

49. Chu S, Brownwell WE, Montrose MH. Quantitative confocal imaging along the crypt-to-surface axis of colonic crypts. *Am J Physiol* 1995; **269**: C1557-1564.

16

Stable isotopes in the study of intestinal metabolism: Digestion, absorption and intestinal nutrient metabolism

S Mahé

Summary

The major stable isotopes used in clinical investigation are [^{13}C], [^{2}H], [^{15}N] and [^{18}O]. The stable-isotope-labelled compounds include amino acids, lipids, sugars, chemicals or drugs as well as isotopic gases, stable metal and mineral isotopes and uniformly-labelled vegetable plants, animal products and yeast. Isotope administration is performed by different routes including oral, gastric, intestinal and intra-venous. Sample collection can be from intestinal effluents, blood, breath and urine. The main application of [^{15}N] is gastrointestinal functional diagnosis and there are two key methods of obtaining information on the metabolic process: end-product analysis and measurement of body samples. The [^{13}C]-O$_2$ breath test is a sensitive method used widely to establish that intestinal bacterial digestion of nonabsorbed foodstuffs is the only source of breath hydrogen in the gastrointestinal tract. The [^{13}C]-labelled breath test is used to measure: (i) gastric emptying rate of solid and liquid test meals based on the characteristics of octanoic acid and (ii) intestinal transit times and rapid changes in gastrointestinal motility under various conditions with [^{13}C]-labelled glycosyl ureides. It can also be used to diagnose small-intestine bacterial overgrowth with [^{13}C]-xylose; lipid malabsorption by the oral administration of [^{13}C]-triolein, [^{13}C]-trioctanoin and [^{13}C]-palmitic acid; and lactose and sucrose deficiency by [^{13}C]-lactose and [^{13}C]-sucrose. Intestinal perfusion techniques are used to quantify nutrient metabolism and absorption in the intestine. Major advances in the uses and availability of labelled compounds have resulted in increased utilization of stable isotopes in human research and diagnosis, these tracers now being extensively used for *in vivo* studies. Their use in physiological and pathophysiological studies in humans and animals can be expected to increase considerably in the near future.

Introduction

The application of stable isotopic tracers in physiological and pathophysiological studies in humans has largely been developed in the last decade, especially in the fields of nutrition and metabolic research into proteins, fats and carbohydrates. Unfortunately, the term 'isotope' is often associated with radiation risks even though this is only true for radioactive isotopes. Stable isotopes do not emit ionizing radiation and are therefore non-toxic at levels used in clinical studies. In addition, their use has the advantage of causing a less significant 'isotope effect': the smaller the relative mass difference between a pair of isotopes, the smaller the expected 'isotope effect'. Therefore, the potential application risk decreases inversely with the size of the isotope used. However, in practice, economic considerations oblige the investigator to keep the dose as small as possible. Finally, stable isotope tracer methodology allows several tracers to be used simultaneously in the same individual. Contrary to magnetic resonance spectroscopy, isotope measurements by mass spectrometry cannot be carried out in or on the organism *in vivo*. A sample which is representative of the compartment pool of interest must be taken from the subject and generally must be prepared prior to the measurement of its isotope content by mass spectrometry.

The most interesting stable isotopes for clinical investigations are listed in Table 16.1. The major stable isotopes are [^{13}C], [^{2}H] and [^{15}N]: the latter is the only convenient nuclide for tracing body nitrogen dynamics. The inventory of stable isotope labelled compounds provides over 6000 products including: [^{15}N], [^{13}C], [^{2}H], [^{18}O] and multi-labelled amino acids, lipids, sugars, chemicals or drugs; uniformly labelled [^{15}N,^{13}C,^{18}O] vegetable plants (wheat, potatoes, peas, soy, beans etc.) animal

Table 16.1 – Principal organic stable isotopes in clinical investigation.

Element/stable isotope	Natural relative abundance (atom-%)	Commercial isotopic enrichment available (atom-%)
^{1}H/^{2}H	99.985/0.014	99.9
^{12}C/^{13}C	98.892/1.108	99
^{14}N/^{15}N	99.634/0.365	99
^{16}O/^{17}O/^{18}O	99.758/0.038/0.204	60/95

products (milk, eggs, meat) and yeast with one or several isotopes and with different isotopic enrichments;[1-7] and isotopic gases, stable metal and mineral isotopes. Several applications not discussed in this chapter use the stable isotopes ^{204}Pb, ^{54}Fe, ^{58}Fe, ^{65}Cu, ^{67}Zn, ^{70}Zn, ^{25}Mg, ^{26}Mg and ^{42}Ca, ^{44}Ca, ^{46}Ca, ^{48}Ca. [8-11]

The main principle of stable isotope application is 'isotope dilution analysis', a quantitative method in which a known amount of tracer is added to an unknown amount of tracee. When isotopic equilibrium is reached (i.e. when the relative isotope abundance is the same throughout the system), the level of isotope is a measure of the previously unknown amount of tracee. To calculate the amount of tracee, only the isotopic enrichment in excess of the naturally occurring isotope component is needed.

This chapter focuses on (i) stable isotope studies of nutrient digestion and absorption in humans and (ii) methods available to investigate gastrointestinal tract diseases, including both malabsorption and intestinal dysfunction syndromes.

Methods

Labelled compound administration, sampling and analysis

Isotopes can be administered by different routes (oral, gastric, intestinal, intravenous) and in different forms (solid or liquid). Moreover, the tracer can be administered as a pulse, continuously or using the 'priming technique', i.e. giving first a bolus injection followed by a slow infusion. The choice of administration route of the tracer is important. The intravenous route is thought to be inappropriate when the oxidation of an amino acid in food is to be measured.[12]

To assess nutrient assimilation by the gut, a large quantity of labelled nutrient is required. Although chemically synthesized compounds for tracer studies are widely available, complex nutrients intrinsically labelled with stable isotope tracers (meat, egg, milk, yeast protein) are expensive. As a result, new approaches to the investigation of nutrient digestion have been developed, such as labelling protein with [^{15}N]. This method is an accurate means of differentiating the endogenous from the exogenous fractions in intestinal effluents, of evaluating the kinetics of protein digestion and absorption and of analysing the secretory nitrogen response to meals in both humans and animals.[13,14]

The sampling compartments available to study nutrient digestion and assimilation are the intestinal lumen, blood, breath and urine. For instance, to measure the isotopic enrichment of a nutrient in plasma, invasive sampling and sophisticated separation and analysis methods are needed. Several different methods have been developed to assess protein metabolism, including the infusion of a stable-isotope-labelled amino acid and the evaluation of its transformation by measuring CO_2 expired (i.e. oxidation), ammonia and urea in urine (i.e. catabolism) and the amino acid itself (or its metabolite) in the plasma (i.e. synthesis). Only in a few cases can the end-products be subject to isotope analysis without prior preparation. This applies to CO_2 (labelled with [^{13}C] from the breath test), NH_3 (labelled with [^{15}N] from the urine test) and [^{2}H]$_2$O (from body water assessment). Compared to [^{15}N] urine tests, [^{15}N] recovery from the plasma is more expensive both in terms of the clinical protocol and biochemical analysis. There has been continued interest in the development of non-invasive methods which might be of practical value in assessing nutrient metabolism under normal living conditions. The 'end-product methods' are ideally suited to this purpose in that the dose of the isotope (most often [^{15}N]-glycine) is taken orally and the enrichment is measured in an end-product of protein metabolism (usually urea and ammonia) excreted in the urine.

Methods using intestinal effluent collection

Collection of intestinal effluents

Studies of intestinal absorption of nutrients in humans by intestinal perfusion are rare. The marker perfusion technique allows a quantitative estimate to be made of the transit time and assessment of the intestinal absorption of specific nutrients without requiring the complete recovery of intestinal contents. Tubes for intestinal perfusion are usually located 80–90 cm from the nose for the ligament of Treitz and 280–350 cm for the ileo-caecal valve, but this depends on individual variation. Studies with short-bowel patients or ileostomists allow complete recovery of the intestinal contents. The digesta samples collected on ice through a tube are treated with a protease inhibitor (e.g. di-isopropylfluorophosphate, 4-(2-aminoethyl)-benzenesulfonyl fluoride) to stop the enzymatic degradation of proteins. Aliquots are used both to measure non-absorbable markers (e.g. polyethylene glycol-4000, phenol red) and to calculate intestinal flow rate and amount of nutrient recovered. The rest of the effluent is frozen at -20°C and lyophilized.

The intestinal flow rate (F ml/min) is calculated according to the formula:

$$F = (F_m \times C_m)/C_d$$

where F_m is the flow rate of the non-absorbable marker; C_m its concentration in the perfusate; and C_d the concentration in the digesta.

Measurement of the luminal labelled nutrient disappearance

In the case of labelled exogenous nutrients, the digestibility is assumed to be the difference between the amount ingested and the amount recovered by the tube in the intestinal lumen. Stable isotope labelling of the nutrient allows direct assessment of digestibility as it can distinguish between endogenous and exogenous origins, particularly for lipids and proteins. For instance, the use of a [15N]-protein allows calculation, from the isotopic $^{15}N/^{14}N$ ratio determined by isotope ratio mass spectrometry in the digesta, of the exogenous and endogenous nitrogen content. In practice, an aliquot of the freeze-dried digesta sample is burned in the presence of purified oxygen in the combustion unit of an elemental analyser at 950°C. The combustion unit is coupled to an isotope ratio mass spectrometer and the isotope ratio of N_2 is measured with reference to a calibrated $^{15}N/^{14}N$ nitrogen tank. The difference between the exogenous and endogenous nitrogen fractions is determined according to the following formula:

$$N_{exo} = N_{tot} \times (APE_d - APE_o)/(APE_m - APE_o)$$

where N_{tot} is the total nitrogen; APE_d, APE_o and APE_m are the enrichment of the digesta, the basal secretions and the ingested meal, respectively.

The endogenous nitrogen in the digesta (N_{endo}) is calculated from the difference:

$$N_{endo} = N_{tot} - N_{exo}$$

Labelling and measurement of luminal endogenous nitrogen

To label the intestinal endogenous nitrogen fraction, a stable-isotope-labelled amino acid is infused intravenously to enrich the amino acid body pool.

This source of nitrogen is used by the tissues (including the gastrointestinal organs) and newly synthesized endogenous proteins will have incorporated this labelled amino acid. The most commonly labelled amino acid is [15N]-leucine. In practice, a small catheter is placed in a forearm vein for blood sampling. Another catheter is placed in a contralateral vein of the other forearm in order to infuse the [15N]-leucine solution (99 % enrichment). At T_0, a priming dose of [15N]-leucine (10 mmol/kg) is given, followed by a constant infusion of [15N]-leucine (10 mmol/kg/h). Blood samples are collected regularly on heparin and the plasma is immediately separated from the whole blood by centrifugation and frozen at -20°C until analysis. The amino acids need to be isolated and derivatized prior to gas chromatography mass spectrometry analysis. Intestinal amino acids (after acid hydrolysis 6 M HCl at 110°C for 24 hours) and plasma-free amino acids (after acidifying the plasma with 1 M acetic acid) are extracted with cation exchange columns (Dowex AG-50×8, Mesh 100; 200, Bio Rad Laboratories, CA, USA). The free amino acids are mixed with 600 μl of an esterification reagent containing acetyl chloride and N-propanol (20% v/v) and then heated at 110°C for 30 min. The reagent excess is evaporated under N_2 and 50 ml of heptafluorobutyric anhydride is added. The mixture is allowed to incubate at 60°C for 30 min and then dried under N_2. The mass spectrometer, interfaced with a gas chromatographer, operates in the positive chemical ionization mode and the enrichment of [15N]-leucine in plasma is determined by single ion monitoring of the ions m/z 282 and 283.

The isotopic dilution method allows calculation of the flow rate of endogenous leucine (Leu_{endo}) using the formula:

$$Leu_{endo} = Leu_{tot} \times (E_i/E_e)$$

where Leu_{tot} is the flow rate of total leucine in the digesta; E_i the [15N]-leucine enrichment in digesta at time i; and E_e the [15N]-leucine enrichment of the endogenous fraction in digesta at the same time and is obtained from a model curve calculated from the experimental curve obtained in the fasting period. Under these conditions, E_e is in the form $E_e = a[1-b.exp(-ct)]$, in which t is the time and the a,b,c parameters are calculated from a non-linear regression model without error correlation and heterocedasticity (Fig. 16.1). Considering that the leucine content of endogenous proteins is constant,[15,16] the endogenous nitrogen flow rate is:

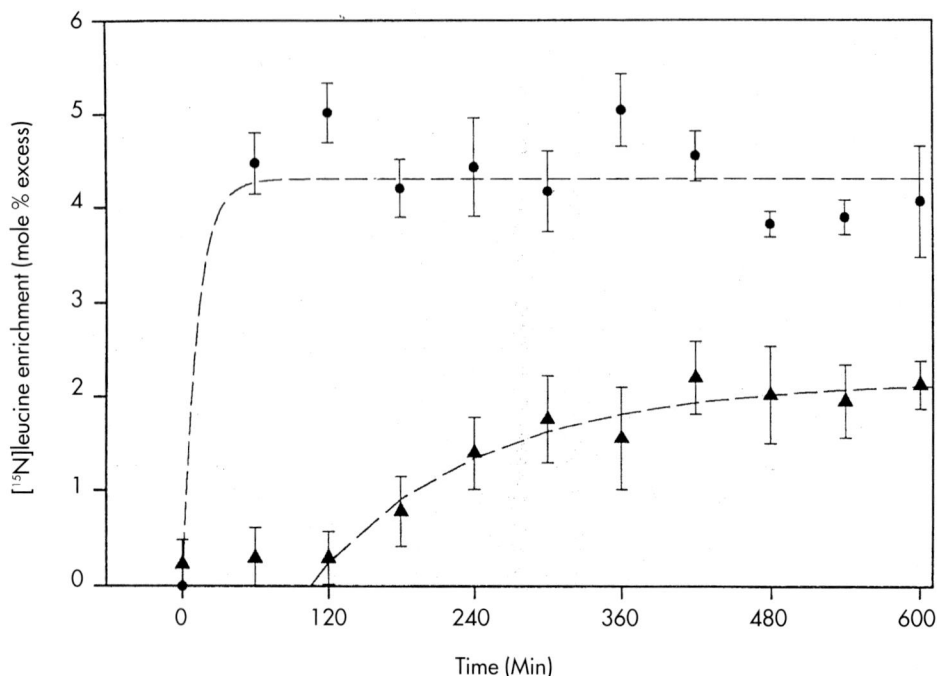

Figure 16.1 – Kinetics of [^{15}N]leucine incorporation in plasma (●) and in jejunal effluents (▲) under fasting conditions in humans following a priming dose of [^{15}N]leucine (10 mmol/kg) at t = 0 and a constant infusion of [^{15}N]leucine (10 mmol/kg/h). Each value represents the mean (SD) of four subjects. The [^{15}N]leucine enrichment of the endogenous secretion (Ee) in the jejunum is fitted by the equation: Ee = 2.18[1 - 2.05 × exp(-0.42 × t)]. The [^{15}N]leucine enrichment in the plasma is fitted by the equation: Ep = 4.31[1 - exp(-0.08 × t)] (From ref 33).

$$N_{endo} = (N_{tot} \times Leu_{endo})/P_{leu},$$

where P_{leu} is the percentage of leucine in endogenous proteins; and N_{tot} the amount of total nitrogen in the digesta.

The P_{leu} value is determined during the fasting period. After meal ingestion, the flow rate of exogenous nitrogen is measured by taking the difference between N_{tot} and N_{endo}.

Methods using blood sample or breath and urine end-product collection

The products of gut absorption and metabolism are measured in blood, breath or urine. Efforts have been made to measure end-products (such as CO_2 in the breath and urinary ammonia and urea) from body excretions, which are available without the need for invasive collection methods.

Blood sample collection

The absorption and metabolism of labelled dietary nutrients could be theoretically investigated by measuring the transfer of the tracer from nutrient to portal plasma. Unfortunately, this pool is not commonly accessible in humans and only peripheral blood samples are available and there is a significant difference between portal and peripheral blood composition due to liver metabolism. To solve this methodological problem, models have been developed to describe the effect of liver metabolism on each nutrient. Also, the development of the euglycaemic clamp represents an approach to inhibit hepatic neoglucogenesis. However, the hepatic metabolism of amino acids, which is particularly important, cannot be by-passed by this kind of technique and strongly limits the use of peripheral blood sampling to determine directly the kinetics of intestinal absorption of labelled proteins and amino acids.

[¹³C]-O₂ breath test end-product test

Breath gas analysis is an important tool in clinical investigation. A number of important metabolic pathways can be monitored by measuring the $^{13}C/^{12}C$ ratio in expired CO_2. This method relies on the fact that a subject with a metabolic disorder may assimilate and oxidize a labelled substrate at a different rate from a subject with normal metabolism. The only source of breath hydrogen in the gastrointestinal tract is that generated by intestinal bacterial digestion of non-absorbed foodstuffs and thus serves to identify malabsorption syndromes. The common characteristic of [¹³C]-O₂ breath test substrates is their chemical structure, including a [¹³C]-labelled functional group which is cleaved during its passage through the stomach or gut or during its absorption. This test offers a number of major advantages over other available methods: it is non-invasive, simple and relatively inexpensive. It is proposed for investigations in pregnancy, infancy and childhood. Moreover, companies provide automated instrumentation for routine analysis. In practice, after overnight fasting the subject is given an oral dose of several mg/kg body weight of the [¹³C]-substrate dissolved in water. Before and for several hours after [¹³C] ingestion, (1-8 hours) breath samples are taken at 15-30 min intervals. The subject is asked to blow into a glass Vacutainer collection tube through a straw.

Urinary [¹⁵N] end-product test

The main application of [¹⁵N] is gastrointestinal functional diagnosis. There are two main methods of obtaining information on metabolic processes: end-product analysis and body sample measurement. Net protein breakdown involves the oxidation of amino acids in which carbons are excreted in the breath as CO_2, Nitrogen is released as ammonia. Ammonia is detoxified by incorporation into the urea in the liver and is excreted in the urine. Approximately 85% of nitrogen excretion is in the form of urea, and consequently the rate of urea production and excretion provides a good indication of the net rate of protein breakdown and oxidation. As a result, the main product of human nitrogen turnover is urea and most metabolic end-products of incorporated nitrogen compounds such as in food are eliminated via urine. Therefore, the metabolism of protein nitrogen has been investigated by measuring the transfer of [¹⁵N] from protein to plasma amino acids and urea. The choice of [¹⁵N]-precursor ([¹⁵N]-amino acids, [¹⁵N]-ammonium chloride, [¹⁵N]-urea, [¹⁵N]-proteins), administration route and

end-product analysis depends on the problem being investigated.

Application to animal studies

Experiments to investigate the digestion and absorption of nutrients are commonly conducted in pigs and rats.

Ileal and faecal nitrogen balance methods

Quantitative assessments of intestinal absorption of specific nutrients require metabolic-balance collection, i.e. complete collections of excreta must be taken to determine the efficiency of absorption of nutrients from different diets. Timed 72-hour metabolic collections are generally accepted as a reliable measure of nutrient absorption. The nutrient absorption is calculated as the difference between the amount consumed and the amount excreted in faeces during the collection period. However, it is now well established that dietary nutrient digestibility should be determined for the ileum rather than the entire digestive tract since the undigested and non-absorbed nutrients entering the colon are metabolized by the microflora and do not represent significant nutritional value.[17,18]

In contrast to human studies where per-oral intubation is needed, intestinal nutrient absorption studies in animals can be done after surgically fitting the animal with re-entry cannulae, permanent ileal T-cannulae, post-valvular T-cannulae or with an end-to-end ileorectal anastomosis isolating the large intestine.[19-21] However, similar to humans, the assessment of protein assimilation by the gut requires the differentiation of exogenous and endogenous nitrogen fractions in the intestinal chyme by using isotopes to mark the alimentary compounds and/or endogenous compounds. With the help of the [¹⁵N]-isotope dilution technique in which endogenous proteins are labelled, undigested dietary and endogenous proteins can be differentiated.[15,22,23]

Portal blood nutrient kinetics

Rérat et al[24] have developed a method in pigs to measure amino acid absorption based on the enrichment of the portal blood following a meal, as shown by the porto-arterial difference in the nutrient concentration, quantified by simultaneous determination of the portal blood-flow rate according to the formulae:

$$q = (C_p - C_a)\ F\ dt \quad \text{and} \quad Q = \sum_{t_o}^{t_1} q$$

where q is the quantity absorbed in the time dt (5 min) during which the factors are considered as constant; C_p the portal concentration; C_a the arterial concentration; F the blood flow rate in the portal vein; and Q the quantity absorbed during the post-prandial period between times t_o and t_1. Q is the net influx of nutrients into the portal blood.

For these calculations, animals are fitted with a micro-electromagnetic flow probe (12-14 mm diameter silicone probe; In Vivo Metic (IVM) Systems CA, USA) to measure the blood flow rate in the portal vein and with two catheters, one placed in the portal vein and the other in the left brachiocephalic artery through the carotid route. These studies have not used a stable isotope technique, but the method could be applied for the precise quantification exogenous amino acid absorption. In less than a decade, the use of new ultrasound transit-time flowmeters has increased (eg Transonic Sstems Inc., NY, USA).

Results and discussion

Digestive function studies in humans

The objective of all methods for evaluating the adequacy of a human diet is to estimate the size of their biologically usable fraction. Thus, the assessment of nutrient assimilation by the gut in order to determine the true intestinal digestibility requires the use of isotopes to mark the alimentary compounds and/or endogenous compounds.

The main application is the concomitant use of labelled substrates and intestinal perfusion techniques to assess a nutrient's bioavailability. These methods have been used particularly with dietary proteins but could also be used with others nutrients (starches, lipids) or drugs. The major difficulty in the study of intestinal protein digestion in humans arises from both the heterogeneity of dietary proteins and the multiplicity of their digestion products present in the lumen. In addition, a further complication arises from the fact that after ingestion, dietary proteins are mixed with endogenous proteins secreted in the lumen. In humans, the true ileal digestibility has been measured using both the intestinal perfusion technique and [15N]-labelled protein. Table 16.2 shows the digestibility and the retention rates of different protein sources (animals and vegetable), and after different treatments (fermentation, purification and concentration). This approach could also be used to assess digestive resistance as well as oral bioavailability of labelled drugs. For instance, immunoglobulin concentrates from bovine colostrum may have the potential to support the host defence system by passive immunization of the gut in humans since they are significantly resistant to digestion by gastric and intestinal enzymes. Moreover, the measurement of [15N] incorporation in different nitrogen pools in the plasma and in the urine has been used to determine the retention, i.e. the metabolic behaviour of [15N]-dietary nitrogen.

Table 16.2 – Estimation of exogenous nitrogen yield in the healthy human intestine.

Test meal	Jejunal absorption (% ingested/4 h)	Ileal digestibility (% ingested/8 h)	NPU[a]	Ref.
[15N]-milk	57	92	75	32
[15N]-yoghurt	51	—	—	32
[15N]-leu/yoghurt[b]	62	—	—	33
[15N]-β-lactoglobuline	62	—	—	34
[15N]-casein	58	—	—	34
[15N]-IgG (colostrum)	—	81	—	35
[15N]-IgM (colostrum)	—	81	—	35
[15N]-pea	69	89	69	36

[a] Net Protein Utilization is calculated using the formula: [(exogenous N absorbed - urinary exogenous N excreted)/ exogenous N ingested] × 100.
[b] Endogenous nitrogen is labelled by intravenous [15N]-leucine perfusion before yoghurt ingestion.

Another approach is to estimate the absorption of $[^{13}C]$-labelled compounds by measuring the $[^{13}C]$-O_2 expired in the breath. This can be applied to the glucidic nutrients, starch, fibre and oligosaccharides.[25,26]

Gastrointestinal clinical applications

Gastric emptying and intestinal transit time

Maes et al[7] have developed a $[^{13}C]$-labelled breath test to measure the gastric emptying rate of solid as well as liquid test meals based on the characteristics of octanoic acid. This test has some advantages over the other techniques (intubation, radioscintigraphic methods, ultrasonographic evaluation): it is non-invasive, causes no radiation; can be performed with minimum stress and is therefore suitable for children and can even be repeated several times within a short period of time.

$[^{13}C]$-labelled glycosyl ureides, which mark the colon microbial flora action, have been used to reflect intestinal transit times and rapid changes in gastrointestinal motility under various conditions.[27] This test could probably be developed to diagnosis a variety of gastrointestinal motility disorders and to study drugs that affect gastrointestinal motility and transit time.

Detection of specific nutrient malabsorption syndromes

Fat malabsorption: In the study of lipid absorption, the $[^{13}C]$-O_2 breath test can replace the need for a specific diet, and collection and analysis of 72 hour faecal fat samples. Contrary to non-absorbed proteins and carbohydrates, non-absorbed fat is not degraded by colonial bacteria. By evaluating the $[^{13}C]$-O_2 breath excretions following oral administration of $[^{13}C]$-triolein, $[^{13}C]$-trioctanoin and $[^{13}C]$-palmitic acid, fat malabsorption due to exocrine pancreatic insufficiency can be differentiated from that due to intestinal mucosal disease or bile salt deficiency.[28] The specific aspect of gut malfunction in steatorrhea should be further clarified by the use of the $[^{13}C]$-palmitic acid absorption test. The free fatty acid must be esterified in the intact intestinal mucus in order to be absorbed. Thus, when this test is used in conjunction with $[^{13}C]$-triolein or $[^{13}C]$-trioctanoin test, differentiation of intestinal mucosal defects, biliary obstruction or liver disease, and pancreatic enzyme deficiency should be possible.

Carbohydrate malabsorption: The assimilation of disaccharides includes two intimately linked stages: hydrolysis followed by transfer of the liberated mono-

saccharides into the blood. The absorption of intact disaccharides is negligible under physiological conditions. Lactose and sucrose are hydrolysed by brush-border disaccharidases of the enterocytes, particularly in the jejunum. $[^{13}C]$-lactose and $[^{13}C]$-sucrose can be used as indicators of lactase and sucrase deficiency, respectively. Moreover, the hexoses $[^{13}C]$-glucose and $[^{13}C]$-fructose are the subject of many investigations on carbohydrate assimilation.[29]

Ileal dysfunction

Bile acids are re-absorbed in the ileum. The breath test involves the use of $[^{13}C]$-glycocholate. Normally, $[^{13}C]$-glycocholate is absorbed and little $[^{13}C]$-O_2 is excreted. If there is bacterial overgrowth of the small intestine or if there has been ileal disease, large amounts of bile acid are exposed to bacteria and are deconjugated, which results in increased $[^{13}C]$-O_2 excretion.[30] In the same way, $[^{13}C]$-xylose, which is preferentially absorbed in the proximal small intestine, is used to diagnosis small-intestine bacterial overgrowth as increased $[^{13}C]$-O_2 excretion is attributable to bacterial overgrowth.

Specific pathologies associated with gastrointestinal deficiency

$[^{13}C]O_2$ breath tests are now the standard non-invasive technique to diagnose and follow treatment efficacy in *Helicobacter pylori* infections. The usefulness of the stable isotope technique is currently being investigated in various intestinal deficiency diseases. For instance, this test seems to be accurate in the diagnosis of pancreatic insufficiency associated with chronic pancreatis.[31]

Major advances in the instrumentation and the availability of labelled compounds have increased the use of stable isotopes in nutrition and metabolism research in humans. These tracers are now extensively used for studies in both humans and animals and can be used repeatedly and in multiple combinations for *in vivo* experiments. However, there are still some disadvantages to the use of stable isotopes as biological tracers: the natural background against which estimation of label must be made (1.1 AP for ^{13}C), and the cost of the labelled compounds and the high-technology measuring equipment needed. Nevertheless, the use of stable isotopes in physiological and pathophysiological studies in humans and animals will increase exponentially. This will be particularly true for the gastrointestinal tract in which stable isotopes represent a non-invasive method of exploration as illustrated by the increasing use of the [^{13}C]-urea breath test for *Helicobacter pylori* diagnosis.

Acknowledgements

The author is grateful to Prof D. Tomé and Dr R. Benamouzig for their advice and critical review of this manuscript.

References

1. Fern EB, Garlick PJ. The rate of nitrogen metabolism in the whole body of man measured with [^{15}N]-glycine and uniformly labelled [^{15}N]-wheat. *Hum Nutr: Clin Nutr* 1983; **37:** 91-107.

2. Wutzke K, Heine W, Drescher U, Richter I, Plath C. ^{15}N-labelled yeast protein - A valid tracer for calculating whole-body protein parameters in infants: A comparison between [^{15}N]-yeast protein and [^{15}N]-glycine. *Hum Nutr: Clin Nutr* 1983; **37C:** 317-327.

3. Lanfer Marquez UM, Lajolo FM. *In vivo* digestibility of bean (*Phaseolus vulgaris L.*) proteins: The role of endogenous protein. *J Agric Food Chem* 1991; **39:** 1211-1215.

4. Kayser B, Acheson K, Decombaz J, Fern E, Cerretelli P. Protein absorption and energy digestibility at high altitude. *J Appl Physiol* 1992; **73:** 2425-2431.

5. Mahé S, Fauquant J, Gaudichon C, Roos N, Maubois JL, Tomé D. [^{15}N]labelling and preparation of milk, casein and whey proteins. *Lait* 1994; **74:** 307-312.

6. Boirie Y, Fauquant J, Rulquin H, Maubois JL, Beaufrère B. Production of large amounts of [^{13}C]leucine-enriched milk proteins by lactating cows. *J Nutr* 1995; **125:** 92-98.

7. Maes BD, Ghoos YF, Geypens BJ, Hiele MI, Rutgeerts PJ. Relation between gastric emptying rate and energy intake in children compared with adults. *Gut* 1995; **36:** 183-188.

8. King JC, Raynolds WL, Margen S. Absorption of stable isotopes of iron, copper and zinc during oral contraceptive use. *Am J Clin Nutr* 1978; **31:** 1198-1203.

9. Schwartz R, Spencer H, Wentworth RA. Measurement of magnesium absorption in man using stable ^{26}Mg as tracer. *Clin Chim Acta* 1978; **87:** 265-273.

10. Turnlund JR, Michel MC, Keyes WR, King JC, Margen S. Use of enriched stable isotopes to determine zinc and iron absorption in elderly men. *Am J Clin Nutr* 1982; **35:** 1033-1040.

11. Fairweather-Tait SJ, Johnson A, Eagles J, Ganatra S, Kennedy H, Gurr MI. Studies on calcium absorption from milk using a double-label stable isotope technique. *Br J Nutr* 1989; **62:** 379-388.

12. Hoerr RA, Matthews DE, Bier DM, Young VR Leucine kinetics from ^{2}H and ^{13}C leucine infused simultaneously by gut and vein. *Am J Physiol* 1991; **260:** E111-E117.

13. Gaudichon C, Roos N, Mahé S, Sick H, Bouley C, Tomé D. Gastric emptying regulates the kinetics of nitrogen absorption from [^{15}N]-labeled milk and [^{15}N]-labeled yoghurt in miniature pigs. *J Nutr* 1994; **124:** 1970-1977.

14. Mahé S, Roos N, Benamouzig R *et al.* True exogenous and endogenous fractions in the human jejunum after ingestion of small amounts of ^{15}N-labeled casein. *J Nutr* 1994; **124:** 548-555.

15. De Lange CFM, Sauer WC, Souffrant WB, Lien K. ^{15}N-leucine and ^{15}N-isoleucine isotope dilution techniques vs ^{15}N-isotope dilution technique for determining the recovery of endogenous protein and amino acids in digesta collected from the distal ileum in pigs. *J Anim Sci* 1992; **70:** 1848-1856.

16. Gaudichon C, Laurent C, Mahé S, Marks L, Tomé D, Krempf M. Rate of [^{15}N]-leucine incorporation and determination of nitrogenous fractions from gastro-jejunal secretion in fasting human. *Reprod Nutr Dev* 1994; **34:** 349-359.

17. De Lange CFM, Sauer WC, Mosenthin R, Souffrant WB. The effect of feeding different protein-free diets on the recovery and amino acid composition of endogenous protein collected from the distal ileum and feces in pigs. *J Anim Sci* 1989; **67:** 746-754.

18. Rowan AM, Moughan PJ, Wilson MN, Maher K, Tasman-Jones C. Comparison of the ileal and fecal digestibility of dietary amino acids in adult humans and evaluation of the pig as a model animal for digestion studies in man. *Br J Nutr* 1994; **71:** 29-42.

19. Phillips WA, Webb KE, Fontenot JP. Isolation of segments of the jejunum and ileum for absorption studies using double reentrant cannulae in sheep. *J Anim Sci* 1978; **46:** 726-732.

20. Green S, Bertrand SL, Duron MJC, Maillard RA. Digestibility of amino acids in maize, wheat and barley meal, measured in pigs with ileo-rectal anastomosis and isolation of the large intestine. *J Sci Food Agric* 1987; **41:** 29-43.

21. Van Leeuwen P, Van Kleef D, Van Kempen G, Huisman J, Verstegen M. The post-valve T-caecum cannulation technique: an alternative method for chyme collection in pigs. *J Anim Physiol Anim Nutr* 1991; **65:** 183-193.

22. Souffrant WB, Rérat A, Laplace JP, Darcy-Vrillon B, Köhler R, Corring T, Gebhardt G. Exogenous and

endogenous contributions to nitrogen fluxes in the digestive tract of pigs fed a casein diet. III. Recycling of endogenous nitrogen. *Reprod Nutr Dev* 1993; **33:** 373-382.

23. Leterme P, Van Leeuwen P, Thewis A, Huisman J, François E. Determination of the true ileal digestibility of pea amino acids by means of ^{15}N-labelled diets or animals. In: *Vth International Symposium on Digestive Physiology in Pigs.* Souffrant-Hagemeister, Bad Doberan, 1994, pp21-24.

24. Rérat A, Vaugelade P, Villiers PA. A new method for measuring the absorption of nutrients in the pig: critical examination. In: Low AG, Partridge IG (Eds) *Current Concepts of Digestion and Absorption in Pigs.* National Institute for Research in Dairying, Hannah Research Institute, Reading, Ayr, *Technical Bulletin* 1980; **3:** 177-214.

25. Tissot S, Normand S, Guilluy R *et al.* Use of a new gas chromatograph isotope ratio mass spectrometer to trace exogenous ^{13}C labelled glucose at a very low level of enrichment in man. *Diabetologia* 1990; **33:** 449-456.

26. Normand S, Pachiaudi C, Khalfallah Y, Guilluy R, Mornex R, Riou JP. [13]C appearance in plasma glucose and breath CO_2 during feeding with naturally ^{13}C-enriched starchy food in normal humans. *Am J Clin Nutr* 1992; **55:** 430-435.

27. Heine WE, Berthold HK, Klein PD. A novel stable isotope breath test: ^{13}C-labeled glycosyl ureides used as noninvasive markers of intestinal transit time. *Am J Gastroenterol* 1995; **90:** 93-98.

28. Watkins JB, Klein PD, Scholler DA, Kirschner BS, Park R, Perman JA. Diagnosis and differentiation of fat malabsorption in children using ^{13}C-labeled lipids: Trioctanoin, triolein, and palmitic acid breath tests.

Gastroenterology 1982; **82:** 911-917.

29. Kien CL, Ault K, McClead RE. *In vivo* estimation of lactose hydrolysis in premature infants using a dual stable tracer technique. *Am J Physiol* 1992; **26:** E1002-E1009.

30. Solomons NW, Schoeller DA, Wagonfeld JB, Ott D, Rosenberg IH, Klein PD. Application of a stable isotope ^{13}C]-labelled glycocholate breath test to diagnosis of bacterial overgrowth and ileal dysfunction. *J Lab Clin Med* 1977; **30:** 431-439.

31. Evenepoel P, Hiele M, Geypens B, Maes B, Rutgeerts P, Ghoos Y. Egg protein assimilation in pancreatic disease studied with a ^{13}C-egg white breath test. *Gastroenterology* 1996; **110:** Abstract A800.

32. Gaudichon C, Mahé S, Roos N *et al.* Exogenous and endogenous nitrogen flow rates and level of protein hydrolysis in the human jejunum after ^{15}N]milk and ^{15}N]yoghurt ingestion. *Br J Nutr* 1995; **74:** 251-260.

33. Gaudichon C, Mahé S, Laurent C *et al.* A ^{15}N]leucine-dilution method to measure endogenous contribution to luminal nitrogen in the human upper jejunum. *Eur J Clin Nutr* 1996; **50:** 261-268.

34. Mahé S, Roos N, Benamouzig R *et al.* Gastro-jejunal kinetics and the digestion of ^{15}N]-b-lactoglobulin and casein in humans: the influence of the nature and quantity of the protein. *Am J Clin Nutr* 1996; **63:** 546-552.

35. Roos N, Mahé S, Benamouzig R, Sick H, Rautureau J, Tomé D. [15]N]-labeled immunoglobulins from bovine colostrum are partially resistant to digestion in human intestine. *J Nutr* 1995; **125:** 1238-1244.

36. Gausserès N, Mahé S, Benamouzig R *et al.* The gastro-ileal digestion of ^{15}N]-labelled pea nitrogen in adult humans. *Br J Nutr* 1996; **76:** 75-85.

17

Studying the basement membrane

Yamina Bouatrouss, Jacques Poisson and Jean-François Beaulieu

Summary

Immunolocalization studies have greatly supported the notion that in the small intestine, epithelial cell proliferation, migration and differentiation are susceptible to various influences along the crypt–villus axis including compositional changes in the basement membrane and differential expression of cellular receptors for these macromolecules. This chapter provides detailed methodology for investigating the epithelial basement membrane composition by indirect immunofluorescent staining in specimens of adult human small intestine. The usefulness of the method is illustrated with laminin $\alpha 1$ and $\alpha 2$ chains and the $\alpha 5$ chain of type IV collagen as two examples of recently discovered and differentially expressed basement membrane components.

Introduction

The basement membrane (BM) is a specialized region of the extracellular matrix that separates parenchymal cells from the interstitial connective tissue. It serves multiple cellular functions during development and at maturity is a dynamic effector of differentiation, adhesion and migration through recognition by specific cell-surface receptors/binding proteins.[1-12] The intestinal epithelium lies on a relatively well-characterized BM containing all the major ubiquitous constituents found in other epithelial BMs (type IV collagens, proteoglycans, laminins, nidogen/entactin) in addition to the interstitial extracellular matrix components tenascin and fibronectin,[13,14] and other macromolecules not yet fully characterized. A number of cell receptors for these macromolecules, namely those of the integrin family, have also been identified.[14]

In the adult small intestine, the continuously renewing epithelium is organized into spatially confined proliferative and differentiated cell compartments, the crypt and the villus respectively.[15] Because of its unique properties, the crypt-villus unit has been used advantageously as a model to analyse, *in vivo*, cell-BM interactions in relation to the cell state.[14] Surprisingly, it was the non-exclusive BM molecules tenascin and fibronectin which were first shown to be differentially expressed along the crypt–villus axis.[16-22] BM components such as type IV collagen and heterotrimeric laminin were detected at the base of all epithelial cells[17,20,22-24] and some of the integrins that use these macromolecules as ligands were found to be expressed under distinctive crypt–villus gradients.[22,25] However, the identification over the last few years of new genetically distinct laminin and type IV collagen chains prompted us, as well as others, to re-investigate the expression of these BM molecules in the small intestine.

This chapter describes the immunofluorescent procedures used in our laboratory to study the expression of type IV collagen $\alpha 1$–$\alpha 5$ chains as well as the constituent chains of laminin-1 and laminin-2 in the adult human small intestine.[26,27]

Methods

Specimens of human small intestine

Small intestinal specimens are obtained from patients with various diseases, mostly inflammatory bowel disease, bowel obstruction, or neoplastic metastases, according to a protocol approved by the Institutional Review Committee on Human Research. Samples from resected adult small intestinal segments are taken from the non-diseased part of each segment (at least 10 cm away from the lesion). Only specimens obtained rapidly should be used and in our experience the overall period required before freezing the tissue after surgery never exceeded 60 min. Segments are then rinsed in phosphate buffered saline (PBS), cut into small fragments (0.5–1.0 cm long), embedded in optimum cutting temperature compound (Tissue Tek, Miles Laboratories, Elkhart, IN), and quickly frozen in liquid nitrogen.[28] These blocks can be kept at -80°C for a number of years without alteration. Fragments of specimens can also be directly frozen in liquid nitrogen for Western blot and reverse transcription-polymerase chain reaction (RT-PCR) analysis.

Primary antibodies

Mono- and polyclonal antibodies directed against laminin, type IV collagen and functional markers of the intestinal crypt-villus axis are used.[26,27] The characteristics and source of these antibodies are summarized in Table 17.1.

Indirect immunofluorescence

Cryosections 2–3 μm thick are cut at -25°C on a Jung Frigocut 2800N cryostat (Leica Canada Inc, Saint-Laurent, Québec, Canada), spread on silane-coated microscope glass slides (3-aminopropyltriethoxy-

Table 17.1 – Characteristics of antibodies.

Antibody	Type	Specificity	Source	Reference
Laminin				
Ab949	P	from EHS tumour	Chemicon Int	26
Ab428004	P	from h placenta	Calbiochem	26
4C7	M	h α1 chain	Dr E Engvall	29
3E5	M	h β1 chain	Dr E Engvall	30,31
2E8	M	h γ1 chain	DSHB	31
5H2	M	h α2 chain	Dr E Engvall	29,32
2G9	M	h α2 chain	Dr E Engvall	29,32
Type IV collagen				
Ab748	P	α1(IV), α2(IV)	Chemicon Int	27,33
M3F7	M	α1(IV)/α2(IV) native	DSHB	34
Mab 17	M	α3(IV)	Dr J Wieslander	35,36
Anti-α3(IV)	P	α3(IV)	Dr J Wieslander	37,38
Anti-α4(IV)	P	α4(IV)	Dr J Wieslander	37
Pale	P	α5(IV)	Dr K Tryggvason	39
Vicky	P	α5(IV)	Dr. K Tryggvason	39
Anti-α5(IV)j	P	α5(IV)		27
Functional markers				
HSI-5	M	mature form of hSI	Dr A Quaroni	40
HMA-3	M	hMGA complex	Dr A Quaroni	41
HAPN-1/2	M	h aminopeptidase N	Dr A Quaroni	42

P = polyclonal; M = monoclonal. EHS = Engelbreth-Holm-Swarm murine tumour. h = human. SI = sucrase-isomaltase; MGA = maltase-glucoamylase complex.

DSHB, Developmental Studies Hybridoma Bank maintained by the Department of Pharmacology and Molecular Sciences, Johns Hopkins University School of Medicine, Baltimore, Maryland, and the Department of Biology, University of Iowa, Iowa City, Iowa, USA.

Chemicon International, El Segundo, CA, USA.

Calbiochem, San Diego, CA, USA

silane solution, Sigma Chemical Co., St Louis, MO, USA), then air-dried for 1 hour at room temperature before storage at -80°C in air-tight containers.

Tissue sections are fixed in either methanol, ethanol or acetone (10 min at -15°C) or in 1% (v/v) paraformaldehyde in 100 mM pH 7.4 sodium phosphate buffer (60 min at 4°C) depending on the antigen.[26,27] Sections are then washed twice in PBS, incubated for 1 hour at 4°C in 100 mM glycine in PBS, and washed twice more with PBS.

The staining procedure with antibodies is performed at room temperature in humid chambers. Sections are first incubated for 1 hour with a blocking solution (2% (w/v) bovine serum albumin (BSA) or 10% (w/v) non-fat powdered milk in PBS) and washed twice in PBS before incubation (60 min at room temperature) with primary antibodies diluted in the blocking solution as follows: anti-α5(IV) antibody is pre-incubated or not with the antigen, 1:500; Ab748, 1:200; all other polyclonal antisera, 1:100; and mono-

clonal antibodies, 1:100 (ascites fluids) or 1:2 (hybridoma-conditioned media). In control reactions, the primary antibodies to be tested are replaced by the appropriate non-immune or pre-immune sera. Sections are then washed three times in PBS and incubated for 60 min with fluorescein-conjugated goat anti-mouse IgG or anti-rabbit IgG (Boehringer Mannheim, Laval, Québec, Canada) used at a final dilution of 1:25 in blocking solution. After a first wash in PBS, sections are stained with 0.01% Evan's blue in PBS, washed again and mounted in glycerol–PBS (9:1) containing 0.1% paraphenylene diamine and viewed with a Reichert Polyvar 2 microscope (Leica Canada) equiped for epifluorescence with 25× and 100× objectives.

For immunolocalization observations, fluorescein isothiocyanate (FITC)-fluorescence is excited with the output of an Osram HBO 100 W/2 lamp filtered with a Reichert B1 module (excitation filter, 450-495 nm; dichroic mirror DS 510; barrier filter, LP 520).

Black and white pictures are taken with Kodak TX-400 film (Kodak Canada, Toronto, Ontario, Canada). For histological observations, selective excitation of Evan's blue is obtained by switching to a Reichert G2 module (excitation filter, 520-560 nm; dichroic mirror DS 580; barrier filter, LP 590). Black and white pictures are taken with Kodak TX-400 films and processed to generate negative prints.[26]

Pretreatment of tissue sections for immunofluorescence

In some experiments designed to expose potentially hidden epitopes, fixed tissues are subjected to various treatments before primary antibody reaction. Each of the following treatments can be performed separately in 30 min: 0.01% collagenase (type I; Sigma) in PBS at 37°C, 10 µg/ml pepsin (Sigma) in 50 mM Tris-HCl (pH 3.0) at 23°C, 10 µg/ml trypsin (Gibco/BRL, Life Technology Inc, Burlington, Ontario, Canada) in PBS at 23°C, 0.25% Triton X-100 (BioRad, Mississauga, Ontario, Canada) in PBS at 23°C, 6 M urea (BioRad) in 100 mM glycine (pH 3.5) at 4°C. After treatment, sections are washed extensively in PBS, incubated with the blocking solution, and subsequently processed for immunofluorescent staining as described above.

Alternative protocols for indirect immunofluorescence

There are a number of commercially available reagents principally designed to replace the classical FITC-conjugated secondary antibody, to allow double labeling experiments and/or to improve the fluorescent signal. Some of these have been used according to the following protocols:

Simple protocols for the co-detection of two antigens

The easiest procedure consists of using, when available, antibodies raised in different species such as the mouse and the rabbit. In this case,[21] the classical protocol described above is used. Primary as well as secondary antibodies (in this case, a fluorescein-conjugated goat anti-mouse IgG and a lissamine–rhodamine-conjugated goat anti-rabbit IgG; Boehringer Mannheim) are diluted together to their respective optimal working concentration in the blocking agent. Additional controls consist of mismatched incubations[21] to verify the absence of cross-reactivity between the two detection systems.

Another procedure has been applied when the primary antibodies are raised in the same species. Under these conditions,[26,44] the classical protocol is used until the application of the first antibody (we generally select the one which gives the weaker signal, in this case the mouse monoclonal 4C7) (60 min). After several washes, we use a lissamine-rhodamine-conjugated goat anti-mouse IgG (Boehringer Mannheim) for the detection of 4C7. Then, for the detection of the second antigen, sections are washed 3 times in PBS and blocked for 30 min with non-immune mouse serum (Sigma), and incubated for 60 min at room temperature with the second monoclonal antibody (HSI-14) biotinylated with sulpho-NHS-biotin (according to the protocol provided by the manufacturer; Pierce, Rockford, IL, USA), followed by FITC-conjugated streptavidine (Boehringer Mannheim) diluted 1:30 in 2% (w/v) BSA in PBS, washed extensively before mounting (without Evan's blue staining) and examined by epifluorescence using B1 and G2 modules as described above.

Amplification procedure with a digoxigenin-conjugated secondary antibody

We have tested a number of procedures in order to improve the intensity of the fluorescent signal obtained for the detection of some antigens. In general, simply raising the final concentration of the primary antibody does not provide acceptable results as it generally increases the background. Similarly, introducing an unconjugated secondary antibody subsequently detected with a fluorescein-conjugated third antibody increases the non-specific labelling of glycoprotein-rich regions (i.e. brush border and goblet cells). Furthermore, the use of a biotin-conjugated secondary antibody (Boehringer Mannheim) detected with FITC-conjugated streptavidin as above does not significantly improve weak signals and produces some background in intestinal epithelial cells (presumably because of endogenous biotin). However, digoxigenin (DIG)-conjugated secondary antibody has been used advantageously to amplify weak signals such as those obtained with antibodies directed to the $\alpha2$ chain of laminin.[26]

The procedure is similar to that described above for the classical protocol except for the introduction of two intermediate antibodies. Indeed, after incubation with the primary antibody (in this case 5G9, 1:100, 60 min) and washes, sections are incubated with an anti-mouse antibody (F(ab')$_2$ fragment) conjugated to DIG (Boehringer Mannheim; 1:200, 45 min) followed by a mouse anti-DIG antibody (clone 1.71.256, 1:400; Boehringer Mannheim). The antibody complex (mouse–sheep–mouse) is finally detected with a fluorescein-conjugated goat anti-mouse IgG antibody and slides are processed as described above.

Application to animal studies

Indirect immunofluorescent staining methods have been used extensively for studying the expression and localization of basement membrane components and associated molecules. For instance, the uniform pattern of staining for the laminin B chains (renamed β and γ chains) and heparan sulphate proteoglycan (presumably perlecan), as well as the gradients of expression of fibronectin and tenascin along the crypt–villus axis, were all first identified in the rodent small intestine.[16,17,19,23]

It must, however, be pointed out that recent studies have revealed fundamental species-specific differences in the expression of laminins and integrins. Indeed, in contrast to the human where laminin-1 and laminin-2 are restricted to the villi and crypts respectively,[26] both laminins are found restricted to the crypts in mice.[45,46] Similarly, as specific antibodies reacting with rat and mouse integrins become available, differ-

ences in patterns of integrin expression between man and rodents appear more and more evident.[45-47] This probably illustrates the fundamental differences in physiology, developmental rate, and sequences that exist between humans and laboratory animals concerning this organ.[14,48,49]

Results and discussion

Functional analysis of the crypt-villus axis

All the specimens used were obtained from partial resection of the small intestine for various pathological reasons. Those obtained from the resection margins were included in the pool of normal specimens based on morphological criteria and after histological analysis. Furthermore, evidence that a typical epithelial cell differentiation gradient was displayed along the crypt-villus axis in these specimens was verified by means of immunostaining with antibodies directed to a villus form of sucrase-isomaltase (mSI), the maltase-glucoamylase (MGA) complex, and aminopeptidase N (APN; see Table 17.1). As expected from previous studies[40,42,43,48] and summarized in Table 17.2, mSI and MGA were restricted at the luminal domain of villus epithelial cells while APN was detected in all enterocytes.

Table 17.2 – Expression of laminin and type IV collagen chains in the normal adult human intestinal mucosa.

Antigen	Expression along the crypt-villus axis				Muscularis mucosa	Reference
	Lower crypt	Upper crypt	Crypt–villus junction	Villus		
Laminin						26
α1 chain	-	+/-	++	+++	+++	Fig. 17.1a
α2 chain	+	+/-	-	-	-	Fig. 17.1b
β1 chain	+++	+++	+++	+++	+++	
γ1 chain	+++	+++	+++	+++	+++	
Type IV collagen						27
α1 chain	+++	+++	+++	+++	+++	
α2 chain	+++	+++	+++	+++	+++	
α3 chain	-	-	-	-	-	
α4 chain	-	-	-	-	-	
α5 chain	+/-	+/-	-	-	-	Fig. 17.2
MGA	-	-	+/-	++	-	43
mSI	-	-	+/-	+++	-	40
APN	++	++	++	++	-	42

a Intensity from strong (+++) to weak (+/-) or absent (-).

mSI = mature form of sucrase-isomaltase; MGA = maltase-glucoamylase complex; APN = aminopeptidase N.

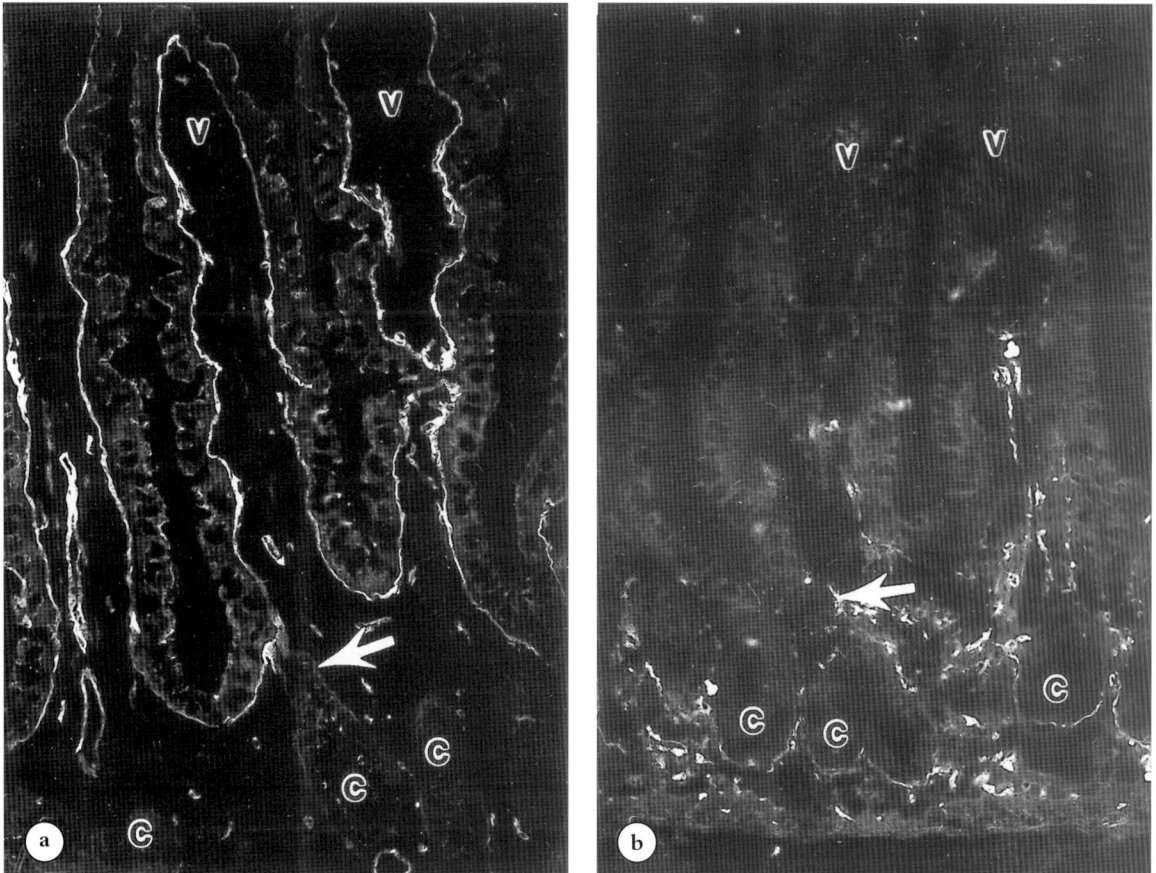

Figure 17.1 – Immunodetection of the α1 and α2 chain of laminin in the adult small intestinal mucosa. Indirect immunofluorescence micrographs from representative fields of cryosections of the ileum from the same patient stained for the detection of the α1 chain with the 4C7 antibody (a) and the α2 chain with the 5H2 antibody (b). The α1 chain was found to be concentrated at the epithelial BM of villi (V) while the α2 chain was found restricted to the bottom of the crypts (C). Arrows denote the crypt-villus junction. ×125

Analysis of the epithelial basement membrane composition

Expression of the two main BM components, laminin and type IV collagen, and their distribution along the crypt-villus axis, were determined with a panel of mono- and polyclonal antibodies (Table 17.1). In all specimens studied, immunodetection of the trimeric laminins and the classical form of type IV collagen ($[\alpha 1(IV)]_2\alpha 2(IV)$) with various antibodies revealed a uniform distribution of these macromolecules at the epithelial BM from the bottom of the crypts to the tip of the villi (Table 17.2).[22, 26 27] Similar patterns of distribution were also observed in the adult intestinal mucosa for other constitutive basement components such as heparan sulphate proteoglycans and entactin/nidogen.[13,14]

More detailed analysis with laminin chain-specific antibodies also revealed a widespread distribution of the β1 and γ1 chains. However, the α1 and α2 laminin chains were found to be expressed in more restricted patterns (Table 17.2). The α1 chain was detected in the villus, from the tip to the crypt–villus junction, but was below detection level in the crypts (Fig. 17.1a). In contrast, the α2 chain was found to be confined to the bottom of the crypts (Fig. 17.1b). These observations, which indicate a differential expression of laminin-1 ($\alpha 1\beta 1\gamma 1$) and laminin-2 ($\alpha 2\beta 1\gamma 1$) along the crypt–villus axis in the normal small intestine, appear to be of functional relevance. Indeed, *in vitro* studies with laminins have shown that specific enterocyte-related gene expression is differentially regulated by variant forms of the molecule.[44]

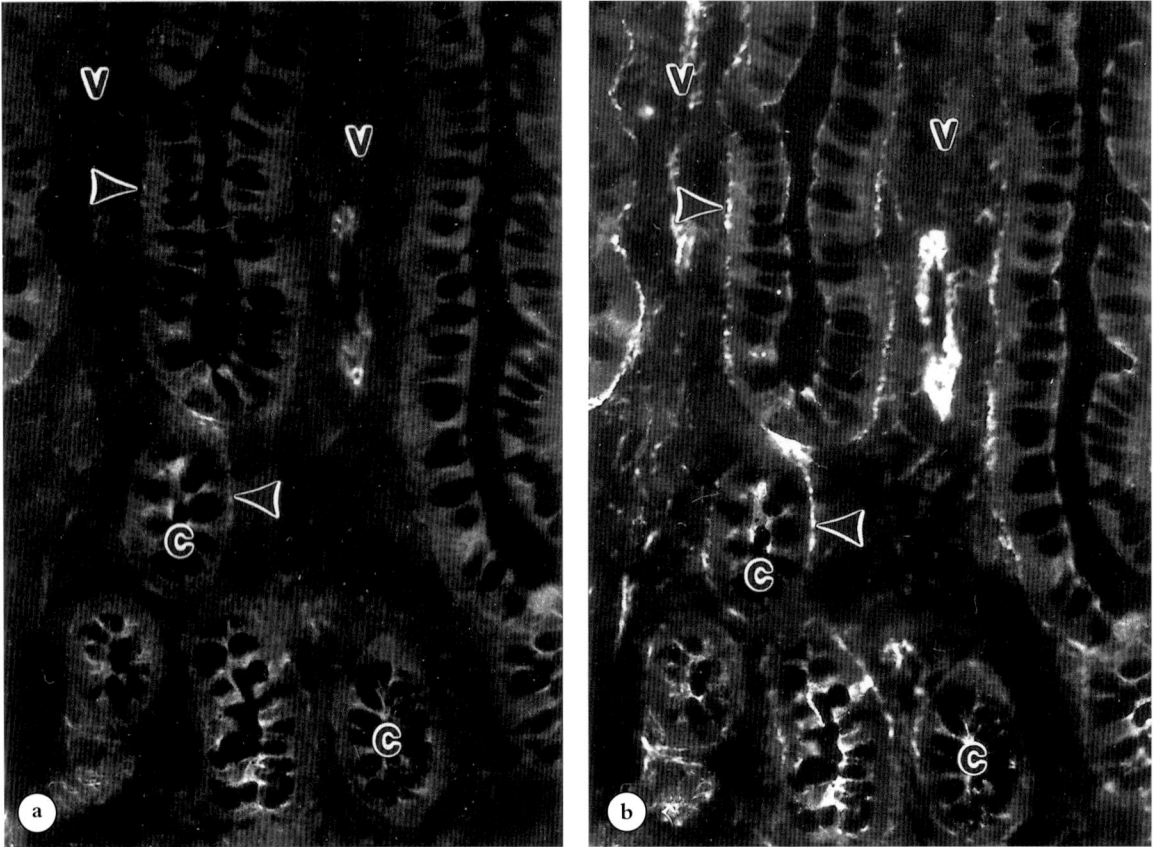

Figure 17.2 – Immunodetection of the α5(IV) chain of collagen in the adult small intestinal mucosa. Serial frozen sections of ileum were stained by indirect immunofluorescence with the anti-α5(IV)j antibody at the dilution of 1:300 (a) and 1:100 (b). At the lower and optimal dilution, the staining (arrowheads) for α5(IV) was below detection level (a) while the antigen was detected in both crypts (C) and villi (V) at the higher concentration (b), suggesting a low level of expression. ×125

The study of type IV collagen chains in the human adult small intestine revealed a clear predominance of the α1(IV) and α2(IV) chains at the epithelial BM. Indeed, the α3(IV) and α4(IV) chains were not detected while the α5(IV) chain was expressed at a relatively low level in the adult (Fig. 17.2), in comparison to the fetal small intestine.[27] Interestingly, in contrast to the α1(IV) and α2(IV) chains which originate from the mesenchymal compartment, the α5(IV) chain was found to be produced by both epithelial and mesenchymal cells.[14,33] The α5(IV) chain was also found to be expressed by a colon carcinoma cell line (Simoneau A, Vachon PH, Beaulieu JF, unpublished observations), suggesting a possible relationship between its expression by intestinal cells and fetal development and cancer progression.

The intestinal epithelial BM is a relatively complex structure, being composed of ubiquitous components but also of relatively minor macromolecules that are subject to specific spatial-temporal patterns of expression. To our knowledge, analysis of these laminin and type IV collagen chains in the intestine under pathological conditions has not yet been investigated. Based on the above observations in the normal intestine, studying laminin-1 and laminin-2 distribution could be of great interest since their expression and therefore their regulatory influences on the epithelium are likely to be altered in intestinal diseases such as chronic inflammation and cancer. Furthermore, analysing α5(IV) chain expression may be of relevance in the study of intestinal tumour progression.

Acknowledgements

The original work and preparation of this article were supported by grants MT-11289 and MT-12904 from the Medical Research Council of Canada and from the "Fonds pour la formation des Chercheurs et l'Aide à la Recherche". The authors thank Drs Eva Engvall, Andrea Quaroni, Karl Tryggvason, Jörgen Wieslander and Peter D Yurchenco who generously provided key antibodies, the members of the Department of Pathology of the CUSE for their co-operation in providing tissue specimens, and N Basora and FE Herring-Gillam for reviewing the manuscript.

References

1. Hay ED. Extracellular matrix. *J Cell Biol* 1981; **91:** 205s-223s.

2. Lin CQ, Bissell MJ. Multi-faceted regulation of cell differentiation by extracellular matrix. *FASEB J* 1993; **7:** 737-743.

3. Kleinman HK, Graf J, Iwamoto Y *et al*. Role of basement membranes in cell differentiation. *Ann NY Acad Sci* 1987; **513:** 134-145.

4. McDonald JA. Matrix regulation of cell shape and gene expression. *Curr Opin Cell Biol* 1989; **1:** 995-999.

5. Paulsson M. Basement membrane proteins: Structure, assembly, and cellular interactions. *Crit Rev Biochem Mol Biol* 1992; **27:** 93-127.

6. Edelman GM. Morphoregulation. *Dev Dynamics* 1992; **193:** 2-10.

7. Hynes RO. Integrins: versatility, modulation, and signaling in cell adhesion. *Cell* 1992; **69:** 11-25.

8. Akiyama SK, Nagata K, Yamada KM. Cell surface receptors for extracellular matrix components. *Biochim Biophys Acta* 1990; **1031:** 91-110.

9. Adams JC, Watt FM. Regulation of development and differentiation by the extracellulair matrix. *Development* 1993; **117:** 1183-1198.

10. Juliano RL, Haskill S. Signal transduction from the extracellular matrix. *J Cell Biol* 1993; **120:** 577-585.

11. Schwartz MA, Schaller MD, Ginsberg MH. Integrins: Emerging paradigms of signal transduction. *Ann Rev Cell Dev Biol* 1995; **11:** 549-599.

12. Timpl R, Brown JC. Supramolecular assembly of basement membranes. *BioEssays* 1996; **18:** 123-132.

13. Simon-Assmann P, Kedinger M, De Archangelis A, Rousseau V, Simo P. Extracellular matrix components in intestinal development. *Experientia* 1995; **51:** 883-900.

14. Beaulieu JF. Extracellular matrix components and integrins in relationship to human intestinal epithelial cell differentiation. *Prog Histochem Cytochem* 1997; **31:** 1-78

15. Leblond CP. The life history of cells in renewing systems. *Am J Anat* 1981; **160:** 114-159.

16. Quaroni A, Isselbacher KJ, Ruoslahti E. Fibronectin synthesis by epithelial crypt cells of rat small intestine. *Proc Natl Acad Sci USA* 1978; **75:** 5548-5552.

17. Simon-Assmann P, Kedinger M, Haffen K. Immunocytochemical localization of extracellular matrix proteins in relation to rat intestinal morphogenesis. *Differentiation* 1986; **32:** 59-66.

18. Aufderheide E, Ekblom P. Tenascin during gut development: appearance in the mesenchyme, shift in molecular forms, and dependence on epithelial-mesenchymal interactions. *J Cell Biol* 1988; **107:** 2341-2349.

19. Probstmeier R, Martini R, Schachner M. Expression of J1/tenascin in the crypt-villus unit of adult mouse small intestine: implication for its role in epithelial cell shedding. *Development* 1990; **109:** 313-321.

20. Beaulieu JF, Vachon PH, Chartrand A. Immunolocalization of extracellular matrix components during organogenesis in the human small intestine. *Anat Embryol* 1991; **183:** 363-369.

21. Beaulieu JF, Jutras S, Durand J, Vachon PH, Perreault N. Relationship between tenascin and α-smooth muscle actin expression in the developing human small intestinal mucosa. *Anat Embryol* 1993; **188:** 149-158.

22. Beaulieu JF. Differential expression of the VLA family of integrins along the crypt–villus axis in the human small intestine. *J Cell Sci* 1992; **102:** 427-436.

23. Laurie GW, Leblond CP, Martin GR. Localization of type IV collagen, laminin, heparan sulfate proteoglycan and fibronectin to the basal lamina of basement membranes. *J Cell Biol* 1982; **95:** 340-344.

24. Trier JS, Allan CH, Abrahamson DR, Hagen SJ. Epithelial basement membrane of mouse jejunum. Evidence for laminin turnover along the entire crypt–villus axis. *J Clin Invest* 1990; **86:** 87-95.

25. McDonald JA, Horton MA, Choy MY, Richman PI. Increased expression of laminin/collagen receptor (VLA-1) on epithelium of inflamed human intestine. *J Clin Pathol* 1990; **43:** 313-315.

26. Beaulieu JF, Vachon PH. Reciprocal expression of laminin A-chain isoforms along the crypt-villus axis in the human small intestine. *Gastroenterology* 1994; **106:** 829-839.

27. Beaulieu JF, Vachon PH, Herring-Gillam E *et al*. Expression of the α5(IV) collagen chain in the fetal human small intestine. *Gastroenterology* 1994; **107:** 957-967.

28. Beaulieu JF, Weiser MM, Herrera L, Quaroni A. Detection and characterization of sucrase-isomaltase in adult human colon and in colonic polyps. *Gastroenterology* 1990; **98**: 1467-1477.

29. Engvall E, Earwicker D, Haaparanta T, Ruoslahti E, Sanes JR. Distribution and isolation of four laminin variants: Tissue restricted distribution of heterotrimers assembled from five different subunits. *Cell Regul* 1990; **1**: 731-740.

30. Gehlsen KR, Dickerson K, Argraves WS, Engvall E, Ruoslahti E. Subunit structure of laminin-binding integrin and localization of its binding site on laminin. *J Biol Chem* 1989; **264**: 19034-19038.

31. Engvall E, Davis G, Dickerson EK, Ruoslahti E, Varon S, Manthorpe M. Mapping of domains in human laminin using monoclonal antibodies: localization of the neurite-promoting site. *J Cell Biol* 1986; **103**: 2457-2465.

32. Leivo I, Engvall E. Merosin, a protein specific for basement membranes of Schwann cells, striated muscle, and trophoblast, is expressed late in nerve and muscle development. *Proc Natl Acad Sci USA* 1988; **85**: 1544-1548.

33. Vachon PH, Durand J, Beaulieu JF. Basement membrane formation and re-distribution of β_1 integrins in a human intestinal co-culture system. *Anat Rec* 1993; **236**: 567-576.

34. Foellmer HG, Madri JA, Furthmayr H. Monoclonal antibodies to type IV collagen: probes for the study of structure and function of basement membrane. *Lab Invest* 1983; **48**: 639-649.

35. Kleppel MM, Santi PA, Cameron JD, Wieslander J, Michael AF. Human tissue distribution of novel basement membrane collagen. *Am J Pathol* 1989; **134**: 813-825.

36. Johansson C, Butkowski R, Wieslander J. Characterization of monoclonal antibodies to the globular domain of collagen IV. *Connective Tissue Res* 1991; **25**: 229-241.

37. Butkowski R, Langeveld JPM, Wieslander J, Hamilton J, Hudson BG. Localization of the Goodpasture epitope to a novel chain of basement membrane collagen. *J Biol Chem* 1987; **262**: 7874-7877.

38. Saus J, Wieslander J, Langeveld JPM, Quinones S, Hudson BG. Identification of Goodpasture antigen as the α3(IV) chain of collagen IV. *J Biol Chem* 1988; **263**: 13374-13380.

39. Hostikka SL, Eddy RL, Byers MG, Höyhtyä M, Shows TB, Tryggvason K. Identification of a distinct type IV collagen a chain with restricted kidney distribution and assignment of its gene to the locus of X chromosome-linked Alport syndrome. *Proc Natl Acad Sci USA* 1990; **87**: 1606-1610.

40. Beaulieu JF, Nichols B, Quaroni A. Posttranslational regulation of sucrase-isomaltase expression in intestinal crypt and villus cells. *J Biol Chem* 1989; **264**: 20000-20011.

41. Cross HS, Quaroni A. Inhibition of sucrase-isomaltase expression by EGF in the human colon adenocarcinoma cells Caco-2. *Am J Physiol* 1991; **261**: C1173-C1183.

42. Quaroni A, Nichols BL, Quaroni E *et al*. Expression and different polarity of aminopeptidase N in normal human colonic mucosa and colonic tumors. *Int J Cancer* 1992; **51**: 404-411.

43. Hauri HP, Sterchi EE, Bienz D, Fransen JAM, Marxer A. Expression and intracellular transport of microvillus membrane hydrolases in human intestinal epithelial cells. *J Cell Biol* 1985; **101**: 838-851.

44. Vachon PH, Beaulieu JF. Extracellular heterotrimeric laminin promotes differentiation in human enterocytes. *Am J Physiol* 1995; **268**: G857-G867.

45. Simon-Assmann P, Duclos B, Orian-Rousseau V *et al*. Differential expression of laminin isoforms and a6-b4 integrins subunits in the developing human and mouse intestine. *Dev Dynamics* 1994; **201**: 71-85.

46. Vachon PH, Basora N, Xu H, Beaulieu JF, Engvall E. Species-specific patterns of laminin variants and laminin-binding integrins in murine and human small intestine. In: *Proceedings Seventh International Symposium on Basememt Membranes*. NIH, Bethesdsa 1995, p87.

47. Menard D, Calvert R. Fetal and postnatal development of the small and large intestine: patterns and regulation. In: Salomon T, Morrisset J (Eds) *Growth of the Gastrointestinal Tract: Gastrointestinal Hormones and Growth Factors*. CRC Press, Boca Raton, 1991, pp. 159-174.

48. Menard D, Beaulieu JF. Human intestinal brush border membrane hydrolases. In: Bkaily G (Ed) *Membrane Physiopathology*. Kluwer Academic Publisher, Norwell, 1994, pp. 319-341.

18

Lipid peroxidation measurement in gastointestinal tissue

Yuji Naito, Toshikazu Yoshikawa and Motoharu Kondo

Summary

There is growing evidence that free radical reactions contribute to the degradation of biological molecules and in turn to the development of gastrointestinal tract disease. Lipids, nucleic acids, enzymes and proteins are important targets of biological damage caused by oxygen free radicals. Unsaturated fatty acids located in the lipophilic section of cell membranes, in particular, are prone to attack by oxygen free radicals which induce a chain reaction of lipid peroxidation. Thiobarbituric acid-reactive substances, an indicator of lipid peroxidation, increase in gastrointestinal mucosa in several pathological conditions, such as acute gastric mucosal injury, ischaemic colitis and inflammatory bowel disease. This chapter reviews the methods to investigate lipid peroxidation *in vivo* and the recent evidence that oxygen free radical-mediated lipid peroxidation is involved in digestive physiology and disease.

Introduction

At their normal rate of generation, some free radicals are useful in the human body. However, when oxygen free radical generation exceeds the capacity of antioxidant defences, the result is oxidative stress. This occurs in many human diseases and can contribute significantly to their pathogenesis, e.g. the superoxide anion and hydroxyl radicals are thought to mediate a large part of the tissue damage produced after inflammation, ischaemia and ischaemia-reperfusion of the small intestine, stomach, heart, kidney, liver and skin, and may also be involved in the pathogenesis of carcinogenesis, transplant rejection, circulatory shock and disseminated intravascular coagulation. Since Itoh & Gruth[1] in 1985 confirmed that ischaemia-reperfusion injures the gastric mucosa, and that these injuries can be ameliorated by the administration of scavengers of reactive oxygen species or free radicals, attention has focused on the involvement of these reactive species in the pathology of gastric mucosal injuries.[2-5]

Free radical and lipid peroxidation

A free radical is defined as a molecule or atom with an unpaired electron. By virtue of their unpaired electron, free radicals are usually unstable and quite reactive. Highly reactive oxygen radicals such as the hydroxyl radical have half lives in the nanosecond to millisecond range. In normal oxidative phosphorylation, molecular oxygen is reduced by four electrons to form H_2O by the following sequence:

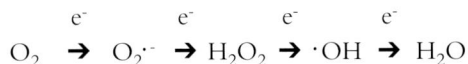

$$O_2 \xrightarrow{e^-} O_2^{\cdot -} \xrightarrow{e^-} H_2O_2 \xrightarrow{e^-} \cdot OH \xrightarrow{e^-} H_2O$$

Both the superoxide anion ($O_2^{\cdot -}$) and hydroxyl radical ($\cdot OH$) have the potential to react with biological radicals and thereby induce tissue damage. Hydrogen peroxide is a less potent oxidizing agent but in the presence of transition metal ions such as iron, $O_2^{\cdot -}$ converts ferric to ferrous iron which can then react with H_2O_2 to generate more reactive hydoxyl radicals ($\cdot OH$). Since most molecules formed under physiological conditions do not have unpaired electrons, free radicals abstract an electron from a stable compound that, in turn, is transformed into a new free radical. Therefore, free radical reactions tend to proceed as chain reactions which will continue until the free radical is deactivated by an antioxidant. The most studied free radical chain reaction in living systems is lipid peroxidation, which is mediated by oxygen free radicals and is believed to be an important cause of cell membrane destruction and cell damage. Biomembranes contain large amounts of polyunsaturated fatty acids (PUFAs) in their phospholipids. PUFAs contain two or more carbon double bonds within their structures which makes them susceptible to oxidative damage by free radical attack.

Experimental evidence suggests that lipid peroxidation reactions on cell membranes may play an important role in free radical-mediated cell injury. *In vitro* studies with purified membrane preparations have shown that lipid peroxidation of biological membranes will cause structural alterations and abnormal membrane functions. The most obvious consequence of membrane lipid peroxidation is the perturbation of various cellular and organellar membrane functions, including transport processes, maintenance of ion and metabolite gradients, receptor-mediated signal transduction, etc. Lipid peroxides, due to their long life, migrate from one site in the body to another and thus propagate the injury. Further support for the toxicity of lipid peroxides comes from the report that increased lipid peroxide in blood provokes injury to the endothelial cells of the artery, and that lipid peroxides produced by burnt skin can injure the gastric mucosa by subsequent lipid peroxidation.[6]

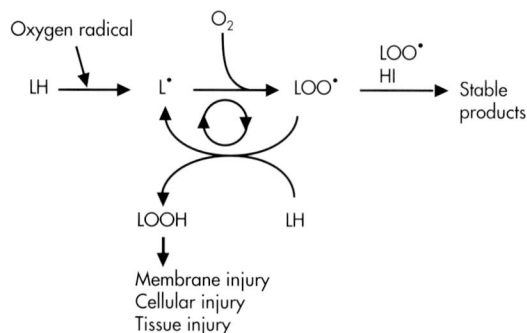

Figure 18.1 – Lipid peroxidation mediated by free radicals.

Mechanism of lipid peroxidation

Free radical-mediated lipid peroxidation has at least three distinct phases (Fig. 18.1). The initial step is the abstraction of an hydrogen atom from a PUFA containing at least two methylene-interrupted double bonds (LH), giving rise to a carbon centred free radical (L·). Hydroxyl and metal-ion free radical complexes probably abstract hydrogen atoms from the hydrocarbon chains of the fatty acids. The greater the number of double bonds, the easier is the removal of hydrogen, which is why PUFAs are particularly susceptible to attack. The second step is the propagation phase in which the lipid radical (L·) reacts with oxygen, generating a peroxyl radical (LOO·). This is usually very fast. The fatty acid peroxyl radical can then abstract a hydrogen atom, either from an adjacent LH, thereby propagating lipid peroxidation, or from another H-donor, resulting in both cases in the formation of a lipid hydroperoxide (LOOH). Hence, a single initiating event can result in the conversion of hundreds of fatty acid side chains to lipid peroxides. In the third step LOOH can undergo further reactions: they can be reoxidized to LOO·, thus reinitiating lipid peroxidation by propagation; and they can be reduced to the alkoxyl radical (LO·), which again can reinitiate lipid peroxidation by abstracting an hydrogen atom from an adjacent LH.

There are a number of cellular and extracellular antioxidative defences which protect cells from the potentially harmful effects of lipid peroxides and their metabolites. The decompositon of both H_2O_2 and lipid peroxides is catalysed by the enzyme glutathione peroxidase. This is a selenium-containing protein which catalyses the decomposition of peroxides at the expense of reduced glutathione (GSH), forming oxidized glutathione (GSSG), H_2O and organic alcohol (LOH). Glutathione is regenerated by glutathione reductase at the expense of NADPH. The NADPH is then regenerated from glucose-6-phosphate by the action of glucose-6-phosphate dehydrogenase. Glutathione peroxidase is found in plasma (extracellular type) and most tissues (cellular and gastrointestinal types) in both the cytosol and mitochondria.

An important membrane and plasma lipoprotein defence against peroxidation is the presence of lipid-soluble antioxidants. Chain-breaking antioxidants can interfere with the propagation of lipid peroxidation damage by trapping LOO· or LO· to form a less active species incapable of reacting with oxygen or LH. The principal chain-breaking lipid-soluble antioxidants in human blood are the four tocopherols, α, β, γ, δ, which together constitute vitamin E. α-Tocopherol is the most active and it localizes into the hydrophobic interior of biological membranes. LOO· generated during lipid peroxidation reacts much faster with α-tocopherol than with adjacent PUFA side chains or membrane proteins and forms a nonreactive tocopherol radical, thereby interrupting the chain reaction of lipid peroxidation.[7]

Methods

Free radicals are extremely reactive and thus short lived. Consequently, free radicals are not amenable to direct assay and activity is usually assessed by indirect methods such as measurement of the various end products of reactions with lipids, proteins and DNA. Table 18.1 lists the methods available for measuring the rate of peroxidation of membrane lipids or fatty acids. Two spectrophotometric methods are commonly used to determine the extent of lipid peroxidation in animal and human tissue extracts: measurement of diene conjugation and thiobarbituric acid (TBA)-reactive substances. Although the latter is not specific for lipid peroxides, it is the easiest method to use and can be applied to crude samples. The assay is based on the reaction of TBA with malondialdehyde (MDA), one of the aldehyde products of lipid peroxidation. There are many variants but basically the sample is heated with TBA under acidic conditions and the amount of pink-coloured MDA-TBA adduct produced is measured by absorbance at 532 nm or by fluorescence at 553 nm (Table 18.2).

Table 18.1 – Methods of measurement of biological lipid peroxides.

1. Uptake of oxygen

2. Titrimetric analysis using iodine release

3. Diene conjugation

4. Hydrocarbon gases

5. Measurement of other end products of peroxidation

6. Loss of fatty acids

7. Light emission

8. Measurement of fluorescene

9. The thiobarbituric acid (TBA) test

10. HPLC-chemiluminescence assay

Table 18.2 – Measurement of thiobarbituric acid (TBA)-reactive substances.

Scrape off the gastrointestinal mucosa using two glass slides
↓ or take two biopsies from the mucosa by endoscopy

Homogenize with 1.5 ml 10mM potassium phosphate
buffer (pH 7.8) containing 30 mM KCl and 0.4%
(v/v) butylated hydroxytoluene in a Teflon Potter-
Elvehjeim homogenizer

The reaction mixture contains:
0.2 ml tissue homogenate
0.2 ml 8.1% (w/v) SDS
1.5 ml 20% (v/v) acetic acid solution (pH 3.5)
1.5 ml 0.8% (w/v) TBA solution
0.6 ml distilled water

Heat at 95°C for 60 min
↓

Cool with tap water
↓

Add 1.0 ml distilled water
5.0 ml of the mixture of n-butanol and pyridine
↓ (15:1, v/v)

Mixture is shaken virgously with vortex
↓

Centrifuge at 3000 rpm for 10 min at room temperature
↓

Measure absorbance of the organic layer at 532 nm

We have measured the concentration of TBA-reactive substances in the mucosa of the gastrointestinal tract using the method of Ohkawa *et al*[8] and in serum by the method of Yagi.[9] In brief, the animals are sacrificed by exsanguination from the abdominal aorta, the stomach or intestine is removed, the mucosa is scraped off using two glass slides and homogenized with 1.5 ml 10 mM potassium phosphate buffer (pH 7.8) containing 30 mM KCl and 0.4% (v/v) butylated hydroxytoluene in a Teflon Potter-Elvehjem homogenizer. TBA-reactive substances can be measured in human tissue specimens obtained by endoscopic biopsy. Two biopsy specimens are taken from the mucosa of the gastrointestinal tract and frozen in phosphate buffered saline containing 0.5% (v/v) butylated hydroxytoluene until measurement of lipid peroxides. It is generally advisable to assay samples as quickly as possible after taking them since there is a tendency for lipid peroxidation to increase with storage.[10] Conversely, lipid hydroperoxides can deteriorate with storage.[11] The assay procedure for lipid peroxide level in mucosal homogenates is as follows: 0.2 ml 8.1% (w/v) sodium dodecyl sulphate (SDS), 1.5 ml 20% (v/v) acetic acid solution adjusted to pH 3.5 with NaOH and 1.5 ml 0.8% (w/v) aqueous solution of TBA are added to 0.2 ml samples of tissue homogenate. The amount ≤ 0.2 ml of 10% tissue homogenate is suitable for the assay of lipid peroxide level in animal tissue. The reactions of lipid peroxides in whole homogenate with TBA are affected by the pH of the reaction mixture: the optimum pH is 3.5. The mixture is made up to 4.0 ml with distilled water and then heated in an oil bath at 95°C for 60 min using a glass ball condenser. After cooling with tap water, 1.0 ml distilled water and 5.0 ml of a mixture of n-butanol and pyridine (15:1, v/v) are added and shaken vigorously. After centrifugation at 3000 rpm for 10 min, the organic layer is taken and its absorbance at 532 nm is measured. When a sample contains bilirubin, fluorometric measurement (excitation: 515 nm; emission: 553 nm) is recommended in place of spectrophotometric measurement. Bilirubin interacts with TBA to interfere with the absorbance at 532 nm at concentrations above 1.0 µg (1.71 nmol) in the reaction mixture. The level of TBA-reactive substances in the mucosal homogenates is expressed as nmol of MDA per g wet weight or per mg protein using 1,1,3,3-tetramethoxypropane as the standard. The total amount of protein in the tissue homogenates is measured by the method of Lowry *et al*.[12] Halliwell & Chirico[13] have suggested modification to the TBA test to avoid artifactual changes.

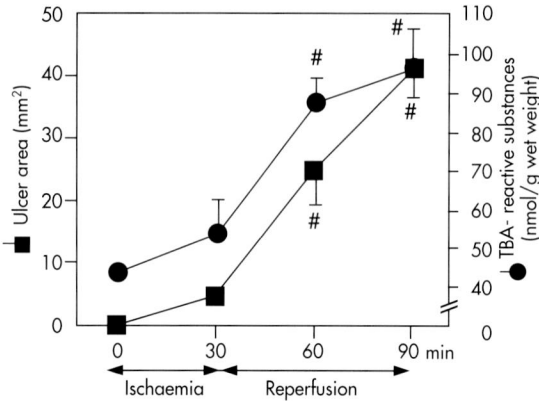

Figure 18.2 – Changes in the total area of erosions and thiobarbituric acid (TBA)-reactive substances in the gastric mucosa after ischaemia-reperfusion. Each point indicates the mean ± SE. #p<0.01 for difference in values of rats before clamping the celiac artery.

First, amplification of peroxidation during assay is prevented by adding the chain-breaking antioxidant butylated hydroxytoluene to the sample before TBA reagents are added. Secondly, high performance liquid chromatography (HPLC) is used to separate the authentic TBA-MDA adduct from other chromogens absorbing at 532 nm.[14,15] Direct assessment of free MDA is more reliably done by HPLC, but MDA is a minor product of lipid peroxidation and is readily metabolized; it is therefore not a promising subject for the analysis of lipid peroxidation *in vivo*.[16]

Various methods have been developed to distinguish specific classes of lipid hydroperoxides. These are based on separation according to lipid class of the various hydroperoxides in a Folch lipid extract or plasma by HPLC and measurement of the chemiluminescence produced during their breakdown in the presence of either luminol[17] or isoluminol.[18] Miyazawa *et al* (1995, personal communication) reported that the level of phosphatidylcholine hydroperoxide in the gastric mucosa increased significantly from a mean basal concentration of 429 pmol/100 mg protein to 516 pmol/100 mg protein 6 hours after water immersion restraint stress in rats. These HPLC tests, although specific and sensitive, are time-consuming in their analysis and preparation of standards and are best used only when information on individual hydroperoxides is required. There have been no reports measuring lipid peroxides in the human gastrointestinal tract using these HPLC methods.

Application to animal studies

Ischaemia-reperfusion injury model in the rat stomach

We have developed an animal model of ischaemia-reperfusion-induced gastric mucosal injury in rats by applying a vascular clamp to the celiac artery and then removing it.[5] The total area of erosions increases gradually after clamping the celiac artery and significantly increases after reperfusion following 30 min of gastric ischaemia (Fig. 18.2). TBA-reactive substances in the gastric mucosa do not increase 30 min after ischaemia but do significantly increase 30 and 60 min after reperfusion. The level of α-tocopherol in the gastric mucosa decreases with time after reperfusion, which suggests that α-tocopherol, a lipid-soluble antioxidant, is consumed in the process of lipid peroxidation in ischaemia-reperfusion to prevent the development of tissue damage. In addition, lipid peroxides accumulate and α-tocopherol consumption closely parallels the development of gastric mucosal injury. This indicates that lipid peroxidation plays a significant role in the pathogenesis of the gastric mucosal lesions induced by ischaemia-reperfusion. The close relationship between lipid peroxidation and gastric mucosal injury has also been observed in other animal models of gastric injury, such as burn shock-, stress- and indomethacin-induced acute gastric mucosal injury.[19,20]

Using an ischaemia-reperfusion-induced gastric injury model, new agents can be tested for their ability to improve the reperfusion injury and to inhibit lipid peroxidation *in vivo*.[21-23] A novel antiulcer agent, rebamipide, significantly reduces the total area of gastric erosion induced by ischaemia-reperfusion and significantly inhibits the increase in TBA-reactive substances of the gastric mucosa (Table 18.3). Rebamipide scavenges hydroxyl radicals *in vitro*, inhibits superoxide production from opsonized zymosan- or platelet activating factor-stimulated neutrophils, and significantly inhibits *Helicobacter pylori*-induced neutrophil activation. The antioxidant action of this agent may be responsible for its antiulcer effect.

Gastric ulcer and lipid peroxidation

To investigate whether oxygen free radicals directly

Table 18.3 – Effect of rebamipide on acute gastric mucosal injury induced by ischaemia–reperfusion in rats

	Total area of erosions (mm²)	TBA -reactive substances (nmol/mg protein)
Control operation	0.0 ± 0.0	0.252 ± 0.019
Ischaemia–reperfusion	38.3 ± 4.6	0.393 ± 0.016
+ rebamipide 30 mg/kg	14.4 ± 3.7**	0.316 ± 0.037*
+ rebamipide 100 mg/kg	6.1 ± 2.3 **	0.302 ± 0.018*

Each value indicates the mean ± SE of 7 experiments. *p<0.05 and **p<0.01 when compared with the ischaemia–reperfusion group.

induce lipid peroxidation of the gastric mucosa *in vivo*, or cause a stomach ulcer that can extend into the muscle proper of the stomach, we have attempted to induce gastric ulcers in rats using a ferrous iron-ascorbic acid (Fe-ASA) reaction system, which is an *in vitro* oxygen radical generating system.[24] A time-course study revealed that the concentration of TBA-reactive substances significantly increased in the gastric mucosa 1 hour after the injection of Fe-ASA solution and remained elevateed after that. These increases preceded grossly evident gastric ulceration. In addition, simultaneous administration of CuZnSOD significantly reduced the area of the gastric ulcer and significantly inhibited the increase in TBA-reactive substances in the gastric mucosa 24 hours after injection of the Fe-ASA solution. These findings suggest that the lipid peroxidation mediated by superoxide radicals, generated by the Fe-ASA system, plays a crucial role in the development of these ulcers. It is highly significant that an experimental ulcer that closely resembles a human gastric ulcer can be attributed to free radical reaction. This ulcer model is useful for the elucidation of the aetiology of human gastric ulcers and can be employed to investigate the pharmacological effects of antiulcer drugs that possess antioxidative activity.

Discussion

Oxygen-derived free radicals are involved in the relapse of duodenal ulceration in patients infected with *Helicobacter pylori*.[25] A recent clinical trial has shown that patients with high levels of TBA-reactive substances in the mucosa of gastric ulcer scars have a relatively higher incidence of ulcer recurrence within 1 year (Fig. 18.3), which suggests that lipid peroxidation is involved in the relapse of gastric ulceration in humans (Naito Y, Yoshikawa T 1996, unpublished observations).

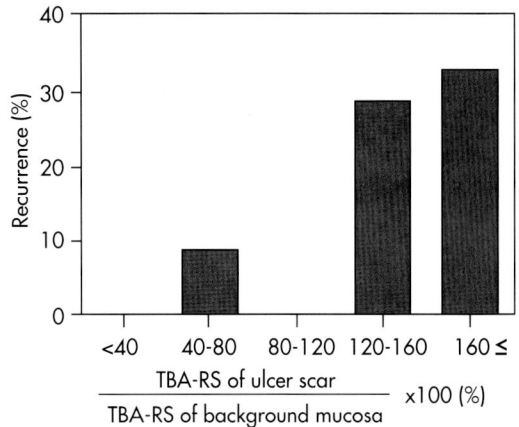

Figure 18.3 – Relationship between lipid peroxide level in the mucosa of gastric ulcer scars and recurrence rate within 1 year. TBA-RS = thiobarbituric acid-reactive substances.

Free radical and lipid peroxidation have been implicated as potential cytotoxic mechanisms responsible for gastrointestinal injury. Measurement of TBA-reactive substances is a simple and valid method to investigate the lipid peroxidation in tissue and to evaluate the pharmacological action of an agent.

References

1. Itoh M, Gruth PH. Role of oxygen-derived free radicals in hemorrhagic shock-induced gastric lesions in rats. *Gastroenterology* 1985; **88:** 1162-1167.

2. Perry MA, Wadhwa S, Parks DA *et al*. Role of oxygen radicals in ischemia-induced lesions in the cat stomach. *Gastroenterology* 1986; **90:** 362-367.

3. Smith SM, Grisham MB, Manci EA *et al*. Gastric mucosal injury in the rat. Role of iron and xanthine oxidase. *Gastroenterology* 1987; **92:** 950-956.

4. Smith MS, Holm-Rutili L, Perry MA et al. Role of neutrophils in hemorrhagic shock-induced gastic mucosal injury in the rat. Gastroenterology 1987; **93:** 466-471.

5. Yoshikawa T, Ueda S, Naito Y et al. Role of oxygen-derived free radicals in gastric mucosal injury induced by ischemia or ischemia-reperfusion in rats. Free Rad Res Commun 1989; **7:** 285-291.

6. Yoshikawa T, Yoshida N, Miyagawa H et al. Role of lipid peroxidation in gastric mucosal lesions induced by burn shock in rats. J Clin Biochem Nutr 1987; **2:** 163-170.

7. Halliwell B, Gutteridge JMC. Lipid peroxidation: a radical chain reaction. In: Halliwell B, Gutteridge JMC (Eds) Free Radicals in Biology and Medicine. Clarendon Press, Oxford, 1985, pp. 139-189.

8. Ohkawa H, Ohnishi N, Yagi K. Assay for lipid peroxides for animal tissues by thiobarbituric acid reaction. Anal Biochem 1986; **95:** 351-358.

9. Yagi K. A simple fluorometric assay for lipid peroxides in blood plasma. Biochem Med 1976; **15:** 212-216.

10. Duthie GG, Morrice PC, Ventresca PG et al. Effects of storage, iron and time of day on indices of lipid peroxidation in plasma from healthy volunteers. Clin Chim Acta 1992; **206:** 207-213.

11. Holley A, Slater T. Measurement of lipid hydroperoxides in normal human blood plasma using HPLC-chemiluminescence linked to a diode array detector for measuring conjugated dienes. Free Rad Res Commun 1991; **15:** 61-63.

12. Lowry OH, Rosenbrough NJ, Farr AL et al. Protein management with the folin phenol reagent. J Biol Chem 1951; **193:** 265-275.

13. Halliwell B, Chirico S. Lipid peroxidation: its mechanism, measurement and significance. Am J Clin Nutr 1993; **57:** 715S-725S.

14. Bird RP, Hung SSO, Hadley M et al. Determination of malonaldehyde in biological materials by high-pressure liquid chromatography. Anal Biochem 1983; **128:** 240-244.

15. Young IS, Trimble ER. Measurement of malondialdehyde in plasma by high performance liquid chromatography with fluorimetric detection. Ann Clin Biochem 1991; **28:** 504-508.

16. Holley AE, Cheeseman KH. Measuring free radical reactions in vivo. Br Med Bull 1993; **49:** 494-505.

17. Miyazawa T, Yasuda K, Fijimoto K. Chemiluminescence-high performance liquid chromatography of phosphatidylcholine hydroperoxide. Anal Lett 1987; **20:** 915-925.

18. Yamamoto Y, Brodsky MH, Baker JC et al. Detection and characterization of lipid hydroperoxides at picomole levels by high-performance liquid chromatography. Anal Biochem 1987: **160:** 7-13.

19. Yoshikawa T, Miyagawa H, Yoshida N et al. Increase in lipid peroxidation in rat gastric mucosal lesions induced by water-immersion restraint stress. J Clin Biochem Nutr 1986; **1:** 271-277.

20. Yoshikawa T, Naito Y, Kishi A et al. Role of active oxygen, lipid peroxidation and antioxidants in the pathogenesis of gastric mucosal injury induced by indomethacin in rats. Gut 1993; **34:** 732-737.

21. Yoshikawa T, Naito Y, Tanigawa T et al. Effect of zinc-carnosine chelate compound (Z-103), a novel antioxidant, on acute gastric mucosal injury induced by ischemia-reperfusion in rats. Free Rad Res Commun 1991; **14:** 289-296.

22. Naito Y, Yoshikawa T, Matsuyama K et al. Effect of rebamipide, a novel anti-ulcer agent, on acute gastric mucosal injury induced by ischemia-reperfusion in rats. Pathophysiology 1994; **1:** 161-164.

23. Naito Y, Yoshikawa T, Matsuyama K et al. Effect of a novel histamine H2 receptor antagonist, IT-066, on acute gastric mucosal injury induced by ischemia-reperfusion in rats, and its antioxidative properties. Eur J Pharmacol 1995; **294:** 47-54.

24. Naito Y, Yoshikawa T, Yoneta T et al. A new gastric ulcer model in rats produced by ferrous iron and ascorbic acid injection. Digestion 1995; **56:** 472-478.

25. Salim AS. The relationship between Helicobactor pylori and oxygen-drived free radicals in the mechanism of duodenal ulceration. Intern Med 1993; **32:** 359-364.

19

Microdialysis as applied to the gastrointestinal tract

Hideo Fukui and Masaki Yamamoto

Summary

Microdialysis, a new bioanalytical sampling technique, enables the measurement of substances in the extracellular space. This technique has been applied to the gastrointestinal tract of dogs to obtain direct evidence for the release of serotonin (5-HT) from the gut wall induced by cisplatin treatment and for the involvement of the released 5-HT in cisplatin-induced emesis. Microdialysis probes were implanted in the ileal wall of anesthetized dogs and perfused with Ringer's solution. The 5-HT levels in the ileal dialysate were increased to 232-294% of the basal level from 100 to 180 min after cisplatin administration (3 mg/kg i.v.), the period when emesis occurs most frequently. The 5-HT levels had then returned to the basal level 280 min after dosing, the time when emetic episodes stop. An increase in 5-HT levels was also detected in the blood dialysate collected from a probe inserted into the cephalic vein in conscious dogs. These results strongly suggest that increased release of 5-HT in the ileum is intimately involved in cisplatin-induced emesis and that the microdialysis technique provides a promising new tool for investigating the pathophysiology of gastrointestinal disorders in both clinical and animal studies.

Introduction

In vivo microdialysis was originally developed as a technique to study cerebral neurochemistry in awake, freely moving animals.[1] A probe placed in the desired tissue is perfused with a physiological solution which is subsequently collected for analysis.[2] The perfusate is contained within the probe and tubing and has access to the tissue only via the semipermeable dialysis membrane. Substances in the extracellular fluid will diffuse into the perfusate while substances in the perfusate will diffuse into the tissue. This technique offers many advantages over earlier methods for investigating biochemical events in the extracellular space. In experimental animals, during the last one and a half decades, the microdialysis technique has been widely used for measuring the extracellular concentrations of many substances in other tissues such as the spinal cord,[3] skeletal muscle,[4, 5] adipose tissue,[4] lung,[5] liver,[5] heart,[6,7] pancreas,[8] adrenal,[9] ovary[10] and plasma[11] as well as the brain.[1, 2] Recently, the technique has been applied to humans, and it has been adapted for use in the brain,[12-14] skin,[15,16] blood[17] and adipose tissue.[18] However, the microdialysis technique has not been applied to the gastrointestinal tract in either animals or humans except for one study with application of the technique to the stomach in rabbits.[19]

It is well known that many anticancer drugs cause nausea and vomiting in patients.[20] In the last decade, a number of studies on the emetic response induced by anticancer drugs, especially cisplatin, have been carried out in various animals, and much evidence suggests that serotonin (5-HT) in the gastrointestinal tract plays a key role in the response.[21,22] In the present study, therefore, microdialysis was applied to the gastrointestinal tract of dogs to obtain direct evidence for the release of 5-HT from the gut wall produced by cisplatin treatment and for involvement of the released 5-HT in cisplatin-induced emesis. In addition, the effects of cisplatin on circulating 5-HT levels were examined using the same technique.

Methods

Microdialysis

As mentioned in the introduction, there are, currently, no applications of microdialysis in clinical studies, though there are no practical reasons why it cannot be applied. The following information therefore pertains to dogs.

Surgery and dialysis in the ileum

The experimental methods for microdialysis and a typical chromatogram of the dog ileum dialysate are shown in Fig. 19.1.

For microdialysis in the gastrointestinal tract, a probe with a fine dialysis fiber is implanted in a selected tissue such as the ileum and perfused with a physiological solution at a slow rate. Low molecular weight compounds such as 5-HT diffuse down their concentration gradients from the extracellular fluid of the ileum into the physiological solution that flows through the fiber. The fluid is collected and analysed. There are many kinds of microdialysis probes which differ in lengths of probe shafts and dialysis fiber, diameters of the fibers and in molecular weight cut-off of the dialysis membrane. The probes are differentially used depending on the tissues dialyzed and the compounds determined. The probes have one of two shapes: the first is a parallel type in which inflow and outflow tubes/cannula are glued side by side and a dialysis fiber is connected to one end of them. The second is a linear type in which

ene tube (PE-50) to a gas-tight glass syringe filled with Ringer's solution (Na+ 147 mM, K+ 4 mM, Ca++ 2.25 mM, Cl- 155.5 mM; Otsuka Pharmaceuticals, Tokyo, Japan) and perfused at 2 μl/min using a microinfusion pump (EP-50, Eicom, Co., Kyoto, Japan).

Animals (beagle dogs of either sex weighing 7.2-11.6 kg and fasted for at least 18 hrs before experiments) are anesthetized with ketamine hydrochloride (50 mg/kg i.m., supplemented with i.v. injection if necessary) after pretreatment with atropine sulfate (0.05 mg/kg s.c.) and xylazine hydrochloride (2 mg/kg s.c.). After cannulation of the cephalic vein and the trachea, a celiotomy is performed under artificial ventilation: animals are placed in a supine

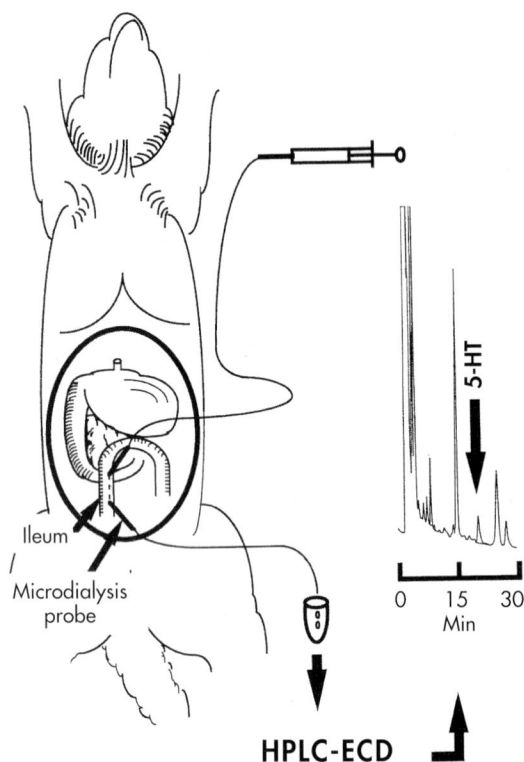

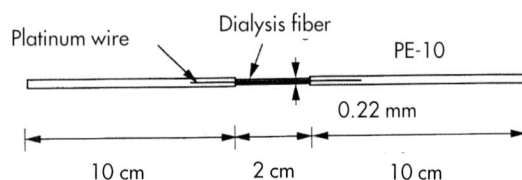

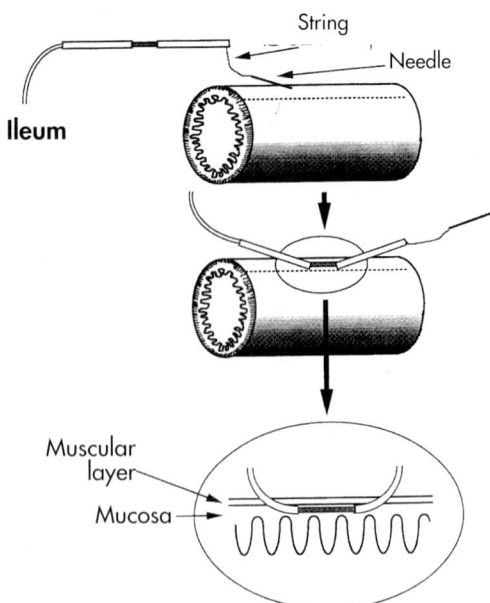

Figure 19.1 – Schematic representation of the experimental methods and a chromatogram of the ileum dialysate.

inflow and outflow tubes are connected to the ends of a dialysis fiber. The probes are available from Eicom, Co., Kyoto, Japan or Carnegie Medicin, Stockholm, Sweden. Eicom, Co. supplies the parallel type for dialysis in the brain and blood and the linear type for dialysis in peripheral tissues, whereas Carnegie Medicin supplies only the parallel type for dialysis in any tissue including peripheral tissues.

In the studies described in this chapter, a linear type microdialysis probe consisting of a single dialysis fiber (20 mm length, 0.22 mm O.D.), two polyethylene tubes (PE-10) and a platinum wire is used (Fig. 19.2). The platinum wire is placed in the dialysis fiber to reinforce it. The dialysis membrane is made of cellulose, and the molecular weight cut-off is below 50 kDa. The length of both the inflow and outflow polyethylene tubes is 10 cm. Before inserting the microdialysis probe into the ileal wall, the inflow polyethylene tube is connected via a larger polyethyl-

Figure 19.2 – Schematic representation of the ileum microdialysis probe and the procedure for insertion of the probe into the ileum.

position, and the abdominal region is shaved after sterilization of the abdominal surface with Povidone-Iodine (Isodine® surgical scrub, Meiji Seika Kaisha, Ltd., Tokyo, Japan). The abdomen is opened approximately 15 cm via a median incision and the ileal region gently pulled out from the abdominal cavity. Operations are carried out under aseptic conditions.

To insert the microdialysis probe into the ileal wall, the outflow polyethylene tube is connected to a needle with a string. Before inserting the needle through the ileal wall, the ileum is cooled for a while with ice in an aseptic bag to shrink the ileum and thicken the ileal wall. The needle is then passed through the ileal wall with the outflow tube, and the outflow tube is pulled through the ileal wall until the dialysis fiber is embedded completely within the ileal wall, as shown in Fig. 19.2. The inflow and outflow tubes are then lightly secured to the surrounding tissue with sutures. After the micro-dialysis probe is implanted, the outflow tube is

connected to a polyethylene tube (PE-50), and the ileum is replaced in the abdominal cavity. Finally, the incision is closed to prevent the ileum from drying. At the end of each experiment, each animal is sacrificed by exsanguination from the common carotid artery, the ileum is dissected out with the probe, and the location of the dialysis probe in the ileal wall is verified macroscopically.

Dialysis in blood

Microdialysis in blood is conducted using conscious dogs. Dogs are placed on a restraining apparatus throughout the experiment. For dialysis in blood, a parallel type probe (Eicom, Co., Kyoto, Japan) consisting of two polyethylene tubes (PE-10) and a single dialysis fiber (10 mm length, 0.22 mm O.D.) is used (Fig. 19.3). The material and molecular weight cut-off of the dialysis fiber are the same as those for dialysis in the ileum. The length of both the inflow and outflow polyethylene tubes is 10 cm. Before inserting the microdialysis probe into the blood vessel, the probe is perfused with Ringer's solution at a rate of 2 µl/min in a way similar to that used for dialysis in the ileum.

To insert the microdialysis probe into the blood vessel, an indwelling needle whose length has been adjusted so that only the dialysis fiber protrudes from the tip of the needle, is inserted into the cephalic vein. The microdialysis probe is then inserted into the indwelling needle, and the microdialysis probe and indwelling needle are fixed together to the forelimb with surgical tape.

In the microdialysis experiment in both the ileum and blood, the microdialysis probe is perfused with Ringer's solution for at least 2 hrs after implantation before collecting baseline samples. This is necessary for stabilization of base-line values, for example the 5-HT levels following the initial damage caused by the insertion of the probe. After taking 4 or 5 baseline samples, the agent under test (e.g. cisplatin) is administered intravenously, and dialysates are collected at regular intervals. Dialysates (40 µl) are collected every 20 min in Eppendorf tubes (500 µl) containing 10 µl of 0.02 M acetic acid or other agent to preserve analytes.

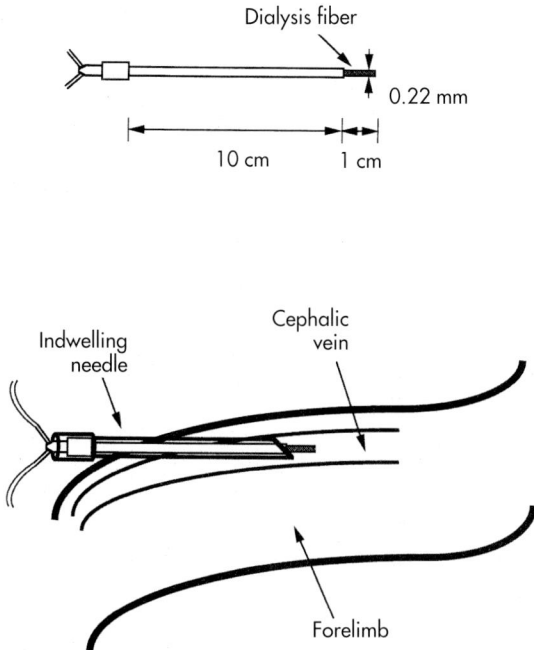

Figure 19.3 – Schematic representation of the blood microdialysis probe and the procedure for insertion of the probe into the cephalic vein.

To estimate the efficiency of the dialysis probes, the recovery of analytes, such as 5-HT is determined *in vitro*: the probes are mounted on a holder, lowered into a solution containing 200 ng/ml of 5-HT and perfused with Ringer's solution at 2 µl/min. For example, the average recoveries are 64.3±1.6% for the dialysis probe for the ileum and 39.8±1.3% for the probe for blood (n=3, mean ± S.E.).

Extraction of 5-HT from ileal mucosa and plasma

To confirm the results of the microdialysis experiments, changes in 5-HT after administration of cisplatin are examined in the ileal mucosa and blood using the extraction method. The ileal mucosa is taken from dogs sacrificed 3 hrs after dosing. Blood samples are collected before dosing and 3 and 5 hrs after dosing.

Assay of 5-HT

5-HT is measured using HPLC with electrochemical detection (ECD). 5-HT is separated on a reverse phase column and detected by a graphite working electrode.

Monitoring of emesis

Emesis is observed in the dogs used for microdialysis in blood. The number of vomiting episodes is counted for 5 hrs after administration of cisplatin.

Drugs and chemicals

Cisplatin (Aldrich Chemical Co., St. Louis, MO.) is dissolved by sonication in physiological saline at 60°C and injected intravenously at a dose of 3 mg/kg in all experiments. The injection volume of cisplatin is 3 ml/kg. Control animals receive the same volume of physiological saline.

Data analysis

In the microdialysis studies, basal amounts of 5-HT in the dialysates varies from dog to dog. Therefore, the average amount of 5-HT in the dialysates of the last three pre-drug samples is taken to be 100%, and all subsequent samples are expressed relative to the basal values. The effect of cisplatin is expressed graphically by taking the mean of the relative value of the corresponding time points.

Results and discussion

Microdialysis techniques have has been applied to the gastrointestinal tract of dogs. Microdialysis probes can be successfully embedded in the ileal wall of the anesthetized dogs and 5-HT in the dialysate of the ileum can be detected clearly by HPLC

(Fig. 19.1). The basal concentration of 5-HT in the dialysate is 1.0±0.4 pmol/20 min (Mean±S.E., n=6). As has already been reported in dogs,[23] vomiting caused by cisplatin occurs in dogs most frequently 2-3 hrs after dosing and stops around 5 hrs after dosing (Fig. 19.4). In the present study, the 5-HT levels in the dialysate increased gradually beginning immediately after cisplatin dosing, and the increase became statistically significant from 100 to 180 min after dosing. The maximum increase in 5-HT levels was 232-294% of the basal level. The 5-HT levels then decreased and returned to the basal level at 280 min (Fig. 19.5). An increase in 5-HT levels following cisplatin treatment was also detected in the dialysate of blood. 5-HT levels in blood showed no marked changes up to 120 min after cisplatin dosing but increased abruptly at 140 min. The 5-HT levels then decreased gradually and had returned to the basal levels 240 min after dosing (Fig. 19.6). The basal concentration of 5-HT in the blood dialysate was 1.4±0.6 pmol/20 min (n=3). The pattern of vomiting was monitored concurrently with microdialysis, and the increase in 5-HT levels in blood was synchronized with the occurrence of emesis. The increases in 5-HT levels in the ileum and blood following cisplatin administration were confirmed using the extraction method, and the concentrations of 5-HT were increased to 271% in the ileal mucosa (Fig. 19.7) and to 478% in plasma (Fig. 19.8) 3 hrs after dosing. These results clearly demonstrate that cisplatin administration causes the release of 5-HT in the ileal wall *in vivo*, correlated well with the occurrence of vomiting, and suggest that the increased release of 5-HT in the ileum is intimately involved in cisplatin-induced emesis. In addition, the results suggest that the microdialysis technique would be very useful for pharmacological and physiological studies of gastrointestinal functions.

As described in the introduction, the microdialysis technique has been applied to humans. Histamine levels in the skin have been studied in relation to cutaneous inflammation.[15,16] It has also been suggested that the technique can be used for continuous long-term monitoring of glucose concentrations in diabetic patients during ordinary daily life.[18] Moreover, cerebral concentrations of amino acids and catecholamines have been measured to study the neurochemical mechanisms of head trauma, ischemia and epilepsy.[12-14] The microdialysis technique has not yet been applied to the human gastrointestinal tract. However, the technique could be applied to the gastrointestinal tract of humans, and it is expected

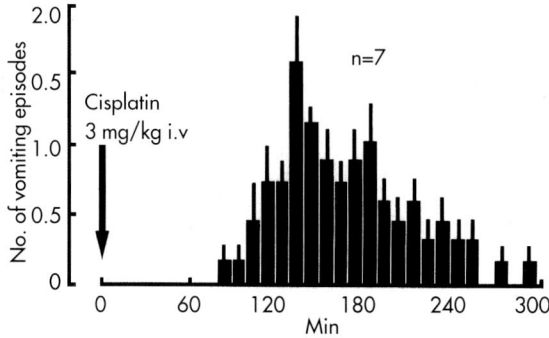

Figure 19.4 – The pattern of vomiting in dogs following cisplatin administration. Each vertical bar represents the mean number of vomiting episodes with S.E. for each 10-min period of the 5-h observation period.

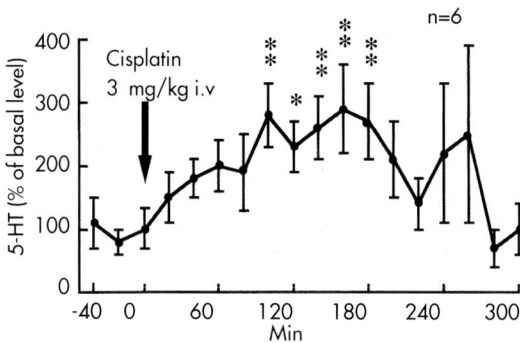

Figure 19.5 – Cisplatin-induced changes in 5-HT levels in the ileum dialysate in anesthetized dogs. Each value is presented as the mean change (%) ±S.E. from the basal level. 5-HT levels in the ileum dialysate were significantly increased from 100 to 180 min after cisplatin dosing and had returned to the basal levels at 280 min. *p<0.05, **p<0.01, compared with the basal level.

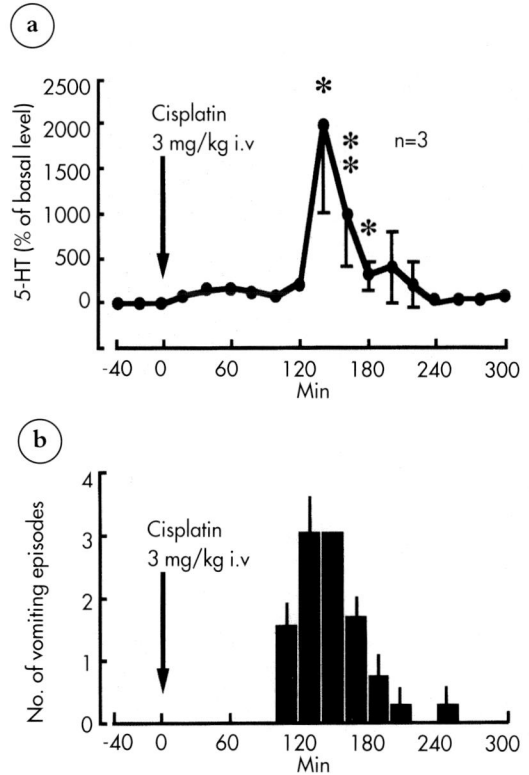

Figure 19.6 – Effects of cisplatin on 5-HT levels in the blood dialysate and vomiting in conscious dogs. Each 5-HT level is presented as the mean change (%) ±S.E. from the basal level. The results of vomiting are the mean±S.E. for the number of vomiting episodes in each 20 min of the total observation period. 5-HT levels in the blood dialysate increased synchronously with the occurrence of emesis. *p<0.05, **p<0.01, compared with the basal level.

to be a promising tool for investigating the pathophysiology of gastrointestinal disorders including nausea and vomiting as indicated by the results in the present study. For example, the pathogenesis of inflammatory bowel diseases (ulcerative colitis and Crohn's disease) has not been fully elucidated yet, but the involvement of the following mediators in the disease has been suggested: cytokines such as interleukin-6 and -8 and tumor necrosis factor α,[24] eicosanoids such as prostaglandin E_2[25] and thromboxane B_2[26] and neuropeptides such as vasoactive intestinal peptide[27,28] and substance P.[27] Therefore, if changes in these mediators in the gastrointestinal tract can be monitored using the microdialysis technique in patients, it should greatly enhance our understanding

of the pathogenesis of these disease. Invasiveness of the technique and the resultant potential for infection may be of concern as risk factors. However, the microdialysis technique is reported to be well tolerated by normal volunteers and patients.[12-18]

Application to animal studies

Regarding the application of the microdialysis technique to the gastrointestinal tract in animals, the technique cannot be applied to the gut of small animals such as rodents and ferrets since the gut wall in these animals is too thin to embed micro-

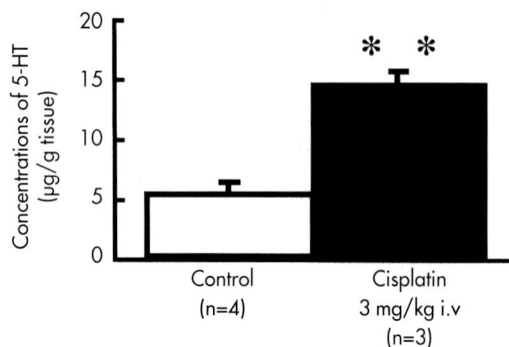

Figure 19.7 – Cisplatin-induced changes in the concentrations of 5-HT in the ileal mucosa (extraction method). The results are the mean±S.E. for the concentrations of 5-HT in the ileal mucosa. The concentrations of 5-HT in the ileal mucosa were significantly increased 3 hrs after injection of cisplatin. **p<0.01, compared with the control.

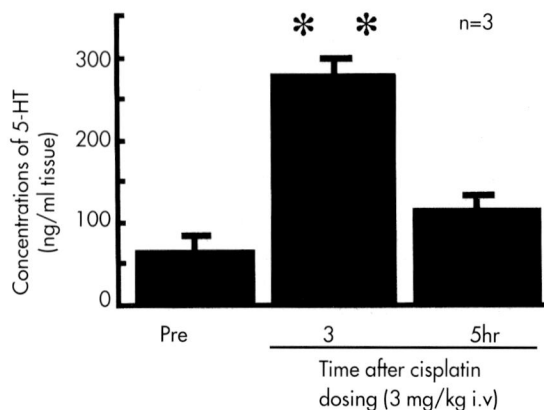

Figure 19.8. – Cisplatin-induced changes in the concentrations of 5-HT in plasma (extraction method). The results are the mean±S.E. for the concentrations of 5-HT in plasma. The concentrations of 5-HT in plasma 3 hrs after dosing were significantly increased compared to the pre-drug value. **p<0.01, compared with the pre-drug value.

dialysis probes. However, application of the technique to the stomach might be possible even in small animals since monoamine concentrations have been successfully determined using the technique in rabbits.[19]

In the studies described in this chapter, an increase in 5-HT levels could be detected in the blood dialysate. Thus, application of the microdialysis technique to blood would also be useful for investigating the pathophysiology of gastrointestinal disorders as an alternative approach instead of dialysis in the gastrointestinal tract, since application of microdialysis to blood is much easier.

In summary, 5-HT levels in the dialysate of the ileum increased synchronously with the occurrence of vomiting following cisplatin injection. In addition, an increase in 5-HT levels was also detected in the blood dialysate. These results strongly suggest that increased release of 5-HT in the ileum is intimately involved in cisplatin-induced emesis and that the microdialysis technique provides a promising new tool for investigating the pathophysiology of gastrointestinal disorders in both clinical and animal studies.

Acknowledgment

The authors thank Mr K. Imai, and Mr T. Kondo for their excellent technical assistance.

References

1. Ungerstedt U. Measurement of neurotransmitter release by intracranial dialysis. In: Marsden CA, ed. *Measurement of neurotransmitter release in vivo*. Chichester, Wiley, 1984; 81-105.

2. Ungerstedt U, Hallström Å. *In vivo* microdialysis - A new approach to the analysis of neurotransmitters in the brain. Life *Science* 1987; **4**: 861-864.

3. Sorkin LS, Hughes MG, Liu D, Willis WD, McAdoo DJ. Release and metabolism of 5-hydroxytryptamine in the cat spinal cord examined with microdialysis. *J Pharmacol Exp Ther* 1991; **257**: 192-199.

4. Fuchi T, Rosdahl H, Hickner RC, Ungerstedt U, Henriksson J. Microdialysis of rat skeletal muscle and adipose tissue: Dynamics of the interstitial glucose pool. *Acta Physiol Scand* 1994; **151**: 249-260.

5. Deguchi Y, Terasaki T, Yamada H, Tsuji A. An application of microdialysis to drug tissue distribution study: *In vivo* evidence for free-ligand hypothesis and tissue binding of beta-lactam antibiotics in interstitial fluids. *J Pharmacobio-dyn* 1992; **15:** 79-89.

6. Timoshin AA, Tskitishvili OV, Serebryakova LI, Kuzmin AI, Medvedev OS, Ruuge EK. Microdialysis study of ischemia-induced hydroxyl radicals in the canine heart. *Experienteria* 1994; **50:** 677-679.

7. Obata T, Hosokawa H, Yamanaka Y. *In vivo* monitoring of norepinephrine and hydroxy free radical generation by ferrous iron in the myocardium with a microdialysis technique. *Comp Biochem Physiol C Comp Pharmacol Toxicol* 1993; **106:** 635-638.

8. Jonsson P, Borgstrom A, Ohlsson K. Measurements of exocrine proteins in the pig pancreas using microdialysis. *Gastroenterology* 1992; **27:** 529-535.

9. Yadid G, Goldstein DS, Pacak K, Kopin IJ, Golomb E. Functional α_3-glycine receptors in rat adrenal. *Eur J Pharmacol Mol Pharmacol Sect* 1995; **288:** 399-401.

10. Hirsch B, Leonhardt S, Jarry H, Reich R, Tsafriri A, Wuttke W. *In vivo* measurement of rat ovarian collagenolytic activities. *Endocrinology* 1993; **133:** 2761-2765.

11. Chen Z, Steger RW. Plasma microdialysis. A technique for continuous plasma sampling in freely moving rats. *J Pharmacol Toxicol Methods* 1993; **29:** 111-118.

12.. Kanthan R, Shuaib A, Goplen G, Miyashita H. A new method of *in vivo* microdialysis of the human brain. *J Neurosci Methods* 1995; **60:** 151-155.

13. Kanthan R, Shuaib A, Griebel R, Miyashita H, Dietrich WD. Intracerebral human microdialysis: *In vivo* study of an acute focal ischemic model of the human brain. *Stroke* 1995; **26:** 870-873.

14. Kanthan R, Shuaib A. Clinical evaluation of extracellular amino acids in severe head trauma by intracerebral *in vivo* microdialysis. *J Neurol Neurosurg Psychiatry* 1995; **59:** 326-327.

15. Anderson C, Anderson T, Anderson RGG. *In vivo* microdialysis estimation of histamine in human skin *Pharmacol* 1992; **5:** 177-183.

16. Petersen LJ, Mosbech H, Skov PS. Allergen-induced histamine release in intact human skin *in vivo* assessed by skin microdialysis technique: Characterization of factors influencing histamine releasability. *J Allergy Clin Immunol* 1996; **97:** 672-679.

17. Stjernstrom H, Karlsson T, Ungerstedt U, Hillered L. Chemical monitoring of intensive care patients using intravenous microdialysis. *Intensive Care Med* 1993; **19:** 423-428.

18. Bolinder J, Ungerstedt U, Arner P. Long-term continuous glucose monitoring with microdialysis in ambulatory insulin-dependent diabetic patients. *Lancet* 1993; **342:** 1080-1085.

19. Meirieu O, Pairet M, Sutra JF, Ruckebusch M. Local release of monoamines in the gastrointestinal tract: An *in vivo* study in rabbits. *Life Science* 1986; **38:** 827-834.

20. Gralla R.J. An outline of anti-emetic treatment. *Eur J Cancer Clin Oncol* 1989; **25:** S7.

21. Andrews PLR, Rapeport WG, Sanger GJ. Neuropharmacology of emesis induced by anti-cancer therapy. *TIPS* 1988; **9:** 334-341.

22. Andrews PLR, Davis CJ, Bingham S, Davidson HIM, Hawthorn J, Maskell L. The abdominal visceral innervation and the emetic reflex: pathways, pharmacology, and plasticity. *Can J Physiol Pharmacol* 1990; **68:** 325-345.

23. Fukui H, Yamamoto M, Sato S. Vagal afferent fibers and peripheral 5-HT3 receptors mediate cisplatin-induced emesis in dogs. *Jpn J Pharmacol* 1992; **59:** 221-226.

24. Murata Y, Yoshida Y, Ishiguro Y. The role of pro-inflammatory cytokines in the pathogenesis of ulcerative colitis. In: Yoshida Y, Murata Y, eds. *Current advances in digestive disease.* Tokyo: Churchill Livingstone. 1994; 103-117.

25. Gould SR. Prostaglandins, ulcerative colitis, and sulphasalazine. *Lancet* 1975; **11:** 988.

26. Vilaseca J, Salas A, Guarner F, Rodriguez R, Malagelada JR. Participation of thromboxane and other eicosanoid synthesis in the course of experimental inflammatory colitis. *Gastroenterology* 1990; **98:** 269-277.

27. Kock TR, Carney JA, Go VLW. Distribution and quantitation of gut neuropeptides in normal intestine and inflammatory bowel diseases. *Dig Dis Sci* 1987; **32:** 369-376.

28. O'Morain C, Bishop AE, McGregor GP, Levi AJ, Bloom SR, Polak JM, Peters TJ. Vasoactive intestinal peptide concentrations and immunocytochemical studies in rectal biopsies from patients with inflammatory bowel disease. *Gut* 1984; **25:** 57-61.

20

Salivary secretion: Investigative techniques

Gordon B Proctor, Deepak K Shori

Summary

Saliva is essential for the maintenance of hard and soft tissues in the mouth and also appears to interact with the other parts of the upper gastrointestinal tract. Although saliva is primarily the product of salivary glands it also contains components derived from the systemic circulation. Whole mouth or mixed saliva is simply collected but contains exogenous contaminants and may thus be unsuitable for studies of salivary biochemistry. The design and application of a number of non-invasive devices which can be used for collecting pure salivas directly from the ducts of salivary glands is described. As saliva is a readily accessible fluid, which can be collected non-invasively and repeatedly without risk to the subject, it is ideally suited for use as a monitor of the mucosal and systemic immune responses and circulating levels of drugs and hormones.

Introduction

As indicated by Mandel[1] saliva appears not to be one of the popular bodily fluids; "It lacks the drama of blood, the sincerity of sweat and the emotional appeal of tears". However, saliva is a readily accessible fluid and has some major advantages for particular types of study, as will become apparent below. Saliva is the product of salivary glands but in addition contains systemic components. Salivary proteins are mainly derived from salivary cells and perform important functions in the mouth. A small proportion of salivary proteins and low molecular weight components are derived from the systemic circulation or, as in the case of IgA, other cells within the gland. Thus saliva can be used in studies of salivary function in man and has great, largely unfulfilled potential, for use in the diagnosis and monitoring of systemic disease.

Salivary secretion is controlled by parasympathetic and sympathetic branches of the autonomic nervous system. The autonomic nerves are the efferent arms of a reflex activated mainly by taste and chewing.[2] The secretory process can be considered in two stages: first the secretion of a primary saliva by acinar cells followed by modification, principally of ionic composition, as it passes through ducts to the mouth.[3] The whole or mixed saliva present in the mouth is the product of three pairs of major salivary glands (the parotid, submandibular and sublingual glands) and various minor glands located in the mucosa of the mouth. Most salivary glands only secrete when reflexly stimulated, e.g. by sucking a lemon drop.

However, in the conscious subject there is a resting secretion which results from background neural activity (in both the peripheral and central nervous systems) in the absence of an overt secretory stimulus.[4]

Much of our knowledge concerning the mechanisms of salivary secretion and its control have been gained from studies in animals and in general terms it appears that the results from animal studies are applicable to man. Animal models have allowed more invasive techniques to be used to uncover precisely how nerves and secretory cells interact. For example, reflex secretion has been studied in the presence of pharmacological blocking drugs or surgical autonomic denervation,[5-7] whilst direct supramaximal electrical stimulation of the nerve supply to salivary glands in terminally anaesthetized animals with or without pharmacological intervention has been performed.[8] Such experiments have provided information on the nerve-mediated mechanisms controlling salivary secretion and its composition and have provided saliva for biochemical analysis in a manner which utilizes physiological neural pathways. This chapter is concerned with the collection and study of saliva in man as limitations of space do not permit detailed consideration of studies on animal models, cell lines and primary cell cultures; recent reviews of these topics elsewhere provide an entrée to the field and more detailed methodological information.[2,9-11]

Methods

Collection of saliva

Whole saliva

Careful consideration should be given to which saliva is required for a proposed investigation. Whole or mixed saliva whilst easy to collect is in reality a 'soup' consisting of saliva and various exogenous components including food, bacteria, exfoliated epithelial cells and their products. If such contamination is acceptable, then whole saliva can be used. Before collection it is important that the subject is comfortable, has had a drink of water if feeling dehydrated and has rinsed out his/her mouth with water to reduce contamination by exogenous substances. A number of collection methods have been used including spitting, drainage, suction and use of absorbent material placed in the mouth. Whichever technique is used, it should be standardized, e.g. spitting accumulated saliva once every 30 seconds into pre-weighed tubes.

If *resting* saliva (i.e. no deliberate secretory stimulus) is to be collected, the subject should keep orofacial movement to a minimum to reduce mechanical stimulation of secretion. It may be necessary to provide wide-top tubes for collection of whole saliva and this can conveniently be achieved by using ordinary test tubes with small funnels placed in them. A period of 5 min should be sufficient to collect enough saliva for most purposes from subjects with a normal flow rate (i.e. 0.3–0.5 ml/min).[12]

If *stimulated* whole saliva is to be collected, a stimulus which does not contaminate the saliva collected should be used. Thus chewing 1 g of inert paraffin wax (Associated Dental Products, Swindon, UK) or of chical (chewing gum base; Wrigley Ltd, Plymouth, UK) is frequently used. Alternatively, swabbing the tongue with a cotton wool roll soaked in citric acid solution (4–5%, w/v) at 30 second intervals for a total of 5 min is a convenient method particularly in edentulous subjects. Whatever stimulus is chosen, it should be standardized throughout the study.

We have collected spitted whole saliva instead of allowing saliva to drain from the mouth. Although the latter reduces the mechanical stimulation associated with spitting, it is often found to be uncomfortable or embarassing for the patient. Suction collection involves continuous aspiration of accumulated saliva from the floor of the mouth which requires active involvement of the researcher. Whole saliva collected by these methods can be cleared by centrifugation at 10,000 g before being stored at -20°C for later analysis; this removes the contaminating components which give it a 'cloudy' appearance.

Much attention has focussed on the use of pre-weighed absorbant cotton wool rolls for collection of mixed saliva. Commercial systems are available, e.g. Salivette® (Sarstedt Ltd, Leicester, UK) utilizes a roll and a centrifuge tube for storage of the saliva-soaked roll and removal of saliva. OraSure® (Epitope Inc., Oregon, USA) contains a preserving solution of unspecified composition and a storage/ transport container. Commercial systems are appealing because of their convenience. However, some caution should be exercised in using the absorbant collection technique depending on the study undertaken. The sample collected should be referred to as oral fluid as quantitative recovery of whole saliva from such rolls is difficult and some proteins/glycoproteins become adsorbed to the roll. For example, nephelometrically determined IgA concentrations were 50% lower in saliva collected by the Salivette® device compared to that collected by

spitting or drainage.[13] To try and avoid such errors polypropylene covered rolls have been developed, but differences are still introduced by such collection.[14]

Ductal saliva

If analyses of salivary constituents are to be performed then it is preferable to collect ductal saliva. The inevitable bacterial contamination in whole saliva may lead not only to the presence of additional proteins but also potentially to modification of salivary proteins/glycoproteins by bacterial proteases and glycosidases. The choice of gland from which saliva is collected may be dictated by the analyses to be undertaken. For example, in studies of salivary mucin it is inappropriate to sample parotid saliva, as little mucin is secreted by these glands, and instead submandibular/sublingual saliva can be collected.

Collection of *parotid saliva* represents an easier option than collection of submandibular/sublingual saliva. The parotid (Stenson's) duct can be cannulated with polyethylene tubing of 0.5–1.5 mm external diameter (Portex Ltd, Hythe, Kent) which has been tapered by heating with a flame and pulling. However, it is technically difficult to cannulate the duct and keep the cannula in place during collection. The procedure frequently leads to discomfort and pain for the subject both during and after collection. The almost universally used collection device for parotid saliva is the suction cup (Fig. 20.1b), also referred to as the Lashley cup[15] or Carlson-Crittenden device.[16] The device is frequently machined from Teflon and consists of two circular chambers, the inner of which is placed over the parotid duct orifice located on the buccal mucosa at the level of the upper second molar (Fig. 20.1a and c). Retention of the cup in position is achieved by applying and maintaining suction to the outer chamber using a 5 ml syringe via a 3-way tap. Correct positioning of the device can be a problem for the inexperienced researcher but can be determined by drying the buccal mucosa with tissue paper before applying a citric acid stimulus to the tongue (as described above) and watching for accumulation of saliva at the ductal orifice as secretion commences. As the outer chamber forms a seal on the mucosa it is possible to stimulate salivary flow with a food of known composition, e.g. sugar-free lemon drop sweets (AL Simpkins Ltd, Sheffield, UK or Vivil Ltd, Thame, UK), without contaminating the saliva collected; such stimulants are convenient for patient studies and appealing to subjects. Alternatively, as with whole saliva, citric acid or chewing can be used as secretory stimuli. The Lashley cup is not

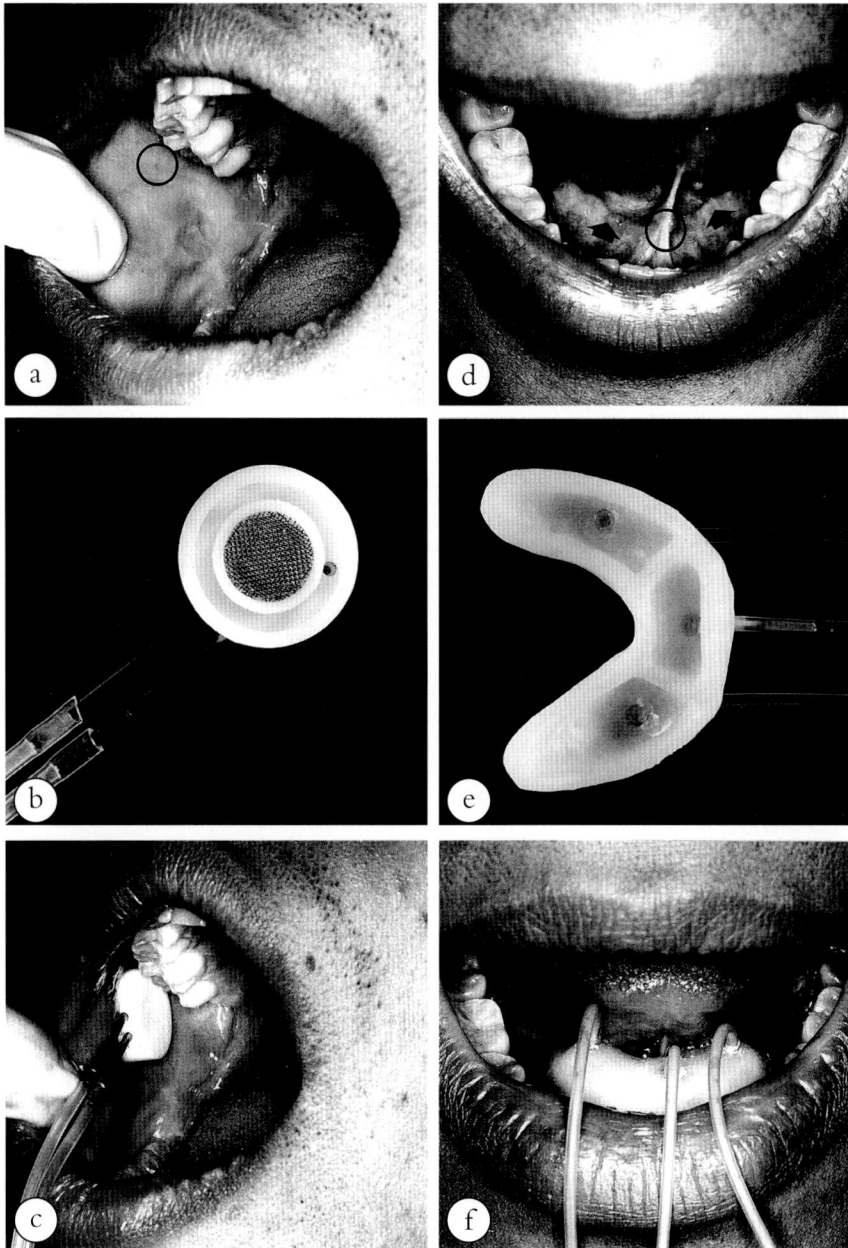

Figure 20.1 − (a) View of location of parotid duct orifice (circled) on the buccal mucosa at the level of the upper second molar. The suction cup is placed over the orifice in order to collect parotid saliva. If difficulty is experienced in finding the ductal orifice then the oral mucosa can be dried and some citric acid applied to the tongue, a droplet of saliva will appear at the orifice as secretion is stimulated. (b) This parotid suction cup has been machined from Teflon. The photograph shows the inner collection and outer suction chambers on the surface which is applied to the buccal mucosa. Suction is applied to the outer chamber, via the tubing, to hold the cup in place over the ductal orifice. Saliva flows from the inner chamber into the tubing and is collected in a test tube. (c) The parotid suction cup is placed over the ductal orifice. (d) View of location of the submandibular (circled) and sublingual (arrowheads) duct orifices on the floor of the mouth under the tongue. (e) A suction cup[22] for the collection of submandibular/sublingual saliva. The photograph shows the surface applied to the mucosa. There is a central collection chamber and the outer suction chambers with associated tubing. (f) View of the submandibular/sublingual suction cup in place.

commercially available but can often be obtained from active research groups (see recent literature in the field) in dental schools. To overcome the need for experienced assistance in parotid saliva collection, simpler non-suction devices have also been designed but remain largely untested on a large scale.[17,18]

A number of different devices have been used to collect *submandibular/sublingual saliva*. It is difficult to obtain separate secretions from these glands as sublingual saliva can enter the mouth not only through a variable number of branching ducts on the floor of the mouth but frequently through the main submandibular (Wharton's) duct (Fig. 20.1d). Separate sublingual saliva has been collected using a segregator appliance,[19] which is cast from plastic and fits onto the floor of the subject's mouth and is retained by attachment to the lower teeth. The device has segregated holes adjacent to the orifices of the sublingual and submandibular glands which allow saliva to flow into attached tubing for collection. The major disadvantage of this device is that it has to be fitted and cast for each subject making patient studies impractical. To obtain such a device a dental school with the necessary expertise should be contacted. To ensure there is no contamination by other salivas the efficiency of the seal between these devices and the mucosa can be tested by introducing a dilute solution of food dye into the mouth. Collection of submandibular/sublingual saliva can also be achieved by direct cannulation of Wharton's duct using tapered polyethylene tubing (see parotid saliva collection). This has the advantage of being applicable to all subjects but carries the same disadvantages as described above for parotid collection. An alternative precast, universal device, like the parotid device, uses suction to hold it in place and was originally employed by Truelove *et al*.[20] and modified by Stephens & Speirs.[21] A further modification of this device using softer materials has been described by Francis & Hector (Fig. 20.1e).[22] The cup is placed on the floor of the mouth under the subject's tongue (Fig. 20.1d and f). Retention of the cup is achieved by suction applied consecutively to each of two 5 ml syringes fitted with 3-way taps. However, this device, like the Lashley cup, is not commercially available but can be made using published information,[20,21] or by contacting researchers active in the field. An alternative precast collection device resembles that of Schneyer[19] but is held in place using rubber-based dental impression material (obtainable from a dental school) which is flexible and can be moulded to the floor of the mouth.[23] This approach has been taken a

step further through the use of dental impression material alone.[24] The material is moulded to the floor of the mouth and then plastic tubing (0.5–1.5 mm external diameter) can be passed through the material to exit close to the submandibular/sublingual gland orifices; this offers the advantage of being quicker than the non-suction precast devices described above. In using all of these devices submandibular/sublingual salivas from both left and right glands are collected simultaneously. Chewing stimuli cannot be used to evoke salivary secretion as the collection tubing is likely to be bitten. Citric acid (see above) is most frequently used as a stimulus although again it is possible to use sugar-free sweets. However, movements of the tongue are more restricted with this device compared to the parotid suction cup.

After collection of parotid or submandibular salivas, precast devices and tubing should be washed by flushing through with distilled water from the suction syringes, and then sterilized. The latter can conveniently be achieved by thorough immersion in a solution of 10% Milton's fluid (Richardson-Vicks Ltd, Egham, UK) overnight.

Minor salivary glands contribute less than 10% of the volume of whole saliva and are present in the mouth on most oral mucosal surfaces. For collection of salivas from these glands 10 µl capillary tubes (Sarstedt Ltd, Leicester, UK) or filter paper (Whatman no.1; Whatman Ltd, Maidstone, UK) discs (0.5 cm diameter) of known weight can be used. For collection of saliva from the minor labial salivary glands the lower lip is everted and dried. After a few minutes droplets of saliva appear on the surface of the lower lip at the ductal orifices of the minor glands and these may be collected.[25] Similarly, for collection from the minor palatine salivary glands, the roof of the mouth is dried and droplets of saliva appearing on the dried mucosa at the ductal orifices are sampled using filter paper discs. Secretion may be stimulated from either labial or palatine salivary glands using citric acid or mechanical stimulation of the hard palate with a round-ended instrument, e.g. a glass rod.[25] Salivas from the minor salivary glands and to a lesser extent those of the the submandibular/sublingual glands can be viscous and difficult to handle due to the high content of mucins. For biochemical analysis they may need to be diluted with water before they can be accurately pipetted.

As mentioned above, whichever saliva is investigated, collection conditions should be standardized throughout the study. A number of physiological factors influence salivary flow and composition including:

Table 20.1 – Protocol for collection of whole mouth or ductal salivas from the major salivary glands

1. Saliva should be collected at approximately the same time of day from all subjects within a study.

2. The subject should be rested (no recent great exertion) and should not have eaten within the last hour. If feeling dehydrated the subject should be given a glass of water.

3. Fit the collection device if ductal saliva is to be collected (see Fig. 20.1 and text).

4. Use weighed vials for collecting saliva. Collect resting saliva (i.e. without a stimulus) first for a period of 5-10 min. Then collect stimulated saliva, a 5-min collection period should be ample for most purposes. Flow can be stimulated using a citric acid swab (4-5%, w/v in distilled water) applied every 30 seconds to the tongue or a sugar-free lemon sweet of known composition (if ductal saliva is being collected). Vials of saliva are re-weighed following collection and salivary volume determined assuming a density of 1.0.

5. For most biochemical analyses saliva can be stored temporarily on ice and then frozen at -20°C for longer-term storage. Whole saliva should be cleared by centrifugation (10,000 *g*) before being stored.

6. Precast collection devices should be washed and sterilized (10% Milton's fluid overnight) after use.

the nature (sweet, sour or salty) and duration of the secretory stimulus; the time of day of collection; recent prior stimulation or dehydration[26] and emotional status.[27] Thus it is important that collections are made using the same secretory stimulus at a similar time of day and if possible at a consistent time after the last meal; subjects should be asked to refrain from eating between the last meal and salivary collection. Table 20.1 shows a standardized collection protocol applicable to the collection of different salivas.

Results and discussion

The functions of many salivary components in the mouth include formation of a protective barrier and lubrication of the oral mucosa, buffering, antibacterial, anti-viral and anti-fungal activities, bacterial aggregation and maintenance of saturated levels of calcium in saliva for remineralization of teeth.[28] Attention is also now being paid to the ways in which saliva interacts with the rest of the gastrointestinal tract, particularly the oesophagus.[29,30] There is growing interest in the potential of saliva as a diagnostic fluid.[31] At present most advances in this field relate to the use of saliva in the diagnosis of systemic disease and monitoring of systemic components as little correlation has been found between the common oral disease, dental caries and periodontal diseases – and changes in salivary composition.[32] The lack of correlation appears to be due primarily to the multifunctionality of many salivary proteins.[32]

The main advantage in using saliva in clinical studies is that collection is non-invasive and can be performed repeatedly without risk to the subject. This also makes it potentially very useful in studies of subjects for whom venepuncture represents a greater risk, e.g. newborns. If it is possible to use whole saliva or oral fluid for studies, then a further major advantage is presented by the ease with which such saliva can be sampled, making it possible for the subject to collect samples repeatedly in his/her own environment. Such sampling has important applications in epidemiological studies and has been used notably in studies of infectious diseases, e.g. the incidence of antibodies to HIV in the saliva of drug abusers.[33] To illustrate the potential of saliva in clinical studies two areas of application will be described.

Use of saliva to monitor systemic levels of steroid hormones and drugs

The movement of any substance from the circulation into saliva depends not only upon a number of molecular characteristics of the substance but also on the way in which saliva is collected. Studies on salivary levels of drugs and hormones have focussed on the use of whole saliva. In general, it appears that such analyses can withstand interference by contaminating components in whole saliva and therefore have a greater range of applications. However, such saliva does present some additional problems for the assay of substances. It should be remembered that some orally administered drugs can bind to oral tissues and then be slowly released in saliva giving falsely high values.[34] One of the main determinants of systemic-salivary movement is the pKa of the substance, and non-ionized lipophilic substances move more easily into saliva. As the pH of saliva increases with stimulation and increasing flow rate, owing to increases in salivary bicarbonate levels,[34] the amount of ionized substance changes with flow rate. In addition, concentrations of some substances in saliva can decrease as flow rate increases owing to a slow movement through the salivary epithelium compared with salivary flow.[34] In theory the latter difficulty can be circumvented by using resting saliva which is formed more slowly. There are a number of other factors influencing the movement of substances from the circulation to saliva, including binding by proteins present in saliva and plasma. As a result of all these influences it is difficult to use salivary levels of substances to predict plasma levels on the basis of mathematical models, although such models do exist.[34] Thus in practice the levels of each substance in saliva and plasma should be determined experimentally.[35] As saliva, unlike blood, is not a routinely sampled fluid there is no broad database to draw upon concerning changes in salivary levels of substances in different subject groups and much work remains to be done.

Despite these problems saliva has proved useful in monitoring systemic levels of unbound steroid hormones and a number of prescribed and proscribed drugs. Use of saliva has enabled monitoring of steroid hormone levels in for example studies of fertility and behaviour.[36-38] The salivary/plasma ratios of a number of drugs have been determined experimentally and the list continues to expand.[35] From these experiments it is clear that a number of different groups of drugs can be usefully monitored using saliva including: theophylline, anti-convulsants (e.g. carbamazepine), digoxin, lithium and anti-cancer drugs (e.g. doxorubicin and 5-fluorouracil). For drugs of abuse qualitative information can frequently be as important as quantitative data and there are a number of applications including forensic medicine, treatment compliance and employment tests. In these areas use of saliva has the important advantage of allowing testing without the invasion of either body (as with blood collection) or privacy (as with urine collection). Data is being accumulated on most drugs of abuse and indicates that there is great potential for salivary-based testing for marijuana, cocaine, barbiturates and opioids.[39] Salivary testing for alcohol intoxication is already established and kits designed for quick, on-site testing of salivary alcohol levels are available.[39]

Monitoring of antibodies in saliva

Unlike serum the predominant immunoglobulin (Ig) in saliva and other mucosal secretions is IgA. It occurs as a dimer which contains in addition the J chain and secretory component.[40] The latter is the cleaved product of a polymeric Ig receptor which is present in epithelial cells and mediates the transport of dimeric IgA across mucosal epithelia and is therefore responsible for its appearance in external secretions.[41] The appearance of antigen-specific sIgA in secretions is subject to a different set of controlling mechanisms compared to circulating antibodies. The balance of experimental evidence indicates that a common mucosal immune system linking the gastrointestinal, respiratory and urogenital tracts exists in man and other species.[42] Antigen-specific sIgA can be detected in mucosal secretions following exposure to antigen at a distant mucosal site.[42] Thus it has been demonstrated that gastrointestinal immunization induces an antigen-specific sIgA response in saliva.[43] A likely mechanism is through the induction of an antibody response in gut-associated lymphoid tissue and seeding of gut-derived IgA producing plasma cells in salivary glands. Saliva can therefore be very conveniently used to monitor mucosal immunity, that is the production of antigen-specific sIgA in response to respiratory and gut infections. Examples include monitoring of antibodies to *Escherichia coli* in neonates, *Bordetella pertussis* in whooping cough and poliovirus.[44-46]

The amounts of IgG and IgM in saliva are small relative to sIgA. However, the development of IgG capture antibody techniques (GACRIA and GACELISA) has enabled the low amounts of antigen-specific IgG and IgM present in saliva to be used as monitors of systemic infection.[47] Thus salivary diagnosis has been used in the diagnosis of measles[48] and should be applicable to many other viral and bacterial infections.[1] Of particular interest is the application of this approach in screening populations for HIV, hepatitis A and B infections.[47]

Acknowledgements

The authors would like to thank Robert Hartley for his splendid photographic assistance and Carol Francis (Dept of Prosthetics, St Bartholomew's and the Royal London School of Medicine and Dentistry) for the provision of a submandibular collection device. Lashley cups were obtained from Dr RWA Linden, Biomedical Sciences Division, King's College London, UK.

References

1. Mandel ID. The diagnostic uses of saliva. *J Oral Pathol Med* 1990; **19:** 119-125.

2. Garrett JR. The proper role of nerves in salivary secretion. *J Dent Res* 1987; **66:** 387-397.

3. Martinez J. Ion transport and water movement. *J Dent Res* 1987; **66:** 638-647.

4. Kerr AC. The physiological regulation of salivary secretion in man. In: *International Series of Monographs on Oral Biology*. Pergamon Press, Oxford, 1961, pp. 24-38.

5. Gjörstrup P. Parotid secretion of fluid and amylase in rabbits during feeding. *J Physiol* 1980; **309:** 101-116.

6. Gjörstrup P. Taste and chewing as stimuli for secretion of amylase from the parotid gland of the rabbit. *Acta Physiol Scand* 1980; **110:** 295-301.

7. Ikawa M, Hector MP, Proctor GB. Parotid protein secretion from the rabbit during feeding. *Exp Physiol* 1991; **76:** 717-724.

8. Burgen ASV. Techniques for stimulating the auriculo-temporal nerve and recording the flow of saliva. In: Sreebny LM, Meyer J (Eds) *Salivary Glands and their Secretions*. Pergamon Press, Oxford, 1964, pp. 303-307.

9. Redman RS, Quissell DO. Isolation and maintenance of submandibular gland cells. In: Dobrosielski-Vergona K (Ed) *Biology of Salivary Glands*. CRC Press, Boca Raton, 1993, pp. 285-306.

10. Oliver C. Culture of parotid acinar cells. In: Dobrosielski-Vergona K (Ed) *Biology of Salivary Glands*. CRC Press, Boca Raton, 1993, pp. 307-318.

11. Patton LL, Wellner RB. Established salivary cell lines. In: Dobrosielski-Vergona K (Ed) *Biology of Salivary Glands*. CRC Press, Boca Raton, 1993, pp. 319-341.

12. Sreebny LM, Broich G. Xerostoma (dry mouth). In: Sreebny LM (Ed) *The Salivary System*. CRC Press, Boca Raton, 1987.

13. Aufricht C, Tenner W, Salzer HR, Khoss AE, Wurst E, Herkner K. Salivary IgA concentration is influenced by the saliva collection method. *Eur J Clin Chem Clin Biochem* 1992; **30:** 81-83.

14. Lenander M, Johansson I, Vilja O, Samaranayake LP.Newer saliva collection methods and saliva composition: a study of two Salivette kits. *Oral Dis* 1995; **1:** 86-91.

15. Lashley KS. Reflex secretion of the human parotid gland. *J Exp Psychology* 1916; **1:** 461-493.

16. Carlson AJ, Crittenden AZ. The relation of ptyalin concentration to the diet and rate of secretion. *Am J Physiol* 1910; **26:** 169-177.

17. Schaeffer ME, Rhodes M, Prince S, Michalek SM, McGhee JR. A plastic intra-oral device for the collection of human parotid saliva. *J Dent Res* 1977; **56:** 728-733.

18. Ericson T, Norland Å. A new device for collection of parotid saliva. *Ann NY Acad Sci* 1993; **694:** 274-275.

19. Schneyer LH. Method for the collection of separate submaxillary and sublingual saliva in man. *J Dent Res* 1955; **34:** 257-261.

20. Truelove EL, Bixler D, Merritt AD. Simplified method for collection of pure submandibular saliva in large volumes. *J Dent Res* 1967; **46:** 1400-1403.

21. Stephens KW, Speirs CF. Methods for collecting individual components of mixed saliva: the relevance to clinical pharmacology. *Br J Pharmacol* 1976; **3:** 315-319.

22. Francis CA, Hector MP. A universal device for collecting submandibular/sublingual saliva. *J Dent Res* 1995; **74:** 844.

23. Block PL, Brottman S. A method of submaxillary saliva collection without cannulation. *NY State D J* 1962; **28:** 116.

24. Oliveby A, Lagerlof F, Ekstrand J, Dawes C. Studies on fluoride concentrations in human submandibular/sublingual saliva and their relation to flow rate and plasma fluoride levels. *J Dent Res* 1989; **68:** 146-149.

25. Söderling E. Collection of saliva. In: Tenovuo JO (Ed) *Human Saliva: Clinical Chemistry and Microbiology*, Vol 1. CRC Press, Boca Raton, 1989, pp. 1-24.

26. Dawes C. Physiological factors affecting salivary flow rate, oral sugar clearance, and sensation of dry mouth in man. *J Dent Res* 1987; **66:** 648-653.

27. Gemba H, Teranaka A, Takemura K. Influences of emotion upon parotid secretion in human. *Neurosci Lett* 1996; **211:** 159-162.

28. Mandel ID. The role of saliva in maintaining oral homeostasis. *J Am Dent Ass* 1989; **19:** 298-304.

29. Valdez IH, Fox PC. Interactions of the salivary and gastrointestinal systems II. Effects of salivary gland dysfunction on the gastrointestinal tract. *Dig Dis* 1991; **9:** 210-218.

30. Sarosiek J, McCallum RW. Do salivary organic components play a protective role in health and disease of the oesophageal mucosa? *Digestion* 1995; **56:** 32-37.

31. Mohamud D, Tabak L. Saliva as a diagnostic fluid. *Ann NY Acad Sci* 1993; **694:** 1-347.

32. Levine MJ. Salivary macromolecules: a structure/function synopsis. *Ann NY Acad Sci* 1993; **694:** 11-16.

33. Johnson AM, Parry JV, Best SJ, Smith AM, De Silva M, Mortimer PP. HIV surveillance by testing saliva. *AIDS* 1988; **2:** 369-391.

34. Haeckel R. Factors influencing the saliva/plasma ratio of drugs. *Ann NY Acad Sci* 1993; **694:** 128-142.

35. Siegal IA. Uses of saliva to monitor drug concentrations. In: Sreebry LM (Ed) *The Salivary System.* CRC Press, Boca Raton, 1987, pp. 58-178.

36. Read GF, Harper ME, Peeling WB, Griffiths K. Charges in male salivary testosterone concentration with age. *Int J Androl* 1981; **4:** 623-627.

37. Lipson SF, O'Rourke MT, Ellison PT. Salivary progesterone profiles: reference data for anthropological studies of reproductive function. *Am J Physiol Anthropol* 1991; **12** (Suppl): 115-116.

38. Dabbs JM Jr, Frady RL, Carr TS, Besch NF. Saliva testosterone and criminal violence in young adult prison inmates. *Pyschosom Med* 1987; **49:** 172-182.

39. Cone EJ. Saliva testing for drugs of abuse. *Ann NY Acad Sci* 1993; **694:** 91-127.

40. Brandtzaeg P. Two types of IgA immunocytes in man. *Nature New Biol* 1973: **243:** 142-143.

41. Brandtzaeg P. Mucosal and glandular distribution of immunoglobin components. Differential localisation of free and bound Secretory Component in secretory epithelial cells. *J Immunol* 1974; **112:** 1553-1559.

42. Mastecky J. The common mucosal immune system and current strategies for induction of immune responses in external secretion. *J Clin Immunol* 1987; **7:** 265-276.

43. Czerkinsky C, Quiding M, Eriksson K *et al.* Induction of specific immunity at mucosal surfaces: prospects for vaccine development. In: Mastecky J (Ed) *Advances in Mucosal Immunology.* Plenum Press, New York, 1995, pp. 1409-1415.

44. Mellender L, Carlsson B, Fehmida J, Soderstrom T, Hanson LA. Appearance of secretory IgM and IgA antibodies to *E. coli* in saliva during early infancy and childhood. *J Pediatr* 1984: **104:** 564-568.

45. Granstrom G, Askelof P, Granstrom M. Specific immunoglobulin A to *Bordella pertussis* antigens in mucosa secretion for rapid diagnosis of whooping cough. *J Clin Microbiol* 1988; **26:** 869-874.

46. Carlsson B, Zaman S, Mellander L, Jalil F, Hanson LA. Secretory and serum immunoglobulin class-specific antibodies to poliovirus after vaccination. *J Infect Dis* 1985; **152:** 1238-1244.

47. Mortimer PP, Parry JV. The use of saliva in viral diagnosis and screening. *Epidem Inf* 1988; **101:** 197-201.

48. Brown DWG, Ramsay MEB, Richards AF, Miller E. Salivary diagnosis of measles: a study of notified cases in the United Kingdom, 1991-3. *Br Med J* 1994; **308:** 1015-1017.

21

Mesenteric lymph node studies

*Dennis S Huang, James Y Wang, Hsin-Min Tsao,
Tracy Karban and Mary B Mazanec*

Summary

As a part of the mucosal immune response, mesenteric lymph nodes (MLN) direct the trafficking of antigen-sensitized B and T cells derived from Peyer's patches (PP), the inductive sites, to the circulation via the lymphatics and thoracic duct. These cells, including intestinal lamina propria (LP) and intraepithelium (IE) lymphocytes, have a predilection for homing to their effector sites to perform immunological defence functions against pathogens. Moreover, invading pathogens from the mucosa may potentially influence trafficking immune cells in MLN. Therefore, study of the alterations of MLN cell functions in accordance with a specific stage of infection is important. This chapter describes immunological techniques to investigate the immune responses in MLN which can also be utilized for other regions involved in the immune response in both human and laboratory animals.

Introduction

Immune responses to foreign antigens at mucosal surfaces are an important adaptive mechanism for the prevention of potentially life-threatening infections.[1] Gut-associated lymphoid tissue (GALT) provides local immune defence against foreign antigens,[2,3] such as viruses,[4] bacteria,[5] parasites,[6] and toxins[7] at the intestinal epithelial surface. MLN located in the mesentery of the intestine, are part of the GALT. MLN direct the migration of antigen-sensitized B and T cells to the thoracic duct and systemic circulation. These cells eventually arrive at mucosal effector sites such as LP and IE lymphocytes. Therefore, MLN are important lymphoid tissues that can be isolated to investigate whether the trafficking B or T cells are functioning normally at a specific stage of infection.

In the GALT, lymphoid cells may be distributed diffusely or occur as follicles with germinal centres, termed PP. The initiation of mucosal immune responses at this inductive site is triggered by the uptake of antigens via microfold (M) cells on the dome region of PP.[8-10] After uptake, antigen is presented to lymphoid follicles located beneath M cells. These lymphoid follicles contain a germinal centre (B cell zone) and a parafollicular region (T cell zone) which are populated by the migration of bone marrow-derived B and T cells, respectively.[11,12]

Commitment to IgA secretion by antigen-sensitized B cells in the germinal centre is influenced by the presence of antigens[6,13] and specialized 'switch' T cells for the production of regulatory cytokines.[14-30] T cell subpopulations contain mature CD3[+] T cells with functional T cell receptors (TCR). Approximately 60% of CD3[+] T cells are CD4[+] T helper cells, which direct the isotype switching event in the inductive and effector sites. After induction, B and T cells preferentially migrate out of the PP via efferent lymphatics to the MLN. Other T cell subpopulations containing mature CD8[+] T cells are also present and provide either suppressor or cytotoxic activity.[31-34] Cytotoxic T cells can kill other target cells that express foreign antigens, whereas T suppressor cells secrete regulatory cytokines. In addition, the T cell population containing the CD3[+]CD4[-]CD8[-] phenotype is a contrasuppressant.[24,35]

MLN are lymphoid tissues which contain migrating lymphocytes that undergo further differentiation and maturation.[12,29,30,36] The cells then leave MLN through the lymphatics and enter the circulation via the thoracic duct. Finally, the cells selectively enter distant mucosal effector areas, such as the LP and IE lymphocyte regions, where they are preferentially retained.[29,30,37] It has been suggested that these lymphocytes possess specific cell surface homing receptors which mediate migration by binding to endothelial cells of the intestinal postcapillary venules, also named high endothelial venules or epithelioid venules.[38-41] At effector sites, antigen-sensitized B cells undergo terminal differentiation into mature IgA-secreting plasma cells with the help of homing T cells.[28-30] Finally, IgA is synthesized, transported, and secreted into the gastrointestinal lumen as secretory IgA.[25,42,43] In addition to promoting B cell maturation, antigen-sensitive T cells secrete cytokines[27,29] and induce cytotoxicity[33,34] at the effector sites as well.

Alterations in the functions of trafficking B and T cells in MLN may indicate that foreign antigens have invaded the epithelium and stimulated a specific mucosal immune response. Elucidation of any effector function changes of MLN cells during an infection may advance our understanding of the influence of antigens on immune cells during their differentiation and maturation. Therefore, we present and discuss in vitro techniques to investigate immune functions of MLN lymphocytes.

Methods

This chapter describes techniques to isolate and purify MLN lymphocytes, to identify lymphocyte subpopulations, and to measure their proliferative responses. In addition, we detail an enzyme-linked immunosorbent assay (ELISA) and an enzyme-linked immunospot (ELISPOT) assay to measure cytokine production, and the reverse transcription-polymerase chain reaction (RT-PCR) which detects the lymphocyte cytokine mRNA level. Finally, cytotoxic T cell functions are examined. The experimental protocols described are for MLN cells in general; however, the techniques can be applied to study the immune cells from other mucosa-associated lymphoid tissues, including other gastrointestinal (PP, LP, and IE), respiratory, and urogenital mucosal tissues.

Collection, separation, and identification of MLN immune cell population

Collection and separation

MLN are removed aseptically and kept in cold complete medium (RPMI-1640; Gibco, Grand Island, NJ, USA) prepared with pyrogen-free deionized distilled water (ddH$_2$O; Baxter, Mountain View, CA, USA) supplemented with 10% (w/v) fetal calf serum (FCS; Hyclone, Logan, Utah, USA), 2 mM L-glutamine, 100 U/ml penicillin, and 100 μg/ml streptomycin (Gibco).[44-46] MLN cells are obtained by gently teasing the tissues through stainless steel wire mesh screens (Sigma, St Louis, MO, USA). Lymphocytes are collected by the Lympholyte-M (SeraLab, Westbury, NY, USA) gradient followed by centrifugation at 400 g for 10 min. Percoll and Ficoll-Paque gradients (Pharmacia, Piscataway, NJ, USA) are also available. Cell viability is determined by trypan blue exclusion.

Most separation techniques utilize the binding of antibodies to cell-surface antigens that are differentially expressed on a given cell subpopulation. To isolate T or B cell subpopulations, one approach is to eliminate undesired cell populations. For instance, a CD8$^+$ T cell subpopulation can be positively selected by an immunomagnetic method.[47] Briefly, MLN cells are incubated with rat anti-mouse CD8$^+$ antibody. Suspensions are washed and incubated with goat anti-rat IgG antibody conjugated to magnetic Dynabeads M-450 (Dynal, Great Neck, NY, USA). Upon exposure to a magnetic apparatus, the cells bound to beads are pulled toward the magnetized side of the tube, allowing unbound cells to be removed and bound cells to be collected. The purity of the desired cell subpopulation can be confirmed by flow cytometry.

Another separation approach is the immunoselection method termed 'panning'.[48] It involves coating plastic surfaces (e.g. petri dishes or flasks) with Protein A or Protein G (Pharmacia), alone or in combination with immobilized monoclonal antibodies. Commercially available AIS MicroCELLector™ cell culture flasks (Applied Immune Sciences, Menlo Park, CA, USA) can also be used. After cells have bound to the immunosorbent surface, unbound cells can be removed and bound cells eluted with a suitable buffer. Flow cytometry can also isolate the desired cell subpopulations by fluorescence-labelled cell sorting.

Identification of a lymphocyte subpopulation by flow cytometry[44]

Cell surface receptors (or antigens) located on the plasma membrane enable cells to recognize self or non-self antigen or receive cytokine messengers. After recognition, cells become activated, resulting in proliferation, differentiation, secretion of cytokines or immunoglobulins, or induction of cell-cell interactions. Use of antibodies specific to cell-surface antigens provides a sensitive approach to investigate the cellular basis of immune responses as well as to identify the immune cell subpopulations present. Antibodies for indirect immunofluorescent staining to study lymphocyte subpopulations are shown in Table 21.1.

The staining of cell-surface antigens is performed as follows. MLN cells (1 × 10^6) are incubated in the presence of 40 μl of the primary antibodies for 30 min at 4°C. After washing with phosphate buffered saline (PBS) and centrifugation (400 g, 10 min), the supernatant is discarded and secondary antibodies are added for another 30 min. After washing with PBS, samples are fixed with 0.5 ml of 2% (w/v) paraformaldehyde solution and kept at 4°C until the analysis of surface IgG, IgA, or IgM cell populations using a FACScan flow cytometer (Becton Dickinson, Mountain View, CA, USA).

Table 21.1 – Primary and secondary antibodies used for indirect and direct immunoflourescent staining (flow cytometry, FC) and enzyme-linked immunosorbent assay (ELISA).

	Source
Unlabelled primary antibodies for FC	
Mouse anti-human CD3, CD4, CD8, IgA and IgM	Sera-Lab, PharMingen, Zymed, Biosource
Rat anti-mouse Thy1, L3T4 (GK 1.5 clone), Lyt2, IgA, IgM and IgG	Sera-Lab, Biosource
Rabbit anti-mouse IgA, IgM and IgG	SBA, Zymed
Goat anti-mouse IgA, IgM and IgG	SBA, Biosource, Zymed
Biotinylated primary antibodies for FC	
Mouse anti-human CD3, CD4, CD8, IgA and IgG	SBA, Sera-Lab, Biosource, Jackson
Rabbit anti-human IgA and IgG	SBA, Jackson
Donkey anti-human IgG and IgM	Jackson
Goat anti-human IgA, IgM, and IgG	SBA, Jackson, Biosource
Rat anti-mouse L3T4, Thy1, Lyt2, IgA, IgM and IgG	PharMingen, Biosource
Goat anti-mouse IgA, IgM and IgG	SBA sera-Lab, Zymed
Florophore (or fluorochrome)-conjugated secondary antibodies for FC	
Goat anti-rat IgG	SBA, Sera-Lab, Jackson
Rabbit anti-mouse IgG	Jackson
Rat ant-mouse IgG	Sera-Lab
Streptavidin	Jackson, ParMingen, Zymed
Florophore (or fluorochrome)-conjugated antibodies for FC	
Rabbit anti-human IgG and IgA	SBA, Jackson, Zymed, Sera-Lab, Cappel
Goat anti-human CD3, CD4, CD5, CD8, IgA, IgM and IgG	PharMingen, Zymed, SBA, Biosource, Jackson
Donkey anti-human IgG anf IgM	Sera-Lab, Jackson, Zymed
Capturing (monoclonal) antibodies for ELISA	
Mouse anti-human IL-2, 4, 5, 6 and 10, IFN-γ, TNF-α, IgA, IgG and IgM	Genzyme, Sera-Lab, Biosource
Goat anti-human IgA, IgG and IgM	Biosource
Rat anti-mouse IL-2, 4, 5, 6 and 10, IFN-γ, TNF-α, IgA, IgG and IgM	PharMingen, Genzyme, Biosource, Endogen
Hamster anti-mouse TNF-α	Genzyme
Goat anti-mouse IgA, IgG and IgM	Sigma, Jackson, Zymed
Rat anti-mouse IL-2, 4, 6 and 10, IFN-γ, TNF-α, IgA, IgG and IgM	Biosource
Standards for ELISA	
Recombinant human IL-2, 4, 5, 6 and 10, IFN-γ, TNF-α	Genzyme
Recombinant mouse IL-2, 4, 6 and 10, IFN-γ, TNF-α, IgA, IgM and IgG	Collaborative, PharMingen, Genzyme, Sigma, SBA
Detecting (monoclonal or polyclonal) antibodies or serum for ELISA	
Rabbit anti-mouse IL-2, 4, 6 and 10, IFN-γ, TNF-α	Genzyme, Collaborative
Biotinylated rat anti-mouse IL-4, 5 and 10	PharMingen
Goat anti-mouse IL-6	R&D
Rabbit anti-mouse IFN-γ and TNF-α	Genzyme, USB, Biosource
HRP-conjugated goat anti-rabbit IgG	Jackson
HRP-donkey anti-goat IgG	Jackson
HRP-conjugated strepavidin	Sera-Lab, Jackson, Sigma, Zymed

BioSource International (Camarillo, CA, USA); Cappel, Organon Teknika Co, USA. (Durham, NC, USA); Collaborative Research Inc, USA. (Bedford, MA, USA); Endogen Inc, USA. (Boston, MA, USA); Genzyme (Cambridge, MA, USA); Jackson ImmunoResearch Lab. (West Grove, PA, USA); PharMingen (San Diego, CA, USA); R&D System (Minneapolis, MN, USA); Sera-Lab, Accurate Chemical & Scientific Co (Westbury, NY, USA); Sigma Chemicals (ST Louis, MO, USA); Southern Biotech Assoc (Birmingham, AL, USA); United States Biochemical Co (Cleveland, OH, USA); Zymed Lab, Inc (San Francisco, CA, USA).

Staining for cytoplasmic IgG, IgM, or IgA is performed somewhat differently. MLN cells are treated with 2% (w/v) paraformaldehyde and 0.25% saponin (w/v) in a 1:1 ratio, followed by immunofluorescent staining. The cells are stored at 4°C until examined by flow cytometry. Data are analysed by Becton Dickinson's Consort 30 program. Another program, Immunocytometry System LYSYS II, version 1.1 (Becton Dickinson), is also commercially available. Ten thousand cells are counted and the absolute cell number of a given subpopulation is calculated by multiplying the total cell number by the percentage of positive cells.

The techniques of multiple immunofluorescent labelling to stain different cell-surface or cytoplasmic antigens are also applicable. However, the selection of proper detecting devices and fluorescence-conjugated antibodies are very important for reliable analysis of cell subpopulations (see below).

Functional studies

Cell culture for immunological studies[44,45,49]

MLN cells (100 µl) in complete medium is added to each well of a 96-well flat-bottom culture plate (Falcon, Oxnard, CA, USA). Subsequently, 100 µl of anti-CD3 antibody (1-3 µg/ml) or mitogen (2-10 µg/ml) (e.g. concanavalin A (ConA) type IV-S (Sigma), lipopolysaccharide (LPS; Difco, Detroit, MI, USA), or phytohemagglutinin (PHA; Sigma)), is added to induce cell proliferation, cytokine secretion, or immunoglobulin production. After a 24-hour (for IL-2, IL-4, and IL-6) or 72-hour (for IL-5, IFN-g, IgA, IgG, and IgM) incubation, the supernatant is collected and stored at -70°C.

Lymphocyte proliferative response studies[44,45]

Lymphocyte proliferative responses are determined by pulsing with methyl-[3H]-thymidine (New England Nuclear, Boston, MA, USA) for the last 4 hours of a 24-hour incubation. The samples are harvested on an automatic cell harvester (Wallac Inc, Gaithersburg, MD, USA). Radioactivity is detected with a liquid scintillation counter. Mean counts per minute (cpm) of quadruplicate samples are recorded. For comparison between groups, results are presented as a stimulation index calculated as the cpm obtained from responding cells cultured with anti-CD3 antibody or mitogen (maximum experimental value) divided by the cpm obtained from the same cells cultured without anti-CD3 antibody or mitogen (background value).

ELISA for cytokine or immunoglobulin quantification[44,45,49-54]

Cytokines play an important role in regulating host immune responses. They stimulate or inhibit the synthesis of other cytokines as well as regulate the expression of a variety of cell surface receptors. As a result, they can enhance T and B cell proliferation which results in further cytokine production or differentiation into antibody-producing cells, respectively. Cytokines can also enhance the development of cytotoxic T cells and the activation of macrophages and other inflammatory cells. Following the differentiation of B cells to antibody-secreting plasma cells, antigen-specific or non-specific immunoglobulins are produced. The quantification of cytokines by bioassay or ELISA is discussed in Chapter 8. In general, *in vivo* or *in vitro* cytokine and immunoglobulin secretion can be conveniently and rapidly detected by an ELISA using specific monoclonal or polyclonal antibodies (Table 21.1). Additionally, ELISA kits are commercially available from, for example, R&D Systems (Minneapolis, MN, USA), Incstar Corporation (Stillwater, MN, USA), Endogen Inc (Boston, MA, USA), Biosource International (Camarillo, CA, USA) and Genzyme Diagnostics (Cambridge, MA, USA).

ELISPOT assay for cytokine or immunoglobulin producing cells[53-56]

The ELISPOT assay can identify cytokine- or immunoglobulin-producing cells and detect or estimate the amount of cytokine or immunoglobulin secretion on a per-cell basis. The technical premise of the ELISPOT assay is similar to that of an ELISA. It involves the use of two different antibodies which recognize different epitopes on a cytokine peptide. In contrast to an ELISA where supernatants are added to an antibody-coated well, in an ELISPOT assay, lymphocytes are co-cultured with a stimulating substance in an antibody-coated well.

Specifically, capturing antibodies (5-20 µg/ml) against specific cytokine proteins are added to a nitrocellulose (or PVDF)-backed microtiter plate for 2 hour at room temperature or overnight at 4°C. After incubation, the plates are washed six times with PBS and allowed to dry briefly. Then, the plates are treated with 5% (w/v) bovine serum albumin (BSA; Sigma) in PBS for 30 min at 37°C to saturate any remaining binding sites. Serially diluted lymphocytes (10^5-10^6 cells/well) in a volume <100 µl are added to each well, followed by the addition of mitogens, antigens, or other stimuli. The plate is incubated at 37°C for

6-24 hour. Unstimulated cells in complete medium are used as a background control. Following incubation, plates are washed extensively 10 times with 0.25% Tween 20 in PBS and once with ddH$_2$O to remove the remaining cells. Detecting antibodies are added to each well at room temperature for 2 hour. Subsequently, horse radish peroxidase (HRP)-conjugated antibody is placed in each well for another 2 hour. Aminoethyl carbazole (AEC) solution (2.5 mg AEC dissolved in 200 μl n,n-dimethylformamide and 9 ml of 0.05 M sodium acetate, pH 5.0, and mixed with 4 μl of 30% (v/v) H$_2$O$_2$ prior to use) in a volume of 50 μl is added to the plate at room temperature for 5-30 min until colour develops. After 3 washes with ddH$_2$O, a dissecting microscope is used to visualize and quantify colour spots on the nitrocellulose filter.

RT-PCR for cytokine mRNA detection

PCR technology can rapidly detect minute quantities of DNA or RNA by amplifying individual nucleotide sequences using primers specific for the sequence. *In vitro* amplification of specific mRNA sequences is performed by using a thermostable DNA polymerase derived from the bacterium *Thermophilus aquaticus* (Taq). The combination of RT and PCR techniques can be used to amplify specific RNA sequences including mRNA specific for cytokines.

RNA isolation[57]

Approximately 1×10^7 cells are washed three times with PBS. RNA is isolated in a single step by adding 1 ml of 4 M guanidinium isothiocyanate (GIT; Gibco) solution to lyse the cells. If tissue is used, 100 mg of tissue is mixed with 1 ml of GIT solution and homogenized in a glass Teflon homogenizer (Corning, NY, USA). After transfer of the homogenate to a clean microcentrifuge tube, 0.1 ml of 2 M sodium acetate (pH 4.0) is added, followed by 1 ml water-saturated phenol and 0.2 ml of 49:1 chloroform/isoamyl alcohol with thorough mixing at 4°C for 15 min. The sample is centrifuged at 10,000 *g* for 20 min. The upper aqueous phase is transferred to a fresh microcentrifuge tube and 1 ml of 100% isopropanol is added to precipitate the RNA. The samples are placed at -70°C for 90 min and centrifuged at 10,000 *g* for 10 min. The RNA pellet is first dissolved in 0.5 ml GIT solution and subsequently precipitated with 0.5 ml 100% isopropanol at -20°C for 30 min. Following centrifugation for 5 min, the pellet is washed once with 75% (v/v) ethanol, dried, and dissolved in 200 μl diethylpyrocarbonate (DEPC)-treated ddH$_2$O.

Samples are stored at -70°C or in ethanol at -20°C until complementary DNA (cDNA) preparation.

cDNA preparation[56-58]

Initially, RNA is reverse-transcribed with a primer that is complementary to the target sequence (antisense primer or poly-T oligonucleotides), creating cDNA copies. The oligonucleotides used to prime the extension of mRNA are designed to amplify unique portions of the RNA which encode the desired cytokine. The sequences are based on published oligonucleotide primers of human or mouse cytokines.[56] Oligonucleotide primers are synthesized by the phosphoramidited method on a "Gene Assembler Plus" DNA synthesizer (Pharmacia). RNA (5 μg/12.5 μl) is boiled at 65°C for 5 min to denature the strands, cooled on ice, and reverse-transcribed into cDNA by adding 1 μl (50 U) RNasin (Promega, Madison, WI, USA), 6 μl 5 x RT buffer (250 mM Tris-HCl, pH 8.3, 15 mM MgCl$_2$, 350 mM KCl, 50 mM dithiothreitol; Promega), 3 μl acetylated BSA (1 mg/ml; Sigma), 3 μl oligo (dT)$_{16}$ (0.5 mg/ml; Sigma), 1.5 μl 2 mM dNTPs (dATP, dCTP, dGTP, and dTTP; Promega), and 1.5 μl RNase-free ddH$_2$O followed by 1.5 μl (300 U) molony-murine leukaemia virus (Mo-MuLV) reverse transcriptase (Boehringer Mannheim, Indianapolis, IN, USA). Mo-MuLV reverse transcriptase is an RNA-dependent DNA polymerase that uses a single-stranded RNA as a template in the presence of a primer to synthesize a cDNA strand. The mixture is overlaid with 50 μl of mineral oil and incubated at 37-42°C for 1-1.5 hours. The reaction is terminated by heating at 65°C for 10 min.

PCR amplification[56,58]

The PCR reaction mixture contains 5 μl of the cDNA product described above, 5 μl 10 × PCR buffer (67 mM Tris-HCl, 16 mM (NH$_3$)$_2$SO$_4$, 2 mM MgCl$_2$, 10 mM mercaptoethanol, 0.17 mg/ml BSA), 4 μl of dNTPs, 2.5 μl of amplification primer (20 μM final concentration), 0.25 μl of 5 U/μl Taq polymerase, and RNase-free ddH$_2$O in a final volume of 50 ml. Amplification is carried out in a DNA Thermal Cycler (Perkin Elmer-Cetus, Montréal, Québec, Canada). Amplification is performed with 30-35 cycles of denaturing at 95°C for 30 seconds, annealing at 60°C for 30 seconds, and elongating at 72°C for 1 min, followed by a final extension at 72°C for 7 min. The amplified samples are electrophoresed on a 2% (w/v) agarose gel in a TBE running buffer (90 mM Tris base, 90 mM boric acid, 2.5 mM EDTA, and 0.1% SDS; Bio-Rad, Hercules, CA, USA) with 1 μg/ml ethidium bromide (Bio-Rad). Individual bands are visualized with a UV light illumination apparatus (Fotodyne, New Berlin, WI, USA). The concentration of PCR products can be determined by comparing unknown sample bands with standard bands of equal intensity.

Cytotoxic T lymphocyte activity studies

To generate a significant antigen-specific cytotoxic T lymphocyte (CTL) response *in vitro*, antigen-reactive CTL precursors should be obtained from a primed *in vivo* source. *In vivo* priming against antigens is performed by injecting the antigen several times into an animal. However, *in vivo* priming is not required for studies employing allogeneic major histocompatibility complex (MHC) antigens since the frequency of alloreactive CTL precursors is sufficient to elicit a primary response *in vitro* against stimulator lymphocytes.

To induce cytolytic activity in CTL precursors, a single-cell suspension is prepared both with responder cells (primed or unprimed) and stimulator cells (allogeneic cells or antigen-exposed syngeneic cells). Responder lymphocytes are plated into 24-well tissue culture plates (Falcon) at 1×10^6 cells/well. Stimulator lymphocytes (2×10^6) irradiated with 10,000 Rads are added to each well and incubated at 37°C for 5 days. Effector lymphocytes are collected by forceful pipetting and plated in triplicate at 1×10^6- 1.2×10^7 cells/well in round-bottomed 96-well plates. Functional assays are performed immediately.

^{51}Chromium-release assay[59-62]
Target cells (e.g. 2×10^6 mouse EL-4, P-815, or human M-548 cells) are labelled with 200 mCi sodium ^{51}Cr (ICN, Costa Mesa, CA, USA) at 37°C for 2 hours. After three washes, target cells are resuspended at a concentration of 10^4-10^5 cells/ml in complete medium. Target cells in 100 µl of medium are added to each well containing effector cells to create various effector:target (E:T) cell ratios. After centrifuging at 600 g for 1 min, the plates are incubated at 37°C for 4 hours (the time varies depending on the activity of effector cells and the susceptibility of target cells to spontaneous ^{51}Cr leakage). The supernatant is then collected using a harvesting apparatus (Skatron, Sterling, VA, USA) and analysed in a gamma counter. Maximal release is determined by lysing target cells with 100 µl of 4% (v/v) Triton X-100. The percentage of specific lysis =

[experimental lysis (cpm) - spontaneous lysis (cpm)] / [maximum lysis (cpm) - spontaneous lysis (cpm)] × 100%

Granule enzyme exocytosis assay[61,62]
During activation by specific target cells, CTL release a large number of cytoplasmic granules that contain serine esterases. The amount of enzyme released during CTL activation can be easily quantified by spectrophotometric measurement of the coloured end product of the enzymatic degradation of a synthetic substrate.

There are several CTL activation methods. First, CTL can be activated by adding them to plates coated with antibodies to all components of T cell receptor (TCR; α or ß and CD3 complex). Secondly, using a mechanism completely independent of the engagement of the TCR complex, CTL can be activated by the addition of PMA and Ca^{2+} ionophores into the culture. Thirdly, CTL can be stimulated by co-culturing them with antigen-bearing target cells. After incubation at 37°C for 4 hours and centrifugation at 200 g, 25 µl of the supernatants are collected. Serine esterase activity is determined by adding 225 µl of the reaction solution containing 0.2 mM substrate (N-α-benzyloxycarbonyl-L-lysine thiobenzyl ester, BLT; Sigma), 0.22 mM colouring agent (5,5'-dithio-bis(2)-nitrobenzoic acid, DTNB; Sigma), and 0.01% Triton X-100 in PBS. Total enzyme content is determined by lysing the effector cells with the addition of 40 µl of 1% Triton X-100. The enzymatic activity of CTL is measured spectrophotometrically at 412 nm. The percentage of antibody-induced esterase secretion =

[experimental secretion - spontaneous secretion] / [total enzyme content - spontaneous secretion] × 100%

Flow cytometric assay[63]
Long incubation periods are unsuitable for the ^{51}Cr-release assay because of the high spontaneous release and possible reutilization of isotopic labels. A novel FACScan-based assay has been developed which allows incubation periods for up to 7 days in a non-radioactive format. In this assay, effector and target cells are stained with red and green fluorescent dye, respectively. At the end of the incubation, a defined number of cell standards are added. The absolute target cell number is determined by FACScan.

More specifically, standard cells are fixed with 2% paraformaldehyde overnight, washed twice with bicarbonate buffer (pH 9.1) and then incubated in the same buffer containing 1 mg/ml fluorescein isothiocyanate (FITC; Sigma) with constant rotation at 25°C for 2-4 hours. After washing four times with PBS, the cells are ready for use. Target cells are washed three times with PBS. To stain the cells, the cell pellet is resuspended in 1 ml diluent and 1 ml 4×10^6 molar green fluorescent dye PKH-2 (Sigma) at 25°C for 10 min with periodical pipetting. Five millilitres of FCS is added to stop the staining reaction and the cells are washed three times. Effector cells are treated similarly except that they are stained with the red lipophilic fluorescent dye PKH-26 (Sigma) at 25°C for 3 min. The stained target and effector cells are mixed at varying E:T cell ratios, and subsequently 3×10^5 mixed cells in 200 µl are added to each well and incubated at 37°C for up to 6 days. The plate is spun at 400 g for 3 min and washed with PBS. Then 50 µl of 0.02% (w/v) EDTA and 0.05% (w/v) trypsin is added to each well at 37°C for 10 min, and the plate is agitated for 3 min on a plate shaker to remove the adherent cell layer. Following agitation, 100 µl of a standard propidium iodide solution (3×10^5 standard cells/ml, 1 mg/ml propidium iodide, and 45% FCS) is added to each well. Cells are dispersed by vigorous pipetting. Cell suspensions are transferred and immediately analysed in a FACScan flow cytometer. Target and standard cells are gated in the green/yellow histogram and analysed in a green/side scatter histogram. The threshold is set on green. Viable target cell number =

[standard cell number] × [cell number in target cell window/cell number in standard window]

Application to animal studies

This chapter focuses on experimental techniques used to study the immunological functions of MLN cells in human and murine models since the mouse immune system is well-characterized and similar to that of humans. Much of our knowledge about immune regulation has been gained from the murine system because mice are relatively inexpensive and easy to house and handle compared with other species. However, these techniques can be adopted for use in human studies with immune cells dissected from gastrointestinal (PP, LP, and IE), respiratory, and urogenital mucosal tissues.

Results and discussion

The GALT, which forms part of the mucosal immune system in the gastrointestinal tract, plays a key role in maintaining health and combatting disease. MLN, a vital part of GALT, have the unique role of directing the migration of antigen-sensitized immune cells, including B and T cells, to their proper destination. The use of cutting-edge experimental techniques to investigate immunological responses within MLN is essential for exploring the mechanisms of a number of immunologically mediated diseases. In addition, there is no single technique that can be used to profile completely immunological events during an infection. As a result, it is necessary to use several different techniques concurrently to define precisely the defence mechanisms employed against pathogens.

Most cell separation and identification techniques of lymphocytes utilize the binding of specific antibodies to cell-surface antigens which are differentially expressed on cells. For cell separation, an immuno-magnetic method in which cells are bound to antibody-coated magnetic beads and sorted with a flow cytometer can be used for both positive and negative selection of a cell subpopulation. Other methods are available, such as the panning method, as well as antibody- and complement-mediated lysis methods. The most effective approach to separating cell subpopulations is to use a combination of these techniques. It is possible that cells that are positively selected on the basis of antibody-mediated binding to particular cell-surface antigens, such as immunoglobulin, MHC class II, Thy-1, CD4, or CD8, may cause cross-linking of the pertinent cell-surface molecules, resulting in potential activation of B or T lymphocytes. This possibility must be considered when interpreting the results of any functional assay which uses antibodies to separate cells. For cell identification, flow cytometry utilizing fluorescein-coupled antibody to cell-surface markers may be used. Not only can cell subpopulations be isolated with sorting techniques, but cell sizes may also be determined by measurement of forward light scatter. Moreover, the activation of cells can be detected by cell cycle analysis. In general, the reactivity of living cells with fluorescence-labelled antibodies to surface antigens is more accurate than that seen by staining histological sections of lymphoid tissues. In addition, background fluorescence is higher with the latter technique, while it is kept to a minimum when staining a cell suspension.

If multiple (double, triple, etc) immunofluorescent labelling is preferentially applied, several aspects need to be evaluated. The set up of detecting devices (light sources, filters and detection systems), the selection of the conjugated antibodies for the degree of colour separation, and the sensitivity of the fluorophore (or fluorochrome), such as lissamine rhodamine sulphonyl chloride (LRSC), Texas red (TR), FITC, tetramethyl rhodamine isothiocyanate (TRITC), indocarbocyanine Cy3 (Cy3), indocarbocyanine Cy5 (Cy5), phycoerythrin (PE), amino-methlcoumarin (AMCA) and allophycocyanin (APC) all need to be carefully considered when desgining experiments. For example, LRSC and TR provide better separation from FITC than TRITC. With the combination of Cy3 and Cy5 for double labelling, a confocal microscope equipped with a krypton/argon laser and infrared detector are required. Moreover, PE has been reported to be the best fluorophore to use with FITC in double labelling since both fluorophores can be excited by a single wavelength (488 nm). The inclusion of a thrid fluorophore with a longer-wavelength-emitting fluorescence, such as AMCA, can be used for a triple labelling effect. Futhermore, careful selction of the host species, fraction (whole or partial molecule) and source of desired antibodies can help eliminate the cross-reactivity of antibody, reduce the non-specific fluorescent background and promote successful multiple immunofluorescent labelling.

Cytokine and immunoglobulin production are regulated by a complex series of events. During the course of an immune response, multiple, pleiotropic cytokines, produced by a variety of cell types, may significantly influence the nature of the immunoglobulin isotype(s) generated. By using different ELISA methods with specific antibodies and standards or known antigens, the production of cytokines or (total or specific) immunoglobulins can be measured. In addition, the amount of antigen in the samples can be detected by ELISA. However, the ELISA technique does not allow quantification of the number of cytokine- or immunoglobulin-secreting cells. The ELISPOT assay offers an alternative approach to quantify specific cell types. For both the ELISA and ELISOPT assays, polyclonal antibodies are useful reagents as capturing antibodies because they react with a wide variety of epitopes on a protein, regardless of denaturation of the protein. Furthermore, cytokine levels, including IL-2 and IL-4 which stimulate target cells to undergo proliferation, can be detected by bioassay.

PCR, which allows exponential amplification of DNA fragments by detection of trace amounts of DNA in a sample has expanded the scope of modern technology significantly. The development of RT-PCR, which uses reverse transcriptase to create a cDNA, has allowed detection and/or quantification of mRNA, thus expanding the limits of detection sensitivity of PCR.

CTL functional assays can detect both the lysis of antigen-expressing target cells by CTL and CTL release of serine esterases upon activation. The latter technique relies on the detection of esterase within cytoplasmic granules of CTL with synthetic substrates. This granule enzyme exocytosis assay has a number of advantages over the ^{51}Cr-release assay since it is very easy to perform and does not depend on another cell (target cell) for a readout system. Moreover, the ^{51}Cr-release assay does not allow long incubation periods since the high spontaneous release and possible reutilization of isotopic labels would render results inaccurate. To overcome this limitation, flow cytometry can be utilized which involves tumour cell killing and allows for a longer incubation period. This application does not require the use of radioactive isotopes.

Other endogenous factors that affect *in vivo* immunological responses may interfere with the results generated from *in vitro* assays. For example, host nutritional status, intestinal microenvironment, enteric-neuroimmune interactions, and endocrine and sex hormone influences can modify immune functions, including antigen uptake and presentation, cytotoxic activity, and cytokine and antibody production. Investigating additional cell-surface markers, including adhesion molecules, and receptors associated with lymphocyte migration during an immune response may also provide insight into the immunological functions of MLN.

Acknowledgements

We would like to thank Frank H Blatnik for his help in preparing the manuscript. This work was supported by National Institute of Health Grant AI-36359 and AI-32588.

References

1. Walker WA, Harmatz PR, Wershil BK. *Immunophysiology of the Gut*. Academic Press, New York, 1993.

2. Castro GA. Gut immunophysiology: Regulatory pathways within a common mucosal immune system. *News Physiol Sci* 1989; **4:** 59.

3. Levine MM, Nataro JP. Intestinal infections. In: Ogra PL, Mestecky J, Lamm ME, Strober W, McGhee JR, Bienenstock J (Eds) *Handbook of Mucosal Immunology*. Academic Press, San Diego, 1994, pp. 505.

4. Amerogen HM, Weltzin R, Farnet CM, Michetti P, Haseltine WA, Neutra MR. Transepithelial transport of HIV-1 by intestinal M cells: a mechanism for

tranmission of AIDS. *J Acq Immune Defic Syndrone* 1991; **4**: 760.

5. Owen RL, Pierce NF, Apple RT, Cray WC Jr. M. Cell transport of *Vibrio cholerae* from the intestinal lumen into Peyer's patches: a mechanism for antigen sampling and for microbial transepithelial migration. *J Infect Dis* 1986; **153**: 1108.

6. Marcial MA, Madara JL. *Cryptosporidium:* cellular localization, structural analysis of absorptive cell-parasite membrane-membrane interactions in guinea pigs, and suggestion of protozoan transport by M cells. *Gastroenterology* 1986; **90**: 583.

7. Shakhlamov VA, Gaidar YA, Baranov VN. Electron-cytochemical investigation of cholera toxin absorption by epithelium of Peyer's patches in guinea pigs. *Bull Exp Biol Med* 1981; **90**: 1159.

8. Owen RL. Sequential uptake of horseradish peroxidase by lymphoid follicle epithelium of Peyer's patches in the normal unobstructed mouse intestine: an ultrastructural study. *Gastroenterology* 1977; **72**: 440.

9. Kabok Z, Ermak TH, Pappo J. Microdissected domes from gut-associated lymphoid tissues: A model for M cell transepithelial transport *in vitro*. In: Jackson S, Kiyono H, McGhee JR *et al* (Eds) *Recent Advances in Mucosal Immunology* (Proceedings of the 7th International Congress of Mucosal Immunology). Plenum Press, New York, 1993.

10. Neutra MR, Kraehenbuhl JP. Transepithelial transport and mucosal defence I: the role of M cells. *Trends Cell Biol* 1992; **2**: 134.

11. Craig, SW, Cebra JJ. Peyer's patches and enriched source of precursors for IgA-producing immunocytes in the rabbit. *J Exp Med* 1971; **134**: 188.

12. Roux ME, McWilliams M, Phillips-Quagliata JM, Lamm ME. Differentiation pathway of Peyer's patch precursors of IgA plasma cells in the secretory immune system. *Cell Immunol* 1981; **61**: 141.

13. Swain SL, Dutton RW, Mckenzie D, Helstrom H, English M. Role of antigen in the B cell response: Specific antigen and the lymphokine IL-5 synergize to drive B cell lymphoma proliferation and differentiation to Ig secretion. *J Immunol* 1988; **140**: 4224.

14. Coffman RL, Shrader B, Carty J, Mosmann TR, Bond MW. A mouse T cell product that preferentially enhances IgA production: I. Biologic characterization. *J Immunol* 1987; **139**: 3685.

15. Harriman G, Kunimoto DY, Strober S, Elliott JF, Pactkau V. The role of IL-5 in IgA B cell differentiation. *J Immunol* 1988; **140**: 3033.

16. Kawanishi H, Saltzman, LE, Strober W. Mechanisms regulating IgA class-specific immunoglobulin produc-

tion in murine gut-associated lymphoid tissues: I. T-cells derived from Peyer's patches that switch sIgM B cells to sIgA B cells *in vitro*. *J Exp Med* 1983; **157**: 433.

17. Kawanishi H, Saltzman L, Strober, W. Mechanisms regulating IgA class specific immunoglobulin production in murine gut-associated lymphoid tissues: II. terminal differentiation of postswitch sIgA-bearing Peyer's patch B cells. *J Exp Med* 1983; **158**: 649.

18. Kawanishi H, Strober W. Regulatory T cells in murine Peyer's patches directing IgA-specific isotype switching. *Ann NY Acad Sci* 1983; **409**: 243.

19. Kiyono H, Cooper MD, Kearney JF, *et al*. Isotype specificity of helper T cell clones: Peyer's patch T cells preferentially collaborate with mature IgA B cells for IgA response. *J Exp Med* 1984; **159**: 798.

20. Kiyono H, McGhee JR, Mosteller LM, *et al*. Murine Peyer's patch cell clones: characterization of antigen-specific helper T cells for immunoglobulin A responses. *J Exp Med* 1982; **156**: 1115.

21. McGhee JR, Mestecky J, Elson CO, Kiyono H. Regulation of IgA synthesis and immune response by T cells and interleukins. *J Clin Immunol* 1989: **9**: 175.

22. Murray P, Mckenzie T, Douglas T, Swain SL, Kagnoff MF. Interleukin 5 and interleukin 4 produced by Peyer's patch T cells selectively enhance immuno globulin A expression. *J Immunol* 1987; **139**: 2669.

23. Sneller MC, Kunimoto DY, Strober W. Molecular aspects of T cells regulations of B cell isotype differen tiation. *Adv Exp Med Biol* 1987; **216A**: 31.

24. Lishimoto T, Hirano T. Molecular regulation of B lymphocyte response. *Ann Rev Immunol* 1988; **6**: 485.

25. Mestecky J, McGhee JR. Immunoglobulin A (IgA): Molecular and cellular interactions involved in IgA biosynthesis and immune responses. *Adv Immunol* 1987; **40**: 153.

26. Tonkonogy SL, McKenzie DT, Swain SL. Regulation of isotype production by IL-4 and IL-5: effects of lymphokines on Ig production depend on the state of activation of the responding B cells. *J Immunol* 1989; **142**: 4351.

27. van Vlasselaer P, Gascan H, de Waal Malefyt R, deVries JE. IL-2 and a contact-mediated signal provided by TCR alpha beta$^+$ or TCR gamma delta$^+$ CD4$^+$ T cells induce polyclonal Ig production by committed human B cells: enhancement by IL-5, specific inhibition of IgA synthesis by IL-4. *J Immunol* 1992; **148**: 1674.

28. Mayer L, Kwan SP, Thompson C *et al*. Evidence for a defect in "switch T cells" in patients with immunode-ficiency and hyperimmunoglobulinemia M. *N Engl J Med* 1986; **314**: 409.

29. McGhee JR, Beagley KW, Taguchi T *et al.* Diversity of regulatory mechanisms required for mucosal IgA responses. In: Kiyono H, Jirillo E, Desimone C (Eds) *Molecular Aspects of Immune Response and Infectious Diseases.* Raven Press, New York, 1990, pp. 67.

30. McWilliams M, Phillips-Quagliata JM, Lamm ME. Mesenteric lymph node B lymphoblasts which home to the small intestine are precommitted to IgA synthesis. *J Exp Med* 1977; **145:** 866.

31. Tomasi TB. Introduction: an overview of the mucosal system. In: Ogra PL, Mestecky J, Lamm ME, Strober W, McGhee JR, Bienenstock J (Eds) *Handbook of Mucosal Immunology.* Academic Press, San Diego, 1994, pp. 4

32. Tomasi TB Jr. Oral tolerance. *Transplantation* 980; **29:** 353.

33. Offit PA, Dudzik KI. Rotavirus-specific cytotoxic T lymphocytes appear at the intestinal mucosal surface after rotavirus infection. *J Virol* 1989; **63:** 3507.

34. Offit PA, Cunningham SL, Dudzik KI. Memory and distribution of virus-specific cytotoxic T lymphocytes (CTL) and CTL precursors after rotavirus infection. *J Virol* 1991; **65:** 1318.

35. Zlotnik A, Godfrey DI, Fischer M, Suda T. Cytokine production by mature and immature CD4-CD8- T cells. Alpha beta-T cell receptor+ CD4-CD8- T cells produce IL-4. *J Immunol* 1992; **149:** 1211.

36. Guy-Grand D, Malassis-Seris M, Briottet C, Vassalli P. Cytotoxic differentiation of mouse gut thymodependent and independent intraepithelial T lymphocytes is induced locally: correlation between functional assays, presence of perforin and granzyme transcripts, and cytoplasmic granules. *J Exp Med* 1991; **173:** 1549.

37. McDermott MR, Bienenstock J. Evidence for a common mucosal immune system. I. migration of B-immunoblasts into intestinal, respiratory and genital tissues. *J Immunol* 1979; **122:** 1892.

38. Gallatin WM, Weissman IL, Butcher EC. A cell-surface molecule involved in organ-specific homing of lymphocytes. *Nature* 1983; **304:** 30.

39. Husband AJ. Kinetics of extravasation and redistribution of IgA-specific antibody-containing cells in the intestine. *J Immunol* 1982; **128:** 1355.

40. Stoolman LM. Adhesion molecules controlling lymphocyte migration. *Cell* 1989; **56:** 907.

41. Butcher EC, Scollay RG, Weissman IL. Organ specificity of lymphocyte migration: mediation by highly selective lymphocyte interaction with organ-specific determinants on high endothelial venules. *Eur J Immunol* 1980; **10:** 556.

42. Bienenstock J, Befus AD. Review: mucosal immunology. *Immunology* 1980; **41:** 249.

43. Lamm ME. Cellular aspects of immunoglobulin A. *Adv Immunol* 1976; **22:** 223.

44. Huang DS, Wang Y, Marchalonis JJ, Watson RR. The kinetics of cytokine secretion and proliferation by mesenteric lymph node cells during the progression to murine AIDS, caused by LP-BM5 murine leukemia virus infection. *Regional Immunol* 1994; **5:** 325.

45. Huang DS, Wang Y, Lung CC, Watson RR. Proliferation responses of spleen and mesenteric lymph node (MLN) cells in retrovirus-induced immunodeficient mice. Adv Biosci 1993; **86:** 325.

46. Lopez MC, Colombo LL, Huang DS, Watson RR. Suppressed mucosal lymphocyte populations by LP-BM5 murine leukemia virus infection producing murine AIDS. *Regional Immunol* 1992; **4:** 162.

47. Leivestad T, Gaudemack G, Ugelstad J, Thorsby E. Positive selection of active T cells of the T8 (CD8) sub-type by immunomagnetic separation. *Tissue Antigens* 1986; **28:** 46.

48. Wysocki LJ, Sato VL. "Panning" for lymphocytes: a method for cell selection. *Proc Natl Acad Sci USA* 1978; **75:** 2844.

49. Wang YJ, Huang DS, Giger PT, Watson RR. The kinetics of imbalanced cytokine production by T cells and macrophages during the murine AIDS. *Adv Biosci* 1993; **86:** 335.

50. Voller A, Bidwell D, Bartlett A. Enzyme-Linked Immunosorbent Assay. In: Rose NR, Friedman H (Eds) *Manual of Clinical Immunology*, 2nd edn. American Society Microbiology, Washington DC, 1980, pp. 359.

51. Wang Y, Huang DS, Eskelson CD, Watson RR. Long-term dietary vitamin E retards development of retrovirus-induced dysregulation in cytokine production. *Clin Immunol Immunopathol* 1994; **72:** 70.

52. Watson RR, Wang YJ, Dehghanpisheh K *et al.* T cell receptor Vß complementarity-determining region 1 peptide administration moderates immune dysfunction and cytokine dysregulation induced by murine retrovirus infection. *J Immunol* 1995; **155:** 2282.

53. VanCott, JL, Staats HF, Pascual DW *et al.* Regulation of mucosal and systemic antibody responses by T helper cell subsets, macrophages, and derived cytokines following oral immunization with live recombinant *Salmonella. J Immunol* 1996; **156:** 1504.

54. Marinaro M, Staats HF, Hiroi T *et al.* Mucosal adjuvant effect of cholera toxin in mice results from induction of T helper 2 (Th2) cells and IL-4. *J Immunol* 1995; **155:** 4621.

55. Taguchi T, McGhee JR, Coffman RL *et al.* Detection of individual mouse splenic T cells producing IFN-g

and IL-5 using the enzyme-liked immunospot (ELISPOT) assay. *J Immunol Methods* 1990; **128:** 65.

56. Coligan JE, Kruisbeek AM, Margulies DH, Shevach EM, Strober W. Current *Protocols in Immunology*. National Institutes of Health. John Wiley & Sons, Inc, New York, 1991.

57. Chomczynski P, Sacchi N. Single-step method of RNA isolation by acid guanidinium thiocyanate-phenol-chloroform extraction. *Anal Biochem* 1987; **162:** 156.

58. Innis MA, Celfand DH, Sninsky JJ, White TJ. *PCR Protocol: A Guide to Methods and Applications*. Academic Press, San Diego, 1990.

59. Huang JH, Greenspan NS, Tykocinski ML. Alloantigenic recognition of artificial glycosyl phosphatidylinositol-anchored HLA-A2.1. *Mol Immunol* 1994; **31:** 1017.

60. Kaplan DR, Griffith R, Braciale VL, Braciale TJ. Influenza virus-specific human cytotoxic T cell clones: heterogeneity in antigenic specificity and restriction by class II MHC products. *Cell Immunol* 1984; **88:** 193.

61. Haecker G, Wagner H. Proliferative and cytolytic responses of human gd T cells display a distinct specificity pattern. *Immunology* 1994; **81:** 564.

62. Taub DD, Ortaldo JR, Turcovski-Corrales SM, Key ML, Longo DL, Murphy WJ. ß chemokine costimulates lymphocyte cytolysis, proliferation, and lymphokine production. *J Leukocyte Biol* 1996; **59:** 81.

63. Flieger D, Gruber R, Schlimok G, Reiter C, Pantel K, Riethmullr G. A novel non-radioactive cellular cytotoxicity test based on the differential assessment of living and killed target and effector cells. *J Immunol Methods* 1995; **180:** 1

22

Measuring cell proliferation

Fabio Farinati, Romilda Cardin and Guido Biasco

Summary

Measurements of epithelial cell proliferation in the digestive system have pointed to the existence of cell kinetic abnormalities which may be involved in the first steps of carcinogenesis. In particular, an expansion of the proliferative compartment, both in quantitative and qualitative terms, has been observed in several diseases which predispose to cancer (i.e. chronic atrophic gastritis, colorectal polyps, ulcerative colitis, cirrhosis and chronic hepatitis). This change in proliferative activity seems to be associated with the presence of cell differentiation defects and can be detected using various methods such as tritiated thymidine or bromodeoxyuridine incorporation. The search for abnormalities in epithelial cell proliferation may be useful in studying the earliest mechanisms leading to cancer, in detecting subjects at a high risk of cancer and for pilot chemoprevention studies, using these abnormalities as intermediate biomarkers of cancer risk in the digestive system.

Introduction

Generally speaking, measuring cell proliferation biomarkers is useful from the clinical point of view in assessing prognosis for patients undergoing loco-regional cancer treatment (particularly surgery) and response to pharmacological treatment.[1]

Cell proliferation is also useful in the research field to: study the natural history of tumours on the basis of the proliferation kinetics of the primary tumour and its synchronous or metachronous metastasis;[2] analyse cell regeneration and the carcinogenic process in different tissues;[3-6] identify patients at risk of developing cancer;[7,8] and discriminate between normal, regenerative and neoplastic tissue changes in cytological or microhistological samples.[9,10] Above all, the biological changes in the mucosa of the gastrointestinal tract can be of interest as intermediate biomarkers of cancer risk in studies designed to test the effect of xenobiotics with possible oncogenic or anti-oncogenic properties.[11]

The normal cell proliferation pattern of the digestive system has certain particular features. In the *gastric mucosa*, proliferating cells are located in the neck of the glands and migrate towards the surface from this stem cell area. As they migrate, they progressively loose their proliferative capacity and undergo differentiation.[12] In the *colon*, the cell proliferative area is located in the lower two-thirds of the glands and, here again, the cytoproliferative pattern is described as abnormal when the upper third of the gland is involved.[13] In the normal *liver*, most of the few hepatocytes showing signs of replication are located in the periportal tract,[14,15] as is the case following partial hepatectomy.[16-18] It is only after massive necrosis or the administration of carcinogens, such as dimethyl-nitrosamine,[6] that an apparent shift in the proliferative compartment towards the perivenular area is observed.

Abnormal cell proliferation is considered an early biological alteration in the multistep process of carcinogenesis. This hypothesis has been supported by several studies,[19-21] but some aspects still need to be expanded and clarified, e.g. which cell kinetic alterations are related to the onset of cancer in the digestive system, how these can be studied and what clinical implications they have.

Methods

The choice of method to study cell kinetics is very important. Several techniques are available for studying cell kinetics in the digestive system, and each of them explores different aspects of cell proliferation and of the cell cycle.

One of the factors affecting the data generated by these studies is the considerable variation in the duration of the different stages in the cell cycle, depending on the organism, its age,[22] cell type, temperature, and other factors.

That part of the cell cycle called the interphase – which excludes the period of mitosis (M), which is relatively short (about 2 hours) – is divided into three parts: G1, S and G2. The interphase is a period of high metabolic activity, during which DNA is synthesized and replicated; it lasts about 22 hours. After mitosis is complete, there is an initial time gap, termed G1 (11 hours), in which the cell grows and performs its metabolic function, metabolizes and performs its functions for the organism. Following G1 there is a period of DNA synthesis, called S (7 hours), in which the DNA is replicated. After the synthesis, another gap phase, G2 (4 hours), occurs, followed by the next mitotic division.

The most important methods for evaluating cell proliferation use tritiated thymidine (^{3}HTdR),

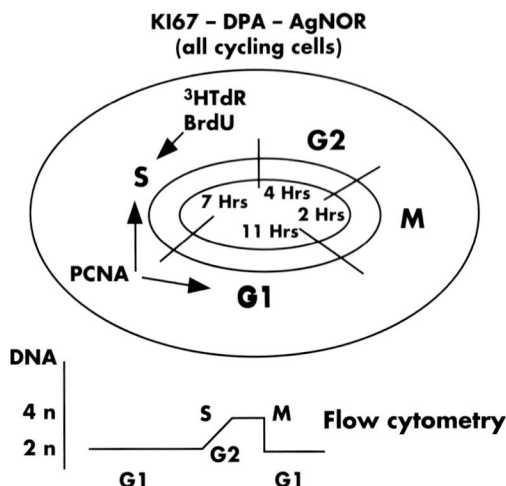

Figure 22.1 – Cell cycle and methodologies for its study

bromodeoxyuridine (BrdU), proliferating cell nuclear antigen (PCNA), nucleolar organizer regions (AgNOR), flow cytometric analysis and Ki67. Some, such as the first two, specifically detect the S phase of the cell cycle; others identify all cycling cells (Ki67) or the G1 and S phase (PCNA). A summary of the cell cycle phases and the different phases identified by each method is given in Fig. 22.1. The choice of method for analysing proliferation depends on several factors, such as the amount and type of material to be analysed (normal, tumour, or cell culture) and the type of information sought (growth rates, complete or partial patterns of growth and ploidy, cell types).

The different approaches to the evaluation of cell proliferative activity can be broadly divided into three categories and these are described below.

1. Incorporation of tritiated pyrimidinic bases or their analogues.
This group includes the use of ³H-thymidine (³HTdR) or bromodeoxyuridine (BrdU), which are selectively incorporated into DNA. For these measurements, autoradiographic or immunohistochemical assays are used and sections of cytological smears are obtained from either surgical or biopsy material. The number of cells in the S phase is expressed as the labelling index, i.e. the ratio between the total number of cells used as the denominator (generally 1000 cells) and the number of cells that have incorporated the different precursors. Possible advantages include feasibility and the opportunity to identify neoplastic and non-neoplastic cells, or at least

different subgroups of cells, under the microscope while determining the labelling index. On the other hand, possible drawbacks include the lack of reproducibility, which makes quality control absolutely necessary, and also the subjective nature of the evaluation, particularly for BrdU.

2. Quantification of the content in nuclear DNA and determination of the fraction of cells in the S phase.
The method known as flow cytometry is based on the fact that each cell has a basal, diploid DNA content during the G0-G1 phase which increases progressively during the S phase, to reach a tetraploid content in the G2 phase. This method can be used on cell suspensions, biopsies or cytohistological samples. A histogram of DNA content frequency is obtained, from which the percentage of cells in the different phases can be established. Flow cytometry enables the automatic evaluation of a high number of cells in a relatively short time. Its main drawbacks include the fact that it is impossible to discriminate normal from neoplastic cells, that it is difficult to obtain an adequate cell suspension from solid tumours, and that the multiclonal nature of human tumours makes it impossible to obtain histograms from single cell populations.

3. Determination of cycle associated nuclear antigens.
This group includes the determination of PCNA, Ki67, AgNOR, DNA polymerase (DPA) and thymidine kinase (TK). These measurements are less accurate than ³HTdR or BrdU incorporation because they are not strictly related to DNA duplication and instead they detect different biological aspects of the cell cycle. However, their use is increasing because they are straightforward, fixed archival material can be used, and a considerable number of samples can be evaluated in a single session.

Thymidine is taken up by cells during DNA synthesis, the S phase of the cell cycle. *In vivo* labelling with ³HTdR followed by autoradiography after its incorporation into the DNA has been used for many years to determine the percentage of S phase cells (or the labeling index). The application of this method, however, is limited by the risk of radiotoxicity and the time it takes to complete (at least 3-6 days).

A more practical approach relies on the use of monoclonal antibodies directed against BrdU, a thymidine analogue, after its incorporation into the DNA of proliferating cells, using an immunoperoxidase technique. This antibody can be used to detect, by immunohistochemistry, the BrdU taken up into the nuclei of cells after *in vivo* or *in vitro* labelling. Several authors have analysed the *in situ* distribution of BrdU-positive cells in human tissues removed after *in vivo* injection of BrdU. [23-25] However, ethical considerations preclude the application of this technique to certain categories of patients, such as healthy volunteers or patients undergoing routine diagnostic procedures.

Other authors suggest that *in vitro* BrdU incorporation methods are as satisfactory as *in vivo* labelling methods.[26] According to the method described by Sasaki *et al*,[27] fragments of fresh tissue are incubated in Dulbecco's modified Eagle medium supplemented with calf serum and BrdU for 1 hour at 37°C. After fixation in cold ethanol, the paraffin sections are prepared in the conventional manner. The sections are dipped in HCl for 20 min at 37°C for partial denaturation of the DNA and treated with pronase. These sections are incubated with anti-BrdU monoclonal antibody (1:250 diluted with PBS) as a primary antibody for 2 hours, with sequentially biotinylated horse anti-mouse IgG for 30 min as a second antibody, then avidin-biotin-peroxidase complex (ABC) solution for 30 min. The percentages of cells found positive for BrdU are determined microscopically by counting more than 1000 nuclei. This index is considered an accurate estimate of the proliferating cell population, but the *in vitro* method of BrdU labelling requires incubation of fresh tissue and thus precludes the use of biopsy material that has not already been treated with the reagent.

Immunohistology is even more useful when antibodies against nuclear proteins, working on routinely-processed parrafin-embedded tissue – such as PC-10 monoclonal antibody – are used.

Proliferating cell nuclear antigen (PCNA) is an intranuclear 36 kDa polypeptide, the expression and synthesis of which is linked with cell proliferation and DNA synthesis. Its expression is modulated during the cell cycle, beginning in the late G1 phase and becoming maximal in the S phase.[28] It is recognized by PC-10 in paraffin-embedded tissue.[29] Hall *et al*[30] proposed a three-step immunoperoxidase method using strept avidin biotin complex to determine PCNA in the S phase of proliferating cells in tissue fixed in 10% formalin solution and embedded in paraffin wax. Sections are cut, mounted on poly-L-lysine-coated glass slides and air dried overnight at room temperature, dehydrated through graded alcohols, and cleared in xylene. PC-10 mouse Ig2a monoclonal antibody is used at a concentration of 1:150 with a 1 hour incubation. The evaluation of

PC-10 immunostaining (PCNA index) is based on the percentage of positive cell nuclei (see Chapter 30).

The nucleolus contains large loops of DNA whose rRNA genes (rDNA) of which are transcribed at an extremely high rate by RNA polymerase I. Such a loop of DNA is known as a nucleolar organizer region (NOR).[31] During the interphase, the fibrillar centres and the surrounding dense fibrillar component are the sites of rRNA localization.[32] Numerous proteins are located in the vicinity of the rRNA. The most studied proteins associated with the NORs are called AgNOR proteins (the silver-stained nucleolar proteins).[31] Silver stainability may be considered a marker of rRNA transcription activity and the one-step silver colloid method has been introduced by Howell & Black[33] for the demonstration of NOR-associated proteins. The usefulness of the method has been increased by means of several modifications.[34]

On AgNOR-stained slides, focusing allows the AgNOR to be seen in the nucleus as black dots under a microscope. AgNOR staining has been used to evaluate the proliferative activity of pre-neoplastic and neoplastic cells and has an advantage over immunohistochemical staining because the one-step AgNOR method is simple and can be applied to routinely-processed paraffin-embedded tissue sections [35,36]

Another method which enables proliferating cells to be treated without pre-treating the sample uses a monoclonal antibody against DNA polymerase alpha (DPA). This enzyme is present in the nuclei of cells in the G1, S and G2 phases of the mitotic cell cycle, and in the cytoplasm of cells in the M phase; the enzyme is absent in the G0 phase.[37] The monoclonal antibody against DPA is produced using the method of Masaki *et al*[38] and the peroxidase-antiperoxidase (PAP) method against the antibody. Cells that react with the monoclonal antibody against DPA stain brown.

Flow cytometric analysis is used to investigate the cellular and nuclear DNA (ploidy) distributions. Samples are centrifuged and the supernatants discarded. The pellet is suspended in a sucrose buffer and stained with propidium iodide for at least 3 hours. The nuclear suspension is then analysed using a flow cytometer equipped with a red fluorescent long-pass 575 nm filter.[39] The level of DNA abnormality is expressed by the DNA index (DI), defined as the ratio of the mean DNA content of the G0/1 atypical peak to the mean DNA content of the normal diploid G0/1 reference cells, according to Hiddemann *et al*.[40]

Cells with a normal diploid karyotype have, by definition, a DI of 1.0.

Ki67 is a monoclonal antibody which reacts with a nuclear protein present in human cells during all active phases of the cell cycle, G1, G2, S and M, but is absent in the resting (G0) phase. Using recombinant sections of the Ki67 antigen as an immunogen, several new monoclonal antibodies have been developed, three of which (MIB1-3), were characterized as true Ki-67 equivalents by immunostaining.[41] The proliferative index is calculated using 5 mm paraffin-embedded sections treated with 6 microwave cycles (750 W) in pH 6 citrate buffer. The Ki67 monoclonal antibody MIB1 is used in a three-step PAP immunohistochemical method.[42] The dilution of MIB1 is 1:50, overnight at 1°C. Treatment of the slides with 6 microwave cycles at 70 W in pH citrate buffer enables the use of fixed, archival tissue.[41]

Thymidine kinase (TK), the enzyme responsible for thymidine phosphorylation before incorporation into DNA, has been used in cell proliferation studies and changes in the enzyme have been correlated with DNA synthesis. Hopkins *et al*[43] showed a valid correlation between thymidine incorporation and TK activity. The enzymatic activity of TK is assayed in the supernatant fractions of tissue homogenized and centrifuged after incubation with the reaction mixture, containing Tris-HCl buffer, ATP, $MgCl_2$, ^3H-thymidine, for 10 min at 37°C.

The radioactivity is measured by a liquid scintillation counter. Results are expressed as counts/min/mg of protein.[44]

Several other methods have been described, such as anti-ribonucleotide reductase,[45] C5F10,[46] p53 transformation-related protein,[47] ornithine decarboxylase activity[48] and the metaphase-arrest method.[49]

Application to animal studies

Accurate measurement of human cell kinetics is one of many aspects for research in gastrointestinal pathophysiology. Methods to measure cell proliferation are often difficult to apply to humans, and often requre that the tissue is cultured *in vitro* immediately after removal from the body. The use of animal models not only overcomes these disadvantages, but also,

and above all, offers the opportunity to investigate the different features and specificities of the various methods when they are applied at different times.

Cell proliferation appears to play a crucial role in several steps in cancer development in many organs and tissues, especially because it represents a necessary condition for the initiation and promotion of chemical carcinogenesis.[50,51] Animal models can prove useful to demonstrate the effect of a specific stimulus on cell proliferation, such as a carcinogen, often in association with other factors such as trace elements or vitamins.

Although material is readily available from human colon cancer patients, there are advantages in using animal material for studying sequential changes and there are a number of models of intestinal carcinogenesis in laboratory rodents, most of which involve the use of parenterally-administered chemical carcinogens. This route of administration can result in a relatively uniform exposure of the tissue to the chemical, and this might be useful in distinguishing changes of a nonspecific toxic nature from changes of importance in the ultimate cancer genesis.

Animal studies are also useful in ascertaining the role of metals and trace elements in chemical carcinogenesis. Siegers *et al*[52] reported an increased incidence of tumour in a mouse model of dimethylhydrazine induced colorectal and intestinal tumourigenesis fed an iron-enriched diet. Lawson *et al*[53] examined the effect of dietary zinc deficiency on the proliferation of epithelial cells (colonocytes) in the large bowel of rats. When compared with feed-restricted rats, the animals with zinc deficiency showed a significant reduction in cell proliferation in the distal colon. Zinc deficiency had no apparent effect on TK activity in the colonocytes.

The process of liver regeneration following partial hepatectomy (PH) is a well-established model of rapidly dividing cells. Experimentally, regeneration can be induced by any acute treatment that will remove or kill a large percentage of the hepatic mass. Loss of parenchyma rapidly induces a wave of cell proliferation so that the total mass of the liver is restored to normal.[54] Using this technique, information about cell growth, transformation and tissue repair after injury can be obtained by various methods.[55,56]

Animal studies have identified an association between the development of gastric carcinoma and alterations in epithelial cell proliferation. In a study to determine the risk of gastric cancer following gastrectomy, Miwa et al[57] identified an increased gastric epithelial cell proliferation in the stomal mucosa of rats which subsequently developed gastric carcinoma, with increased cell count in the proliferative zone, a longer duration of the S phase and an increased cell cycle time.

Results and discussion

It is impossible to summarize the abundance of studies on cell proliferation in the digestive system and what follows represents only a selection.

Oesophagus

The study of cytoproliferation has been used mostly in assessing the biological properties and neoplastic risk in Barrett's oesophagus. Aneuploid cell populations, with an increase in the S phase fraction, have been demonstrated in patients with this lesion,[58,59] and particularly in cases revealing other DNA abnormalities and/or histological changes, such as dysplasia or cancer. These abnormalities in cell DNA content also correlate with an increased Ki67 expression, a fact that testifies to an overall increase in cycling cell fraction.[58,59]

Stomach

In the stomach too, epithelial cell proliferation has been used as an indicator of the risk of gastric carcinoma. Increased cell proliferation has been shown in association with gastric cancer[60] and in patients with gastric cancer precursors, such as atrophy and intestinal metaplasia.[61] These findings have been confirmed in studies using [3]HTdR or BrdU, which have shown the expansion of the proliferative compartment towards the apex of the gastric pit as the most relevant change.[60,62,63]

The fraction of cells in the S phase has been investigated as a prognostic factor for survival in gastric cancer with no extranodal metastasis, but no correlation has been found.[64,65]

More recently, interest has focused on the study of the mechanisms underlying the risk of cancer epidemiologically correlated with *Helicobacter pylori* infection. Studies using various methods[66-69] have shown that *Helicobacter pylori* infection correlates with increased cell proliferation, and this has been confirmed by *in vitro* studies.[70]

Colon

In the colon, many proliferation markers have been used to assess the risk of cancer in patients with lesions considered to be potential cancer precursors, such as ulcerative colitis[71] and colonic polyps.[72,73] BrdU, PCNA and [3]HTdR are the most frequently used markers, again with specific attention to the gland crypt compartment involved in hyperproliferation.

The evaluation of colonic epithelial cell proliferation has been the intermediate goal or intervention studies, based on the administration of calcium or omega-3 fatty acids in the chemoprevention of colon cancer. Using [3]HTdR, Anti et al[74] demonstrated that the administration of omega-3 fatty acids induces normalization of the abnormal cell proliferation patterns in patients with sporadic adenomatous colorectal polyps. These findings could not be reproduced by other authors using BrdU,[75] thus confirming that the results of these studies should be evaluated with caution as they frequently conflict.

In animal models, calcium administration proved capable of steadily decreasing the rectal cell hyperproliferation induced by bile acid administration.[76]

Finally, rectal cell proliferation has been assessed to evaluate the mechanisms underlying the increased risk of colorectal cancer due to exposure to xenobiotics, as in alcoholics.[77,78] Animal studies have confirmed increased rectal cell proliferation in chronically ethanol fed rats.[79]

Studies in humans and animal models suggest that, despite certain limitations and with all due precautions and caveats, cell proliferation abnormalities can be proposed as intermediate biomarkers of gastrointestinal cancer risk. These biomarkers can be useful in evaluating cancer risk at an individual level and, perhaps more importantly, the effect of exogenous and endogenous factors in human carcinogenesis or in intervention studies.

References

1. Tannock I. Cell kinetics and chemotherapy, a critical review. *Cancer Treat Rep* 1978; **62:** 1117-1133.

2. Risio M, Lipkin M, Candelaresi GL *et al*. Correlations between rectal mucosa cell proliferation and the clinical and pathological features of nonfamilial neoplasia of the large intestine. *Cancer Res* 1991; **51:** 1917-1921.

3. Seki S, Sakaguchi H, Kawakita N *et al*. Identification and fine structure of proliferating hepatocytes in malignant and non-malignant liver disease by use of a

monoclonal antibody against DNA polymerase alpha. *Human Pathol* 1990; **21**: 1020-1030.

4. Tanaka T, Takeuchi T, Nishikawa A *et al*. Nucleolar organizer regions in hepatocarcinogenesis induced by N-2-fluorenylacetamide in rats: comparison with bromodeoxyuridine immunohistochemistry. *Jpn J Cancer Res* 1989; **80**: 1047-1051.

5. Vemuru RP, Aragona E, Gupta S. Analysis of hepatocellular proliferation: study of archival liver tissue is facilitated by an endogenous marker of DNA replication. *Hepatology* 1992; **16**: 968-973.

6. Paolucci F, Mancini R, Marucci L, Benedetti A, Jezequel AM, Orlandi F. Immunohistochemical identification of proliferating cells following dimethylnitrosamine-induced live injury. *Liver* 1990; **10**: 278-281.

7. Tarao K, Shimizu A, Harada M et al. Difference in the *in vitro* uptake of bromodeoxyuridine between liver cirrhosis with and without hepatocellular carcinoma. *Cancer* 1989; **64**: 104-109.

8. Tarao K, Shimizu A, Ohkawa S *et al*. Development of hepatocellular carcinoma associated with increases in DNA synthesis in the surrounding cirrhosis. *Gastroenterology* 1992; **103**: 595-600.

9. Ojanguren I, Ariza A, Llatjos M, Castella' E, Mate Jl, Navas-Palacios JJ. Proliferating cell nuclear antigen expression in normal, regenerative, and neoplastic liver: a fine-needle aspiration cytology and biopsy study. *Human Pathol* 1993; **24**: 905-908.

10. Shimuzu A, Tarao K, Takemiya S, Harada M, Inoue T, Ono T. S-phase cells in diseased human liver determined by an in-vitro BrdU-anti-BrdU method. *Hepatology* 1988; **8**: 1535-1539.

11. Lipkin M. Biomarkers of increased susceptibility to gastrointestinal cancer: new application to studies of cancer prevention in human subjects. *Cancer Res* 1988; **48**: 235-245.

12. Willems G, Lehy T. Radioautographic and quantitative studies on parietal and peptic cell kinetics in the mouse. *Gastroenterology* 1975; **69**: 416-426.

13. Lipkin M, Sherlock P, Bell B. Cell proliferation kinetics in the gastrointestinal tract of man. II. Cell renewal in stomach, ileum, colon, and rectum. *Gastroenterology* 1963; **45**: 721-729.

14. Arber N, Zajicek G, Ariel I. The streaming liver. II. Hepatocyte life history. *Liver* 1988; **8**: 80-87.

15. Benedetti A, Mancini R, Giulioni G, Orlandi F, Jezequel AM. Immunocytochemical localization of S-phase cells in normal rat liver. In: Dianzani MU, Gentilini P (Eds) *Chronic Liver Damage*. Excerpta Medica, Amsterdam, 1990, pp. 87-92.

16. Fabrikant JL. The kinetics of cellular proliferation in regenerating liver. *J Cell Biol* 1968; **36**: 551-565.

17. Zajjicek G, Schwartz-Arad D, Bartfeld E. The streaming liver. V. Time- and age-dependent changes of hepatocyte DNA content, following partial hepatectomy. *Liver* 1989; **9**: 164-171.

18. Edwards JL, Koch A. Parenchymal and littoral cell proliferation during liver regeneration. *Lab Invest* 1964; **3**: 32-43.

19. Ponz de Leon M, Roncacci I, Di Donato P *et al*. Pattern of epithelial cell proliferation in colorectal mucosa of normal subjects and of patients with adenomatous polyps or cancer of the large bowel. *Cancer Res* 1988; **48**: 4121-4126.

20. Biasco G, Paganelli GM, Miglioli M *et al*. Rectal cell proliferation and colon cancer risk in ulcerative colitis. *Cancer Res* 1990; **50**: 1156-1159.

21. Risio M. Mucosal cell proliferation in colorectal neoplasia. In: Rossini FP, Lynch HT, Winawer S (Eds) *Recent Trends in Colorectal Cancer: Biology and Management of High Risk Groups*. Elsevier Science Publisher BV, Amsterdam, 1992, pp.155-158.

22. Roncucci L, Ponz de Leon M, Scalmati A *et al*. The influence of age on colonic epithelial cell proliferation. *Cancer* 1988; **62**: 2373-2377.

23. Hoshino T, Nagashima T, Murovic J, Levin ME, Levin VA, Rupp SM. Cell kinetic studies of in situ human brain tumors with bromodeoxyuridine. *Cytometry* 1985; **6**: 627-632.

24. Hoshino T, Nagashoma T, Cho KG *et al*. S-phase fraction of human brain tumors in situ measured by uptake of bromodeoxyuridine. *Int J Cancer* 1986; **38**: 369-374.

25. Shuttle B, Reinders MMJ, Bosman FT, Blijham GH. Studies with antibromodeoxyuridine antibodies. II. Simultaneous detection of antigen expression and DNA synthesis by *in vivo* labeling of mouse intestinal mucosa. *J Histochem Cytochem* 1987; **35**: 371-374.

26. Shimizu A, Tarao K, Takemiya S, Harada M, Inoue T, Ono T. S-phase cells in diseased human liver determined by an *in vitro* BrdU-anti-BrdU method. *Hepatology* 1988; **8**: 1535-1539.

27. Sasaki K, Ogino T, Takahashi M. *In vitro* BrdUrd labeling of solid tumors and immunological determination of labeling index. *J Histotechnol* 1987; **10**: 47-49.

28. Ogata K, Ogata Y, Nakamura RN, Tan EM. Purification and N-terminal amino acid sequence of proliferating cell nuclear antigen (PCNA/cyclin) and development of ELISA for anti-PCNA antibodies *J Immunol* 1985; **135**: 2623-2627.

29. Garcia RL, Coltera MD, Gown AM. Analysis of proliferative grade using antiPCNA/cyclin monoclonal antibodies in fixed embedded tissues. Comparison with flow cytometric analysis. *Am J Pathol* 1988; **154:** 223-235.

30. Hall PA, Levison DA, Woods AL *et al.* Proliferating cell nuclear antigen (PCNA) immunolocalization in paraffin sections: an index of cell proliferation with evidence of deregulated expression in some neoplasms. *J Pathol* 1990; **162:** 285-294.

31. Fakan S, Hernandez-Verdun D. The nucleolus and nucleolar organizer regions (collective review). *Biol Cell* 1986; **56:** 189-206.

32. Hernandez-Verdun D, Derenzini M, Bouteille M. The morphological relationship in electron microscopy between NOR-silver proteins and intra-nuclear chromatin. *Chromosoma* 1982; **85:** 461-473.

33. Howell E, Black DA. Controlled silver staining of nucleolar organising regions with protective colloidal developer: a one step method. *Experentia* 1980; **36:** 1014.

34. Ploton D, Menager M, Jeannesson P, Himber G, Pigeon F, Adnet J-J. Improvement in the staining and in the visualization of the argyrophilic proteins of the nucleolar organizer region at optical level. *Histochem J* 1986; **18:** 5-14.

35. Suarez V, Newman J, Hiley C, Crocker J, Collins M. The value of NOR numbers in neoplastic and non-neoplastic epithelium of the stomach. *Histopathology* 1989; **14:** 61-66.

36. Tanaka T, Takeuchi T, Nishikawa A, Takami T, Mori H. Nucleolar organizer regions in hepatocarcinogenesis induced by N-2-Fluorenylacetamide in rats: comparison with Bromodeoxyuridine immunohistochemistry. *Jpn J Cancer Res* 1989; **80:** 1047-1051.

37. Nakamura H, Morita T, Masaki S *et al.* Intracellular localization and metabolism of DNA polymerase alpha in human cells visualized with monoclonal antibody. *Exp Cell Res* 1984; **151:** 123-133.

38. Masaki S, Tanabe K, Yoshida S. Large polypeptides of 10S DNA polymerase alpha from calf thymus: Rapid isolation using monoclonal antibody and tryptic peptide mapping analysis. *Nucleic Acids Res* 1984; **12:** 4455-4467.

39. Roncalli M, Borzio M, Brando B, Colloredo G, Servida E. Abnormal DNA content in liver-cell dysplasia: a flow cytometric study. *Int J Cancer* 1989; **44:** 204-207.

40. Hiddemann W, Schumann J, Andreeff M *et al.* Convention on nomenclature for DNA cytometry. *Cytometry* 1984; **5:** 445-446.

41. Cattoretti G, Becker MHG, Key G *et al.* Monoclonal antibodies against recombinant parts of the Ki67 antigen (MIB-1 and MIB-3) detect proliferating cells in microwave-processed formalin-fixed paraffin sections. *J Pathol* 1992; **168:** 357-363.

42. Sternberger LA. The unlabeled antibody (PAP) method. *J. Histochem Ctyochem*, 1997; **27:** 1657-1659.

43. Hopkins HA, Campbell HA, Barbirolli B *et al.* Thymidine kinase and deoxyribonucleic acid metabolism in growing and regenerating livers from rats on controlled feeding schedules. *Biochem J* 1973; **136:** 955-966.

44. Kahn D, Stadler J, Terblanche J, Van Hoorn-Hickman R. Thymidine kinase: An inexpensive index of liver regeneration in a large animal model. *Gastroenterology* 1980; **79:** 907-911.

45. Engstrom Y. Monoclonal antibodies against mammalian ribonucleotide reductase. *Acta Chem Scand Ser B Org Chem Biochem* 1982; **36:** 343-344.

46. Lloyd RV, Wilson BS, Varani J, Gaur PK, Moline S, Makari JG. Immunocytochemical characterization of a monoclonal antibody that recognized mitosing cells. *Am J Pathol* 1985; **121:** 275-283.

47. Dippold WG, Gilbert J, DeLeo AB, Khoury G, Old LG. p53 transformation related protein: detection by monoclonal antibody in mouse and human cells. *Proc Natl Acad Sci USA* 1981; **8:** 1695-1699.

48. Rao CV, Nayini J, Reddy BS. Effect of oltiprax [5-(2-pyrazinyl)-4-methyl-1,2-dithiol-3-thione] on azoxymethane-induced biochemical changes related to early colon carcinogenesis in male F344 rats. *Proc Soc Exp Biol Med* 1991; **197:** 77-84.

49. Matthew JA, Pell JD, Prior A *et al.* Validation of a simple technique for the detection of abnormal mucosal cell replication in humans. *Eur J Cancer Prev* 1994; **3:** 337-344.

50. Columbano A, Rajalakshami S, Sarma DSR. Requirement of cell proliferation for the initiation of liver carcinogenesis as assayed by three different procedures. *Cancer Res* 1981; **41:** 2079-2083.

51. Argyris TG. Regeneration and the mechanisms of epidermal tumor promotion. *Crit Rev Toxicol* 1985; **14:** 211-258.

52. Siegers CP, Bumann D, Trepkau HD, Schadwinkel B, Baretton G. Role of iron in cell proliferation and tumorigenesis. In: *Chemically Induced Cell Proliferation. Implications for Risk Assessment.* Wiley-Liss, New York, 1991, pp. 439-444.

53. Lawson MJ, Butler RN, Goland GJ *et al.* Zinc deficiency is associated with suppression of colonocyte proliferation in the distal large bowel of rats. *Biol Trace Element Res* 1988; **18:** 115-121.

54. Michalopoulos GM. Liver regeneration: Molecular mechanisms of growth control. *FASEB* 1990; **4:** 176-187.

55. Lanier Tl, Berger EK, Eacho PI. Comparison of 5-bromo-2-deoxyuridine and [³H]thymidine for studies of hepatocellular proliferation in rodents. *Carcinogenesis* 1989; **10:** 1341-1343.

56. Teocharis SE, Skopelitou AS, Margeli AP, Pavlaki KJ, Kittas C. Proliferating cell nuclear antigen (PCNA) expression in regenerating rat liver after partial hepatectomy. *Dig Dis Sci* 1994; **39:** 245-252.

57. Miwa K, Kamata T, Miyazaki I, Hattori T. Kinetic changes and experimental carcinogenesis after Billroth I and II gastrectomy. *Br J Surg* 1993; **80:** 893-896.

58. Blount PL, Meltzer SJ, Yin J, Huang Y, Krasna MJ, Reid BJ. Clonal ordering of 17p and 5q allelic losses in Barrett dysplasia and adenocarcinoma. *Proc Natl Acad Sci* 1993; **90:** 3221-3225.

59. Reid BJ, Sanchez CA, Blount PL Levine DS. Barrett's esophagus: cell cycle abnormalities in advancing stages of neoplastic progression. *Gastroenterology* 1993; **105:** 119-129.

60. Brito M, Filip MI, Morris RW. Cell proliferation study on gastric carcinoma and non-involved gastric mucosa using a bromodeoxyuridine (BrdU) labelling technique. *Eur J Cancer Prev* 1992; **1:** 429-435.

61. Cahill RJ, O'Morain. Gastric epithelial cell proliferation. *Eur J Cancer Prev* 1994; **3 (Suppl 2):** 55-60.

62. Lipkin M, Correa P, Mikol YB *et al.* Proliferative and antigenic modifications in epithelial cells in chronic atrophic gastritis. *J Natl Cancer Inst* 1985; **75:** 613-619.

63. Biasco G, Paganelli GM, Miglioli M, Barbara L. Cell proliferation biomarkers in the gastrointestinal tract. *J Cell Biochem* 1992; **16G:** 73-78.

64. Rugge M, Sonego F, Panozzo M *et al.* Pathology and ploidy in the prognosis of gastric cancer with no extranodal metastasis. *Cancer* 1994; **73:** 1127-1133.

65. Wyatt JI, Quirke P, Ward DC *et al.* Comparison of histopathological and flow cytometric parameters in prediction of prognosis in gastric cancer. *J Pathol* 1989; **158:** 195-201.

66. De Koster E, Buset M, Fernandes E *et al.* Influence of HP and gastritis on gastric antrum and corpus mucosal cell proliferation status. *Acta Gastroenterol Belg* 1993; **56:** 61-66.

67. Cahill R, Xia H, Sant S, Beattie S, Hamilton H, O'Morain C. Effect of *Helicobacter pylori* on gastric cell proliferation. *Ir J Med Sci* 1992; **161 (Suppl 10):** 31-35.

68. Brenes F, Ruiz B, Correa P *et al. Helicobacter pylori* causes hyperproliferation of the gastric epithelium: pre- and post-eradication indices of proliferating cell nuclear antigen. *Am J Gastroenterol* 1993; **88:** 1870-1875.

69. Lynch D, Mapstone NP, Clarke AMT *et al.* Cell proliferation in *Helicobacter pylori* associated gastritis and the long term effect of eradication therapy. *Gut* 1994; **35 (Suppl 2):** S4.

70. Tsujii M, Kawano S, Tshigami Y *et al.* Ammonia produced by *Helicobacter pylori* accelerates cell proliferation of human gastric mucosa. *Gastroenterology* 1991; **100:** A177.

71. Biasco G, Lipkin M, Minarini A, Higgins P, Miglioli M, Barbara L. Proliferative and antigenic properties of rectal cells in patients with chronic ulcerative colitis. *Cancer Res* 1984; **44:** 5450-5454.

72. Risio M, Coverlizza S, Ferrari A, Canderalesi GL, Rossini FP. Immunohistochemical study of epithelial cell proliferation in hyperplastic polyps, adenomas, and adenocarcinomas of the large bowel. *Gastroenterology* 1988; **94:** 899-904.

73. Risio M, Lipkin M, Canderalesi GL, Bertone A, Coverlizza S, Rossini FP. Correlations between rectal mucosa cell proliferation and clinical and pathological features of nonfamilial neoplasia of the large intestine. *Cancer Res* 1991; **51:** 1917-1921.

74. Anti M, Marra G, Armelao F *et al.* Effect of omega-3 fatty acids on rectal mucosal cell proliferation in subjects at risk for colon cancer. *Gastroenterology* 1992; **103:** 883-891.

75. Bartram H-P, Gostner A, Reddy BS *et al.* Missing anti-proliferative effect of fish oil on rectal epithelium in healthy volunteers consuming a high-fat diet: potential role of the n-3:n-6 fatty acid ratio. *Eur J Cancer Prev* 1995; **4:** 231-237.

76. Piard F, Martin M, Boutron M-C, Hillon P, Hammann A, Martin F. Effect of different doses of dietary calcium on murine colonic cell proliferation. *Eur J Cancer Prev* 1994; **3:** 215-221.

77. Pollack ES, Nomura AMY, Heilbrun LK, Stemmermann GN, Green SB. Prospective study of alcohol consumption and cancer. *N Engl J Med* 1984; **310:** 617-621.

78. Wu AH, Paganini-Hill A, Ross RK, Henderson BE. Alcohol, physical activity and other risk factors for colorectal cancer: a prospective study. *Br J Cancer* 1987; **55:** 687-694.

79. Simanowski UA, Seitz HK, Baier B, Kommerell B, Schmidt-GayK H, Wright NA. Chronic ethanol consumption selectively stimulates rectal cell proliferation in the rat. *Gut* 1986; **27:** 278-282.

23

Isolation of intestinal smooth muscle cells

H Ohashi and S Komori

Summary

Cell isolation from the longitudinal muscle layer of guinea-pig ileum involves two major processes, digestion of the tissue pieces with a combination of collagenase and papain and dispersion into smooth muscle cells by agitating the enzyme-treated tissue pieces. Prepared single muscle cells were shown to preserve their individual function using whole-cell patch clamp techniques. Under current clamp mode, they discharged action potentials spontaneously or in response to electrical stimulation and, under voltage-clamp mode, responded with membrane currents to a variety of stimuli. Furthermore, the cells exhibited increases in the cytosolic Ca^{2+} concentration reflecting Ca^{2+} entry through Ca^{2+} channels in the plasma membrane and Ca^{2+} release from intracellular stores. The procedures for cell isolation are substantially applicable to other intestinal smooth muscle tissues from both animal and human preparations. Studies in single muscle cells have the potential to elucidate new membrane-mediated mechanisms of action of drugs and toxins and bring therapeutic advances in gastrointestinal disorders in both humans and animals.

Introduction

Many studies on isolated muscle tissues and segments of the intestine, in which tension (or shortening, or pressure) and electrical activity are recorded, have made a relevant contribution to our understanding of smooth muscle function in intestinal movements. Currently, intense efforts have been made to understand the characteristics of the ion channels of the cell membrane and the mechanism of intracellular signal transduction in smooth muscle cells. The whole-cell patch-clamp technique has been used for such studies. With this technique, membrane currents within single cells can be monitored, thereby allowing the effects of drugs, toxins and ions to be examined. Simultaneous ratiometric quantification of Ca^{2+} concentrations can be made within the cells using fluorescent dyes such as fura-2. The patch-clamp technique can be applied to single isolated smooth muscle cells and makes it possible to alter ionic environments inside as well as outside the cell and to introduce different agents such as putative intracellular messengers. One problem with this technique however, occurs in the preparation of single smooth muscle cells which retain *normal* properties.

In this chapter, we will describe how to disperse the longitudinal muscle layer of intestinal tissues into its constituent smooth muscle cells by digesting away the collagenous matrix. Some of the physiologically relevant properties of the enzymatically dispersed cells are also described.

Methods

Since, theoretically, exactly the same principles for preparation of single smooth muscle cells are applicable to intestinal tissues from animal and clinical preparations,[1-15] the following pertains to guinea-pig ileum. Male guinea-pigs, weighing 350-450g, were stunned and exsanguinated, and a length of 10-15 cm of the ileum was removed. The isolated intestine was placed in a Petri dish containing physiological salt solution (PSS) of the following composition (mM): NaCl : 126, KCl : 6, $CaCl_2$: 2, $MgCl_2$: 1.2, glucose: 14 and HEPES: 10.5 (titrated to pH 7.2 with NaOH), and divided into several segments (each 2-3 cm long). The lumen of the intestinal segments was flushed with PSS to remove the content, and the adhering tissues were trimmed away.

Cell isolation

To obtain single smooth muscle cells, the following procedures were performed with care at room temperature (20-25°C), except where indicated.

Preparation of muscle sheets of the longitudinal muscle layer

Each intestinal segment was pulled over a glass tube with a diameter of 8 mm (to fit the lumen), and the longitudinal muscle layer was separated from the underlying tissue by stroking away the muscle layer from its mesenteric attachment along its whole length and then along its circumference over the whole area, using cotton wool moistened with PSS. Alternatively, after freeing it from its mesenteric attachment, the longitudinal muscle layer was peeled from the underlying circular muscle layer over the whole area of the segment using a pair of fine tweezers. Muscle sheets of the longitudinal muscle layer were cut into small pieces of 3×3 mm square on a rubber board moistened with PSS, placed in a test tube containing 2 ml Ca^{2+}-free PSS (PSS to which no $CaCl_2$ was added), and incubated at 37°C for 10 min before moving on to the next procedure.

Some fragments of the circular muscle layer as well as nerve plexuses clinging to the obtained muscle sheets difficult to remove. However, they are small in amount and may be dispersed readily into their constituent cells early in the process of enzymatic digestion (see below).

Enzymatic digestion

After incubation at 37°C for 10 min (see above), the Ca^{2+}-free solution in the test-tube was replaced with 1 ml of 30 μM Ca^{2+}-added PSS containing collagenase (Sigma, type XI; 0.2-0.6 mg/ml), papain (Sigma, from papaya latex; 0.3-0.6 mg/ml) and bovine serum albumin (2-5 mg/ml), and left to stand at 37°C for 15 min to allow enzyme digestion of the tissue pieces. Enzyme digestion in this manner was repeated once more and the enzyme solution was then removed by replacing twice with 2-3 ml of a low-Ca^{2+} PSS, (120 μM Ca^{2+}). The concentrations of both enzymes can be determined at one's own discretion in the two successive incubations and for different tissues.

The solutions of collagenase and papain were made up in distilled water to give a concentration of 30 mg/ml for the former and 60 mg/ml for the latter, and stored at -20°C in volumes of 100 to 200 μl. The same lot of either enzyme was only used for 5 days from its first thawing to avoid possible reduction of the enzyme activity by repeating freezing and thawing.

In many studies,[9-13] a trypsin inhibitor has been used with these enzymes. However, the role of the enzyme inhibitor in the enzymatic digestion has not been described; it might serve to protect smooth muscle cells against trypsin, as a trace of it is contained in collagenase. In our experiments, a tripsin inhibitor was not used, since no appreciable improvement in the cell dispersion was demonstrated, and cell damage was suspected.

Dispersion into single cells

To disperse into single smooth muscle cells, the enzyme-treated tissue pieces were agitated in 2-3 ml of 120 μM Ca^{2+}-added PSS by drawing in and out of a Pasteur pipette, the internal diameters at the tip of which was large enough for the tissue pieces to pass the bore without friction, 50-70 times. The agitation was repeated at an interval of about one second. When the solution became cloudy with cells and debris from the tissues, it was retained in a new test-tube. The tissue agitation and subsequent collection of cells suspended in the solution were repeated ten to twelve times. To ascertain the distribution of muscle cells in the retained solution, a small aliquot from the solution of each of the test tubes was examined under a microscope with a magnitude of ×100 or ×200. In general, muscle cells were present richly with less debris in the solution of the 4th to 8th test-tubes. Therefore, the solution of these test-tubes was combined, filtered through a fine nylon mesh to remove debris and then centrifuged at about 600 r.p.m. for 2 min. The cells were resuspended in 2-5 ml of 0.5 mM Ca^{2+}-added PSS, placed on cover-glasses as a small aliquot (approx. 0.1 ml) and kept in a moist atmosphere at 4°C, for 1 to 10 hours until used.

Muscle cells derived from the circular muscle layer are difficult to contain, since the tissue is far smaller in amount (see above) and exposed more readily to the enzymes, so that the enzymatically-dispersed components from it can appear in the solution of the first to third test-tubes.

Muscle cells which can be used for electrophysiological experiments (see below) appear in the retained solution with such a bell-shaped distribution pattern that they increase in number to a peak in the 4th to 6th test-tube solution and then gradually decrease. A prominent appearance of muscle cells with debris in the solution of the first to third test-tubes can be taken as an indication of "overcooking" of the tissues with the enzymes. No progressive increase in the number of muscle cells may indicate insufficient digestion of the tissues.

Alternatively, the relevance of dispersed muscle cells can be assessed by their ability to attach themselves to the surface of a cover-glass. A cover-glass with cells, after storage at 4°C for 30 min or more, was placed on the bottom of an organ bath (0.8 ml in volume) fixed on the stage of a microscope, and then the organ bath was perfused with 10 ml or so of PSS in a short time (10-15 sec) using a pair of syringes, one for injection and the other for suction. If many muscle cells are missing from the glass surface after the bath perfusion, this may indicate a lack of success in obtaining muscle cells in a reliable state.

Favourable cells

Microscopic observations of cells attached to the cover-glass revealed that single muscle cells have heterogenous morphological appearances, which are virtually similar to those previously described and illustrated for the enzymatically-isolated cells of the longitudinal muscle layer of rabbit jejunum[10] and ileum.[12] Muscle cells are in a relaxed, elongated state (100-300 μm long and 3-5 μm wide) or in a contracted situation to different extents, with some lysed or ghost cells.

Relaxed, elongated cells were unfavourable for studies in which the membrane potential and membrane current are measured using a conventional whole-cell patch-clamp technique[14] or a nystatin-perforated patch-clamp technique,[15] and the cytosolic Ca^{2+} concentration ([Ca^{2+}]i) measured using a Ca^{2+}-sensitive dye, fura-2.[16] They produce a strong contraction in response to an undesirable but unavoidable stimulus, resulting from handling a patch pipette. The contraction scarcely allows the seal resistance between the tip of the patch pipette and the cell membrane to reach a gigaohm level. Even if they have been held under the whole-cell patch-clamp, they cause a strong contraction in response to a test drug such as carbachol (10-100 μM) which dislocates the patch pipette or the cell site from which the fura-2 signal is recorded. Finally, such cells have disadvantages in that they are not readily dialysed with patch-pipette solution and are thus unfavourable to the establishment of isopotentiality throughout the cell membrane using a conventional patch-clamp technique.[12]

Partially contracted cells, especially with a wide region in the central part (see Plate 2 in ref. 10 and Fig. 2B & C in ref. 12), are favourable for the whole-cell patch clamp. It is essential to apply the patch pipette to the wide, central part. Such cells, held under the current clamp mode, discharge action potentials spontaneously or in response to depolarising current pulses.

Cell damage

Some damage is inevitable in preparing the single muscle cells, although it is difficult to know what extent of their normal function is preserved. One may find that only a very small fraction of single muscle cells respond to an agonist, whereas most cells respond to another, as is the case with histamine and carbachol in the same cell type.[1] An apt explanation for this is that it is due to cell damage that may occur with prolonged exposure to the enzymes, although how

receptors for the former agonist and/or their signal transduction systems are impaired cannot be ascertained, nor the distribution of the receptors in such a small population of the cells.[1]

Results and discussion

Single muscle cells prepared in this isolation procedure, when dialysed with a K$^+$-based pipette solution and held under the current clamp, responded to depolarising current pulses with discharges of action potentials with an overshoot of 10-30 mV, the action potential discharge being followed by a rise in cytosolic Ca^{2+} concentration [Ca^{2+}]i (Fig.23.1A). Nicardipine, a Ca^{2+} channel blocker, abolished the action potential discharge and [Ca^{2+}]i rise and TEA, a K$^+$ channel blocker, increased the total duration and overshoot of action potentials and the size of [Ca^{2+}]i rises (Fig.23.1B). Under the voltage-clamp, a depolarising step from the holding potential of -50 or -60 mV evoked a fast, brief inward Ca^{2+} current followed by a slow, long outward K$^+$ current (Fig. 23.2A-left). Therefore, inclusion of a Cs$^+$ - based solution into patch pipettes resulted in elimination of the K$^+$ current and potentiation of the Ca^{2+} current (Fig. 23.2A-right). On application of carbachol, a brief, large K$^+$ current occurred as a result of activation of K$^+$ channels by a rapid, massive release of Ca^{2+} from intracellular stores brought about by increased formation of inositol 1, 4, 5, - trisphosphate (InsP$_3$) an intracellular Ca^{2+}- releasing messenger (Fig. 23.2B). The cells also responded to the agonist with a non-selective cationic current, as shown in Fig. 23.2C, which is fundamental to the depolarisation of the cell membrane in the muscle tissue.[19-21] Thus, the single muscle cells retain their membrane excitability and receptor-operated signal transduction systems.

The cell isolation procedure which produces such physiologically relevant cells is theoretically applicable to other intestinal tissues including clinical preparations, e.g., rabbit ileum,[22,23] and jejunum,[18,24,25] rat ileum,[26] chicken rectum [27,28] and human jejunum[14] and colon.[15] However, to obtain reasonably functional muscle cells, it may be necessary to practice the procedure and become familiar with it.

It is of interest that in guinea-pig taenia caeci, the membrane hyperpolarization mediated by adrenoceptors is markedly reduced or blocked after treatment with collagenase at concentrations required for cell

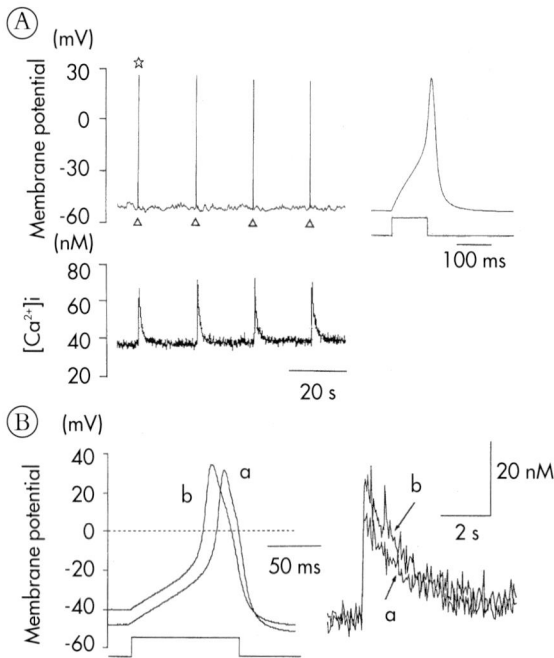

Figure 23.1 - Action potentials (APs) accompanied by [Ca^{2+}]i increases. Simultaneous records of changes in membrane potential and [Ca^{2+}]i were made in a single longitudinal smooth muscle cell isolated from guinea-pig ileum. The cell was bathed in normal PSS, patch clamped with a pipette filled with a KCl-based solution and held under the current clamp mode. The patch clamp was achieved by the nystatin-perforated technique.[17] For measuring [Ca^{2+}]i, the cell, before being patch-clamped, was loaded with a Ca^{2+}—sensitive dye, fura-2, by extracellular application of its membrane-permeable analogue.[8] *A)* APs (upper trace) and rises in [Ca^{2+}]i (bottom trace) evoked by a train of four depolarising current pulses of 100 msec duration at 30 pA intensity, as indicated by Δ below the upper trace. The inset to the right shows a time-expanded trace of the action potential asterisked (✰). *B)* superimposed records of APs (left panel) and Ca^{2+} rises (right panel) evoked by a depolarising current pulse (30 pA, 100 msec) from another cell before (a) and after (b) application of 2 mM TEA, a K$^+$- channel blocker.

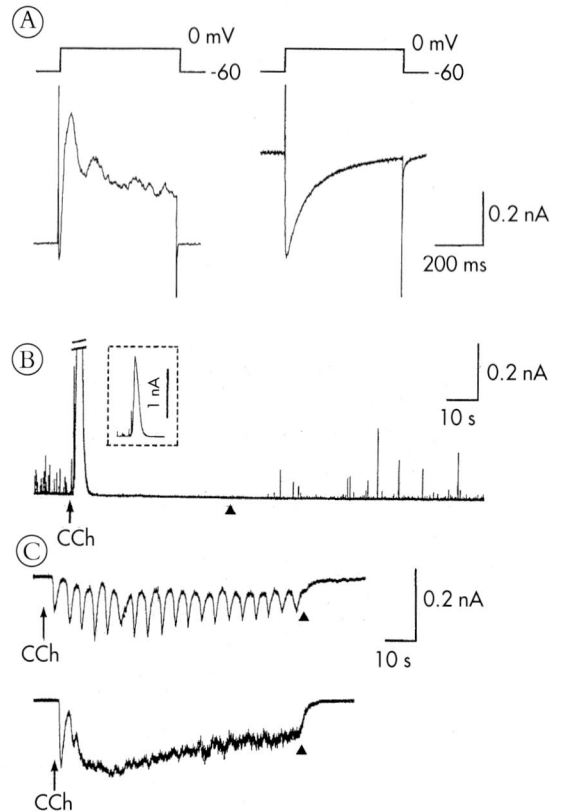

Figure 2 - Whole-cell membrane current records from single ileal muscle cells. Cells were bathed in normal PSS and held under voltage clamp using a conventional whole-cell patch clamp technique.[16] *A)* a brief inward Ca^{2+} current followed by a sustained, but gradually relaxed, outward K$^+$ current (left panel) evoked by a depolarising step to 0 mV from the holding potential of -60 mV in a cell dialysed with a KCl-based pipette solution, and an inward Ca^{2+} current (right panel) in another cell dialysed with a CsCl-based pipette solution to block K$^+$ channels. *B)* a brief, large outward current evoked by carbachol (CCh, 100 μM) in a cell held at 0 mV using a patch pipette filled with a KCl-based solution. The inset shows the CCh-evoked current with its full size. The CCh-evoked current is due to opening of Ca^{2+} - activated K$^+$ channels caused by a rapid, massive release of Ca^{2+} from internal stores.[1,18] The closed triangle indicates the removal of CCh (also in C). *C)* inward currents evoked by 2 μM (upper trace) and 10 μM CCh (lower trace), respectively with and without a sustained oscillatory component in different cells held at -50 mV with a pipette filled with a CsCl-based solution. The inward current arises from opening of non-selective cationic channels[1,20,21] The oscillatory component is caused by periodic release of Ca^{2+} from the stores regulated by InsP$_3$- and extracellular Ca^{2+} dependent mechanisms.[2,3,8]

isolation.[29] Furthermore, in single muscle cells isolated from the same muscle tissue with collagenase, catechol and drugs containing the catechol moiety, such as adrenaline, noradrenaline and isoprenaline, all potentiate voltage-gated Ca^{2+} current with an equipotency and these effects are resistant to both α - and β -adrenoceptor antagonists.[30] The broad effect has been suggested to be mediated by enzyme - modified adrenoceptors. Adrenoceptors, especially in intestinal smooth muscles, might be prone to enzyme-induced modification.

In conclusion, a means of preparing single longitudinal smooth muscle cells of guinea-pig ileum has been described, although care must be taken to prevent cell damage that might occur during handling for the preparation. The single muscle cells preserve their individual function and are useful for analysis of single channel activity, characterisation of receptor-coupled signal transduction systems and their mutual interactions as well as clarification of the biomolecular mechanisms of Ca^{2+} mobilisation. Thus, studies in the single muscle cells have the potential to provide new insights into the effects of drugs and toxins on gut motility.

References

1   Komori S, Kawai M, Takewaki T, Ohashi H. GTP-binding protein involvement in membrane currents by evoked carbachol and histamine in guinea-pig ileal muscle. *J Physiol* 1992; **450**: 105-126.

2   Komori S, Kawai M, Pacaud P, Ohashi H, Bolton TB. Oscillations of receptor-operated cationic current and internal calcium in single guinea-pig ileal smooth muscle cells. *Pflügers Arch* 1993; **424**: 431-438.

3. Komori S, Iwata M, Unno T, Ohashi H. Modulation of carbachol-induced $[Ca^{2+}]i$ oscillations by Ca^{2+} - influx in single intestinal smooth muscle cells. *Br J Pharmacol* 1996; **119**: 245-252.

4. Ohashi H, Takewaki T, Unno T, Komori S. Mechanical and current responses to neurotensin in the smooth muscle of guinea-pig intestine. *J Auton Pharmacol* 1994; **14**: 239-251.

5. Zholos AV, Komori S, Ohashi H, Bolton TB. Ca^{2+} inhibition of inositol trisphosphate-induced Ca^{2+} release in single smooth muscle cells of guinea-pig small intestine. *J Physiol* 1994; **481**: 97-109.

6. Unno T, Komori S, Ohashi H. Inhibitory effect of muscarinic receptor activation on Ca^{2+} channel current in smooth muscle cells of guinea-pig ileum. *J Physiol* 1995; **484**: 567-581.

7. Unno T, Komori S, Ohashi H. Some evidence against involvement of arachidonic acid in muscarinic suppression of voltage-gated calcium channel current in guinea-pig ileal smooth muscle cells. *Br J Pharmacol* 1996; **119**: 213-222.

8. Kohda M, Komori S, Unno T, Ohashi H. Carbachol-induced $[Ca^{2+}]i$ oscillations in single smooth muscle cells of guinea-pig ileum. *J Physiol* 1996; **492**: 315-328

9. Momose K, Gomi Y. Studies on isolated smooth muscle cells. VI. Dispersion procedures for acetylcholine-sensitive smooth muscle cells of guinea-pig. *Jpn. J. Smooth Muscle Res* 1980; **16**: 29-36

10. Benham CD, Bolton TB. Patch-clamp studies of slow potential-sensitive potassium channels in longitudinal smooth muscle cells of rabbit jejunum. *J Physiol* 1983; **340**: 469-486

11. Bolton TB, Lang RJ, Takewaki T, Benham CD. Patch and whole-cell voltage clamp of single mammalian visceral and vascular smooth muscle cells. *Experientia* 1985; **41**: 887-894

12. Ohya Y, Terada K, Kitamura K, Kuriyama H. Membrane currents recorded from a fragment of rabbit intestinal smooth muscle cell. *Am J Physiol* 1986; **251**: C335-C346

13. Nakao K, Inoue R, Yamanaka K, Kitamura K. Actions of quinine and apamin on after-hyperpolarization of the spike in circular smooth muscle cells of the guinea-pig ileum. *Naunyn-Schmiedeberg's Arch Pharmacol* 1986; **334**: 508-513

14. Farrugia G, Rich A, Rae JL, Sarr MG, Szurszewski JH. Calcium currents in human and canine jejunal circular smooth muscle cells. *Gastroenterology* 1995; **109**: 707-717.

15. Xiong Z, Sperelakis N, Noffsinger A, Fenoglio-Preiser C. Fast Na- current in circular smooth muscle cells of the large intestine. *Pflügers Arch* 1993; **423**: 485-491.

16. Hamill OP, Marty A, Neher E, Sakmann B, Sigworth FJ. Improved patch-clamp techniques for high-resolution current recording from cells and cell-free membrane patches. *Pflügers Arch* 1981; **391**: 85-100.

17. Horn R, Marty A. Muscarinic activation of ionic currents measured by a new whole-cell recording method. *J Gen Physiol* 1988; **92**: 145-159.

18. Komori S, Bolton TB. Calcium release induced by inositol 1,4,5 trisphosphate in single rabbit intestinal smooth muscle cells. *J Physiol* 1991; **433**: 495-517.

19. Bolton TB, Clark JP, Kitamura K, Lang RJ. Evidence that histamine and carbachol may open the same ion channels in longitudinal smooth muscle of guinea-pig ileum. *J Physiol* 1981; **320**: 363-379.

20. Benham CD, Bolton TB, Lang RJ. Acetylcholine

activates an inward current in single mammalian smooth muscle cells. *Nature* 1985; **316:** 345-346.

21. Inoue R, Isenberg G. Acetylcholine activates non-selective cation channels in guinea pig ileum through a G protein. *Am J Physiol* 1990; **258:** C1173-C1178.

22. Nagasaki M, Komori S, Tamaki H, Ohashi H. Effect of trimebutine on K⁺ current in rabbit ileal smooth muscle cells. *Eur J Pharmacol* 1993; **235:** 197-203.

23. Nagasaki M, Komori S, Ohashi H. Effect of trimebutine on voltage-activated calcium current in rabbit ileal smooth muscle cells. *Br J Pharmacol* 1993; **110:** 399-403.

24. Komori S, Bolton TB. Role of G-proteins in muscarinic receptor inward current and calcium store release in rabbit jejunal smooth muscle. *J Physiol* 1990; **427:** 395-419.

25. Komori S, Bolton TB. Inositol trisphosphate releases stored calcium to block voltage-dependent calcium channels in single smooth muscle cells. *Pflügers Arch* 1991; **418:** 437-441.

26. Ito S, Ohta T, Nakazato Y. Inward current activated by carbachol in rat intestinal smooth muscle cells. *J Physiol* 1993; **470:** 395-409.

27. Komori S, Matsuoka T, Kwon S-C, Takewaki T, Ohashi H. Membrane potential and current responses to neurotensin in the longitudinal muscle of the rectum of the fowl. *Br J Pharmacol* 1992; **107:** 790-796.

28. Matsuoka T, Komori S, Ohashi H. Membrane current responses to externally-applied ATP in the longitudinal muscle of the chicken rectum. *Br J Pharmacol* 1993; **110:** 87-94.

29. Tokuno H, Tomita T. Collagenase eliminates the electrical responses of smooth muscle to catecholamines. *Eur J Pharmacol* 1987; **141:** 131-133.

30. Muraki K, Bolton TB, Imaizumi Y, Watanabe M. Receptor for catecholamines responding to catechol which potentiates voltage-dependent calcium current in single cells from guinea-pig taenia caeci. *Br J Pharmacol* 1994; **111:** 1154-1162.

24

Use of argyrophilic nucleolar organizer region (AgNOR) staining techniques

Edda Vuhahula and Ikuko Ogawa

Summary

The nucleolar organizer regions (NOR) are loops of DNA present in the nucleoli of cells that transcribe ribosomal RNA. Active cell proliferation is accompanied by NOR dissociation resulting in NOR dispersed throughout the nucleus. The study of NOR, a parameter that reflects the functional metabolic differentiation and cell cycle phase of normal and neoplastic cells, may be useful for the evaluation of biological behaviour of some tumours. The silver staining NOR (AgNOR) technique is a relatively new method which has been applied extensively in normal, hyperplastic and malignant tissue of several lesions and a difference in quality and/or quantity of AgNOR has been demonstrated between high- and low-grade tumours and between benign and malignant counterparts of tumours of various origin, including those of gastrointestinal tract. The AgNOR dots in high-grade malignancies are numerous, highly irregular and less distinct. In contrast, in low-grade tumours these dots are larger, fewer in number and regular in shape. Since the AgNOR method is specific, simple and inexpensive, it is recommended as a routine diagnostic and prognostic parameter for the grading and/or classification of tumours of the gastrointestinal tract and also as a discriminatory parameter in borderline lesions and in tumours with similar histological patterns but different biological behaviour. This chapter describes the staining procedures and the results obtained from different laboratories.

Introduction

Nucleolar organizer regions (NOR) are loops of ribosomal DNA which occur in nuclei and direct ribosome and protein synthesis. They are localized on the short arms of acrocentric chromosomes, i.e. chromosomes 13, 14, 15, 21 and 22. The AgNOR technique has been used on chromosomal preparations to study the chromosomes in certain genetic disorders, including trisomy 21. NOR are transcribed by RNA polymerase 1 to ribosomal DNA which are assembled in the ribosomes where they are required for protein synthesis.[1-12] The NOR can accurately be demonstrated by the silver staining technique performed at room temperature on paraffin embedded tissue specimens and can be visualized with an optical microscope.[1] The technique is based on argyrophilia of non-histone NOR-associated proteins, namely RNA polymerase 1, C23 protein (nucleolin 110 kDa), B23 phosphoprotein, 78 kDa protein and C23-related protein.[1-3,13-18] The function of these proteins is uncertain; however, a role in ribosomal DNA transcription or in maintaining the conformation of DNA in the NOR is postulated.[1,2-10]

The argyrophilia of NOR proteins appears to be a good cytochemical marker of both the ribosomal DNA and the level of the actual or potential transcription of the ribosomal DNA; hence their quantity and quality seem to relate to such variables as cell proliferation rate, cell ploidy, cell transcriptional activities and tumour malignancy potential.[1-5,11,12,16-18] Moreover, AgNOR count has been shown to correlate with other methods of analysis for proliferative activity such as mitotic rate, immunohistochemistry for p53,[5] Ki-67,[6,7] PCNA,[8] expression and cell ploidy by DNA cytometry.[5,9]

Since NOR reflects the level of cell metabolism and proliferative activities, information on the biological aggressiveness - as reflected by growth rate (in this case as determined by the number or conformity of the AgNOR), may allow closer evaluation of behaviour and its possible clinical outcome.

The staining technique is simple and inexpensive, and more importantly, it is remarkably specific for detecting NOR as confirmed by ultrastructure studies.[10-12,19] The method has been suggested for use in routine tumour histology.[1,11-15]

Methods

Tissue preparation

AgNOR staining can be used on different types of tissue preparation such as frozen sections, smears, chromosomes, semi-thin sections of a plastic-embedded specimen and paraffin-embedded specimens.[1] This chapter focuses mainly on paraffin-embedded specimens which are available in most laboratories and are useful in retrospective studies. Nevertheless, the staining procedure for the different types of preparations is essentially the same.

The selection of study material and type of fixatives is very important as AgNOR stainability is known to be influenced by the methods of tissue preparation, sampling of specimens and staining procedures. Attention should be paid to rigorous technique and resolution of intranucleolar AgNOR. Smith *et al*[4] have shown that certain fixatives are highly deleterious to the AgNOR reaction. Most researchers agree that conventional 10% formal saline is a satisfactory fixation method. Alcoholic fixative may give stronger staining but this makes no difference in relation to AgNOR numbers.

For decalcified specimens, remnants of decalcifying agent may be precipitated by silver nitrate solution and therefore mistaken for AgNOR, particularly when the precipitates lie on the nucleolus. Thorough washing of tissue specimen before processing and adequate rinsing of sections during the staining process may counteract any adverse effects. Also, prolonged fixation time in formalin or any other fixative, may cause aggregation of NOR within the nucleoli. Griffiths *et al*[20] reported that AgNOR number from palatal tonsil tissue fixed for 24 hours was lower than that from tissue fixed for 30 min. Tissues fixed for 12-18 hours seem to give best results.[11,12]

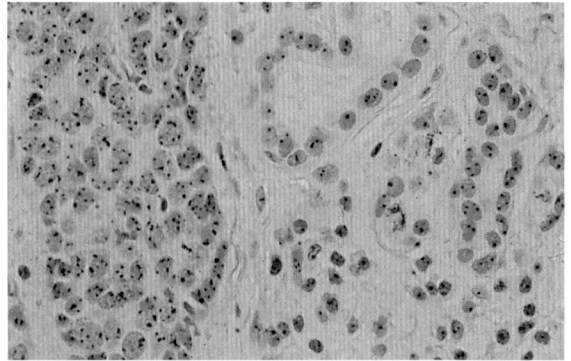

Figure 24.1 – AgNOR staining pattern in neoplastic and non-neoplastic tissue. Numerous and irregular AgNOR dots are seen in neoplastic area (left side) and are quite different from those few AgNOR with regular contour in the non-neoplastic (but hyperplastic) area (right side).

Staining procedure

For paraffin embedded blocks, 3-4 mm thick sections are suitable. For the purpose of orientation, one section should be routinely stained by hematoxylin and eosin. It must be appreciated that absolute numbers of NOR will not be resolved in the 3-4 μm thickness. The staining steps for AgNOR technique are as follows:

1. deparaffinize in xylene, 3 changes, 10 min each;
2. rehydrate through ethanol (100%, 99%, 95% and 80%), 3 min each;
3. rinse in running deionized distilled water for 10 min;
4. post-fix in ethanol/acetic acid solution (3:1) for 30 min;
5. incubate in AgNOR solution for 30 min under 20°C in the dark. (Preparation of AgNOR solution: A solution + B solution = 1:2; A solution: 2% gelatin + 1% aqueous formic acid; B solution: 50% aqueous silver nitrate);
6. rinse in the running deionized distilled water for 10 min;
7. treat with 2% gold chloride (for gold toning) for 10 min;
8. post fix with ×5 diluted photographic solution (FujiFix, Tokyo, Japan);
9. rinse in running deionized distilled water, 10 minutes.
10. counterstain with Mayer's haematoxylin, or 1% methyl green, for 30 seconds;

11. wash well in running deionized distilled water for 10 mins;
12. dehydrate in ethanol, clear in xylene and mount.

Analysis of AgNOR

The observer(s) should decide how many fields per section to examine and how many nuclei to analyse. Under the light microscope, a magnification of more than 100 is needed and therefore oil immersion should be employed. AgNOR are visualized as well-defined black or brown dots arranged individually or in clusters as shown in Figs 24.1-24.3. In the examination of AgNOR an eye piece graticule helps to minimize the re-evaluation of the dots.

The two commonest parameters evaluated are quantification of AgNOR[1,7,11,12,15] and determination of morphological changes of AgNOR conformity.[7,16,17,18] In the latter, size, shape and/or distribution of AgNOR within the nucleolus, inside and outside the nucleoli are evaluated. Crocker *et al*[15] proposed a standardized method for counting AgNOR which appears simple and reproducible in different laboratories.[11,12] Furthermore since the evaluation of NOR is subjective in nature, any method of analysis adopted should be validated. Inter-observer and intra-observer variation should be sought.

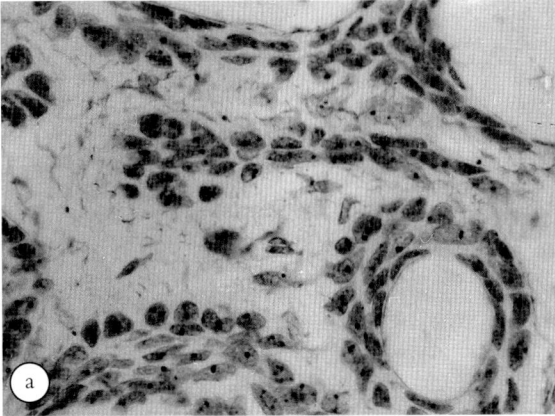

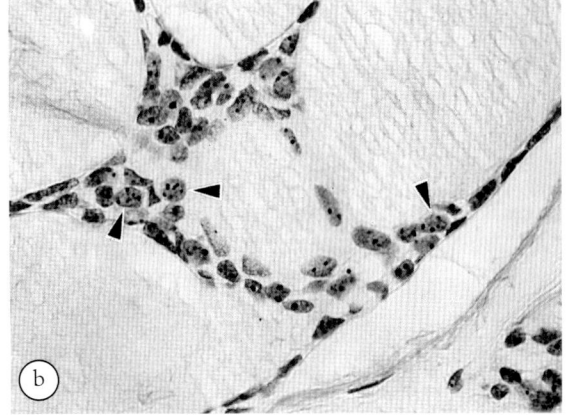

Figure 24.2 – AgNOR staining pattern in two adenoid cystic carcinomas with well-differentiated pattern. (a) Tumour with 1-3 AgNOR dots/nucleus. The patient was well after 16 years of follow-up. (b) Many AgNOR dots (arrow heads) are seen. The patient had lymph node and lung metastases and died 6 years after initial diagnosis.

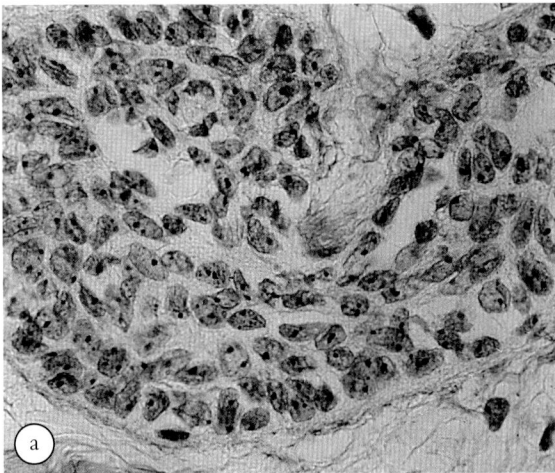

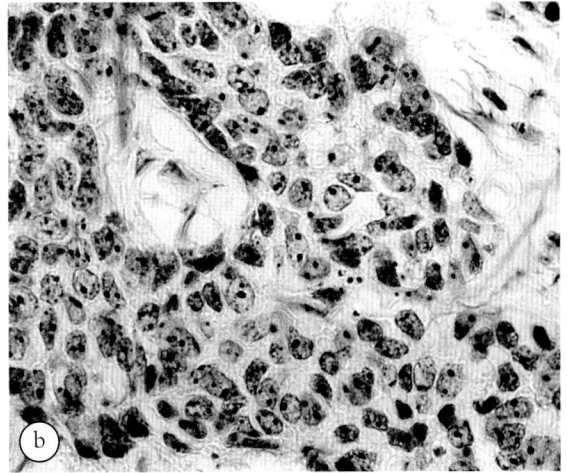

Figure 24.3 – AgNOR staining pattern in two solid tumours of salivary adenoid cystic carcinoma (i.e. poorly differentiated). (a) Few AgNOR dots are seen in a tumour which had a favourable course over a 9-year follow-up period. (b) Numerous AgNOR dots in a tumour which had an unfavorable course. The patient had lung metastasis and died 3 years after initial diagnosis.

Application to animal studies

Although the significance of NOR in experimental carcinogenesis is not yet clear, several investigators[16-18] have published promising results on the use of AgNOR evaluation in studying the process of carcinogenesis as well as in distinguishing benign from malignant tumours. Yoshimi *et al*[16] used hamster cheek pouches to study AgNOR morphological changes after inducing 7,12-dimethlybenzyl [a]anthrax, whereas Deleener *et al*[17] and Tanaka *et al*[18] used rats to analyse the AgNOR changes in the process of carcinogenesis. This promises the possibility of designing animal models for further studies of nucleolar structure and variations in nucleolar activity using the AgNOR technique in normal and pathological lesions.

Results and discussion

There appears to be greater variation in size and configuration of the AgNOR in malignant compared with normal or hyperplastic cells. Fig. 24.1 shows a section of salivary glandular tissue: the non-neoplastic part with normal tissue exhibits one or two well-defined AgNOR, whereas in the adjacent neoplastic area and in the tumours shown in Figs 24.2 and 24.3, there are numerous AgNOR dots with greater variability in size and shape. The exact biochemical nature of NOR and the mechanisms for their increased numbers in a neoplastic tissue are not fully understood. It is speculated that, whereas in a normal or relatively inactive cell the NOR are not discernible because they are tightly aggregated in the one or two nucleoli normally present in the nucleus, an increase in transcriptional activity may result in a quantitative increase of NOR from dissociation of activated NOR, and/or impaired association of NOR resulting in disorderly dispersion of NOR throughout the nucleus.[2,4-7,11-12] Moreover in the tumour with increased ploidy, such as aneuploidy tumour, an increase in NOR is expected due to an abnormal increase in NOR-bearing chromosomes. Also, an increase in transcriptional activity may result in increased prominence of NOR and the normally inconspicuous NOR may be more readily discernible. Alternatively, the disorganized NOR in the actively proliferating cells may be accompanied by association of actively NOR and/or dispersion of multiple nucleoli resulting in larger aggregates of NOR with bizarre configurations.

There has been a progressive increase in studies to validate the diagnostic and prognostic usefulness of AgNOR in certain neoplasms including tumours of gastrointestinal tract and these have met with varying degree of success.[3,5,13,14] This method promises to be a useful and accurate microscopic approach that can define cellular and/or nuclear alterations associated with degree of malignancy and which can benefit the classification, grading, diagnostic and prognostic processes, and hence influence the planning and management procedures of the patient.

The analysis of AgNOR count has been used with success to discriminate benign from malignant lesions of various origins. Studies on the predictive value of AgNOR on different types of gastrointestinal tract tumours and other sites[4,8,11,12] have provided promising results on the use of AgNOR count as a prognostic parameter. In some carcinomas such as oral squamous cell carcinoma,[13] salivary adenoid cystic carcinoma,[11,12] carcinoma of sigmoid colon and rectum[3] and advanced colorectal carcinoma,[14] the AgNOR method has been credited with providing additional prognostic advantages over histology. It is interesting to note in Vuhahula *et al's* report[12] that irrespective of histological pattern, AgNOR count corresponded well with the biological behaviour of the cases shown in Figs 24.2 and 24.3.

Fig. 24.4 shows AgNOR count in different histological patterns of salivary adenoid cystic carcinoma with respect to clinical outcome.[12] A general trend towards increased AgNOR count in association with higher grades is observed, and the difference is statistically significant ($p<0.005$) between Grade 1 and Grade 3 tumours. Higher counts were more likely to be found in poorly differentiated or solid tumours (Grade 3) with most of them exhibiting poor prognosis, whereas low counts were mainly seen in well differentiated or glandular tumours (Grade 1). However, the striking finding is that, regardless of other prognostic factors, each AgNOR count correlated well with the respective clinical behaviour of the tumour. Similar results have been published for the analysis of AgNOR count in sigmoid and colon, and advanced colorectal carcinomas.[3,14] In colorectal carcinoma, NOR were the single most reliable

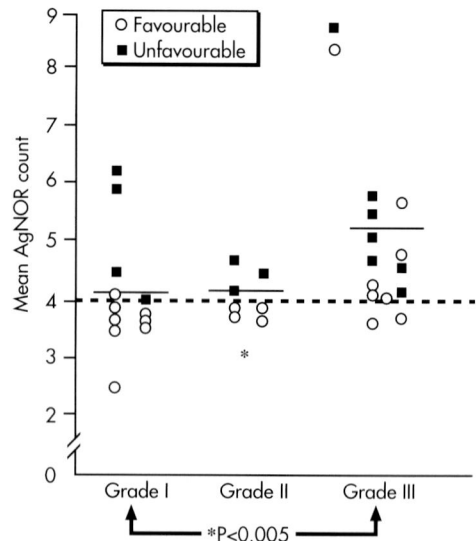

Figure 24.4 – Distribution of mean AgNOR counts per patient with different histological patterns in relation to prognosis. represents mean AgNOR count for each grade; *Wilcoxon's test.

prognostic variable for predicting the survival and correlated with decreasing degree of histological differentiation and with the presence of metastasis.

The AgNOR technique has also been credited with discriminating salivary adenoid cystic carcinoma from other tumours with low grade malignancy characteristics, e.g. polymorphous low-grade carcinoma, epithelial myoepithelial carcinoma and basal cell adenocarcinoma.[19] Significant differences in the quantity and quality of AgNOR were obtained between adenoid cystic carcinoma and the other tumours. The method is now being suggested for use in routine tumour histopathology.

Despite the usefulness of this method in tumour pathology, some drawbacks have been encountered. The overlap of AgNOR value between different lesions is to be expected, since the absolute numbers of AgNOR in nuclei cannot be evaluated in 3 or 4 μm section. On occasion this overlap may prohibit the use of this technique as an absolute criterion for establishing the final diagnosis. Also, the evaluation of AgNOR is still not yet universally standardized and is time consuming. Computer programs to assess the AgNOR would allow objective evaluation and standardization of the technique, thus eliminating variation in NOR scores reported from different laboratories and allowing meaningful comparison of different studies.

The AgNOR technique is a useful adjunct in the classification and grading of tumours, differential diagnosis between benign and malignant lesions, establishing prognosis, predicting the behaviour of the lesion and giving nucleus and nucleolar details. The method is reproducible and can be interpreted with ease.

Acknowledgement

The authors are grateful to Prof. Hiromasa Nikai, Chairman and Head of Department of Oral Pathology, Hiroshima University, School of Dentistry, who supervised this research work, and to all members of the department for their inestimable support. A great deal is owed to the sponsor of the research, the Ministry of Education, Culture and Science of Japan.

References

1. Ploton D, Meneger M, Jeannesson P, Himber G, Pigeon F, Adnej J. Improvement in the staining and visualization of the argyrophilic proteins of nucleolar organizer region at the optical level. *Histochem J* 1986; **18**: 5-14.

2. Ruschoff J, Plate K, Bittinger A, Thomas C. Nucleolar organizer (NORs). Basic concepts and practical application in tumor pathology. *Pathol Res Pract* 1989; **185**: 878-885.

3. Ruschoff J, Bittinger A, Neumann K, Schimitxz-Moorman P. Prognostic significance of nucleolar organizer in carcinoma of sigmoid colon and rectum. *Pathol Res Pract* 1990; **186**: 85-91.

4. Smith R, Crocker J. Evaluation of nucleolar organizer-associated protein in breast malignancy. *Histopathology* 1988; **12**: 113-125.

5. Derenzini M, Romagnoli T, Mingazzini P, Marinozzi V. Interphasic nucleolar organizer region distribution as a diagnostic parameter to differentiate between benign from malignant epithelial tumors of human intestines. *Virchow Arch Cell Path* 1988; **54**: 334-340.

6. Ishii K, Nakajima T. Evaluation of malignant grade of salivary gland tumor. Studies by cytofluometric nuclear DNA analysis, histochemistry for nucleolar organizer region and immunohistochemistry for p53. *Pathol Internal* 1994; **44**: 287- 296.

7. Di Stephano D, Mingazzini P, Sauchi I, Donnet M, Marinozzi V. A comparative study of histopathology, hormone resptors, peanut lectin binding, Ki-67 immunostaining and nucleolar organizer region-associated proteins in human breast cancer. *Cancer* 1991; **67**: 463-471.

8. Kawase N, Shiokawa, Ota H, Saitoh T, Yoshida H, Kazama K. Nucleolar organizer region and PCNA expression in prostatic cancer. *Pathol Internal* 1994; **44**: 213-222.

9. Giri DD, Nottngham JF, Lawry J, Dundas AC, Underwood JCE. Silver binding nucleolar regions (AgNORs) in benign and malignant breast lesions: correlation with ploidy and growth phase by DNA flow cytometry. *J Pathol* 1989; **157**: 307-313.

10. Hernandez-Verdun D, Hubert J, Bourgeouis CA, Bouteille M. Ultrastructure localization of AgNOR stained proteins in the nucleolus during the cell cycle and in other nucleolar structures. *Chromosoma* 1980; **79**: 349-362.

11. Vuhahula EAM, Nikai H, Ogawa I, Miyauchi M, Takata T, Ito H. Prognostic value of agyrophilic nucleolar organizer regions (AgNOR) count in adenoid cystic carcinoma of salivary glands.

12. Vuhahula EAM, Nikai H, Ogawa I et al. Correlation between argyrophilic nucleolar organizer region (AgNOR) counts and histologic grades with respect to biologic behavior of salivary adenoid cystic carcinoma.

J Oral Pathol Med 1995; **24**: 437–442.

13. Sano K, Takahashi H, Fujita *et al*. Prognostic implication of silver-binding nucleolar organizer regions (AgNORs) in oral squamous cell carcinoma. *J Oral Pathol Med* 1991; **20**: 53–56.

14. Moran K, Cook T, Forster G *et al*. Prognostic value in advanced colorectal cancer. *Br J Surg* 1986; **76**: 1152–1155.

15. Crocker J, Boldy, DAR, Egan MJ. How should we count AgNORs? Proposals for a standardized approach. *J Pathol* 1989; **158**: 185–188.

16. Yoshimi N, Gimenez-Canti IB, Slaga TJ. Morpholigical changes of the nucleolar organizer regions induced by 7, 12- dimethylbenz[a]anthracene in the hamster cheek pouch. *J Oral Pathol Med* 1993; **22**: 97–100.

17. Deleener A, De-Gerlache J, Lans M, Kirsch-Volders M. Nucleolar changes during the first steps of experimental hepatocarcinogenesis in rats. *Cancer Genet Cytogenet* 1985; 151–157.

18. Tanaka T, Takeuchi T, Nishikawa A, Takami T, Mori H.Nucleolar organizer regions in hepatocarcinogenesis induced by N-2-fluorerylacetamide in rats. Comparison with bromodeoxyuridine immunohistochemistry. *Jpn J Cancer Res* 1989; **80**: 1047–1051.

19. Vuhahula E. *The Prognostic Implication of Argygrophilic Nucleolar Organizer Regions (AgNOR) Count in Adenoid Cystic Carcinoma of Salivary Glands*. Thesis: Submitted in partial fulfillment of the requirements for the PhD in Dentistry and Oral Pathology, 1995.

20. Griffiths AP, Butler CW, Roberts P, Dixon MF, Quirke P. Silver stained structures (AgNORs): Their dependence on tissue fixation and absence of prognostic relevance in rectal adenocarcinoma. *J Pathol* 1989; **159**: 121–127.

25

In situ hybridization techniques as applied to the gastrointestinal tract

A Gillessen, T Pohle, M Shahin and W Domschke

Summary

Modern endoscopy gives almost complete access to the gastrointestinal tract with the option to take biopsies from the mucosa. The tissue obtained can be investigated with several methods. *In situ* hybridization requires careful handling of the tissue and organ-specific modification of the technique. This chapter highlights the problems specific to *in situ* hybridization of tissue from the gastrointestinal tract and gives detailed instructions for the application of radioactive and non-radioactive techniques. The expression of extracellular matrix protein mRNAs in healing gastric ulcers in rats is used as an example to demonstrate the use of different *in situ* hybridization techniques and the pros and cons of these techniques are evaluated.

Introduction

In situ hybridization was first described in 1969 by Gall and Pardue[1] and has been applied to the localization of DNA sequences, mRNA and chromosomal mapping. It is based on the fact that labelled single-stranded fragments of DNA or RNA containing complementary sequences (probes) under appropriate conditions hybridize *in situ* to cellular DNA or RNA forming stable hybrids. This technique enables the morphological localization of cells marked in this way in tissue sections. Specific problems may occur in applying *in situ* hybridization to tissues of the gastrointestinal (GI) tract. Cell turnover in GI mucosa is rapid. Frequent changes at the cellular and subcellular level are found in this tissue, so that even minor trauma may cause a significant change in the mucosal structure. RNases are found in high concentrations in the mucus and this causes additional problems for the *in situ* hybridization technique. Excellent organization is required to guarantee instant fixation after tissue sampling. The mucus may also be responsible for some artificial binding of probes and antibodies during the *in situ* hybridization procedure, which possibly necessitates special pretreatment of the slides.

In the human GI tract, tissue is collected by biopsy via endoscopy in almost all cases. The size of biopsy specimens, type of instrument employed and investigators' accuracy are critical in determining the quality of the collected material. The more detailed investigation of the whole thickness of the gastric wall needs surgical operation sections or animal models which give, in addition, the possibility to study experimentally-induced pathological changes during time-course experiments.

Different *in situ* hybridization techniques can be used for different parts of the GI tract. To demonstate the diversity of methods available, this chapter describes the expression of extracellular matrix protein mRNAs in healing gastric ulcers using *in situ* hybridization in rats as well as human gastric biopsies.

Methods

*Radioactive in situ hybridization using *^{35}*S-labelled single-stranded RNA probes*

Preparation of tissue sections and fixation

The aim is to retain the maximum level of cellular target RNA, maintain optimum morphological detail and enhance probe penetration. Therefore, ulcer samples are immediately frozen in liquid nitrogen and stored at -70°C until used. Tissue sections (5 μm) collected on glass slides, pretreated with 2% (v/v) aminopropyltriethoxysilane/acetone, to avoid loss of tissue during the hybridization process, are dried briefly on a hot plate at 80°C and fixed in 4% (v/v) paraformaldehyde/phosphate buffered saline (PBS; 0.1 M, pH 7.2) for 20 min. The slides are subjected to three washes in PBS and dehydration in graded ethanol (50%, 70%, 96%, 100%, (v/v)) and short air drying. The sections are packed in air-tight boxes containing desiccant and stored at -70°C.

Construction of radiolabelled (^{35}S-UTP) cRNA probes

RNA probes are obtained by inserting a specific cDNA sequence into an appropriate transcription vector (mM each), containing an RNA polymerase promotor. Hence, cDNA fragments of rat α1(I) procollagen (pα1R1) and mouse α1(III) and α1(IV) procollagens (pHf-934 and pHT21, respectively) are subcloned into the plasmid pGEM1 (Promega Biotec, Heidelberg, Germany) at the appropriate restriction sites with the exception of pHT21 which is a pGEM1-derived plasmid.[2-4]

Linearization

For transcription, the circular plasmids are linearized by a restriction endonuclease digestion, *Eco*R1 or *Hind*III (Gibco-BRL, Karlsruhe, Germany), according to the type of collagen investigated. Linearization is then tested using agarose gel-electrophoresis and λ-DNA phage, HindIII fragments as size standards.

Transcription

To obtain run-off transcripts of either the antisense (complementary to mRNA) or sense (anticomplementary, negative controls) strands, the appropriate RNA-polymerase (SP6 or T7, Gibco-BRL) is used, under optimal reaction conditions, to incorporate free ribonucleotides into single-stranded cRNA transcripts of the DNA insert. The enzyme copies certain DNA sequences from a specific promotor to generate a series of radioactively labelled ribonucleotide triphosphates into an RNA probe. This is performed using 80-100 μCi ^{35}S-uridine 5′(α-thio) triphosphate (1250 Ci/mmol; New England Nuclear, Dreieich, Germany) as previously reported.[5] Briefly, 10 μl reaction mixture (0.5 mM each adenosine-, cytidine- and guanosine-5′-triphosphate/1 mM dithiothreitol/10 units human placental RNase inhibitor/6 mM $MgCl_2$/10 mM Tris-HCl, pH 7.5/ 2 mM spermidine/10 mM NaCl), including 1 μg linearized plasmid and 16 units of either SP6 or T7 polymerase, is added to an Eppendorf tube containing the ^{35}S labeled uridine-triphoshate after lypholysation using a vacuum concentrator. The plasmid DNA is removed by digestion with 25 μg/ml RNase-free DNase I in a mixture containing 2.5 mg/ml yeast tRNA and 10 units RNase inhibitor (Promega, Heidelberg, Germany) for 10 min at 37°C. Free ribonucleotides are removed by phenol-chloroform extraction followed by ethanol precipitation.

To enhance penetration into tissue the size of the RNA probes is adjusted to 50-200 bases by controlled alkaline hydrolysis in 80 mM $NaHCO_3$/120 mM Na_2CO_3, pH 10.2/10 mM dithiothreitol (DTT) at 60°C. The reaction is then stopped with 0.2 M sodium acetate, pH 6.0/1% (v/v) acetic acid/10 mM DTT. After ethanol precipitation the incorporated radioactivity is assessed.

Prehybridization treatment of tissue sections

This step is designed to enhance accessibility of target mRNA to the probe and to decrease background labelling. The components of the prehybridization mix saturated sites in the tissue section that might otherwise bind non-specifically to nucleic acid. Briefly, basic proteins in tissue sections are neutralized with 0.2 M HCl for 20 min and rehydrated in PBS. After digestion with 0.125 mg/ml pronase

(Boehringer Mannheim, Mannheim, Germany) for 10 min, sections are quickly rinsed in 0.1 M glycine/PBS to stop the reaction and fixed in 4% (v/v) paraformaldehyde/PBS, pH 7.0 for 20 min. Slides are then washed in PBS for 3 min, acetylated with 0.25% (v/v) acetic anhydride in triethanolamine (0.1 M, pH 8.0) for 10 min to minimize non-specific binding, washed again in PBS for 5 min, dehydrated in graded ethanol and air dried prior to hybridization.[6,7]

Hybridization

25 μl of a hybridization mixture containing 5×10^5 cpm of ^{35}S-labelled RNA probe (positive or negative strand RNA probe) in 50% (v/v) formamide, 10% (v/v) dextran sulphate /10 mM DTT /10 mM Tris-HCl, pH 7.5/10 mM $NaPO_4$/ 0.3 M NaCl/5 mM ethylene diaminetetra-acitic acid (EDTA)/0.002% (v/v) Ficoll 400/0.002% (v/v) polyvinylpyrolidine/0.002% (v/v) bovine serum albumin/0.2 mg/ml yeast tRNA are applied to each section, covered with a siliconized 22 mm^2 coverslip and incubated over night (16-18 hours) in a sealed humid chamber at 50°C.

Posthybridization washing

This step must be extensive (up to several hours) as it is necessary to induce dissociation of imperfect hybrids and to reduce non-specific background signals. Excess probe is removed by gentle agitation for 5 hours at 52°C in posthybridization washing solution (0.1 M Tris-HCl, pH 7.5/0.1 M $NaPO_4$ /0.3 M NaCl/50 mM EDTA/1× Denhard's solution/10 mM DTT).

Denhardt's solution is:

1% (w/v)	polyvenylchloride
1% (w/v)	pyrrolidone
2% (v/v)	BSA

To decrease background, slides are digested with 20 μg/ml RNase A in 0.1 M Tris-HCl, pH 7.5 /1 mM EDTA/0.5 M NaCl for 30 min at 37°C, then rinsed for 30 min in the same buffer without the enzyme. Further washing by gentle agitation in descending concentrations of standard saline citrate (SSC; 300 mM NaCl/1.5 mM sodium citrate), 2×SSC, 0.1×SSC, for 30 min each at room temperature, is followed by brief dehydration in graded ethanol (30, 70, 90, 100% v/v) containing 0.3 M ammonium acetate and air drying.

Autoradiography

The slides are dipped into the photographic emulsion (e.g. Ilford G5 nuclear emulsion, Ilford, Mobberley Cheshire, UK) after being equilibrated at 43°C and diluted 1:1 with 0.6 M ammonium acetate. After drying for 2 hours, slides are stored in light-proof boxes containing desiccant and kept in the refrigerator at 4°C for exposure, which varies from 5-20 days according to the type of probe used. The exposed slides are then developed in Kodak D19 developer (Kodak, Hemel Hempstead, UK) diluted with deionized water (1:1, v/v) for 3 min with intermittent agitation, rinsed in 1% acetic acid (v/v), then fixed in Kodak Fixer diluted with deionized water (1:3, v/v) for 6 min. All steps must be carried out in total darkness or with minimal exposure to a red safelight. Finally, the sections are washed extensively in tap water, counterstained in haematoxylin-eosin, mounted in Corbitt balsam and evaluated.

Controls

The specificity of the probes is assessed by Northern blot analysis of polyadenylated RNA from normal and diseased tissue.[7] Control hybridization with sense probes is performed to assess non-specific RNA-RNA hybridization.

Non-radioactive in situ hybridization using digoxigenin-labelled riboprobes

All buffers and glassware used for the detection of RNA are made RNase-free according to standard protocols.[8] If not otherwise stated, all procedures are performed at room temperature and all chemicals are of highest purity (e.g. from Sigma).

Preparation of tissue sections and fixation

Ulcers as well as corresponding areas of intact gastric wall are dissected out and immediately placed separately in freshly prepared 4% (v/v) paraformaldehyde solution in PBS (127 mM NaCl; 2.7 mM KCl; 8.1 mM Na_2HPO_4; 1.5 mM KH_2PO_4; pH 7.4)/50 mM EDTA at 4°C. The tissues are kept in the fixative over night, followed by standard paraffin embedding.

RNA probes

Various RNA probes can be used depending on the field of study. We have used fragments of cDNA of rat pro α1(I) collagen (pα1R1) (kindly provided by

Dr D Rowe, Philadelphia, USA)[2] and human (1αIV) procollagen probe (pHT21) (kindly provided by Dr K Tryggvason, Oulu, Finland),[9] each subcloned into the PstI-restriction site of the vector pGEM 1 (Promega Biotec). The suitability of the human (1αIV) procollagen probe for rat tissues has been confirmed previously.[10]

Preparation of run-off transcripts

Sense and anti-sense RNA probes are transcribed *in vitro* from linearized plasmid containing either pα1R1 or pHT21 using digoxigenin-labelled UTP (Dig-UTP) propriate RNA polymerase (SP6 or T7) (DIG RNA Labeling Kit SP6/T7; Boehringer Mannheim, Germany). Briefly, 1 μg of linearized template DNA is incubated with 1 mM ATP, 1 mM CTP, 1 mM GTP, 0.65 mM UTP, 0.35 mM DIG-UTP, 20 units RNase inhibitor, and 40 units of the appropriate polymerase for 2 hours at 37°C. Template DNA is removed by DNase treatment (20 units DNase I, RNase-free, for 15 min at 37°C). The reaction is stopped by adding EDTA to a final concentration of 16 mM. Synthesized RNA is purified by precipitation with LiCl (0.1 mol/liter) and chilled ethanol (75% v/v); finally it is dissolved in an appropriate volume of diethylpyrocarbonate-treated distilled water. Labelling efficiency is proved by direct detection on nylon membranes as suggested by the manufacturer. The size of the probes is reduced to fragments of approximately 150 bases by alkaline lysis.[11]

Prehybridization

Tissue sections of 5 μm on aminopropyltriethoxysilane-coated glass slides are deparaffinized with xylene and rehydrated in graded ethanol (100%, 96%, 70%, 50%, (v/v)). To avoid non-specific binding of RNA probes to gastric mucus, 0.1% (v/v) xylometazoline (Zyma, Munich, Germany) is applied to the specimens.[12] The sections are immersed in 0.2 M HCl / 0.8% (v/v) pepsin A at 37°C for 20 min, refixed with 4% (v/v) paraformaldehyde solution in PBS for 20 min and acetylated with 0.1 M triethanolamine/0.25% (v/v) acetic anhydride for 10 min. The specimens are covered with prehybridization buffer (50% (v/v) formamide, 2×SSC (0.3 M NaCl; 0.03 M sodium citrate), 1×Denhardt's solution,[13] 0.5 mg/ml denatured salmon sperm DNA, 0.25 mg/ml yeast tRNA, 10% (w/v) dextran sulphate) and incubated in a humid box for approximately 2 hours at 50°C.

Hybridization

Hybridization is performed under the same conditions for 16 hours after adding a labelled probe to a final concentration of approximately 1.5 µg/ml.

Posthybridization

Procedures include two 20 min washes in a solution of 50% (v/v) formamide; 2×SSC; 1% (v/v) β-mercaptoethanol at 50°C; 20 min washes in 2×SSC and 0.1×SSC, respectively, at 50°C; and the destruction of unhybridized probe by RNase A (20 µg/ml) digestion.

Immunological detection

The detection of the probe-mRNA hybrids is performed according to Miller *et al*,[14] with some modifications. Briefly, the sections are blocked with 2% (v/v) normal sheep serum (NSS) and 0.05% Triton X-100 (Boehringer Mannheim) in 2×SSC for 1 hour at room temperature. The slides are washed twice for 5 min with buffer 1 (50 mM Tris-HCl; 225 mM NaCl; pH 7.5) before antibody solution (alkaline phosphatase-conjugated F(ab) fragments of anti-digoxigenin antibody (Boehringer Mannheim) at a dilution of 1:1000; 1% (v/v) NSS; 0.3% (v/v) Triton X-100 in buffer 1) is applied in a humid chamber at 37°C for 2 hours. Unbound antibody conjugate is removed by two 5 min washes in buffer 1; then the slides are equilibrated in buffer 2 (100 mM Tris-HCl, 100 mM NaCl; 50 mM $MgCl_2$; pH 9.5) for 10 min. Non-specific alkaline phosphatase activity is blocked by 5 mM levamisole; the digoxigenin-anti-digoxigenin conjugates are visualized with 0.15 mg/ml 5-bromo-4-chloro-3-indolyl phosphate/0.3 mg/ml nitro blue tetrazolium (BCIP/NBT) in 100 mM Tris buffer and 5 mM $MgCl_2$, pH 9.5. Then the slides are dehydrated and observed without nuclear counterstain. Photomicrographs are taken with a differential interference microscope (Leitz, Wetzlar, Germany).

Controls

Controls for specificity include the omission of probe (to exclude the possibility of non-specific binding of the anti-digoxigenin antibody) and the anti-digoxigenin antibody (to check for non-specific alkaline phosphatase activity) and the destruction of target mRNA by incubating the sections with RNAse A (100 µg/ml; Sigma) prior to detection (to exclude binding of probe to tissue components other than RNA), or hybridization with the sense probe (to assess non-specific RNA-RNA hybridization).

Application to animal studies

The technique of acid induction of gastric ulcers in rats is widespread and well accepted. After laparotomy in deep narcosis, male Wistar rats (body weight 200-220 g) receive a single application of acetic acid on the serosa of the stomach.[15] Groups of 10 animals are sacrificed after 2, 5, 7, 9, 12, 15, 20, 30 and 60 days. The stomachs are removed and ulcers as well as corresponding areas of intact gastric wall are dissected and immediately stored in fixation medium. Control animals are treated in the same manner but without the application of acid.

Results and discussion

Both *in situ* hybridization techniques bind specifically to the target mRNAs in the tissue regardless of the type of fixation. In specimens from control rat stomachs, only a very few signals are detectable. In ulcer tissue, the stroma of the submucosa and the lamina propria next to the ulcer contain many cells expressing procollagen α1(I), procollagen α1(III), as well as α1(IV) collagen mRNA. The signals are restricted to mesenchymal cells, while epithelial cells show no reactivity. Type I, III and IV collagen mRNA are expressed in cells of the granulation tissue beneath the ulcer craters (Figs. 25.1 and 25.2). A pronounced expression of α1(IV) collagen mRNA is found along the serosal cell layer and perivascular sites of normal and ulcer specimens (Fig. 25.3). In the ulcer area, both probes for procollagen type I showed the clearest signals, while the type III probes are found in almost the same distribution, but with slightly weaker intensity. The increase of collagen mRNA expression starts on day 3 and continues up to day 20. Interestingly, procollagen mRNA for type I and III is also detectable in certain layers of the muscularis propria (Fig. 25.4).

Regarding the choice of label for *in situ* hybridization, many investigators apply radioisotopes because of their higher sensitivity due to the variability of autoradiographic exposure time.[16-18] A large body of evidence has accumulated suggesting that non-radioactive labels, especially digoxigenin, yield comparable results.[19,20]

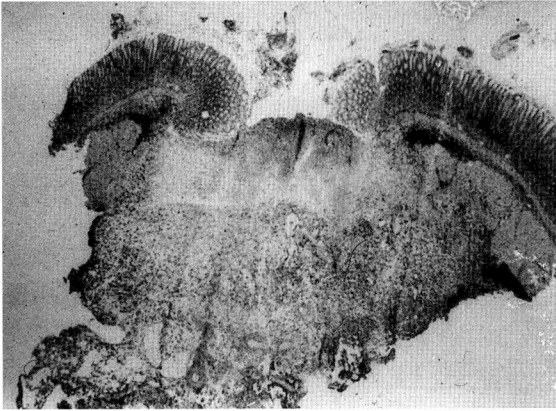

Figure 25.1 - In situ hybridization with ³⁵S-labelled α(I) procollagen anti-sense RNA probe on rat gastric ulcer on day 3. Strong cellular labelling predominantly in the submucosa at the ulcer margin indicates a remarkable upregulation of collagen synthesis as early as 3 days after ulcer induction. Magnification ×160.

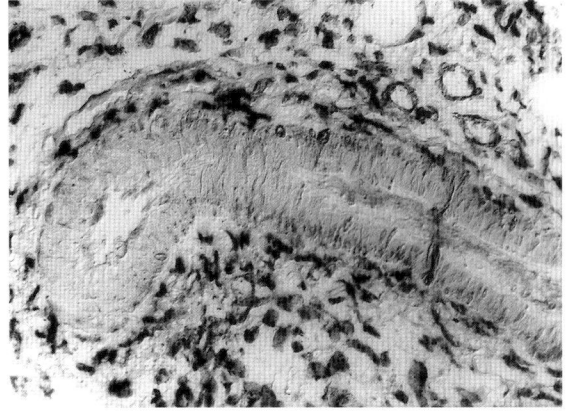

Figure 25.3 - The perivascular region in the submucosa next to the ulcer crater from a 5-day-old rat. Collagen type IV-mRNA (digoxigenin-labelled pro α(IV) collagen RNA probe) is highly expressed in the stroma cells of this area. Magnification ×350.

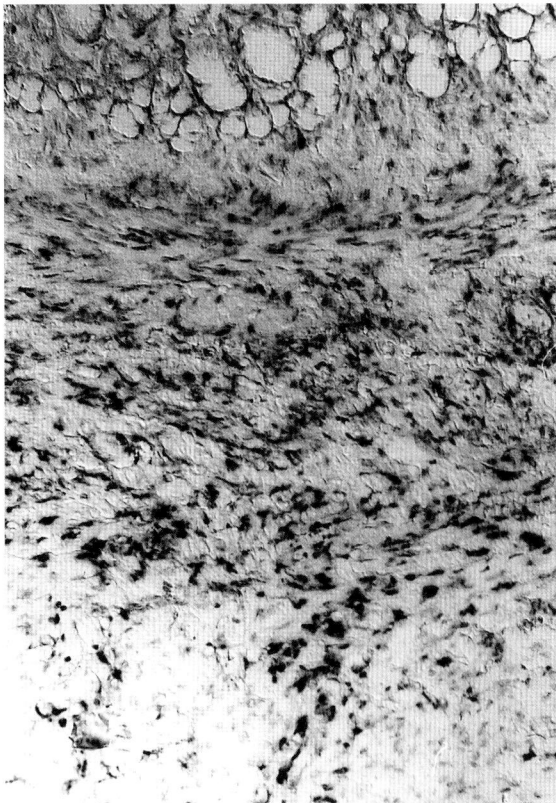

Figure 25.2 - Microphotogram of a 12-day-old rat gastric ulcer subject to *in situ* hybridization with a digoxigenin-labelled pro α(I) collagen RNA probe. Signals are distributed in the submucosa beneath cystically dilated glands which cover the former ulcer; few signals are present in the mesenchymal component of the mucosa. Magnification ×187.

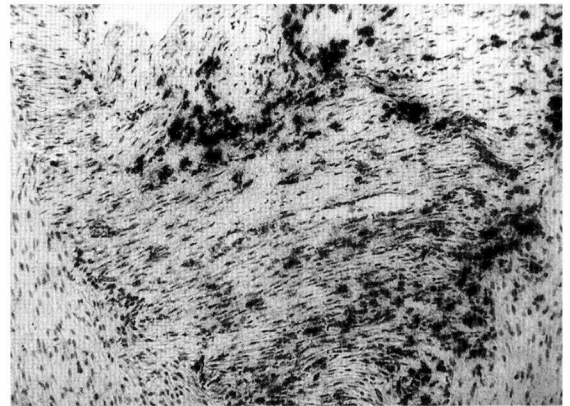

Figure 25.4 - In situ hybridization with ³⁵S-labelled α(III) procollagen anti-sense RNA probe on a rat gastric ulcer on day 7. Strong cellular labelling is seen in certain layers of the muscularis propria underneath the ulcer. Magnification ×160.

Non-radioactive *in situ* hybridization has gained importance because labels are independent of the half-life of radioisotopes and can yield results within 2 days. Further advantages are the lack of radiation and the visualization of hybridization signals at the level of the section (and not in an emulsion layered on top).[21]

Regarding the sensitivity and specificity of the applied digoxigenin system, the use of BCIP/NBT as substrate for alkaline phosphatase is said to be superior to most other substrate systems[22] as well as to other immunological detection methods.[23]

Although the possibility of a semiquantitative assessment of gene expression by counting the grains might favour the use of isotopes in some research settings, first attempts are being made to quantitate hybridization signals of non-radioactive labels by microphotometric measurement of the mean optical densities of the alkaline phosphatase reaction product using a computer-controlled scanning microscope photometer.[24]

The physiology of the human GI tract may pose some difficulties for the application of non-isotopic *in situ* hybridization to tissues of this origin, as brush-border membranes of the epithelial lining cells contain high amounts of alkaline phosphatase which cannot be inhibited by levamisole. Therefore, the acidic depurination step of the pretreatment procedure should be included, because acid treatment inactivates these phosphatases. Another problem inherent to gut tissue is the mucus covering the luminal surface. Mucus components may bind the labelled probe in a non-specific manner. If this problem should occur and cannot be overcome by modification of the conventional pretreatment procedures, the inclusion of a digestion step utilizing xylometazoline 0.1% (v/v) may be helpful.[12] Although not documented, another cause of non-specific staining may be the cross-reactivity of the commonly used polyvalent anti-digoxigenin-antibody with pharmacologically

applied digoxin (see ordering information supplied by Boehringer Mannheim,). In addition, digoxigenin is one of the commonest metabolites of digoxin.[25] In tissues containing high amounts of digoxin, such as the myocardium, digitalis may be demonstrable by immunohistochemistry.[26]

In summary, for highly expressed mRNAs like procollagen type I the non-radioactive *in situ* hybridization technique is favoured while the radioactive method with ^{35}S-labelled riboprobes is the more sensitive method and should be reserved for mRNAs with weak expression (Table 25.1). With the modifications mentioned above, *in situ* hybridization is an effective tool in several diagnostic procedures applied to the GI tract.

Acknowledgments

We are grateful to Dr D Rowe, Philadelphia, Dr D Schuppan, Berlin, Dr D Rowe, Farmington, Dr DJ Prockop, Philadelphia, and Dr K Tryggvason, Oulu, for providing the cDNA of rat pro (1(I) collagen (p(1R1) and human pro (1(IV) collagen (pHT21), respectively. We also wish to acknowledge the excellent technical assistance of Mrs M Humberg and Mrs G Puls.

References

1. Gall JC, Pardue ML. Formation and detection of RNA-DNA hybrid molecules in cytological preparations. *Proc Natl Acad Sci* USA 1969; **63:** 378-383.

2. Genovese C, Rowe D, Kream B. Construction of DNA sequences complementary to rat α1 and α2(I) collagen mRNA and their use in studying the regulation in type I collagen synthesis by 1,25-dihydroxyvitamin D. *Biochemistry* 1984; **23:** 6210-6216.

3. Liau G, Yamada Y, de Crombrugghe B. Coordinate regulation of the level of type III and type I collagen mRNA in most but not all mouse fibroblasts. *J Biol Chem* 1985; **260:** 531-536

4. Nath P, Laurant M, Horn E, Sobel ME, Zon G, Vogeli G. Isolation of an α1 type IV collagen cDNA clone using a synthetic oligodeoxynucleotide. *Gene* 1986; **43:** 301-304.

5. Haffner R, Willson K. *In situ* hybridization to messenger RNA in tissue sections. In Monk M (ed) *Mammalian Development.* IRL Press, Oxford, 1987, pp. 199-215.

6. Hogan B, Costantini F, Lacy E. *Manipulating the Mouse Embryo. A Laboratory Manual.* Cold Spring Harbor

Table 25.1 – Comparison of advantages of radioactive and non-radioactive *in situ* hybridization (ISH) techniques.

Radioactive ISH	Non-radioactive ISH
Higher sensitivity	Faster (2 vs 5-20 days)
"Gain up" with longer autoradiography	Signal in the cells
Silver grains to count	No radioactivity

Laboratory, Cold Spring Harbor, 1986, pp. 228–242.

7. Milani S, Herbst H, Schuppan D, Hahn EG, Stein H. *In situ* hybridization for procollagens type I, III and IV mRNA in normal and fibrotic rat liver. Evidence for predominant expression in non-parenchymal liver cells. *Hepatology* 1989; **10**: 84–92.

8. Sambrook J, Fritsch EF, Maniatis T. *Molecular Cloning: A Laboratory Manual*, 2nd edn. Cold Spring Harbor Laboratory, Cold Spring Harbor, 1989.

9. Pihlajaniemi T, Tryggvason K, Myers JC *et al.* cDNA clones coding for the pro-α1 (IV) chain of human type IV procollagen reveal an unusual homology of amino acid sequences in two halves of the carboxyl-terminal domain. *J Biol Chem* 1985; **260**: 7681–7687.

10. Cleutjens JPM, Havenith MG, Beek C, Vallinga M, Ten Kate J, Bosman FT. Origin of basement membrane type IV collagen in xenografted human epithelial tumor cell lines. *Am J Pathol* 1990; **136**: 1165–1172.

11. Cox KH, DeLeon DV, Angerer LM, Angerer RC. Detection of mRNAs in sea urchin embryos by *in situ* hybridization using asymmetric RNA probes. *Dev Biol* 1984; **101**: 485–502.

12. Van den Berg FM, Zijlmans H, Langenberg W, Rauws E, Schipper M. Detection of campylobacter pylori in stomach tissue by DNA *in situ* hybridisation. *J Clin Pathol* 1989; **42**: 995–1000.

13. Denhardt DT. A membrane-filter technique for the detection of complementary DNA. *Biochem Biophys Res Comm* 1966; **23**: 641–646.

14. Miller MA, Kolb PE, Raskind MA. A method for simultaneous detection of multiple mRNAs using digoxigenin and radioisotopic cRNA probes. *J Histochem Cytochem* 1993; **41**: 1741–1750.

15. Okabe S, Roth JLA, Pfeiffer CJ. A methods for experimental, penetrating gastric and duodenal ulcers in rats. *Dig Dis Sci,* 1971; **16**: 277–284.

16. Li J, Stefaneanu L, Kovacs K, Horvath E, Smyth HS. Growth hormone (GH) and prolactin (PRL) gene expression and immunoreactivity in GH- and PRL-producing human pituitary adenomas. *Virchows*

Arch A Pathol Anat 1993; **422**: 193–201.

17. Stefaneanu L, Kovacs K, Horvath E, Lloyd RV. *In situ* hybridization study of pro-opiomelanocortin (POMC) gene expression in human pituitary corticotrophs and their adenomas. *Virchows Arch A Pathol Anat* 1991; **419**: 107–113.

18. Wilcox JN. Fundamental principles of *in situ* hybridization. *J Histochem Cytochem* 1993; **41**: 1725–1733.

19. Komminoth P, Merk FB, Wolfe HJ, Roth J. Comparison of ^{35}S and digoxigenin-labeled RNA and oligonucleotide probes for *in situ* hybridization. *Histochemistry* 1992; **98**: 217–228.

20. Xerri L, Monges G, Guigou V, Parc P, Hassoun J. Detection of gastrin mRNA by *in situ* hybridization using radioactive- and digoxigenin-labelled probes: a comparative study. *APMIS* 1992; **100**: 949–953.

21. Wiethege T, Voss B, Pohle T, Fisseler-Eckhoff A, Müller KM. Localization of elastase and tumor necrosis factor mRNA by non-radioactive *in situ* hybridization in cultures of alveolar macrophages. *Pathol Res Pract* 1991; **187**: 912–915.

22. Ehrlein J, Wanke R, Weis S, Brem G, Hermanns W. Sensitive detection of human growth hormone mRNA in routinely formalin-fixed, paraffin-embedded transgenic mouse tissues by non-isotopic *in situ* hybridization. *Histochemistry* 1994; **102**: 145–152.

23. Cremers AFM, Jansen in de Wal N, Wiegant J *et al.* Non-radioactive *in situ* hybridization. A comparison of several immunocytochemical detection systems using reflection-contrast and electron microscopy. *Histochemistry* 1987; **86**: 609–615.

24. Asan E, Kugler P. Qualitative and quantitative detection of alkaline phosphatase coupled to an oligonucleotide probe for somatostatin mRNA after *in situ* hybridization using unfixed rat brain tissue. *Histochemistry* 1995; **103**: 463–471.

25. Gault MH, Longerich LL, Loo JC *et al.* Digoxin biotransformation. *Clin Pharmacol Ther* 1984; **35**: 74–82.

26. Sotonyi P. Morphological examination of cardiac glycoside in myocardial cells. *Tokai J Exp Clin Med* 1990; **15**: 227–233.

26

Diagnostic morphological methods: Use of immunomorphological and enzymohistochemical methods for a single disease entity

Luigi Maiuri

Summary

Primary adult-type hypolactasia is the most common form of genetically determined disaccharidase deficiency. The analysis of the expression and distribution of lactase mRNA, protein and activity by a multi-faceted morphological approach (immunohistochemistry, enzymohistochemistry, non-isotopic *in situ* hybridization) reveals that in the proximal jejunum of adults with persistent high lactase activity, lactase mRNA, protein and activity are uniformly expressed in all villous enterocytes. In contrast, in all individuals with adult-type hypolactasia two populations of enterocytes (lactase positive and lactase negative) are present in the villous. The lactase positive enterocytes of hypolactasic tissues also have comparatively lower lactase activity than enterocytes from individuals with persistently high activity. Therefore the presence of villous enterocytes lacking lactase mRNA and/or protein or activity is a useful diagnostic marker of adult-type hypolactasia. The correlation between the number of enterocytes that express lactase and the levels of lactase-specific activity in hypolactasic tissues shows that morphological criteria are an alternative method for the diagnosis of adult-type hypolactasia in human biopsy specimens from the proximal small jejunum.

Introduction

The diagnosis of many diseases is facilitated by the detection of the expression and distribution of antigens (proteins) in different tissues. The lack (or the abnormal expression) of different antigens may be the hallmark of different pathologies and may represent either the primary defect or a consequence of an impaired metabolic pathway. In some circumstances these abnormally expressed proteins may have an enzymatic function and consequently an abnormal enzyme activity may be detected. Usually the diagnosis of several enzyme deficiencies is performed by biochemical analysis of the gene product (assessment of enzyme activity) or by molecular characterization of the gene defect and in some cases by the detection only of products of the impaired metabolic pathways. In this chapter it is demonstrated that, under some circumstances, genetically determined enzyme dificiencies may be easily revealed by the detection of abnormal expression and distribution of RNA, protein or enzyme activity at the pathological site by morphological techniques.

This is the case for adult-type hypolactasia. In such a disease a multi-faceted morphological approach may be useful diagnostically and from analysis of the localization of the gene transcript as well as of the gene product, reveal the pathogenic mechanisms causing disease.

Primary adult-type hypolactasia is the most common form of genetically determined disaccharidase deficiency. In most humans and mammals, intestinal lactase activity declines, on weaning, to about 5-10% of the activity at birth. In a very high proportion of the population of northern Europe, however, and many other milk-drinking areas of the world, lactase activity persists into adult life.[1] These two phenotypes, namely lactase persistent and lactase non-persistent (adult hypolactasia), are genetically determined[1,2] and are attributable to different alleles at one autosomal locus. Lactase deficiency in adults is the recessive phenotype.[3]

Individuals are classified as hypolactasic or lactase persistent by determining the ratio between sucrase and lactase activity in mucosal scrapings of jejunal biopsies. In an extended survey of individuals in southern Italy, which contained mainly hypolactasic subjects, many of whom had very low levels of lactase activities, a lactase/sucrase ratio of 0.17 was considered a convenient benchmark to discriminate the two groups.[4]

The cellular basis of adult-type hypolactasia has been widely investigated by biochemical, molecular and histological approaches. Lactase-phloryzin-hydrolase (LPH) is synthesized as a single chain 115-145 kDa precursor, with subsequent proteolytic processing into the 150-160 kDa mature form which is inserted into the brush-border membrane.[1] *In vitro* biosynthetic studies have shown a markedly reduced synthesis of the precursor of the lactase protein in duodenal and jejunal peroral or surgical biopsy specimens from most individuals with adult-type hypolactasia;[5-8] slower processing of the protein[6,8] or higher label incorporation of [^{35}S]-methionine into lactase protein have been found in a few hypolactasic tissues,[8] thus demonstrating that adult-type hypolactasia is a heterogeneous condition.

Heterogeneity of adult-type hypolactasia has also been shown at the messenger RNA level. In most samples, there was apparently a marked reduction of lactase mRNA,[7,9] whereas in some subjects, high levels of transcripts encoding the LPH protein were found.[9]

In recent years a morphological approach has been used to define the physiological mechanisms leading to lactase deficiency in mammals and man. These morphological studies have provided an understanding of the pathogenesis of adult-type hypolactasia; moreover, they form a simple diagnostic approach to this disease entity.

Methods

Morphological studies are performed on jejunal biopsies, from around the Treitz region, from subjects with persistent high lactase activity or with adult-type hypolactasia. In all samples assessment of disaccharidase activities is performed as previously reported.[1,10-12] Similar experiments have also been carried out on the small intestine from white New Zealand rabbits of different ages (15-day-old suckling animals, which show high levels of lactase activity in the small jejunum, and 8-month-old adult animals, showing adult-type hypolactasia). In rabbits, the jejunum and ileum is divided in three equal parts, corresponding to the proximal, middle and distal small intestine.[13] Part of the tissue from each intestinal region is fixed in 4% (w/v) buffered paraformaldehyde and paraffin embedded according to routine histological procedures; another part is embedded in OCT compound (Tissue Tek, Miles Lab, Elkhart, IN, USA), snap frozen in isopenthane cooled in liquid nitrogen and then stored at -70°C until used; a third part is fixed in 4% buffered paraformaldheyde and then processed for surface immuno- and enzymo-histochemistry.[13]

Immunohistochemistry

Eight monoclonal antibodies to human lactase are used to detect the human lactase protein (kindly donated by Dr Dallas Swallow, MRC, University College, London, UK).[14,15] Four monoclonal antibodies can also be used to detect rabbit lactase protein.[16] A monoclonal antibody to human sucrase is used in human tissues as control antibody (kindly donated by Dr Quaroni, Cornell University, Ithaca, USA).

Three μm paraffin embedded deparafinized sections are repeatedly washed at room temperature in Tris buffered saline (TBS) and then incubated with 0.3% H_2O_2 for 30 min followed by incubation with 0.004% protease XXIV (Sigma Chem Co, St Louis,

MO, USA) for 30 min. The sections are then individually incubated with different monoclonal antibodies against human lactase overnight at 4°C, followed by biotinylated rabbit anti-mouse Ig (Dako, Copenhagen, Denmark, 1:300 for 1 hour) and peroxidase-conjugated streptavidin (Dako, 1:600 for 1 hour). The peroxidase is visualized by 0.01% H_2O_2-diaminobenzydine-tetrahydrocloride (Sigma), and the sections are then counterstained with Mayer's hematoxylin and mounted.

Enzymohistochemistry

Ten μm cryostat sections are collected on slides and air dried at room temperature. The experiments are carried out according to the procedure described by Lojda & Kraml.[17] Briefly, the sections are incubated in a medium containing 3 mg 5-Br-4-Cl-3-indolyl-β-D-fucoside (Sigma) as a substrate dissolved in 0.3 ml dimethylformamide: 6 ml 0.1 M citrate phosphate buffer, pH 6 are added and shaken well: 0.5 ml 0.05 M potassium ferricyanide and 0.5 ml 0.05 M potassium ferrocyanide are added. The mixture is shaken and filtered.[17] The sections are incubated for 5, 15, 30, 45, 60 and 120 min at 37°C.[4] The reaction is stopped by washing in saline and fixing in 4% formaldheyde. The sections are then mounted and analysed under the microscope. The reaction is considered positive when a blue colour appears on the brush-border membranes.

The same sectons are then submitted to quantitative analysis of lactase expression.[4,18] The amount of indigo formed by hydrolysis of the substrate is determined by using an IBAS 2000 microphotometer set (Zeiss, Germany) at 660 nm. The absorbance of the sample is expressed as optical density integrated for the examined area, allowing a homogeneous evaluation of the sample. Five cells of three different sections are examined for each sample and the mean value is calculated.

Surface immunohistochemistry

The procedure is as described by Schmidt et al.[13,19]. After fixation human and rabbit samples are treated with DL-dithiothreitol (Sigma) for 1 hour at 4°C to remove mucin. A single layer of villi is dissected and the muscle of the gut wall removed under the microscope. The villous layer is then incubated in Petri dishes with 0.1% phenylhydrazine HCl (Sigma) in PBS for 30 min to remove endogenous peroxidase and then with monoclonal anti-lactase antibodies (diluted 1:5 in PBS, overnight at 4°C). This is followed by incubation with peroxidase-conjugated rabbit Ig directed against mouse Ig (Dako; 1:100 in PBS containing 0.5% bovine serum albumin, for 1 hour at room temperature) and then peroxidase-antiperoxidase complex (Dako; 1:100 in PBS containing 0.5% bovine serum albumin, for 1 hour at room temperature). Peroxidase is subsequently detected as for conventional immunohistochemistry. The microscopic observation is perfomed on whole preparation at 40× magnification using a stereomicroscope (Zeiss, Germany).

Surface enzymohistochemistry

Samples are processed as for surface immunohistochemistry.[13] A single layer of dissected villi is incubated in Petri dishes with 5Br-4Cl-3indolyl-β-D-fucoside, as for conventional enzymohistochemistry. The reaction is carried out at 37°C for 24 hours and stopped by washing in saline and fixing in 4% (w/v) formaldehyde. The reaction is considered positive when a blue colour appears on the villous wall.

Detection of lactase mRNA by non-isotopic in situ hybridization

The lactase DNA template used for *in vitro* transcription is a small genomic segment containing all of exon 12 (203 base pairs (bp)) and a total of 97 additional flanking nucleotides cloned into the *Hind*II and *Sma*I sites of the vector pGEM-3, which was subcloned from a clone λ chr lac 19 (kindly supplied by Dr Ned Mantei, Laboratorium fur Biochemie, ETH Zentrum, Zurich, Switzerland).[20] The plasmid is linearized with *Hind*III for T7 transcription and *Eco*RI for the SP6 transcription. The transcription with digoxygenin-uridine triphosphate (Boehringer Mannheim, Indianapolis, IN, USA) using T7 polymerase (BRL, Bethesda, MD, USA) as antisense probe and SP6 polymerase (BDH) sense probe is performed as recommended by Boehringer Mannheim in their non-radioactive *in situ* hybridization manual. Digoxygenin incorporation is measured by dot blot analysis of serial dilutions of the probe and detection with anti-digoxygenin. The amount of RNA transcribed is determined using ethidium bromide by the 'Saran-wrap' serial dilution method and compared with dilutions of a standard RNA solution.[21]

Four µm paraffin embedded sections are mounted on aminoalkylsilane-treated slides.[22,23] The slides are then deparafinized, hydrated and incubated in 0.3% Triton-X-100-PBS for 15 min and 0.1 M glycine-PBS for 5 min. The RNA is unmasked by exposing the sections to 10 µg/ml proteinase K (BDH, Poole, UK) in 0.1 M Tris-HCl (pH 8.0) and 50 mM ethylenediamonetetraacetic acid at 37°C for 30 min. After proteolysis, sections are quickly rinsed in PBS and distilled water, postfixed in 4% (w/v) paraformaldehyde in PBS for 5 min and immersed in 0.25% acetic anhydride (BDH) in 0.1 M triethanolamine (BDH) for 10 min. The sections are then prehybridized in 50% formamide, 2×SSC, 0.3% bovine serum albumin and 250 µg/ml denatured salmon sperm DNA at 45°C for 30 min, dehydrated through a graded ethanol series up to 99% ethanol and left to air dry. Hybridization is performed at 45°C for 16 hours. The hybridization buffer contains 50% formamide, 2×SSC, 10% dextran sulphate, 0.25% bovine serum albumin, 0.25% Ficoll 400 (Sigma), 0.25% polyvinyl pyrrolidone-360 (BDH), 10 mmol/l Tris-HCl (pH 7.5), 0.5% sodium dodecyl sulphate, and 250 mg/ml denatured salmon sperm DNA. The probe concentration is 5 ng/µl in hybridization buffer. Next, 20 µl of the solution is carefully applied on the section, which is covered with a coverslip. After hybridization, the coverslips are gently removed in 2×SSC; then the sections are washed by placing the slides vertically in a rack and immersing the rack in 4 litres of 2×SSC for 30 min at 45°C. The wash is stirred continuously with a magnetic stirrer; followed by a wash in 0.2×SSC (15 min at 45°C) and finally with 0.1×SSC (15 min at 45°C). The sections are then transferred to PBS (2 × 10 min at 37°C) and finally incubated with 3% normal goat serum for 20 min and then with TBS. The probe is visualized by the peroxidase immunodetection method (see above) by incubating the sections with peroxidase-conjugated sheep anti-digoxygenin (Boehringer Mannheim) for 2 × 1 hour (working dilution, 1:50), The peroxidase is visualized as for immunohistochemistry. Hybridization with the sense probe under the same experimental conditions serves as the control.

Morphometric analysis

The number of enterocytes expressing the lactase mRNA and/or protein or activity is independently calculated by counting 300 villous enterocytes and is expressed as a percentage of the total number of absorptive cells. Statistical evaluation of each variable is calculated by the Wilcoxon rank test.

Results and discussion

Immunomorphological analysis with monoclonal antibodies to human lactase reveals that all the villous enterocytes express the lactase protein in the proximal jejunum of subjects with persistent high lactase activity.[14] In contrast, in hypolactasic samples the lactase protein is patchily distributed on the villous with some enterocytes expressing the lactase protein surrounded by a majority of negative cells (Fig. 26.1), whereas sucrase and isomaltase proteins show uniform distribution.[14]

The presence of two populations of enterocytes (lactase-positive and lactase-negative) is a constant phenomenon in proximal small intestine of hypolactasic subjects. The number of enterocytes which express the lactase protein significantly correlates with the lactase-specific activity in the hypolactasic tissues which show reduced synthesis of lactase proteins.[23]

Patchy expression of lactase protein is also observed in the small intestine of rabbits after weaning,[16] whereas in small intestine from suckling rabbits a uniform expression of lactase is evident in all villous enterocytes. However, in adult mammals an unexpected degree of complexity in the expression of the lactase protein has been found along the villous and proximal-distal axis of the small intestine. In proximal and distal regions the lactase protein is present only in patches of positive enterocytes principally located on the lower part of the villous, whereas other enterocytes contain no detectable protein;[16] in the mid small intestine, there is uniform distribution of lactase protein. Two populations of enterocytes (lactase positive and lactase negative) are therefore present in proximal and distal regions of the adult mammalian intestine, whereas only lactase positive enterocytes are present in the mid small intestine. In humans the patchiness of the expression of lactase is probably limited to the proximal and distal parts of the small intestine. The presence of enterocytes without lactase appears to be one cause of adult-type hypolactasia.

Enzymohistochemical analysis of frozen tissue reveals that in subjects with persistent high lactase activity, the lactase activity is detected in all villous enterocytes, whereas in tissues with adult-type hypolactasia and reduced *in vitro* biosynthesis of lactase protein the lactase activity shows the same patchy distribution as the lactase protein.[13] Moreover, differences in lactase positive enterocytes also exist between lactase persistent and hypolactasic individuals. Assessment of lactase activity in single enterocytes by quantitative enzymocytochemistry[4] demonstrates that activity increases linearly over time in both persistent and hypolactasic samples; however, absorbance is greater in the former at all incubation times (p<0.001). At 60 min of incubation the lactase activity in persistent tissues is 4.6 times higher than in hypolactasic tissues. Moreover, in persistent tissues lactase activity is detected after only 5 minutes of incubation with the substrate, whereas in hypolactasic tissues it is still undetectable after 15 min and appears only after 30 min of incubation. These findings suggest that lactase-positive enterocytes of hypolactasic tissues have less lactase activity than enterocytes of persistent individuals.

Surface immunohistochemical and enzymohistochemical analysis[13] reveal that in tissues with persistent high lactase activity a uniform expression of both lactase protein and lactase activity is evident on the villous wall from the base to the top of the villi (Fig. 26.2a).[13] Hypolactasic subjects show scattered areas of enterocytes which express lactase protein and lactase activity randomly distributed on the villous wall and there are no continuous ribbons or sheets of positive cells (Fig. 26.2b), as would be expected if the origin of this phenomenon were clonal.[13]

In the proximal jejunum of adult rabbits a few vertical continuous sheets of lactase positive enterocytes arise from the base of the villi and stop at different levels along the villous wall (Fig. 26.2c); in contrast in the mid small intestine lactase protein and lactase activity

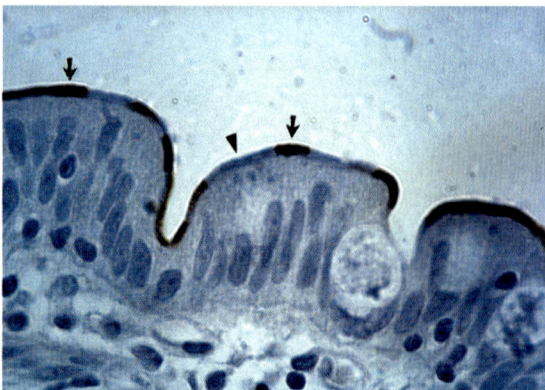

Figure 26.1 - Lactase protein expression in villous enterocytes in the proximal jejunum of human subjects with adult-type hypolactasia. The lactase protein is patchily distributed. Note that lactase expression is present in some villous enterocytes (arrows), whereas others fail to show any staining (arrowhead). Immunohistochemistry, peroxidase staining technique, original magnification ×800.

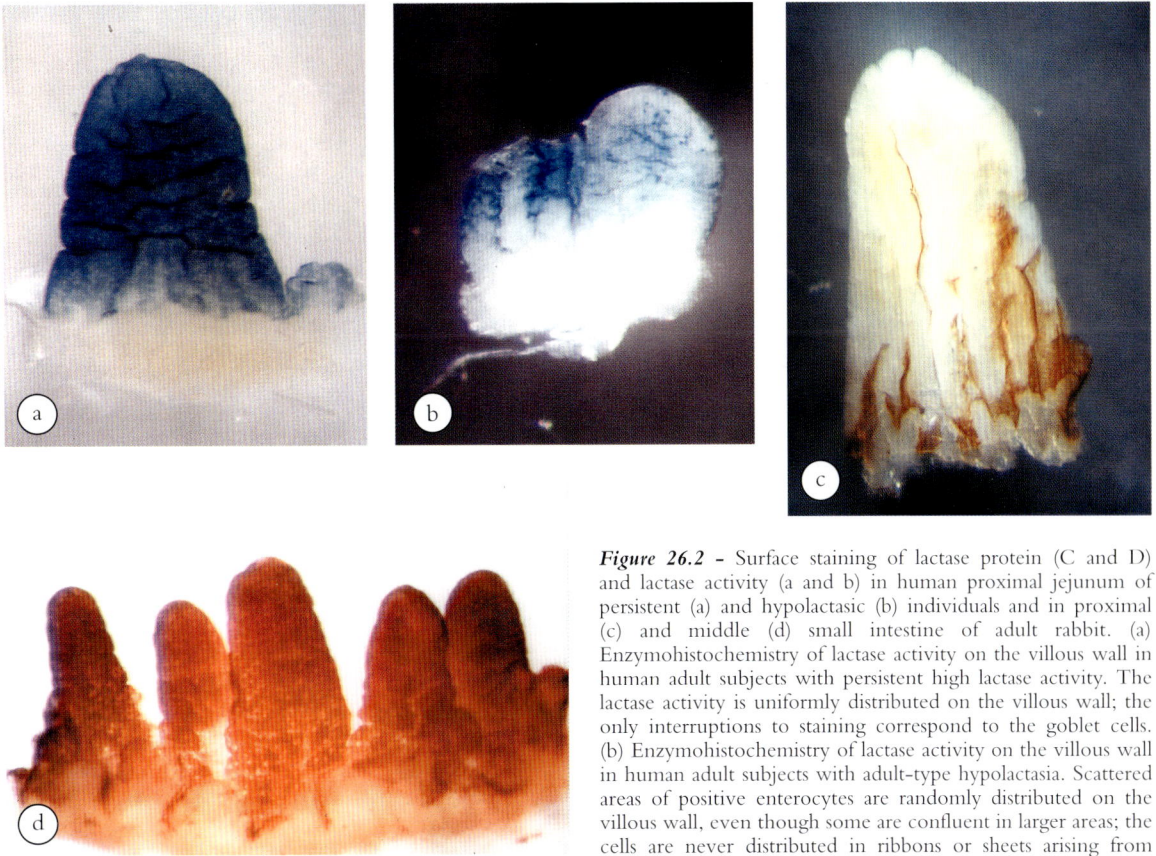

Figure 26.2 – Surface staining of lactase protein (C and D) and lactase activity (a and b) in human proximal jejunum of persistent (a) and hypolactasic (b) individuals and in proximal (c) and middle (d) small intestine of adult rabbit. (a) Enzymohistochemistry of lactase activity on the villous wall in human adult subjects with persistent high lactase activity. The lactase activity is uniformly distributed on the villous wall; the only interruptions to staining correspond to the goblet cells. (b) Enzymohistochemistry of lactase activity on the villous wall in human adult subjects with adult-type hypolactasia. Scattered areas of positive enterocytes are randomly distributed on the villous wall, even though some are confluent in larger areas; the cells are never distributed in ribbons or sheets arising from the base of the villi. Surface enzymohistochemistry, original magnification ×50 (a and b). (c) Expression of lactase protein on the villous wall in the proximal jejunum of adult rabbit. Sheets or ribbons of lactase immunoreactive enterocytes are present on the villous wall. The areas of positive enterocytes arise from the base of the villi and stop at different levels along the villous wall. (d) Expression of lactase protein of villous wall in the mid small intestine of the adult rabbit. The lactase protein is uniformly distributed on the villous wall; the only interruptions to staining correspond to the goblet cells. Surface immunohistochemistry, peroxidase staining technique (DAB substrate (c), aminoethyl-carbazole substrate (d)), original magnification $\times 64$ (c), $\times 50$ (d).

are uniformly distributed in all villous enterocytes of the villous wall (Fig. 26.2d).[13]

Therefore in the proximal small intestine of the adult rabbit a clonal origin may explain the mosaic expression of lactase along the villous,[13] but in hypolactasic human intestine, a clonal origin of these two populations of enterocytes (lactase positive and lactase negative) does not explain the observed patchy pattern.

Immunohistochemistry, enzymohistochemistry and *in situ* hybridization techniques reveal that in persistent tissues, lactase mRNA, protein and activity are present in all villous enterocytes.[23] In hyplactasic tissues, lactase mRNA is detected only in some villous enterocytes (Fig 26.3); some also express protein and activity, whereas others do not.[23] In some hypolactasic subjects, which show high label incorporation of [^{35}S]-methionine in biosynthetic studies,[8] a variable number of villous enterocytes with

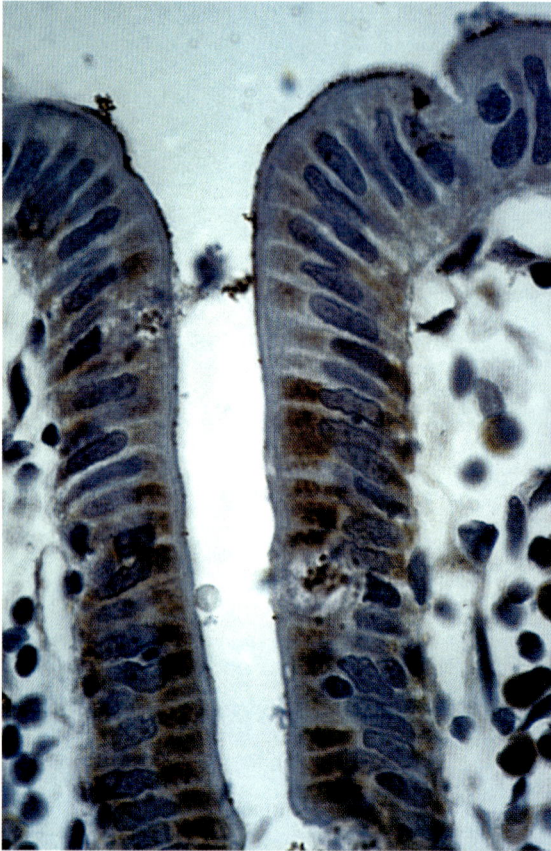

Figure 26.3 - In situ hybridization of lactase mRNA in the proximal jejunum of subjects with adult-type hypolactasia. Only some villous enterocytes express lactase mRNA, whereas others do not show any staining. The negative enterocytes are present as a group of cells or as single negative enterocytes interspersed within large positive areas. In positive enterocytes, the lactase mRNA is detected in the cytoplasm, whereas the nuclei and the brush border are negative. Non-isotopic *in situ* hybridization, immunoperoxidase detection, original magnification × 800.

lactase mRNA and protein do not express lactase activity.[23] Various types of enterocytes are, therefore, present even on a single villous in human proximal intestine from individuals with adult-type hypolactasia: enterocytes without detectable lactase mRNA; with mRNA and without detectable lactase protein on the brush border; with lactase protein and devoid of lactase activity; and, finally with lactase mRNA, protein and activity[23] and suggests that different mechanisms control lactase expression in enterocytes on the same villous.

Together morphological studies demonstrate a mosaic regulation of lactase in human adult-type hypolactasia, and various control mechanisms are involved, including transcription, mRNA stability and the rate of protein turnover. The existence of cell-to-cell differences even within one villous of a single individual suggests that expression can be compromised at several different stages. The dominant mutation(s) that lead(s) to lactase persistence, whatever the mechanism, clearly obscures this cell-to-cell heterogeneity.

A multi-faceted morphological approach is therefore able to clarify the mechanisms leading to adult-type hypolactasia: the simultaneous analysis of the expression and distribution of mRNA, protein and lactase activity at the site of its expression provides direct evidence of the pathophysiological mechanisms leading to disease.

Furthermore, this morphological method may be implemented for diagnostic purposes. In adult type hypolactasia, in fact, the mosaic distribution of lactase along the villous is a constant feature of hypolactasic intestinal samples and it is absent in all the persistent tissues; the presence of villous enterocytes lacking lactase mRNA and/or protein is therefore a useful diagnostic marker of adult-type hypolactasia. Finally, diagnosis of adult-type hypolactasia may be easily performed a short time after explants. In fact, the detection of expression and distribution of lactase activity by enzymohistochemistry is a very simple procedure and the absence of staining after 5 minutes excludes a condition of persistent high lactase activity. The morphological diagnosis of adult-type hypolactasia is also useful in excluding, by histological analysis of biopsies, any intestinal pathologies resulting in mucosal damage which could be responsible for secondary enzyme deficiency.

This evidence supports the claim that immunohistochemistry, enzymohistochemistry and *in situ* hybridisation techniques may once again become essential tools for the diagnosis of several gastrointestinal diseases.

References

1. Semenza G, Auricchio S. Small intestinal disaccharidases. In: Scriver CR, Beaudet AL, Sly WS *et al.* (Eds) *The Metabolic Basis of Inherited Diseases*, 6th edn. McGraw-Hill, New York, 1989, pp. 2975-2997.

2. Auricchio S, Rubino A, Landolt M, Semenza G, Prader A. Isolated lactase deficiency in the adult. *Lancet* 1963; **ii:** 324-326.

3. Ellestead-Sayed JJ, Haiworth JC, Hildes JA. Disaccharidase consumption and malabsorption in Canadian indians. *Am J Clin Nutr* 1977; **30:** 698-703.

4. Maiuri L, Rossi M, Raia V *et al.* Morphological method for the diagnosis of human adult-type hypolactasia. *Gut* 1994; **35:** 1042-1046.

5. Witte J, Lloyd M, Lorenzson V, Korsmo H, Olsen W. The biosynthetic basis of adult lactase deficiency. *J Clin Invest* 1990; **86:** 1338-1342.

6. Sterchi EE, Mills PR, Fransen JAM *et al.* Biogenesis of intestinal lactase- phlorizin hydrolase in adults with lactose intolerance. *J Clin Invest* 1990; **86:** 1329-1337.

7. Lloyd M, Mevissen G, Fisher M *et al.* Regulation of intestinal lactase in adult hypolactasia. *J Clin Invest* 1992; **89:** 524-592.

8. Rossi M, Maiuri L, Fusco MI, Danielsen EM, Auricchio S. The human adult-type hypolactasia is a heterogeneous condition in *in vitro* biosynthetic studies. In: Auricchio S, Semenza G (Eds) *Dynamic Nutrition Research 3.* Common Food Intolerances 2: Milk in human nutrition and adult-type hypolactasia. Karger, Basel, 1993, pp. 174-187.

9. Sebastio G, Villa M, Sartorio R *et al.* Control of lactase in human adult-type hypolactasia and in weaning rabbits and rats. *Am J Hum Genet* 1989; **45:** 489-497.

10. Asp NG, Dahlqvist A. Human small intestinal β-galactosidases. Specific assay of three different enzymes. *Anal Biochem* 1972; **47:** 527-538.

11. Sebastio G, Huzinker W, Ballabio A, Auricchio S, Semenza G. On the primary site of control in the spontaneous development of small intestinal sucrase-isomaltase after birth. *FEBS Lett* 1986; **208:** 460-464.

12. Ciccimarra F, Starace E, Vegnente A. Osservazioni sul metodo di dosaggio delle attivita' disaccaridasiche nella mucosa intestinale umana. *Boll Soc Ital Bio Sper* 1968; **45:** 336-339.

13. Maiuri L, Rossi M, Raia V, Paparo F, Garipoli V, Auricchio S. Surface staining of lactase protein and lactase activity in adult-type hypolactasia. *Gastroenterology* 1993; **105:** 708-714.

14. Maiuri L, Raia V, Potter J *et al.* Mosaic pattern of lactase expression by villous enterocytes in human adult-type hypolactasia. *Gastroenterology* 1991; **100:** 359-369.

15. Green FR, Greenwell P, Dickson L, Griffiths B, Noades J, Swallow DM. Expression of the ABH, Lewis, and related antigens on the glycoproteins of the human jejunal brush border. In: Harris JR (Ed) *Subcellular Biochemistry*; vol 12, Immunological aspects. Plenum Press, New Press, New York, 1988, pp. 119-153.

16. Maiuri L, Rossi M, Raia V *et al.* Patchy expression of lactase protein in adult rabbit and rat intestine. *Gastroenterology* 1992; **103:** 1739-1746.

17. Lojda Z, Kraml J. Indigogenic methods for glycosidases III. An improved method with 4-Cl-5-Br-3-indolyl-β-D-fucoside, and its application in studies of enzymes in the intestine, kidney and other tissues. *Histochemie* 1971; **25:** 195-207.

18. Gutschmidt S, Emde C. Early changes in brush border disaccharidase kinetics in rat jejunum following subcutaneous administration of tetraiodothyronine. *Histochemistry* 1981; **71:** 189-198.

19. Schmidt GH, Wilkinson MM, Ponder BAJ. Cell migration pathway in the intestinal epithelium: as *in situ* marker system using mouse aggregation chimaeras. *Cell* 1985; **40:** 425-429.

20. Mantei N, Villa M, Enzler T *et al.* Complete primary structure of human and rabbit lactase-phlorizin hydrolase: implications for biosynthesis, membrane anchoring and evolution of the enzyme. *EMBO J* 1988; **9:** 2705-2713.

21. Sambrook J, Fritsch EF, Maniatis T. *Molecular Cloning: A Laboratory Manual*, 2nd edn. Cold Spring Harbor Laboratory, Cold Spring Harbor, NY, 1989.

22. Rentrop M, Knapp B, Winter H, Schweizer J. Aminoalkylsilane-treated glass slides as support for in situ hybridization of Keratin cDNAs to frozen tissue sections under varying fixation and pretreatment conditions. *Histochem J* 1986; **18:** 271-276.

23. Maiuri L, Rossi M, Raia V *et al.* Mosaic regulation of lactase in human adult-type hypolactasia. *Gastroenterology* 1994; **107:** 54-60.

Immuno electron-microscopy in gastro-entero-pancreatic cells with reference to connexins 32 and 26

Masao Yamamoto, Kazuhiko Fujiki and Toshifumi Ohkusa

Summary

Gastric surface mucous cells, pancreatic acinar cells, and hepatocytes have large gap junctions (GJ) consisting of Cx 32 and 26 molecules. In immuno-electron microscopy for GJs, two methods are used; the LTPE method with freezing and thawing after paraformaldehyde-glutaraldehyde fixation, and the LTPE method with frozen section of unfixed tissue. In both methods, 5 nm gold particles labelled with anti-Cx 32 antibody easily approach and combine with the epitopes at the inner surface of the GJs, and are uniformly distributed along the GJs. Cx 32 and 26 co-localized in a GJ. Non-specific reactions were few and negligible.

In the non-cancerous gastric mucosa of human, the positive values against anti-Cx 32 were 100% in the body and less in the antrum (64%). The positive value against anti-Cx 26 was less (45% in the body and 36% in the antrum). In cancerous tissue, however, the GJs were lost, and only a specimen (9%) showed a positive reaction to Cx 32 and Cx 26. Therefore, the loss of cell-to-cell communication (CCC), especially Cx 26 as a product a cancer suppressing gene of cancer, may be involved in growth and differentiation, and the pathological behaviour of cancer cells.

Introduction

Evidence for cell-to-cell communication (CCC) between every cell, (with the exception of skeletal muscle, neurones, spermatozoa and blood cells), has been documented using a variety techniques.[1-3] CCC through gap-junction (GJ) channels has been postulated to play a growth-regulatory role in cell differentiation and morphogenesis[4-7] through positional information,[8] and carcinogenesis.[9-11] The GJs in the alimentary tract comprise a family of connexin (Cx) molecules; Cx 43, 26, 32, 37 and also ductin.[12,13] Cx 26 and 32 are produced by the epithelial cells, while Cx 43 molecules localize in smooth muscles and pericytes.

The morphology and development of GJs, as a model to observe the behaviour of integral protein molecules in the plasma membrane, have been studied in detail beacause of their well-known localization in GJ plaques, their functional states, the molecular events associated with them (i.e. phosphorylation, open and closing of channels, channel formation), and the fine structure of connexon which is formed from larger hexamer of Cx[7,8,14-17] GJs are therefore a suitable model with which to study the functions of integral membrane proteins with immuno-electron microscopy.

Methods

General preparation of tissues and cells for antibody application with immuno-electron microscopy involves membrane-permeabilisation to allow entry of the primary and secondary antibodies into the cells and fixation to stabilise cellular structures during subsequent incubations and washes. In practice, four basic approaches are used to treat antibodies:

1. *Gentle detergent extraction* (Triton X-100, Nonidet or Tween 20 which must be used in concentrations ranging from 0.1% to 1% v/v for 10 min at 25°C) followed by mild paraformaldehyde (3.7% w/v paraformaldehyde, 30 min, 25°C) fixation that preserves antigenic determinants. This procedure removes many soluble proteins from cells, leaving structures that can then be visualised against a reduced background signal.

2. *Mild formaldehyde fixation* (3.7% w/v paraformaldehyde, 30 min, 25°C) prior to detergent permeabilization. This fixation stabilises both soluble and insoluble proteins at their native locations in cytoplasm.

3. *Concurrent permeabilization and fixation* by cold (-20°C) organic solvents such as methanol and/or acetone (1:1 in mixed solution) for 5 min in the freezer (-20°C). This procedure precipitates proteins and allows detection of both soluble and insoluble proteins and Cx molecules, at their native locations in light microscopy.[18] However, in electron microscopy, cytoplasmic changes caused by the precipitation and extraction of lipids from cell membrane are so severe that one can not observe the fine structure of the cytoplasm.

4. *Rapid freezing* by attachment to a metal block (copper or gold) cooled in liquid nitrogen (-196°C) or helium (-269°C).[19] This method preserves, almost perfectly, the molecular structure and location in cells until just before the incubation of primary antibody or fixation. However, it is difficult to stop enzymatic reactions (such as proteolysis) during incubation with the primary antibodies, if anti-protease treatment or fixation is not conducted before incubation. Another difficulty of the method is that good fixation can be obtained only 30-50 μm in depth from a cooled metal.

Cx molecules, other membrane proteins, some enzymes and hormones, even after the mild fixation, lost their binding epitopes during incubation at room temperature.[19] Therefore, for immuno-electron-microscopic observations in this chapter, we recommend the use of the low-temperature-pre-embedding (LTPE) method with the lower concentration of fixation by paraformaldehyde-glutaraldehyde and with fresh-tissue-frozen-sections.

Antibodies

Cx 32 antibody, as used in the following procedures, can be provided by Prof. Y Kanno and Dr C Hirono (Department of Physiology, Hiroshima University School of Dentin, Hiroshima 734, Japan). The monoclonal antibody (14-84-A1) is made from purified GJ fraction of rat liver and the epitope was the C-terminal of the Cx. Another type of anti-Cx 32 monoclonal antibody (6-3G-11) is provided by Prof. T Shimazu, Department of Biochemistry, Ehime University School of Medicine, Shigenobu-Cho 791-02, Japan, and the epitope is also C-terminal.[20] Anti-Cx 26 polyclonal antibody (#17), rabbit polyclonal antibody, whose epitope is a.a.101-a.a.119, can be provided by Profs W R Loewenstein and B Rose (Marine Biological Laboratory, Woods Hole, NM 02543, USA). Another anti-Cx 26 antibody, rabbit polyclonal antibody, whose epitope is a.a. 113-a.a.123, can be provided by Prof. H Ohta (Department of Biochemistry, Kyorin University School of Health Sciences, Tokyo 192, Japan). Anti-Cx 43 antibody (HL-1063), rabbit polyclonal antibody, can be provided by Profs W R Loewenstein and B Rose. Another anti-Cx 43, rabbit polyclonal antibody, is produced by Dr Ueda (Nippon Shinnyaku, First Research Section of Pharmacology, Kyoto, Japan). The commercial monoclonal and polyclonal antibodies for Cxs can be obtained from Zymed Lab. Inc., CA 94080, USA.

Secondary antibodies are anti-rabbit IgG antibody (Goat) conjugated by FITC (Biomed. Tech. Inc., Stoughton, MA 02072, USA), anti-mouse F(ab')$_2$ fragment -Rhodamine (Goat) (Boehringer Mannheim Biochem. Philadelphia, USA), anti-rabbit IgG antibody conjugated 5 nm colloidal gold and anti-mouse IgG antibody conjugated 5 nm colloidal gold (Goat) (Polysciences, Inc., Warrington, Pennsylvania 18976-2590, USA).

Immunohistochemistry with doubly stained-frozen sections

Fresh tissue blocks (5×5×2 mm) of stomach, intestine, pancreas and liver are quickly embedded into O. C. T compound (Miles Inc. Diagnostics Division, Elkhart, IN 46515, USA) in Cryomold I for Biopsy (Tissue-Tek II, Lab-Tek Division, Miles Laboratories, Naperville, IL 60540, USA), frozen in liquid nitrogen, and subsequently 4 μm-thick sections are cut with a cryostat (Histostat microtome 2200, Reichert, Wien, Austria). The sections are placed on a slide glass coated with poly-L-lysine solution (Sigma, St. Louis, MO 63178, USA), melted by the warm finger touched on the opposite glass surface of the sections, then freeze-dried for 1 to 2 day at -20°C, and rinsed three times in cooled PBS at 4°C to exclude O. C. T compound.

Phosphate buffered saline (1 litre)

$NaH_2PO_4 \cdot 2H_2O$	1.2 g
$Na_2HPO_4 \cdot 12H_2O$	10.4 g
NaCl	8.0 g

adjusted to pH 7.3 by either of the phosphates.

These are blocked for 30 min at 4°C in 20% (v/v) of Block Ace (Yukijirushi KK, Sapporo, Japan) in a moisture box, incubated with anti-Cx 32 and 26 antibodies diluted at 1/100 (v/v) over night at 4°C in a refrigerator, washed three times with PBS and incubated with 1/100 diluted FITC and Rhodamine conjugated secondary antibody for 1 hour at room temperature.

After staining, sections are washed three times for each 10 min in PBS. These are immersed in anti-bleaching reagent (Perma Fluor, Lipshaw Immunon, Pittsburgh, PA 15275, USA), fixed in a cover slip by a manicure and photos are taken by double exposure with a fluorescent microscope (Nikon, Tokyo, Japan).

There are two simple and easy ways to verify the specificity of the anti-serum by fluorescent microscopy. The negative and positive control tests of the anti-serum. Prepare the tissue section without the antigen as a negative control; for example, if you stain the tight junction in intestinal absorbed cells, one should stain the blood cells or the skeletal muscle. As a positive control, stain the gastric mucosa or pancreatic exocrine tissue. One should always be sure of the reliability of the staining technique and the antibodies.

The LTPE method: Fixed-tissue-block-pre-embedding with freezing and thawing for immuno-electron microscopy

A dozen small pieces (approximately 0.5 × 0.5mm) of gastric, intestinal, pancreatic and liver tissue are fixed in fresh 2% (w/v) paraformaldehyde (EM grade; Nacalai Tesque, Inc. Kyoto, Japan) and 0.2% (v/v) glutaraldehyde (TAAB Lab. Equip. Ltd., Berks, RG7 4OW, England) in 0. 1M cacodylate buffer, pH 7.3, for 1 hour at 4°C and washed three times for each 10 min in PBS to remove extra-fixatives and other soluble components.

Composition of 0.2M cacodylate buffer (litre):

Sodium cacodylate (Na(CH$_3$)$_2$AsO$_2$) 42.8 g

Distilled water   700 ml

Adjust by 0.2M HCl at pH 7.3
   and make up to l litre.

2% (w/v) paraformaldehyde and 0.2% (v/v)
   glutaraldehyde (100 ml):

Paraformaldehyde powder   2.0 g

Distilled water   40 ml

The milky solution is heated to 40-60°C and 2-5 drops of 1M NaOH added. 1ml of 25% glutaraldehyde solution and 50 ml of 0.2M cacodylate buffer is added, and the final volume is made up to 100 ml.

Freeze the tissue in liquid nitrogen at -196°C and thaw at 4°C repeating this cycle three times in PBS. The pieces of tissue are blocked for 30 min at 4°C in 20% (v/v) of Block Ace, incubated with anti-Cx 32 or 26 antibodies diluted at 1/100 (v/v), overnight at 4°C, washed three times each for 2 min with PBS at room temperature, and incubated with 1/50 diluted colloidal gold conjugated secondary antibody for 6 h at 4°C on a Mini Disk Rotor (BC-710; Bio Craft KK, Tokyo, Japan). For observation of non-specific reactions of the secondary antibody, some tissue blocks are incubated only in 1/50 diluted colloidal gold conjugated secondary antibody without prior antibody staining. They are fixed again by 2% (v/v) glutaraldehyde containing 0.1 M cacodylate buffer, pH 7.3 for 1h at 4°C, washed with cacodylate buffer, postfixed by 1% (w/v) osmium tetroxide containing 0.1M cacodylate buffer, pH 7.3, for 30 min at room temperature, dehydrated by graded ethanol, washed by the propylene oxide and embedded in Epon 812 (TAAB Lab. Equip. Ltd, Berks, England).

Ultrathin sections are cut by a Diamond knife fitted in an auto-ultramicrotome (Reichert-Nissei Ultracuts: Leica, Wien, Austria), mounted on copper grids and stained with saturated uranyl acetate for 20-40 min at room temperature, followed by lead citrate (Reynold solution) for 20 min at room temperature, then washed in distilled water, dried at room temperature, coated by carbon, and examined at 100 kV with an H-7000 electron microscope (Hitachi, Tokyo, Japan).

Reynold solution and the lead staining method

1) Pb(NO$_3$)$_2$ 1.33 g
   Na$_3$(C$_6$H$_5$O$_7$)-2H$_2$O   1.76 g
   Distilled water   30 ml

   Shake vigorously for 1 min and leave for 30 min.

2) Add approximately 8 ml of IN-NaOH, adjust at pH 12.0 and make up to 50 ml by the addition of distilled water.

3) Stain the thin sections for 10 to 20 min in above solution.

   When it is over-stained, destain in 0.02N NaOH for a few seconds.

Immunohistochemical staining to human cancer tissue

Tissue specimens are taken from a tumorous lesion of the gastric carcinoma, and ideally from the peripheral area away from the carcinoma in the gastric body and antral mucosa, using biopsy-forceps (FB-25K, Olympus, Tokyo, Japan). The specimens are dipped into O.C.T. compound for embedding and quickly frozen in liquid nitrogen. Subsequently, 6 μm-thick sections are cut with a cryostat (Leica CM 1900 Leica Inst. GmbH, Nussloch, Germany). The sections on slide glass are blocked with 1 ml of normal 10% (w/v) goat serum (Rockland, Gilbertsville, PA USA) for 20 minutes, incubated with 1 ml of the primary antibody (100 mg/ml) for 1 hour, and washed three times in 10 ml of 10 mM PBS at room temperature. Then, 1 ml of biotin-conjugated goat anti-mouse IgG antibody (Fab specific, Sigma Chemical Co., St Louis, MO, USA) diluted 1/100 in PBS is applied to the section for 1 hour at room temperature. After washing three times with 10 ml of PBS, sections are incubated with avidin-biotin complex (Vectastain ABC-GO Standard Kit, Vector Labo., Inc., Burlingame, CA, USA) for 30 min at room temperature, washed three times with PBS, stained by a working solution of 3,3'-diaminobenzidine (DAB Substrate Kit for Peroxidase, Vector Labo., Inc., Burlingame, CA, USA) for 3 minutes. After washing for 5 minutes in distilled water, the sections are counterstained by Mayer's haematoxylin solutions[21] and washed in tap water until the nuclei turn dark blue. The sections are observed under a microscope, ×400-1000 (Olympus, Tokyo, Japan). Histopathological examinations are made of the same specimens by haematoxylin - eosin staining.

Mayer's haematoxylin solutions:

1) Dissolve 1.0 g of haematoxylin in 1000 ml of distilled water;

2) Add 0.2 g of sodium iodate and 50 g of aluminium potassium sulphate;

3) Add 50 g of chloral hydrate and 1 g of citric acid;

4) Leave for two weeks.

To investigate non-specific reactions arising from the first antibody with fluorescent microscopy and electron microscopy, it is desirable that the Absorbing Test is performed as follows.

1. Prepare a ready absorbed - first - antibody - solution containing an overdose of antigen (peptides or isolated molecules).

2. Stain some blocks or sections with the absorbed-first-antibody-solution, and proceed with the same method as above. If the antibody shows no nonspecific reaction, one should observe a negative reaction in the preparation of the Absorbing Test.

Application to animal studies

Animals

Male Sprague-Dawley rats and ICR mice were anaesthetised by ether and the stomach, duodenum, jejunum, ileum, pancreas, and liver were resected. These tissues were washed using a cool saline or PBS at 4°C to remove the contents of their lumens and any residual blood.

Double staining of frozen sections and LTPE preparation with frozen section in unfixed rat tissues

Gastric, intestinal, pancreatic and liver tissue blocks were frozen in O.C.T. compound with liquid nitrogen after resection from rats. 10 μm frozen tissue sections were taken using a cryostat (Histostat microtome 2200, Reichert, Wien, Austria) and some frozen sections were doubly stained by the double-staining method described above.

The other sections were immersed in the paraformaldchyde-glutaraldehydc fixative for 5 min at 4°C and washed three times in cooled PBS at 4°C by centrifugation at 300 g for 2 min at 4°C. The pellets of the sections were processed by primary antibody staining as described in the LTPE method.

Cx 32 and 26 distribution in alimentary system

The family of Cxs consists of Class I (Cx 31, 31.1, 26, 32) and Class II (Cx 43, 33, 37, 46, 40).[22-25] Generally, Cx 26 and 32 are found in most epithelial cells, while Cx 43 is confined to circular and vascular smooth muscle, endothelial cells, pericytes, pancreatic islet cells and myoepithelial cells (Table 27.1).[26-29]

In this animal study, hepatocytes, gastric surface mucous and pancreatic acinar cells had large GJs. Mucous neck, chief and intestinal crypt cells had medium to small GJs. The gastric cells except parietal cells, also expressed Cx 32 and 26, but Cx 26 was less well expressed.[17,26]

General GJ morphology and co-localization of Cx 32 and 26

To form a channel which is approximately 20 nm in width, a connexon makes contact with a connexon of a partner cell (Fig. 27.1A). In both LTPE preparations, a large GJ was labelled by colloidal gold conjugated with anti-Cx 32 (Fig. 27.1B), which was uniformly distributed along the GJ plaques. Non-specific reactions were few and negligible in all observations.

Table 27.1 – Cxs expression in the alimentary system of adult mammals. Localization data are from references 1, 2, 13, 22, 26, 27, 28 and 32 . #4: Studied in ref. 26 using freeze fracture; Cx types could not be detected.

Anatomical region	Expression of mRNA	Type of connexin molecules
Esophagus	Cx 32, Cx 26, Cx 43	
Epithelium		Cx 26, Cx 43
Smooth muscle		Cx 43
Stomach	Cx 32, Cx 26, Cx43	
Surface mucous cell		Cx 32, Cx 26
Mucous neck cell		Cx 32, Cx 26?
Parietal cell		no GJP
Chief cell		Cx 32, Cx 26
Smooth muscle		Cx 43
Small intestine	Cx 32, Cx 26, Cx 43, Cx 37	
Absorptive cell		no GJP
Goblet cell		no GJP
Crypt cell		Cx32, Cx 26
Paneth cell		Cx32, Cx 26
Duodenal gland cells		Cx32, Cx 26
Endocrine cells		no GJP
Circular smooth muscle		Cx 43
Longitudinal smooth muscle		--#4
Pancreas	Cx 32, Cx 26, Cx 43	
Exocrine cell		
Duct cell		no GJP
Acinar cell		Cx 32, Cx 26
Endocrine cell		Cx 43, Cx 26
Liver	Cx 32, Cx 26, Cx 43, Cx 37	
Hepatocyte		Cx 32, Cx 26
Ito cell		Cx 43
Salivary gland	Cx 32, Cx 26, Cx 43	
Sero-mucous cell		Cx 32, Cx 26
Mucous cell		Cx 32, Cx 26
Myoepithelial cell		Cx 43

To observe the distribution of both Cxs, double staining with anti-Cx 32 and 26 was performed in the exocrine pancreas and photographs taken using the double exposure methods. The focus of FITC spots moved to just below the Rhodamine spots, meaning that both Cxs belonged to a GJ plaque (Fig. 27.lC). Other types of cells also showed same co-localization, except for hepatocytes (Table 27.1).

Results and discussion

Cx 32 and 26 in human gastric cancer

The expressive ratio of Cx 32 and 26 was immunohistochemically studied in human gastric tissues (Table 27.2). Cancerous and non-cancerous tissue of the body and antrum of eleven Japanese patients (aged

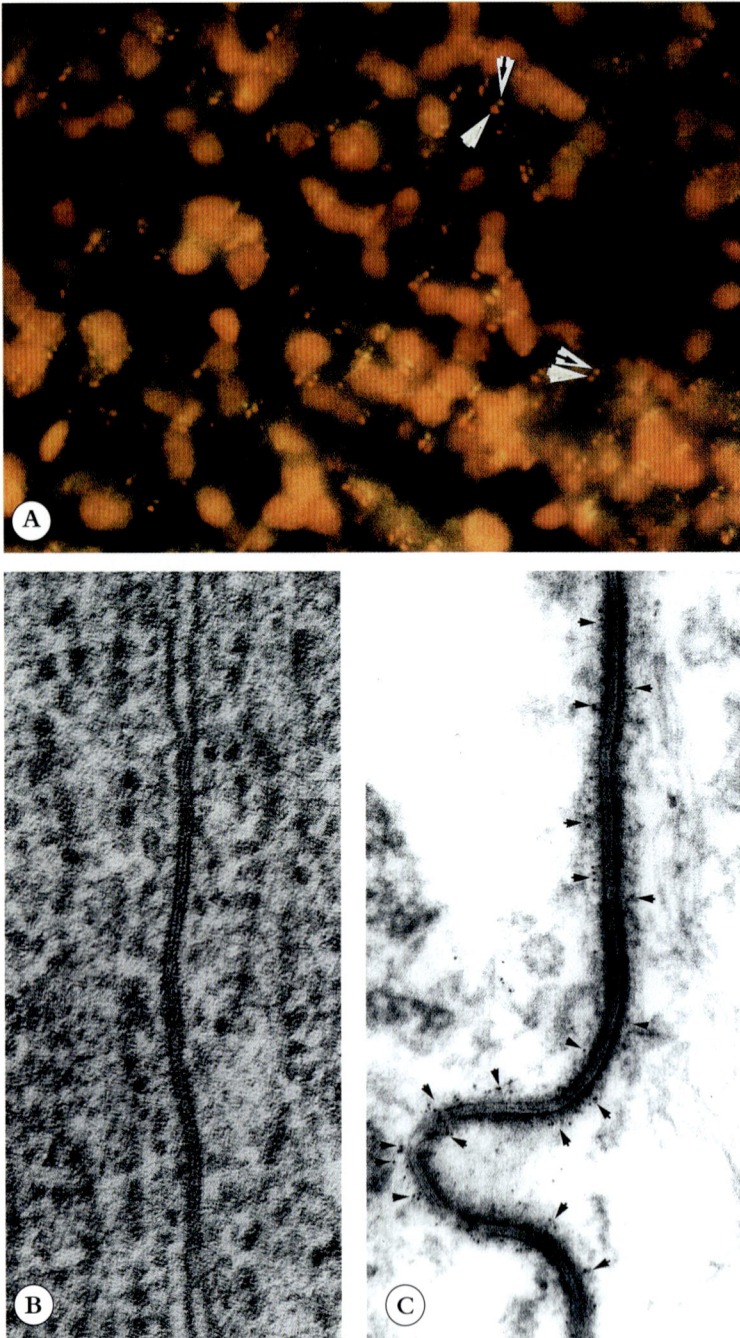

Figure 27.1 –
A) Double-staining and double-exposure of rat pancreatic acinar tissue. Both Cx 32 (green FITC spots; white arrow-heads) and Cx 26 (orange Rhodamine spots; small black arrow-heads) spots always array as a set of spots at short distance. This is due to the change of focus when exchanging the filter for FITC and Radiomen. It shows that both Cx molecules distribute in a GJ plaque. ×3,000.

B) Transverse view of a GJ plaque of two adjacent pancreatic acinar cell in adult rat. The high magnification picture of GJ shows a pentalamellar structure which is separated by a prominent central dense strata or gap (5 nm thickness) between the external leaflets of two aposed GJ membranes. The dense strata has a regular periodicity, spaced 8-10 nm apart. ×114,000.

C) In LTPE preparations with freezing-thawing, the immuno-electron microscopy of GJ of acinar cell in adult rat pancreas. Many Cx 32 molecules are labelled by the dot of colloidal gold particles (arrow-heads) which are located at the inner surface of the GJ membrane. ×100,000.

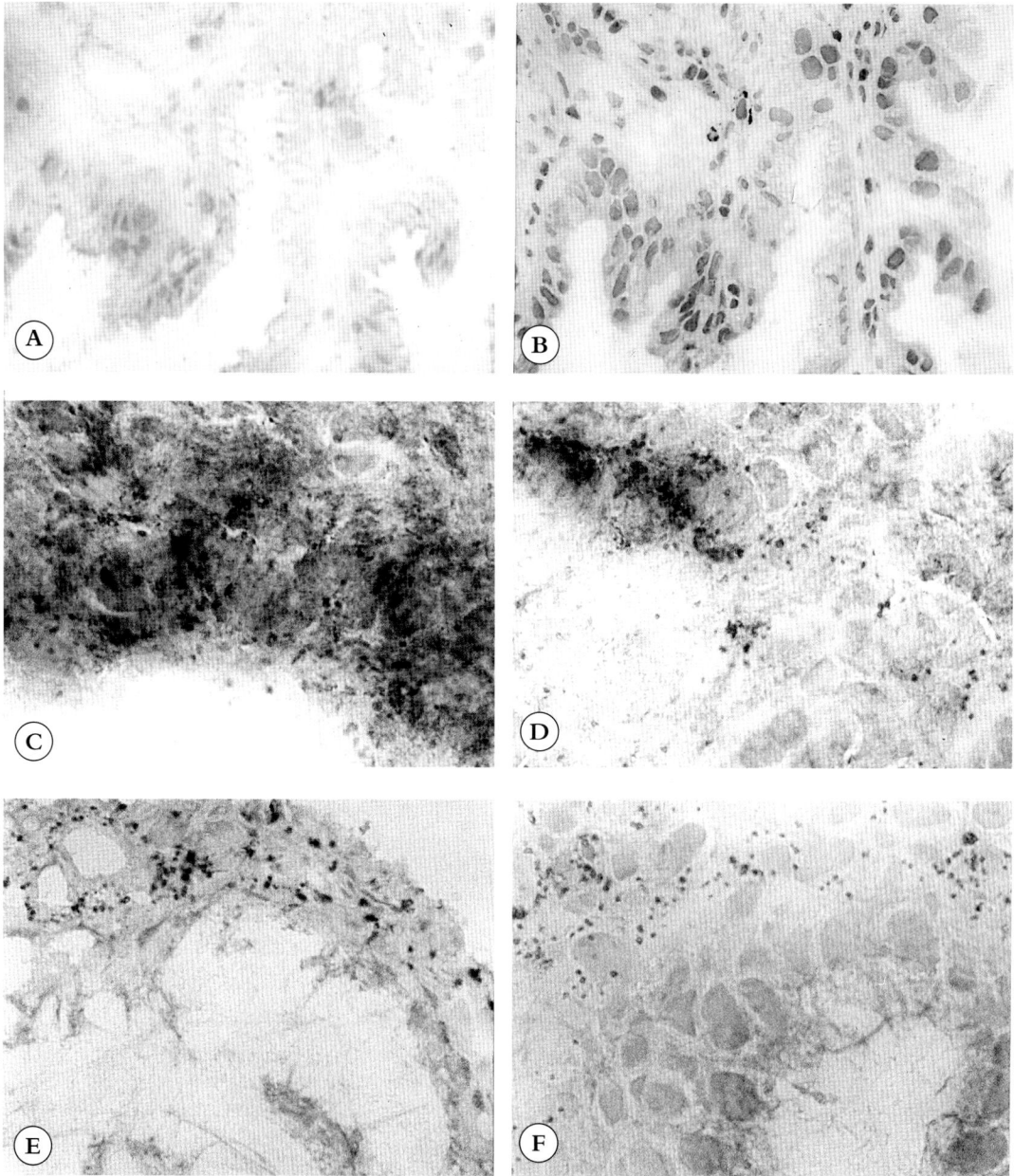

Figure 27.2 – Immunohistochemical localization of Cx 32 and 26 in surface mucous cells of gastric cancer.

A) A non-cancerous mucosa of the body in a patient with gastric cancer stained with anti-Cx 32, showing many staining spots. × 3,200.

B) A non-cancerous mucosa of the body in a patient with gastric cancer stained with anti-Cx 26, showing many staining spots.× 3,200.

C) Positive cells of a cancerous mucosa in a patient with gastric cancer stained with anti-Cx 32, showing no staining spots. × 3,200.

D) Positive cells of a cancerous mucosa in a patient with gastric cancer stained with anti-Cx 26, showing no staining spots. × 3,200.

E) Negative cells of a cancerous mucosa in a patient with gastric cancer stained with anti-Cx 32, showing no staining spots. × 2,300.

F) Negative cells of a cancerous mucosa in a patient with gastric cancer stained with anti-Cx 26, showing no staining spots. × 2,300.

Table 27.2 – The frequency of Cx 32 and 26 detection in gastric mucosa of patients with gastric cancer.

		Carcinoma	Body	Antrum
Cx 32	+	1	11	7
	–	10	0	4
Frequency		9%	100%	64%
Cx 26	+	1	5	4
	–	10	6	7
Frequency		9%	45%	36%

52±14 years, Male/Female: 8/3) was pinched off during gastroendoscopy for gastric cancer and classified histopathologically as the intestinal-type in 5 patients and the diffuse-type in 6 patients. The study was approved by the Ethics Committee, and informed consent was obtained from all patients.

In the non-cancerous tissue, positive reactions for anti-Cx 32 (Fig.27.2A) were found in the entire gastric body and in 64% of the antrum. However, anti-Cx 26 positive staining (Fig.27.2B) was found in only 45% of the non-cancerous body and 36% of the antrum. Among these, positive values for *both* anti-Cxs were 44% in the body and 27% in the antrum.

On the other hand, in the cancerous tissue, only one case (9%) showed positive spots for anti- Cxs but all other tissues (Figs. 27.2C and D) were negative. The frequency in the cancerous mucosa is significantly lower than that in the non-cancerous mucosa (p<0.02, analysed by Fisher's exact test).

Loss of CCC and carcinogenesis

CCC is considered to be important for growth, differentiation, and also carcinogenesis.[4,30,31] Some studies[32,33] indicated less expression of Cx in breast cancer, and others[34] showed that the gastric surface mucous cells communicated electrically and that cellular uncoupling occurs in cancerous cells. Tumour promoters and nongenotoxic carcinogens inhibited CCC or GJ growth. This evidence demonstrates that the loss of CCC is a feature of carcinogenesis.[31,35-37]

Studies[35,37] have also shown that up-regulation of CCC between transformed and normal cells gradually eliminated the former and suppressed tumour growth. In addition, it has also been demonstrated[36] that the incorporation of Cx gene into transformed cells also led to normalisation of growth. Therefore, the Cx gene plays a role as a suppressor gene of cancer,[11] and less expression of Cx 26 would be indicative of carcinogenesis in the gastric mucosa and also in other GEP cells.

Acknowledgments

The authors wish to thank Profs W R Loewenstein and B Rose for providing the anti-Cx 43 and 26 antibodies, and for advice on double-staining. We also thank Prof. Y Kanno, Dr C Hirono, Dr A Takeda and Prof. H Ohta for making and providing anti-Cx 32 and 26 monoclonal antibodies.

References

1. Dermietzel R, Spray DC. Gap junctions in the brain: where what type, how many and why? *TINS* 1993; **16:** 186-192.

2. Bennett MVL, Barrio LC, Bargicello TA Spray DC, Hertzberg E, Sa'ez JC. Gap junctions: new tools, new answers, new questions. *Neuron* 1991; **6:** 305-320.

3. Larsen WJ. Biological implications of gap junction structure, distribution and composition: A review. *Tissue cell* 1983; **15:** 645-671.

4. Loewenstein WR. Junctional intercellular communication and the control of growth. *Biochem Biophys Acta* 1979; **560:** 1-65.

5. Loewenstein WR. Junctional intercellular communication: The cell-to-cell membrane channel. *Physiol Rev* 1981; **61:** 829-913.

6. Yamamoto M, Kataoka K. Large particles associated with gap junctions of pancreatic exocrine cells during embryonic and neonatal development. *Anat Embryol* 1985; **171:** 305 -310.

7. Yamamoto M, Kataoka K. Electron microscope observation on the formation of primitive villi in rat small intestine with special reference to intercellular junctions. *Arch Histol Cytol* 1992; **55:** 551-560.

8. Wolpert L. Positional information and spatial pattern of cellular differentiation. *J Theor Biol* 1969; **25:** 1-47.

9. Mesnil M, Yamasaki H. Cell-cell communication and growth control of normal and cancer cells: evidence and hypothesis. *Mol Carcinog* 1993; **7:** 14-17.

10. Loewenstein WR, Kanno Y. Intercellular communication and the control of growth: lack of communication between cancer cells. *Nature (Lond)* 1966; **209:** 1248-1249.

11. Yamasaki H. Gap junctional intercellular communication and carcinogenesis. *Carcinogenesis* 1990; **11:** 1051-1058.

12. Finbow ME, Pitts JD. Is the gap junction channel -the connexon-made of connexin or ductin? *J Cell Sci* 1993; **106:** 463-472.

13. Willecke K, Heynkes R, Dahl E *et al.* Mouse connexin 37: cloning and functional expression of a gap junction gene highly expressed in lung. *J Cell Biol* 1991; **114:** 1049-157.

14. Yamamoto M, Kataoka K. An electron microscope study on development of the exocrine and endocrine pancreas with special reference to intercellular junctions. *Arch Histol Jpn* 1988; **51:** 315-325.

15. Yamamoto M, Kataoka K. Cytodifferentiation of pancreatic acinar and intestinal absorptive cells accompanied by rapid formation of gap junction plaques. *Prog Cell Biol* 1995; **4:** 305-308.

16. Ohkusa T, Yamamoto M, Kataoka K *et al.* (1993) Electron microscopic study of intercellular junctions in human gastric mucosa with special reference to their relationship to gastric ulcer. *Gut* 1993; **34:** 86-89.

17. Ohkusa T, Fujiki K, Tamura Y, Yamamoto M, Kyoui T. Freeze-fracture and immunohistochemical studies of gap junctions in human gastric mucosa with special reference to their relationships to gastric ulcer and gastric carcinoma. *J Microscope Tech* 1995; **31:** 226-233.

18. Melan MA, Sluder G. Redistribution and differential extraction of soluble proteins in permeabilized culture cells: implications for immunofluorescence microscopy. *J Cell Sci* 1992; **101:** 731-743.

19. Fujimoto K. Freeze-fracture replica electron microscopy combined with SDS digestion for cytochemical labeling of integral membrane proteins: Application to the immunogold labeling of intercellular functional complexes. *J Cell Sci* 1995; **108:** 3443-3449.

20. Takeda A, Kanoh M, Shimazu T, Takeuchi N. Monoclonal antibodies recognizing different epitopes of the 27-kDa gap junctional protein from rat liver. *J. Biochem* 1988; **104:** 901-907.

21. Lce AB, Mayer P. Grundzüge der Mikroskopischen Technik für Zoologen und Anatomen. 1910; **4:** 515.

22. Haefliger JA, Bruzzone R, Jenkins NA, Gilbert DJ, Copeland NG, Paul DL. Four novel members of the connexin family of gap junction proteins: molecular cloning, expression and chromosome mapping. *J Biol Chem* 1992; **267:** 2057-2064.

23. Beyer EC, Paul DL, Goodenough DA. Connexin 43, a protein from rat heart homologous to a gap junction protein from liver. *J Cell Biol* 1987; **105:** 2621-2629.

24. Demietzel R, Leibstein A, Frixen U, Janssen-Timmen U, Traub 0, Willecke K. Gap junctions in several tissues share antigenic determinants with liver gap junctions. *EMBO J* 1984; **3:** 2261-2270.

25. Nicholson B, Derrnietzel R, Teplow D, Traub O, Willecke K, Revel J-P. Two homologous components of hepatic gap junctions. *Nature* 1987; **329:** 732-734.

26. Yamamoto M. (unpublished observations).

27. Meda P, Pepper MS, Traub O, Willecke K, Gross D, Beyer E, Nicholson B, Paul D, Orci L. Differential expression of gap junction connexins in endocrine and exocrine glands. *Endocrinology* 1993; **133:** 2371-2378.

28. Reed KE, Westphele EM, Larson DM, Wang H-Z, Veenstra RD, Beyer EC. Molecular cloning and Functional expression of human connexin 37, an endothelial cell gap junction protein. *J Clin Invest* 1993; **91:** 997-1004.

29. Kyoui T, Ueda F, Kimura K, Yamamoto M, Kataoka K. Development of gap junctions between gastric surface mucous cells during cell maturation in rat. *Gastroenterol* 1992; **102:** 1930-1935.

30. Takeichi M. Cadherin cell adhesion receptor as a morphogenetic regulator. *Science* 1991; **251:** 1451-1455.

31. Yamasaki H, Katoh F. Further evidence for the involvement of gap junctional intercellular communication in induction and maintenance of transformed foci in BALB/c 3T3 cells. *Cancer Res* 1988; **48:** 3490-3495.

32. Wilgenbus KW, Kirkpatrick CJ, Knuechel R, Willecke K, Traub O. Expression of Cx 26, Cx 32 and Cx 43 gap junction proteins in normal and neoplastic human tissues. *Int J Cancer* 1992; **51:** 522-529.

33. Fentiman IS, Hurst J, Ceriani RL, Taylor-Papadimitriou J. Junctional intercellular communication pattern of cultured human breast cancer cells. *Cancer Res* 1979; **39:** 4739-4743.

34. Kanno Y, Matsui Y. Cellular uncoupling in cancerous stomach epithelium. *Nature* 1968; **2118:** 775-776.

35. Klauning JE, Ruch RJ. Biology of disease: Role of inhibition of intercellular communication in carcinogenesis. *Lab Invest* 1990; **62:** 135-146.

36. Metha PP, Hotz-Wagenblatt A, Rose B, Shalloway D, Loewenstein WR. Incorporation of the gene for a cell-cell channel protein into transformed cells leads to normalization of growth. *J Memb Biol* 1991; **124:** 207-225.

37. Metha PP, Bertrum JS, Loewenstein WR. Growth inhibition of transformed cells correlates with their Functional communication with normal cells. *Cell* 1986; **44:** 187- 196.

28

Immunocytochemical investigation of paraffin-embedded tissue

Tadashi Terada and Yukisato Kitamura

Summary

Immunocytochemistry (ICC) study of paraffin-embedded tissue is a powerful tool for detection and elucidation of the *in situ* tissue distribution of certain antigens, such as peptides, proteins and carbohydrates. The principle behind ICC is antigen–antibody binding. The antigen–antibody complex is visualized by several methods, including the use of fluorescent materials, metal and enzyme–substrate complexes. The unlabelled antibody–enzyme ICC method is widely used because of its high specificity, sensitivity and convenience. It consists of three steps: 1) the tissue antigen is bound by the primary antibody; 2) the antigen–antibody complex is bound by the secondary antibody raised to the primary antibody; 3) the complex is bound by the enzyme-linked antibody raised to the secondary antibody or by avidin–biotin– enzyme complex. The enzyme-linked complex is then visualized by conversion of the substrates into visible substances by the enzyme. There are three different ICC methods using this unlabelled antigen– antibody method: peroxidase– anti-peroxidase (PAP), avidin-biotin–enzyme complex (ABC), and alkaline phosphatase–anti-alkaline phosphatase (APAAP) methods. In ICC, the specificity of antibody and immunostaining must be defined by Western blot analysis.

Introduction

Immunocytochemistry (ICC) or immunohistochemistry is a powerful method for detecting antigens in tissues *in situ* and investigating their distribution and intracellular localization. The antigens include peptides, proteins and carbohydrate residues of glycoproteins. The principle behind ICC is the specific binding between antigens and antibodies and the subsequent visualization of the antigen–antibody complex by various methods. Although ICC using fresh frozen sections is superior to and more reliable than that using paraffin sections, the latter generally result in good staining with excellent tissue architecture preservation. The ICC study of paraffin sections is not suitable for immunoelectron microscopic analysis.

Methods

General features of ICC studies of paraffin-embedded tissues

This technique consists of two sequential procedures: first, tissue antigens are bound by antibodies (primary antibodies); and secondly, the antigen–antibody complex is visualized by various procedures, including the immunofluorescent method (fluorescent dye), the metal-labelling method (metal such as gold) and the enzyme-antibody method (enzyme-linked antibodies). Among these, the latter is an excellent, reproducible and sensitive method, and therefore it is usually performed in routine ICC.

There are three enzyme-linked antibody ICC methods: a direct method, an indirect method and an unlabelled antibody-enzyme method. In the direct method, a labelled primary antibody is applied directly to the tissue preparation. This method is specific but it is not sensitive. In the indirect method, the primary antibody is unlabelled and the antigen–antibody complex is identified by a labelled secondary antibody raised to the immunoglobulins of the species providing the primary antibody. This method is more sensitive than the direct method. In the unlabelled antibody-enzyme method, sections are treated with a primary antibody and then by an unlabelled secondary antibody against the primary antibody. The antigen–primary antibody–secondary antibody complex is bound by enzyme-labelled antibodies against the secondary antibody or by enzyme-labelled avidin–biotin complex. This method is much more sensitive than the direct or indirect methods, and therefore is widely used in ICC of paraffin sections.

Although several techniques for this unlabelled antibody–enzyme method have been developed, the peroxidase–anti-peroxidase (PAP),[1] avidin-biotin–peroxidase complex (ABC),[2] and alkaline phosphatase–anti-alkaline phosphatase[3] methods are regarded as sensitive and easily performed, and these are described below.

Tissue fixation

Many fixatives can be used, including 4% (w/v) formaldehyde solution (10% formalin), aldehyde, car-

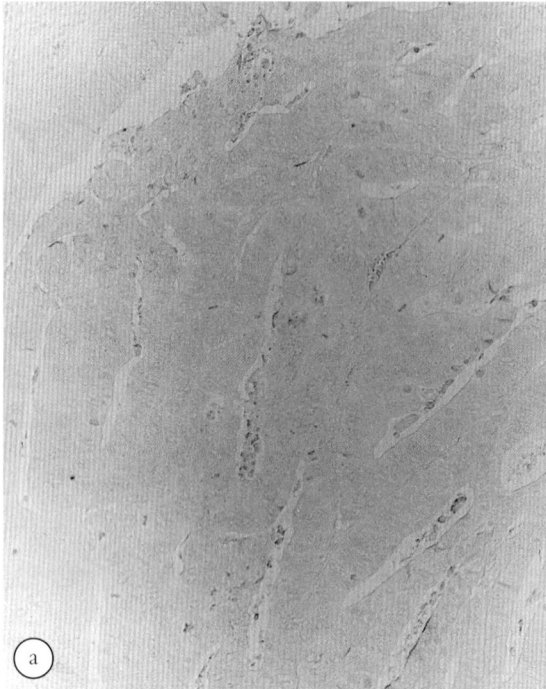

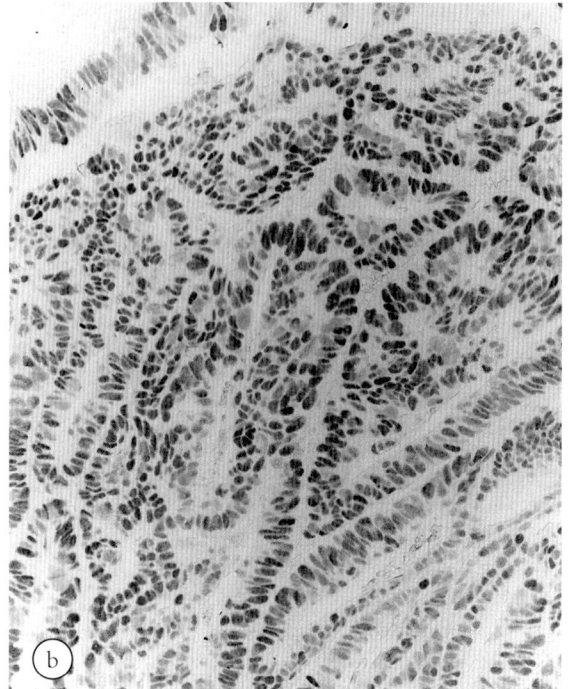

Figure 28.1 – Antigen retrieval using microwave oven heating of tissue sections a) No microwave treatment shows no staining. Immunostaining for p53 protein in colon carcinoma, ×200. b)

Serial section of a. Pretreatment of microwave results in clear nuclear staining of p53 protein. Immunostaining for p53 protein, ×200.

boimide, alcohol, acetone, citrate and Bouin solution. However, the most commonly used fixative is neutral-buffered 10% formalin. Formalin fixation usually results in excellent tissue architecture preservation, while other fixatives may be excellent for the preservation of antigenicity but relatively poor in maintaining tissue architecture. The archival tissue specimens in most laboratories have been fixed with formalin. In prospective studies, however, the most appropritae fixative can be used. For example, alcohol fixation is good for the detection of cytokeratins and Bouin fixative for peptide hormones. Fixation time is important for preservation of antigenicity and ranges from 3-24 hours, depending on fixative. Long fixation usually inactivates or unmasks tissue antigens, resulting in a false negative reaction in ICC. In addition, long fixation may cause diffusion of certain antigens such as serum proteins onto other sites, resulting in a positive reaction at the wrong sites.

Preparation of tissue sections

Tissue sections of 3-5 μm are made from paraffin-embedded specimens by a microtome. The tissue sections should be adhered to glass slides coated with poly(L-lysine) (PL) (formaldehyde, citric acid and pictric acid) (Sigma, St. Louis, USA) to prevent them from becoming detached from the glass side during immunostaining.

Antigen retrieval

In ICC studies of paraffin sections, it must always be borne in mind that some antigens may be hidden or unmasked by cross-linkage or coagulation caused by fixatives or paraffin-embedding procedures. Therefore, a negative reaction does not necessarily indicate that the antigen is absent in the tissue and it is possible that the antigen has simply been unmasked. Antigen exposure is necessary. For this, protease predigestion is a useful method. Deparaffinized sections are incubated at 37°C for 30 min in 0.1% (w/v) trypsin in Tris-HCl buffer (tris aminomethane-HCI, pH 7.0 Sigma), 0.4% (w/v) pepsin in phosphate buffered saline (PBS), or 0.05% (w/v) protease in Tris-HCl buffer. Boiling of the tissue sections in citrate buffer (10 nmol/L citric acid, pH 6.0) twice for 5 min each in a microwave is another excellent method and may be particularly useful for antigens such as p53 protein (Fig. 28.1), proliferating cell nuclear antigen, Ki-67 and bcl-2 protein.[4]

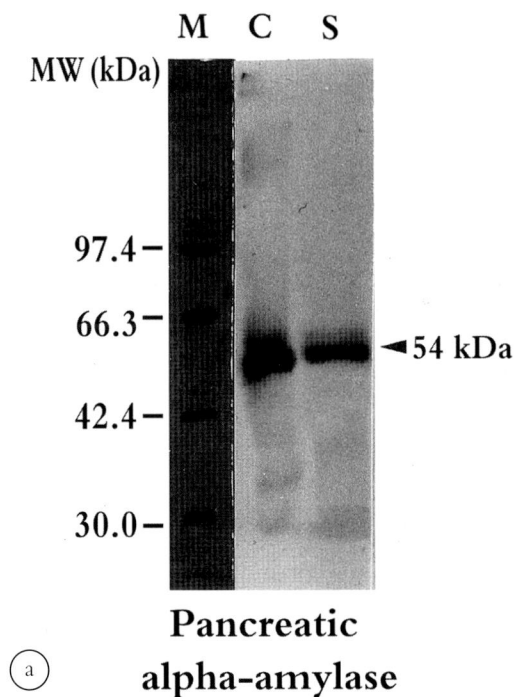

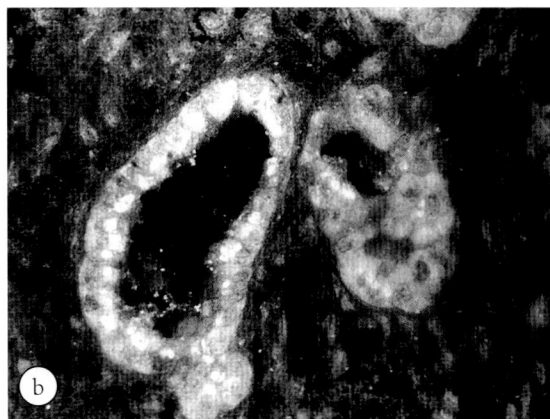

Figure 28.2 – Western blot analysis for pancreatic α-amylase in human bile (a) and immunocytochemical demonstration of pancreatic α-amylase in intrahepatic bile ducts (b). (a) Control (purified α-amylase) and sample bile show band of 54 kDa of pancreatic α-amylase. M, molecular marker. C, control. S, sample bile. (b) Confocal laser scanning microscopical analysis of immunocytochemical specimens of intrahepatic bile ducts shows immunoreactive pancreatic α-amylase in the bile duct cells and in the lumen, ×300.

Eradication of 'background staining'

The antigen-antibody reaction is highly specific. However, observers are occasionally dogged by mild non-immunological staining called 'background staining' or 'non-specific staining'. This results mainly from weak non-immunological antigen-antibody binding. To avoid or reduce 'background staining', before applying the primary antibody, sections should be treated for 20 min with 5% normal serum (diluted by PBS) of the animal species used in the secondary antigens. In addition, sections should be treated with 0.3% (v/v) H_2O_2 in methanol to quench endogenous peroxidase activity in the immunostaining using peroxidase-labeled secondary antibodies.

Primary antibodies

There are two types of primary antibody: polyclonal (anti-serum or IgG fraction) and monoclonal. The Fab or F(ab') fraction of IgG can be used as primary antibody. Polyclonal antibody recognizes many epitopes in an antigen, but ICC using a polyclonal antibody occasionally results in rather high background staining. In contrast, a monoclonal antibody reacts with only one epitope of the antigen, and ICC using a monoclonal antibody results in clear and low background staining. However, the monoclonal antibody may crossreact with the same epitope of different antigens. Therefore, specificity of ICC using monoclonal antibodies must be defined using Western blot analysis.

A large number of primary antibodies, both polyclonal and monoclonal, are available from commercial sources. When primary antibodies are not available commercially, they may be developed by immunizing animals with the antigen for polyclonal antibodies or by the myeloma cell hybridoma technique for monoclonal antibodies.

Every antibody must be optimally diluted with PBS containing 1% (w/v) bovine serum albumin, giving rise to working primary antibody solution. To determine the optimal dilution, variable dilution primary antibody solutions must be examined using positive control tissues.

Specificity of primary antibodies

To test that the primary antibody specifically binds with a particular antigen, Western blot analysis may be necessary to confirm the specificity (Fig. 28.2). In practice, the purified or recombinant antigen, homogenate of positive control tissue and homogenate of tested tissue are electrophoresed in sodium dodecyl sulphate polyacrylamide (SDS-PAGE) gel. Then, the proteins are electrically transferred onto nitrocellulose membrane and subjected to the immunostaining procedure. When a discrete band of predicted molecular weight antigen is recognized, it can be concluded that the primary antibody is specific for the given antigen. For further details, please refer to reference 5.

Secondary antibodies

Secondary antibodies (usually IgG fraction) raised against immunoglobulins of the primary antibodies are now mostly available from commercial sources. In the ABC method, biotinylated secondary antibodies are used and are available from commercial sources. Fab or F(ab') fragments of IgG are also available. These small fragments of immunoglobulins are useful for detecting some hidden antigens.

Detection of antigen–antibody complex

The antigen–antibody complex is detected by enzyme-conjuctated (peroxidase or alkaline phosphatase) anti-secondary antibody in the PAP and APAAP methods and by enzyme-conjugated (peroxidase or alkaline phosphatase) avidin–biotin complex or streptavidin–biotin complex in the ABC method. Detection of the antigen-antibody complex is performed by enzymatic conversion of invisible substrates into visible substances. Fast red, Texas red or fast blue are used as the substrate for the alkaline phosphatase-mediated visualization, and 3,3'-diaminobenzidine tetrahydrochloride (DAB) or aminoethyl carbazol (AEC) are used for the peroxidase-mediated procedure. Fluorescent dyes such as Texas red are applicable to confocal laser scanning microscopic analysis (Fig. 28.2b).

Other reagents

Buffers, normal serum, moist chambers, substrates and enzyme-labelled antibodies are available commercially. ICC kits containing almost all reagents for the whole ICC procedure are available from commercial sources (Dako, Glostrup, Denmark) in detecting systems for frequently used antigens.

Specificity of immunostaining

To confirm that the immunostaining is specific for the particular antigen, several procedures should be performed. First, positive control tissue and nega-

tive control tissue should be used in each immunohistochemical run. Secondly, non-immune serum and PBS should be used instead of the primary antibodies followed by immunostaining; no staining should result with this procedure. Thirdly, an absorption test should be performed.[6] That is, the primary antibody is mixed with the purely extracted or recombinant antigen. The mixed solution is incubated at 4°C overnight with agitation, followed by centrifugation at 60 000 rpm for 10-20 min at room temperature. The supernatant is used as 'primary antibody', followed by immunostaining. This procedure should lead to no staining. Finally, if possible, the presence of mRNA for the antigen should be investigated by in situ hybridization, Northern blot hybridization or reverse transcription-polymerase chain reaction (RT-PCR).[7,8]

Practical procedures of immunostaining

The PAP, ABC and APAAP procedures consist of three steps: 1) the tissue antigen is bound by the primary antibody; 2) the antigen-bound primary antibody is bound by the secondary antibody; 3) the antigen-primary antibody-secondary antibody complex is detected by the third antibody against the secondary antibody or ABC complex. All reaction procedures should be done in a moist chamber except for washing in PBS.

Peroxidase–anti-peroxidase (PAP) method

(Fig. 28.3)

1. Sections 3 μm are mounted on PL slides;

2. Deparaffinization by xylene and rehydration by graded methanol;

3. Proteinase predigestion or microwave oven pretreatment (when necessary);

4. Eradication of endogenous peroxidase activity by immersing the sections for 30 min in absolute methanol containing 0.3% (v/v) H_2O_2;

5. Application of 5% (v/v) normal serum (serum of animals in secondary antibodies diluted by PBS) to the sections for 20 min at room temperature;

6. Treatment with primary antibody solution (optimally diluted) for 30 min at room temperature to overnight at 4°C;

7. Washing three times with PBS for 20 min;

8. Treatment with secondary antibodies (optimally diluted) for 30 min-1 hour at room temperature;

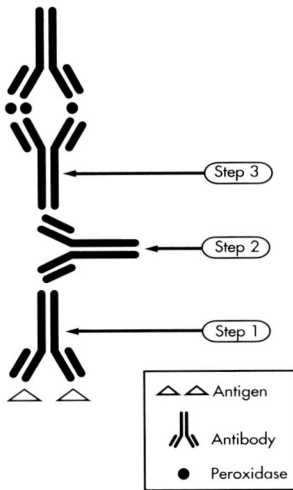

Figure 28.3 – Schematic diagram of the principle of PAP procedure

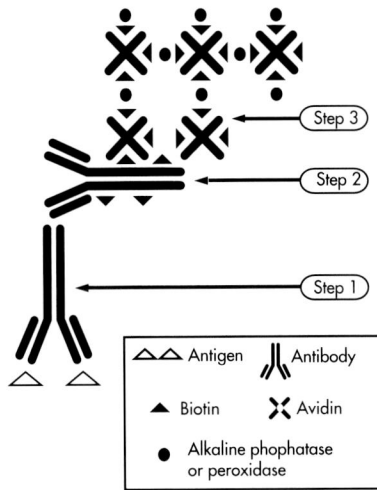

Figure 28.4 – Schematic diagram of the principle of ABC procedure

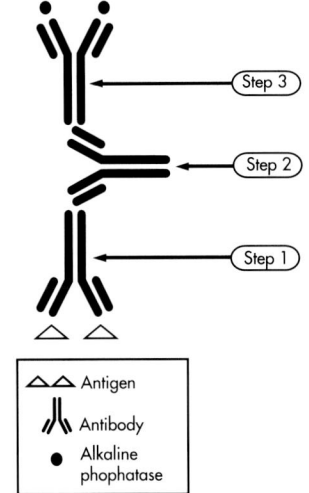

Figure 28.5 – Schematic diagram of the principle of APAAP procedure

9. Washing three times with PBS for 20 min;

10. Incubation with PAP complex for 30 min to 1 hour at room temperature;

11. Treatment of sections with 0.02% (w/v) DAB containing 0.03% (v/v) H_2O_2;

12. Washing in tap water for 5 min;

13. Nuclear stain (haematoxylin or methyl green);

14. Washing in tap water for 10 min;

15. Dehydration by graded alcohol and xylene;

16. Mount with cover slip.

Avidin–biotin–peroxidase complex (ABC) method

(Fig. 28.4)

1. Repeat steps 1-7 as above;

2. Treatment with biotinylated secondary antibodies (optimally diluted) for 30 min to 1 hour at room temperature;

3. Washing three times with PBS for 20 min;

4. Incubation in ABC complex or streptABC complex for 30 min-1 hour at room temperature;

5. Repeats steps 11-16 as above.

Alkaline phosphatase anti-alkaline phosphatase (APAAP) method

(Fig. 28.5)

1. Repeat steps 1-3 and 5-7 as above;

2. Treatment with biotinylated secondary antibodies (optimally diluted) for 30 min to 1 hour at room temperature;

3. Washing three times with PBS for 20 min;

4. Incubation in APAAP complex for 30 min to 1 hour at room temperature;

5. Treatment of sections by fast red and levamisole;

6. Repeat steps 12-16 as above.

Double immunostaining

To identify two antigens in a given section, double immunostaining provides considerable information. This procedure requires two sequential immunocytochemical steps. For example, the ABC and APAAP methods are combined. First, the ABC method is performed with DAB development (brown colour), and then the APAAP method is applied to the secton with fast red (red colour) or fast blue (blue colour) development.

Evaluation of immunostaining

The localization of reaction products should be carefully evaluated under a microscope. In ICC studies of extracellular matrix antigens such as collagen and laminin, reaction products should be observed in the extracellular space. In ICC of intracellular membraneous antigens such as growth factor receptors, reaction products are seen in the cytoplasm with membraneous accentuation. For ICC examinations of intracellular antigens such as intermediate filaments, reaction products are seen in the cytoplasm with accentuation in certain positions such as cytosol, Golgi apparatus, subnuclear, mitochondria or lysosomes. For ICC investigations of nuclear proteins such as certain oncogene products, reaction products should be localized to the nucleus.

ICC studies of paraffin sections occasionally yield heterogenous staining; some cells are positive and others negative. This negative reaction may be a false negative due to fixation or paraffin-embedding artifact. However, in such heterogenous staining, observers should semiquantitate or quantitate the positive cells to evaluate the overall appearance of the ICC results.

Application to animal studies

In ICC investigations in animals, ICC of cryostat fresh sections is more suitable than ICC of paraffin sections, because fresh tissue specimens are readily available and provide more specific and reliable results. In addition, fresh tissues are suitable for immunoelectron microscopic analysis as well as molecular biochemical methods. However, epoxy resin or paraffin embedding of tissues after favourable fixation is necessary for permanent tissue antigen preservation.

In ICC using cryostat sections, tissues obtained from animals are unfixed, frozen and embedded in OCT compound. Cryostat sections 10 μm thick are directly, or after postfixation with acetone, subjected to ICC. Alternatively, fresh tissues are briefly fixed with paraformaldehyde or periodate-lysine-paraformaldehyde (PLP), frozen and embedded in OCT compound, followed by sectioning and ICC. ICC of fresh frozen sections has the advantage of reliable antigen expression with minimal artifact, but has the disadvantage of poor tissue architectural preservation. However, the use of fresh frozen sections is the best ICC method. OCT compound-embedded tissues can be stored at -80°C. When there are numerous tissue specimens to be examined, the fresh tissues can be snap frozen in liquid nitrogen and stored at -80°C until used.

For permanent storage of tissues and antigens, paraffin-embedding is a useful method and antigen expression can be examined retrospectively. In addition, ICC of paraffin-embedded tissues gives rise to sections with excellent tissue architecture, and conventional stains such as haematoxylin and eosin are more suitable in paraffin-embedded sections than in cryostat sections. However, fresh sections are more useful than paraffin-embedded sections for the molecular analysis of protein and nucleic acid.

Results and discussion

ICC studies of paraffin sections have the advantages of excellent tissue architecture, permanent observation of stained sections, and permanent preservation of embedded tissue. However, in ICC of paraffin-embedded sections, it should always be taken into consideration that tissue antigens may be unmasked during fixation and the paraffin-embedding procedure. Therefore, negative immunostaining does not always denote that the antigens are absent in the tissues. In addition, positive immunostaining does not always confirm that the antigens are present in the tissues; positive immunostaining implies that there are epitopes with which the primary antibody reacts. Moreover, polyclonal and monoclonal antibodies derived from ascites occasionally contain other non-specific antibodies. Therefore, in every ICC study, the specificity of the antibodies must be examined by various methods including absorption test and Western blot analysis.

It has recently been indicated that ICC alone is not a reliable method for detecting antigens. Western blot analysis using fresh tissue is now a necessary adjunct to ICC. In addition, analysis of the mRNA and DNA encoding the antigens is frequently used in recent morphological studies.[7,8] Although fresh tissues are far superior to paraffin-embedded materials for RNA and DNA analysis, paraffin sections can be analysed for these mRNA and DNA.[7,8] In particular, DNA and mRNA can occasionally be extracted from paraffin sections.[7,8] The extracted DNA and mRNA can be analysed by Southern and Northern blot analyses. The polymerase chain reaction (PCR) and RT-PCR methods using specific primers and probes are useful methods for detecting certain DNA genes and mRNA, respectively. The determination of a base sequence can be done using PCR products. Recent studies have combined ICC with these molecular techniques and strengthen the data significantly.

References

1. Sternberger LA, Hardy PH, Cuculis JJ. The unlabeled antibody-enzyme method of immunohistochemistry: Preparation and properties of soluble antigen-antibody complex (horseraddish peroxidae-antihorseraddish peroxidase) and its use in identification of spirochetes. *J Histochem Cytochem* 1970; **18:** 315-333.

2. Hsu SM, Raine L, Fanger H. Use of avidin–biotin–peroxidase complex (ABC) in immunoperoxidase techniques: A comparison between ABC and unlabelled antibody (PAP) procedures. *J Histochem Cytochem* 1981; **29:** 577-580.

3. Cordel JL, Falini B, Erber WN *et al.* Immunoenzymatic labeling of monoclonal antibodies using immune complexes of alkaline phosphatase and monoclonal anti-alkaline phosphatase (APAAP) complexes. *J Histochem Cytochem* 1984; **32:** 219-229.

4. Shi SR, Key ME, Kalra KL. Antigen retrieval in formalin-fixed, paraffin embedded tissues: An enhancement method for immunohistochemical staining based on microwave oven heating of tissue sections. *J Histochem Cytochem* 1992; **39:** 741-748.

5. Tedara T, Morita T, Hoso M, Nakanuma Y, Pancreatic enzymes in epithelium of intrahepatic large bile ducts and in hepatic bile in patients with extrahepatic bile duct obstruction. *J Clin Pathol* 1994; **47:** 924-927

6. Terada T, Nakanuma Y. Expression of pancreatic enzymes (α-amylase, trypsinogen and lipase) during human liver development and maturation. *Gastroenterology* 1995; **108:** 1236-1245.

7. Montgomery EA, Hartmann DP, Carr NJ, Holterman DA, Sobin LH, Azumi N Barrett esophagus with dysplasia. Flow cytometric DNA analysis or routine, paraffin-embedded mucosal biopsies. *Am J Clin Pathol* 1996; **106:** 298-304

8. Dakhama a, Macek V, Hogg JC, Hegele RG. Amplification of human beta-actin gene by the reverse transcriptase-polymerase chain reaction: implications for assessment of RNA from formalin-fixed, paraffin-embedded material. *J Histochem Cytochem* 1996; **44:** 1205-1207.

29

Fluorescent microscopy of immune cells in the Peyer's patches and small intestines in immunodeficiency

María C López, María E Roux and Ronald R Watson

Summary

Peyer's patches are the main source of IgA B cell precursors that home to the intestinal lamina propria and other secretory sites where they terminally differentiate into IgA plasma cells that synthesize and secrete IgA. It has been demonstrated that IgA B cells require the presence of functional T cells in order to achieve terminal differentiation. In this chapter, the use of fluorescence microscopy to identify and quantitate lymphoid cells is described. We present data using two different models of secondary immunodeficiency, where T cell functionality is severely compromised, to demonstrate the techniques and their application. In the first study, we show that severe protein deficiency affects IgA B cell differentiation and then even when rats are adequately re-fed, the immunodeficiency cannot be completely abrogated. In the second study, we show a similar picture in mice infected with a retrovirus producing murine AIDS. From these two different studies, we can conclude that when immunodeficieny affects T cells, mucosal immunity will also be affected.

Introduction

The small intestine is an important and extended body defence barrier against pathogenic bacteria and viruses, but it also harbours commensal friendly bacteria that live associated with the mucous secretions that cover the intestinal surfaces. These secretions contain secretory immunoglobulins (IgA and IgM) bound to the polyimmunoglobulin receptor, and IgG transported by passive diffusion.[1-3] In the normal intestine, antigen is processed within the M cells - specialized antigen-presenting cells - at the Peyer's patches (PP). In the PP, M cells present antigen to highly specialized T cells known as switch T cells, mucosal T cells or Th3 cells. These PP helper cells, and environmental factors, give the signals required for IgM B cells to switch to IgA B cells.[4-6] Meanwhile other T cells provide the signals for IgA B cell proliferation and migration from the PP into the mesenteric lymph nodes.[7-10] IgA B cells further mature in the mesenteric lymph nodes (MLN)[11] before reaching the thoracic duct, entering the blood stream and homing back to secretory sites such as the intestinal lamina propria, uterine cervix and salivary glands. Here, the T cells will once more provide help to facilitate the final step in B cell differentiation into IgA plasma cells, therefore completing the 'IgA cell cycle'.[3]

In immunodeficiency secondary to severe protein deficiency or to retrovirus infection, the failure of IgA B cell differentiation leaves the host incapable of producing the large amounts of blocking antibodies required, not only to neutralize pathogenic bacteria, but also to control the number of commensal bacteria.[12-15] Moreover, the overall failure in cell-mediated immunity facilitates bacteria, parasite and virus invasion of the host's mucosal surfaces and spread through the whole body depending on the severity of the immunodeficiency.

Methods

To investigate PP and the small intestine in humans the difficulty must be realized of accessing the tissue to obtain the desired sample. Large enough samples for multiple studies can always be obtained from cadaveric donors or from normal tissues from surgical patients undergoing partial intestinal resections. Unfortunately, the main source of samples for human studies are intestinal biopsies which provide only a limited amount of very precious tissue.

Samples can be processed in different ways that will either render isolated cells[16-18] or tissue sections. Isolated cells can either be stained to define their phenotype or cultured in the presence of specific mitogens and/or antigens to determine their ability to produce and release into the supernatant specific cytokines, or their ability to proliferate by incorporating ^{3}H-thymidine. The incorporation of ^{3}H-thymidine into the cell nucleus in response to mitogen stimulation indicates that cells are responsive and not anergized. Moreover, ^{3}H-thymidine incorporation in *in vitro* studies in the presence of specific antigens (food, bacteria or virus) indicates the cells have been sensitized *in vivo* towards the challenge and can recognise it *in vitro*. Isolated cells can be further purified to obtain pure T cell subsets (either CD4 or CD8 cells) and cultured in the presence of irradiated antigen-presenting cells and antigen in order to generate antigen-specific T cell clones.[19]

The methods described here to study the small intestine can also be applied to the large intestine.

Cell isolation and purification from fresh tissue

The resected tissue or biopsy must be manipulated in sterile conditions and placed in either phosphate buffered saline (PBS; Gibco, Grand Island, NJ, USA) or in Hank's balance salt solution (HBSS; Sigma, St Louis, MO, USA), and with antibiotics (penicillin-G 10 000 U/l and streptomycin 1g/l; Sigma). A biopsy is immersed in 3-5 ml of PBS or HBSS, while a piece of resected intestine measuring 10×10 cm requires at least 300 ml. The tissues must be kept at 4°C until processed. An intestinal resection sample should be cut in at least 1 cm^2 sections, and repeatedly washed in PBS or HBSS at room temperature to remove the mucus. To perform this step the intestinal segments are tranferred to a sterile conical flask containing at least 100 ml PBS or HBSS, the flask is gently shaken two or three times and the washing solution is aspirated carefully to avoid losing tissue. A further 5 min wash, in similar conditions, but with magnetic stirring and in 1 mM dithiothreitol (Sigma) in PBS or HBSS is highly recommended to eliminate the remaining mucus. To isolate the intestinal intra-epithelial lymphocytes (IEL), two 30 min incubations at 37°C, with magnetic stirring, in 100 ml of either PBS or RPMI 1640 (Sigma) supplemented with 10 mM (N-[2-hydroxyethyl] piperazine -N'-[2-ethane-sulphonic acid]) (HEPES; Sigma), 1 mM ethylene diaminotetra-acetic acid (EDTA; Sigma), 2-5% (v/v) heat inactivated fetal calf serum (FCS; Gibco) and 40 mg/ml DNAse (Boehringer Ingelheim, Heidelberg, Germany) are required. The incubation medium, containing the IEL, is then carefully collected leaving the intestinal segments behind. These segments are retained for isolation of lamina propria lymphocytes (LPL). The medium containing the IEL is filtered through a 90 μm mesh (Bellco Biotechnology, Vineland, NJ, USA), glass wool, cotton wool or nylon wool columns to eliminate dead cells and debris, and is collected in 50 ml tubes at room temperature. Then, the IEL are spun down at 4°C at 400 g for 10 min, washed with the same medium as before, spun down again, resuspended in medium containing HBSS, 10 mM HEPES and 5% (v/v) FCS, and counted. Then, the cell suspensions are adjusted to no greater than 1×10^7 cells/ml. The IEL are now ready for the last purification step through a 60%-40% Percoll gradient (Pharmacia, Uppsala, Sweden). Percoll dilutions must be prepared following strictly the instructions provided by the manufacturer. If cells are resuspended in HBSS it is advisable to prepare Percoll dilutions in HBSS. The gradients are prepared in 50 ml tubes, 15 ml of a 60% Percoll solutions is deposited in the bottom of the tube, followed by 15 ml of a 40% Percoll solution, and by 15 ml IEL cell suspension. The number of tubes required depends on the number of cells obtained. The gradients are spun

down at 600 g for 20 min at 20°C. IEL are collected from the interface between 60% and 40% Percoll. They are washed twice in cold medium containing RPMI 1640 10 mM HEPES and 10% (v/v) FCS, at 400 g for 10 min. Then the cells are counted and viability is determined using trypan blue exclusion. Cell suspensions with a viability higher than 80% are kept in the cold until further use. If the viability is lower, the cells are discarded.

After collecting the medium containing the IEL, the remaining small intestine segments are incubated with an equal amount of medium as used in the previous step but containing: RPMI 1640, 10 mM HEPES, 5% (v/v) FCS and 10 U/ml collagenase (Sigma, catalogue number C-6885). The LPL are collected after incubation at 37°C for 90 min with continuous stirring. The cell suspensions are filtered through a 90 μm mesh, nylon wool or cotton wool columns to eliminate dead cells and debris and are further purified in a Percoll gradient as described above for IEL. These cells are ready for staining and analysis either under the microscope or using a flow cytometer. Purified T and B cell subsets can be obtained following the panning technique,[20] or using nylon wool columns specially designed for T cell purification.[21]

The panning technique[20] involves coating plastic Petri dishes with specific monoclonal antibodies and incubating the dishes with lymphoid cells. After incubation, those cells bearing markers recognised by the antibodies are attached to the dishes, while the other cells are recovered from the incubation medium. Attached cells require energetic pipetting to be released. The technique permits the isolation of T cell subsets, while isolation using nylon wool columns[21] only permits the purification of total T cells. Moreover, the preparation of nylon wool is extremely time consuming. Although some authors still use these methods, nowadays it is much easier to obtain specific columns that render total T, or CD4 or CD8 pure cells (R&D Systems, Abingdon, UK).

Cell staining

To stain live cells it is extremely important that the cell suspensions are kept at 4°C after isolation and throughout the staining procedure in order to slow down metabolism and avoid the internalization and co-capping of surface markers. The cell suspensions are adjusted to between 1×10^6 to 1×10^7 cells/ml in PBS containing 1% (w/v) bovine serum albumin (BSA; Sigma) and 0.01% (w/v) sodium azide

(SA; Sigma). 100 µl of the cell suspension is deposited in each well of a 96-well V bottom plate (Costar, Cambridge, MA, USA). The specific primary purified monoclonal antibody or directly conjugated monoclonal antibody is diluted in 50 µl of the same medium used to resuspend the cells, and the ideal dilution - that the researcher must check personally - would be around 1 µg antibody/1 × 10^6 cells. The cells are incubated for 30 min to 1 hour at 4°C, using a plate shaker where available. Then, the cells are washed with 50 µl of PBS/BSA/sodium azide (SA), spun down at 600 g for 4 min at 4°C. The plate is inverted and the supernatant discarded. Then the cells are resuspended in 200 µl of PBS/BSA/SA, and spun down again under the same conditions. Finally, cells are resuspended in 100 µl of PBS/BSA/SA and a fluorochrome-conjugated secondary antibody is added where necessary and the incubation procedure and washes are repeated. At the end of the staining procedure, in order to preserve the staining, the cells must be fixed with 2% (w/v) paraformaldehyde (Sigma) in PBS, pH 7.4. When the samples are analysed in a flow cytometer, 300-500 µl of fixative are used to resuspend and fix the cells, but if the cells are analysed under a fluorescence microscope it is convenient to use 1500-2000 µl of fixative. To analyse the cells under fluorescence microscopy it is convenient to prepare cytospins using super frosted slides (BDH, Poole, UK) or precoated slides, that must be coated by the user following the instructions provided by the manufacturer (e.g. Biobond, British BioCell, Cardiff, UK). The cytospins are prepared by depositing 200-300 µl of cells in fixative in the conical insert attached to the slide in the cytocentrifuge, and spinning down at 400 rpm for 4 min. Then, the slides are air dried. Once the cells are firmly adhered to the slides it is necessary to cover the cytospins with a drop of mounting medium - generally PBS/glycerol 10:90 (v/v) - (glycerol; Sigma) and a coverslip. The edges of the coverslip are sealed with nail polish for permanent preservation of the sample. It is important to keep the slides in darkness at 4°C to preserve the staining.

Whether the cells are analysed under the fluorescence microscope or using a flow cytometer, secondary antibodies conjugated with different fluorochromes can be selected. It is possible to detect up to three colours simultaneously using fluorescence microscopy and secondary antibodies conjugated with the following fluorochromes: 7-amino-4- methyl-coumarin-3 acetic acid (AMCA, blue), fluorescein or fluorescein isothiocyanate (FITC, green) and rhodamine or Texas Red (red). Several brands of microscopes permitting the detection of fluorochromes are available: Leica (Heidelberg, Germany), Leitz (Wetzlar, Germany), Zeiss (Jena, Germany), Olympus (Hamburg, Germany) among others.

Tissue sections

Tissue sections can be obtained after processing the tissues in different ways. To study lymphocyte surface markers (CD antigens), snap freezing of the sample and cryostat sectioning is generally performed. However, studies using archival samples or studies performed in developing countries - where liquid nitrogen or freezer cooling to a least -70°C are not always available - need alternative techniques. For archival samples processed through the conventional formalin fixation and paraffin- embedding technique, the microwave antigen retrieval technique[22-24] seems to be the ideal option. Alternatively, where cryopreservation of the sample is not possible, fixation in 95% ethanol following the technique of Sainte-Marie,[25] is an option if adequate monoclonal antibodies recognizing the cluster differentiation (CD) antigens in these conditions are available.

Staining of tissue sections

Sections obtained from paraffin-embedded tissues require deparaffinization in xylene for 5 min and several steps of rehydration in decreasing concentrations of ethanol in water (100%, 90%, 70%, 50% and 30%: 5 min each) and a final rehydration step in PBS or water, before proceeding with the staining. On the other hand, frozen sections only need a short fixation in cold acetone (10 min at 4°C) and rehydration in PBS. The whole staining procedure is generally performed in a humid chamber at room temperature. The primary antibody is applied for 30 min to 1 hour. In special situations, where the only antibodies available have low affinity for the cell marker, an overnight incubation at 4°C could be the best option although some authors prefer an hour incubation at 37°C. The primary antibodies are generally used as purified antibodies or biotin-conjugated antibodies and prepared in PBS 1% (w/v) BSA, using 50 µl diluted antibody. After incubation with the primary antibody, the slides are transferred to coplin jars where two or three washes of at least 5 min each in PBS are recommended. Then, the slides are transferred back to the humid chamber, and 50 µl of the secondary antibody labelled with a fluorochrome (e.g. FITC-goat anti-rat) or fluorochrome-conjugated streptavidin are used as second-step reagents. This incubation is generally performed at room temperature for 30 min and followed by three washes in PBS. After this step, the sections are covered with mounting medium (described above) and a coverslip. The slides must be kept at 4°C in the dark.

Where high non-specific background is observed there are several possible solutions: a 10 min block with 50 μl PBS 20% (w/v) BSA followed by one wash in PBS before incubating with the primary antibody; or preparation of the primary antibody in PBS with 5-10% (v/v) serum from the same species where the secondary antibody was raised; or preparation of the primary antibody (biotinylated one) in PBS with 5-10% (v/v) serum from the same species where the primary antibody was raised; or preparation of the primary and secondary antibodies in PBS with 10% (v/v) serum from the same species under study (e.g. AB human serum for human tissue). In all these examples the incubations are performed at room temperature, for 30 min and the volume of diluted antibody added is 50 μl.

There are several commercial sources of monoclonal antibodies to use in human studies; we recommend the primary antibodies provided by Becton Dickinson (Mountain View, CA, USA) and Immunotech (Westbrook, ME, USA). For fluorochrome-labelled secondary antibodies the best options are: Southern Biotechnology Associates (Birmingham, AL, USA), Dako A/S (Glostrup, Denmark) for FITC, rhodamine and Texas Red-conjugated secondary antibodies, and Bioprobes (Molecular Probes, Eugene, OR, USA) for AMCA-conjugated secondary antibodies.

Application to animal studies

The methods described above can be used in rodent studies with minor modifications. The most important factor to take into account is that in rodents work is carried out predominantly on the whole small intestine. Therefore, it is very important to remember to isolate the PP even if they were to be discarded later on, and to clean the outside of the intestine of blood vessels, lymphatics and fat tissue. Then, the intestine is opened longitudinally and washed with 10 μl PBS, before cutting it into smaller segments (0.5 × 0.5 cm) and continuing with the procedure as described for human intestines above. For the final step of cell purification either Percoll gradients or

mouse or rat lymphocyte separation medium (Cedarlane, Hornby, Ontario, Canada) can be used.

Preparation of single cell suspensions from mouse or rat PP

Mice have approximately 12 PP in their small intestine, the diameter ranging between 1 and 2 mm. Rats may have up to 18-20 PP and their diameter can reach 4 mm. It is standard procedure to dissect out all PP and place them in medium (RPMI 1640, 10% (v/v) FCS, 10 mM HEPES, and antibiotics as described previously)[12,15] on ice until they are processed. To isolate single cells the PP are placed on a plastic cell strainer (Falcon, Becton Dickinson, Bedford, MA, USA) or a 80 μm stainless steel wire mesh (Bellco Biotechnology) previously wet with medium. A plastic syringe plunger is used to press the cells through the mesh. The cells must be washed twice with 5 ml medium, resuspended in 1-2 ml medium and kept on ice until use. Cell number and viability are determined as described above: if the viability is >80%, the cell suspension is adjusted as indicated above, and is ready for cell-surface marker staining (see above). If cytoplasmic markers are of interest (as alpha or mu immunoglobulin heavy chains, detectable in B cells) a cytospin is prepared (see above). The cytospins must be air dried, fixed for 30 min by dipping in cold methanol (4°C) and again air dried. They can either be stained immediately or kept dessicated at -20°C for several weeks. The staining for cytoplasmic markers is as described for tissue sections above, beginning with a rehydration in PBS.

To evaluate T and B cell populations in rat studies, tissues are processed either by snap freezing or by Sainte Marie's protocol[25] with similar results. According to the latter protocol, tissues are fixed by dropping them into pre-cooled (4°C) 95% (v/v) ethanol and kept in the fridge overnight to 24 hours; this is the main difference when compared with conventional paraffin embedding where tissues are fixed in formalin. Then, tissues are dehydrated in four changes of pre-cooled absolute ethanol, 1 hour each. The tissues are cleared by passing through three changes of pre-cooled xylene, 1 hour each. Finally, the tissues are embedded in four consecutive baths in paraffin at 56°C, 1 hour each.

In rat studies, we use monoclonal antibodies anti-T cell markers (SeraLab, Crawley Down, Sussex, UK) followed by either affinity-purified fluorescein or rhodamine-conjugated goat anti-mouse IgG (Cappel,

Division of Oregon Teknika Corp, Durham, NC, USA). To determine B cell markers, we use affinity-purified polyclonal antibodies anti-rat immunoglobulin heavy chains (Cappel), followed by affinity-purified fluorescein-conjugated rabbit anti-goat antibody (Cappel).

To evaluate T and B cell populations in mouse studies we have used snap frozen tissues. In mouse studies, monoclonal antibodies anti-T cell markers (PharMingen, San Diego, CA, USA; SeraLab, distributed by Accurate Chemicals, Westbury, NY, USA) followed by FITC-labelled goat anti-rat immunoglobulins (Southern Biotechnology Associates, Birmingham, AL, USA), or affinity-purified rhodamine-conjugated goat anti-rat F(ab')$_2$ (Cappel) or affinity-purified FITC-labelled goat anti-hamster immunoglobulins (Caltag, San Francisco, CA, USA). To analyse B cells containing μ or α immunoglobulin heavy chains, we use affinity-purified polyclonal antibodies (Cappel) followed by affinity-purified FITC or rhodamine-conjugated rabbit anti-goat antibody (Cappel) or Texas Red-conjugated rabbit anti-goat antibody (Jackson ImmunoResearch, West Grove, PA, USA).

Results and discussion

Applicabilty of the methods to human data

The studies performed in coeliac patients by Per Brandtzaeg's group,[26-28] represent the best example of applying the methods described above to human subjects.

Aquired immuodeficiency after HIV infection is the most important human immunodeficiency. As HIV infected patients suffer a great variety of gastro-intestinal infections that become life threatening and require precise diagnosis, duodenal and colonic biopsy material has become more easily available.[29] The studies have shown alterations in the immuno-architecture of the small intestine, even when secondary infections are absent.[30] A decrease in villous height, villous surface area and in the number of mitotic figures was observed in the duodenal mucosa.[31] An increased number of CD3+ and CD8+ cells associated with a decreased number of CD4+ cells gave an inverted CD4/CD8 ratio in the ILP.[32] Moreover, the number of CD25+ cells (activated lymphocytes) was also decreased.[32] These results are

confirmed using flow cytometric techniques.[33,34] Similar results were obtained studying biopsies of large intestines.[35,36] The loss of CD4+ cells in both intestines is even more marked than in peripheral blood.[34] Other authors studied B cell populations in the ILP of HIV infected individuals and found a decreased number of IgA1+, IgA2+, IgM+ and IgG4+ cells in the duodenal lamina propria and of IgA2+ and IgG2+ in the colonic lamina propria.[37] Taken together these results indicate that HIV infection induces a loss of functional T cells that provide help for B cell differentiation, reducing the amount of neutralizing antibodies and, therefore, favouring opportunistic infections.

Immunodeficiency due to protein deficiency in rats

We studied severe protein deficiency after considering the central role that protein has in every metabolic pathway. We used weanling rats in an attempt to model children's mucosal immune system. Severe protein deficiency was induced by feeding rats with a protein-free diet for 13-16 days.[38] Protein deficiency provoked a dramatic decrease in the number of B cells in PP (Table 29.1).[12,13] Double staining studies showed the presence of a pre-B cell population[12] in the PP, indicating the step of B cell differentiation where the breakdown took place. Concomitantly, B and T cell numbers were also decreased in the ILP (Table 29.2).[14] We also evaluated the possibility of immune restoration by re-feeding protein-deprived rats with an adequate diet. Unfortunately, sIgA+ B cells could not reach control values in the PP of re-fed rats (Table 29.1).[12,13] As severe protein deficiency also affected the thymus, in a partially reversible fashion,[39] a decreased number of mature T cells was found in the PP of re-fed rats (Table 29.1). Moreover, successful maturation of IgA B cell precursors in the MLN had not taken place, since an inadequate number of IgA plasma cells was observed in the ILP.[40] Other studies have also shown that MLN blasts derived from rats suffering protein calorie malnutri-tion and vitamin A deficiency were not able to repopulate the ILP as could blasts from normal rats.[41]

These studies indicate that T and B cell differentiation are affected by severe protein deficiency and suggest that although differentiation can be partially restored after protein re-feeding, a certain level of damage will continue to affect the host even if protein deficiency is completely reversed.

Table 29.1 – Absolute number of T and B Cells in the Peyer's patches of rats with severe protein deficiency.

Experimental groups	T cells[*]		B cells[*]		
	CD4[*]	CD8[+]	cytμ	sIgM[+]	sIgA[+]
39-day control	2.9 ± 0.3	2.1 ± 0.4	6.5 ± 1.1	9.4 ± 0.9	4.9 ± 0.9
SPD	2.6 ± 0.4	2.2 ± 0.3	4.2 ± 0.3[§]	2.0 ± 0.6[§]	1.3 ± 0.2[§]
60-day control	8.3 ± 0.9	7.5 ± 1.5	10.9 ± 0.3	5.4 ± 2.0	15.4 ± 1.9
RFR	3.6 ± 0.8[§]	3.6 ± 0.9[§]	5.4 ± 1.6[#]	7.9 ± 1.5	5.0 ± 0.7[§]

T and B cell subsets were analysed in the Peyer's patches of rats suffering severe protein deficiency (SPD), after protein re-feeding (RFR), and in their respective age-matched controls. [*] Data are presented as absolute number of cells × 10^{-5} ± SE. Experimental vs age-matched control: [§]$p < 0.01$; [#]$p < 0.05$. Reprinted from ref. 12 with kind permission of Elsevier Science Ltd.

Table 29.2 – T and B cells in the intestinal lamina propria of rats with severe protein deficiency.

Experimental groups	CD4[*]	CD8[+]	IgA[+]
39-day control	136.3 ± 13.0	141.4 ± 18.3	137.4 ± 8.7
SPD	46.6 ± 10.9[§]	53.0 ± 9.9[§]	6.6 ± 1.5[¶]
60-day control	183.4 ± 7.9	158.5 ± 4.7	230.9 ± 19.2
RFR	216.8 ± 14.7	188.1 ± 19.5	94.6 ± 13.2[§]

T and IgA B cell were analysed in the intestinal lamina of rats suffering severe protein deficiency (SPD), after protein re-feeding (RFR) and in their respective age-matched controls. Data are presented as number of positive cells ± SE per 30 high powered fields. Experimental vs age-matched control: [§]$p < 0.001$; [¶]$p < 0.0005$. Modified from ref. 14 with kind permission of John Wiley & Sons, Inc.

Table 29.3 – Absolute number of T and B cells in the Peyer's patches of murine AIDS infected mice.

Experimental groups	CD4[*]	CD8[+]	sIgA[+]
Control	6.7 ± 4.9	6.2 ± 5.1	10.9 ± 4.3
LP-BM5 infected	0.9 ± 0.6[§]	0.6 ± 0.4[§]	0.7 ± 0.9[§]

T and B cells from the Peyer's patches of murine AIDS infected mice (LP-BM5 infected, 4 months after infection) and control mice were analysed. Data are presented as absolute number of cells × 10^{-5} ± SD. Experimental vs. control: [§]$p < 0.01$. Modified from ref. 15 with kind permission of John Wiley & Sons, Inc.

Table 29.4 – T and B cells in the intestinal lamina propria of murine AIDS infected mice.

Experimental groups	CD4[*]	CD8[+]	sIgA[+]	IgA[+]CD5[+]
Control	30.3 ± 9.1	11.1 ± 6.1	34.4 ± 19.0	5.1 ± 2.5
LP-BM5 infected	10.6 ± 3.6[§]	7.4 ± 3.5	11.7 ± 3.1[§]	1.6 ± 0.6[#]

T and B cells from the intestinal lamina propria of murine AIDS infected mice (LP-BM5 infected, 4 months after infection) and control mice were analysed. Data are presented as number of positive cells ± SD per 20 high power fields. Experimental vs. control: [§]$p < 0.01$; [#]$p < 0.05$. Modified from ref. 15 with kind permission of John Wiley & Sons, Inc.

Immunodeficiency due to retrovirus infection

When susceptible strains of mice are infected with LP-BM5 murine leukaemia virus, an immunodeficiency state, with many features in common with HIV infection in humans, is rapidly achieved.[42,43] One of the more dramatic outcomes of HIV infection is the variety of secondary infections that can affect the host, including pathogenic organisms for immunocompetent hosts such as *Mycobacterium tuberculosis*, or other agents such as *Pneumocistis carinii* and *Cryptosporidium parvum* that could only severely affect an immunocompromized host.[44-46]

We successfully reproduced *Cryptosporidium parvum* infection in mice infected with LP-BM5 murine leukaemia virus for 4 months.[47] Moreover, we also showed an impairment in T-cell differentiation in LP-BM5 infected mice.[48,49] We investigated the changes induced by retrovirus infection in T and B cell populations in the PP and ILP that could have facilitated parasite infection. We observed a decreased number of CD4[+], CD8[+] and sIgA[+] cells in the PP (Table 29.3, data obtained using flow cytometry)[15] and a decreased number of CD4[+], IgA[+] cells (total IgA[+] cells compromise IgA B1 and IgA B2 cells) and IgA[+] CD5[+] (IgA B1 cells only) cells in the ILP (Table 29.4).[15] Our data indicate that mice infected with LP-BM5 for 4 months were unable to mount an adequate secretory response as observed in AIDS patients.[50-52]

From the two types of secondary immunodeficiency described above, it can be concluded that when immunodeficiency affects T cells, mucosal immunity will be further affected.

Acknowledgements

The studies presented were supported by grants PID 3-0212 and 3-0007 from the National Council for Scientific and Technical Research (CONICET) to ME Roux and NIH grants AA08037 and DA04827 to RR Watson.

References

1. Brandtzaeg P. Basic mechanisms of mucosal immunity - A major adaptive defense system. *Immunologist* 1995; **3**: 89-96.

2. Brandtzaeg P. History of oral tolerance and mucosal immunity. *Ann NY Acad Sci* 1996; **778**: 1-27.

3. Lamm ME. Cellular aspects of immunoglobulin A. *Adv Immunol* 1976; **22**: 223-290.

4. Gearhart PJ, Cebra JJ. Differentiated B lymphocytes. Potential to express particular antibody variable and constant regions depends on site of lymphoid tissue and antigen load. *J Exp Med* 1979; **149**: 216-227.

5. Kawanishi H, Satzman LE, Strober W. Mechanisms regulating IgA class-specific immunoglobulin production in murine gut-associated lymphoid tissues. I. T-cells derived from Peyer's patches that switch sIgM B cells to sIgA B cells *in vitro*. *J Exp Med* 1983; **157**: 433-450.

6. Chen Y, Kuchroo VK, Inobe J-I, Hafler DA, Weiner HL. Regulatory T cell clones induced by oral tolerance: suppression of autoimmune encephalopathies. *Science* 1994; **265**: 1237-1240.

7. Kawanishi H, Strober W. Regulatory T cells in murine Peyer's patches directing IgA-specific isotype switching. *Ann NY Acad Sci* 1983; **409**: 243-257.

8. Kiyono H, McGhee JR, Mostellar LM *et al*. Murine Peyer's patch T cell clones. Characterization of antigen-specific helper T cells for immunoglobulin A responses. *J Exp Med* 1982; **156**: 1115-1130.

9. Kiyono H, Cooper MD, Kearney IF *et al*. Isotype specificity of helper T cell clones. Peyer's patch T cells preferentially collaborate with mature IgA B cells for IgA response. *J Exp Med* 1984; **159**: 718-811.

10. Kawanishi H, Saltzman L, Strober W. Mechanisms regulating IgA class-specific immunoglobulin production in murine gut-associated lymphoid tissues. II. Terminal differentiation of postswitch sIgA-bearing Peyer's patch B cells. *J Exp Med* 1983; **158**: 649-669.

11. Roux ME, McWilliams M, Phillips-Quagliata JM, Lamm ME. Differentiation pathway of Peyer's patch precursors of IgA plasma cells in the secretory immune system. *Cell Immunol* 1981; **61**: 141-153.

12. Lopez MC, Roux ME. Impaired differentiation of IgA-B cell precursors in the Peyer's patches of protein depleted rats. *Dev Comp Immunol* 1989; **13**: 253-262.

13. Lopez MC. *Alterations in the IgA Cell Cycle in Immunodeficiency due to Protein Malnutrition*. Thesis, Faculty of Pharmacy and Biochemistry, University of Buenos Aires, Buenos Aires, 1987.

14. Gonzalez Ariki S, Lopez MC, Roux ME. IgA B lymphocytes and subpopulations of T lymphocytes in the intestinal villi of immunodeficient Wistar rats. *Reg Immunol* 1992; **4**: 41-45.

15. Lopez MC, Colombo LL, Huang DS, Watson RR. Suppressed mucosal lymphocyte populations by LP-BM5 murine leukemia virus infection produing murine AIDS. *Reg Immunol* 1992; **4**: 162-167.

16. Lyscom N, Brueton MJ. Intraepithelial, lamina propria and Peyer's patch lymphocytes of the rat small intestine: isolation and characterization in terms of immunoglobulin markers and receptors for monoclonal antibodies. *Immunology* 1982; **45:** 775-783.

17. Davies MDJ, Parrot DMV. Preparation and purificaton of lymphocytes from the epithelium and lamina propria of murine small intestine. *Gut* 1981; **22:** 481-488.

18. Cerf-Bensussan N, Guy-Grand D, Griscelli C. Intraepithelial lymphocytes of human gut: isolation, characterisation and study of natural killer activity. *Gut* 1985; **26:** 81-88.

19. Lundin KEA, Scott H, Hansen T *et al.* Gliadin-specific, HLA-DQ(α1*0501,β1*0201) restricted T cells isolated from the small intestinal mucosa of celiac disease patients. *J Exp Med* 1993; **178:** 187-196.

20. Wysocki L, Sato VL. Panning for lymphocytes: a method for cell selection. *Proc Natl Acad Sci USA* 1978; **75:** 2844-2848.

21. Julius MF, Simpson E, Herzenberg LA. A rapid method for the isolation of functional thymus-derived murine lymphocytes. *Eur J Immunol* 1973; **3:** 645-649.

22. Cattoretti G, Pileri S, Parravicini C *et al.* Antigen unmasking on formalin-fixed, paraffin-embedded tissue sections. *J Pathol* 1993; **171:** 83-98.

23. Lan HY, Mu W, Nikolic-Paterson DJ, Atkins RC. A novel, simple, reliable, and sensitive method for multiple immunoenzyme staining: use of microwave oven heating to block antibody crossreactivity and retrieve antigens. *J Histochem Cytochem* 1995; **43:** 97-102.

24. Shi SR, Key ME, Kalra KL. Antigen retrieval in formalin-fixed, paraffin-embedded tissues: an enhancement method for immunohistochemical staining based on microwave heating of tissue sections. *J Histochem Cytochem* 1991; **39:** 741-748.

25. Sainte-Marie G. A paraffin-embedding technique for studies employing immunofluorescence. *J Histochem Cytochem* 1962; **10:** 250-256.

26. Halstensen TS, Brandtzaeg P. Phenotypic characteristics of human intraepithelial lymphocytes. In: Kiyono H, McGhee J (Eds) M *Mucosal Immunity: Intraepithelial Lymphocytes. Advances in Host Defense Mechanisms.* Raven Press, New York, 1994, pp.147-161.

27. Brandtzaeg P, Halstensen TS, Hvatum M, Kvale D, Scott H. The serologic and mucosal immunologic basis of celiac disease. In: Walker WA, Harmatz PR, Wershil BK (Eds) *Immunophysiology of the Gut.* Academic Press, London, 1993, pp. 295-333.

28. Halstensen TS, Scott H, Farstad IN, Michaelsen TE, Brandtzaeg P. *In situ* two- and three-color immuno-fluorescence staining of mucosal T-cells in celiac disease. In: Graumann W, Drukker J (Eds) *Progress in Histo and Cytochemistry*, vol 26. Fischer Verlag, Stuttgart, 1992, pp. 201-210.

29. Ullrich R, Heise W, Bergs C, L'Age M, Riecken EO, Zeitz M. Gastrointestinal symptoms in patients infected with human immunodeficiency virus: relevance of infective agents isolated from gastrointestinal tract. *Gut* 1992; **33:** 1080-1084.

30. Ullrich R, Zeitz M, Heise W *et al.* Mucosal atrophy is associated with loss of activated T cells in the duodenal mucosa of human immunodeficiency virus (HIV)-infected patients. *Digestion* 1990; **46(Suppl 2):** 302-307.

31. Ullrich R, Riecken EO, Zeitz M. Human immuno-deficiency virus-induced enteropathy. *Immunol Res* 1991; **10:** 456-464.

32. Zeitz M, Ullrich R, Riecken EO. The role of the gut-associated lymphoid tissue in the pathogenesis of the acquired immunodeficiency syndrome (HIV-infection). In: MacDonald TT, Challacombe SJ, Bland PW, Stokes CR, Heatley RV, Mowat AMcI (Eds) *Advances in Mucosal Immunology.* Kluwer Academic Publishers Dordrecht, 1990, pp. 655-659.

33. Schneider T, Ullrich R, Jahn HU *et al* and the Berlin Diarrhea/Wasting Syndrome Study Group. Loss of activated CD4-positive T cells and increase in activated cytotoxic CD8-positive T cells in the duodenum of patients infected with human immunodeficiency virus. *Adv Exp Med Biol* 1995; **371B:** 1019-1021.

34. Schneider T, Jahn HU, Schmidt W, Riecken EO, Zeitz M, Ullrich R. Loss of CD4 T lymphcytes in patients infected with human immunodeficiency virus type 1 is more pronounced in the duodenal mucosa than in the peripheral blood. *Gut* 1995; **37:** 524-529.

35. Schneider T, Ullrich R, Bergs C, Schmidt W, Riecken EO, Zeitz M. Abnormalities in subset distribution, activation and differentiation of T cells isolated from large intestine biopsies in HIV infection. *Clin Exp Immunol* 1994; **95**: 430-435.

36. Ullrich R, Schneider T, Bergs C *et al.* Loss of CD4 positive T cells and evidence for impaired differen-tiation by both CD4 and CD8 positive T cells in the large intestine of patients infected with human immunodeficiency virus (HIV). *Adv Exp Med Biol* 1995; **371B:** 1015-1017.

37. Lennartz EG, Herbst EW, Peter HH. Immunohistologische charakterisierung des intestinalen immunsystems bei patienten mit AIDS. *Immun Infekt* 1994; **22:** 26-27.

38. Lopez MC, Roux ME, Langini SH, Rio ME, Sanahuja JC. Effect of severe protein deficiency and refeeding on precursor IgA-cells in Peyer's patches of growing rats. *Nutr Rep Int* 1985; **32:** 667-674.

39. Roux ME, Slobodianik NH, Lopez MC et al. Etude de al cinétique de récuperation du thymus et des plaques de Peyer, chez des rats carencés en protéines au sevrage après l'administration de caséine. In: Lemonnier D, Ingenbleek Y (Eds) Les Carences Nutritionnelles dans les Pays en Voie de Développement. Karthala-ACCT, Paris, 1989, pp. 241-250.

40. Lopez MC, Slobodianik NH, Roux ME. Impaired maturation of IgA B cell precursors in the mesenteric lymph nodes due to protein deficiency. Immunologia 1988; **7:** 133-137.

41. McDermott MR, Mark DA, Befus AD, Baliga BS, Suskind RM, Bienenstock J. Impaired intestinal localization of mesenteric lymphoblasts associated with vitamin A deficiency and protein-calorie malnutrition. Immunology 1982; **45:** 1-5.

42. Mosier DE, Yetter RA, Morse III HC. Retroviral induction of acute lymphoproliferative disease and profound immunosuppression in adult C57BL/6 mice. J Exp Med 1985; **161:** 766-784.

43. Chattopadhyay SK, Makino M, Hartley JW, Morse III HC. Pathogenesis of MAIDS, a retrovirus induced immunodeficiency disease in mice. In: Wu B-Q, Zheng J (Eds) Immunodeficient Animals in Experimental Medicine. Karger, Basel, 1989, pp. 12-18.

44. Pantaleo G, Fauci AS. New concepts in the immunopathogenesis of HIV infection. Annu Rev Immunol 1995; **13:** 487-512.

45. Miedema F. Immunobiology of HIV infection. From latency and reactivation to protection and perturbation. Immunologist 1995; **3:** 228-230.

46. Flanigan TP. Human immunodeficiency virus infection and cryptosporidiosis: protective immune responses. Am J Trop Med Hyg 1994; **50(Suppl):** 29-35.

47. Darban H, Enriquez J, Sterling CR et al. Cryptosporidiosis facilitated by murine retroviral-infection with LP-BM5. J Inf Dis 1991; **164:** 741-745.

48. Lopez MC, Colombo LL, Huang DS, Wang Y, Watson RR. Modifications of thymic cell subsets induced by long-term cocaine administration during murine retroviral infection producing AIDS. Clin Immunol Immunopathol 1992; **65:** 45-52.

49. Lopez MC, Chen G-J, Colombo LL. Spleen and thymus cell subsets modified by long-term morphine administration and murine AIDS - II. Int J Immunopharmacology 1993; **15:** 909-918.

50. Sweet SP, Rahman D, Challacombe SJ. IgA subclasses in HIV disease: dichotomy between raised levels of serum and decreased secretion rates in saliva. Immunology 1995; **86:** 556-559.

51. Belec L, Meillet D, Gaillard O et al. Decreased cervicovaginal production of both IgA1 and IgA2 subclasses in women with AIDS. Clin Exp Immunol 1995; **101:** 100-106.

52. Belec L, Dupre T, Prazuck T et al. Cervicovaginal overproduction of specific IgG to human immuno-deficiency virus (HIV) contrasts with normal or impaired IgA local response in HIV infection. J Inf Dis 1995; **172:** 691-697.

30

Flow cytometry: Clinical and experimental applications to intestinal pathologies

Hsin-Min Tsao, Fen-Fang Huang and Dennis S Huang

Summary

Flow cytometry is a widely used method that offers several advantages over other conventional methodologies. It can be used for simultaneous quantitation of antigenic, biochemical and biophysical characteristics of individual cells. Its merits are underscored by its capacity to perform phenotyping, cell sorting, coordinate regulation analysis, cell-cycle analysis and various metabolic activity analysis rapidly and correlatively on a single cell basis from a heterogeneous population of cells. Flow cytometry has become an indispensable tool in every field and has made substantial contributions to gastrointestinal studies. This chapter discusses several useful clinical and experimental appplications of flow cytometry.

Introduction

Flow cytometers use excitation light(s) to exicte fluorescent dyes (also called fluorochromes) that "stain" cells. When a stained cell intercepts with the excitation light, the fluorochromes are excitable and emit fluorescent emissions. Based on their wavelengths, these emissions and scattered excitation light are routed, split and detected by detectors placed behind various band-pass filters. For example, the detector behind a 530 nm band-pass filter detects green light; while that behind a 580 nm band-pass filter detects orange light. The detectors then translate the flourescence intensities into digitized brightness levels, which reflect cellular properties such as metabolic activities or the abundance of a certain molecule.

Lymphoid cells responding to immunological insults in the gastrointestinal tract can be separated into several compartments including lymphoid follicles (e.g. Peyer's patches), lamina propria lymphocytes (LPL) and intraepithelial lymphocytes (IEL), which can be differentiated by anatomical location, cell phenotype and function. When studying intestinal diseases, including infections, inflammatory reactions and tumours, these lymphocyte populations must be analysed. For example, antigen-stimulated LPL, which have migrated from lymphoid follicles such as Peyer's patches, preferentially home to the mucosal lamina propria, where they are retained to perform their immunological functions; IEL, adhering to intestinal enterocytes in the mucosal intraepithelium, exhibit constitutive cytotoxic T lymphocyte (CTL) activity[1,2] against infected epithelial cells (EC)[3] and stressed autologous cells[4] by cytolytic action in addition to cytokine production.[5,6]

In this context, flow cytometric analysis is used to study the expression profiles of T cell differentiation antigens on LPL,[7] the effects of bacterial, viral and parasitic infections on IEL subset composition,[8-10] the adhesion molecules expressed by IEL for enterocyte interaction,[11] and the phenotype of parasite-specific cytotoxic effector IEL induced after oral infection.[12] Flow cytometry is also capable of detecting multiple intracellular cytokines simultaneously and correlating them with surface phenotype on a single cell basis.[13]

This chapter describes several useful flow cytometric applications and lists the fluorescent properties of various types of fluorochromes (Table 30.1) as well as the theoretical bases of their applications (Table 30.2). Details are also provided on phenotype analysis utilizing multicolour staining, with emphasis on direct versus indirect immunostaining and correlated analysis for cell-surface marker and intracellular antigens. DNA content-cell cycle analysis, one of the most popular flow cytometric applications clinically, flow cytometric applications for several metabolic activity assays, including analysis of intracellular calcium, pH and cellular membrane potential changes, and ways for identifying apoptotic cells and documenting cytotoxic activity are also described.

Methods

Cell collection and preparation for flow cytometric analysis[7,14-16]

Dissected mucosa is incubated in $Ca^{2+}Mg^{2+}$-free Hanks' balanced saline solution (HBSS, Sigma, St Louis, MO, USA) containing 1 mM dithiothreitol (Calbiochem, La Jolla, CA, USA) and 2 mM ethylene dinitrilo-tetra-acetic acid (EDTA) at 37°C for 20 min to remove mucus and debris. The mucosa is then tumbled freely in HBSS containing 2 mM EDTA by a rotating mixer at 37°C for 60-75 min to detach the epithelium. The resulting supernatants (EC and IEL) are collected and passed through a glass wool column to remove cell debris.

The supernatant is centrifuged over a Percoll discontinuous density gradient (Pharmacia, Piscataway, NJ, USA) at 500 *g* for 30 min. EC are collected from the 20-44% interface and IEL are recovered from the 44-67% interface. Cell viability is scored by trypan blue exclusion.

The remaining mucosal fragment is incubated at 37°C overnight in an orbital shaker in RPMI 1640 medium

Table 30.1 – Commonly used fluorochromes and their fluorescent properties [15, 24-26]

◄- - - - UV - - - - ►|◄- Violet -►|◄-Blue - ►|◄---Green - -►|◄- Orange -►|◄- - - - - Red - - - - - - ►

Immunoconjugates

Cascade Blue	|◄HC - -Ar- - - -►|420
AMCA (7-amino-4 methylcoumarin-3-acetate)	|◄-HC-Ar- - - - - ►| 450
FITC (fluorescein isothiocyanate)	|◄-HC - - - -Ar►|520
TRITC (tetramethylrhodamine)	|◄- - - -HN- - ►|590
PE (R-phycoerythrin)	|◄- - - - -Ar- - - - ►| 590
Duochrome (tandem PE-Texas Red)	|◄- - - - -Ar- - - - ►| 613
Texas Red	|◄- - HN - -Kr- -HN►| 620
APC (allophycocyanin)	|◄- - - HN -Kr- -HN►|660
Cychrome (Tandem PE-Cy5.18)	|◄- - - -Ar- - - - - - -HN - - - - -►|670
PerCP (peridinin chlorophyll A protein)	|◄- - - - -HC - - - -Ar- - - - - -HN►| 672

Nucleic acid stains

Hoechst 33342	|◄- - -HC - -Ar- - - - -HC ►460 (HO-DNA)
DAPI (4',6-diamidino-2-phenylindole)	|◄- - -HC - -Ar- - - - -HC - ►|470 (DAPI-DNA)
MI (mithramycin)	|◄ Ar- - - - - - - -HC- - - - - -Ar►| 575
PY (pyronin Y)	|◄- Ar- - - - - - - - HN►|570 (PY-dsRNA)
EB (ethidium)	|◄- - - HC - -Ar- - - - - - HN - Kr- ►| 595
PI (propidium iodide)	|◄- HC - -Ar►| |◄- - - HC- - - - -Ar- - - - HN - Kr- - ►| 620
7AAD (7-amino-actinomycin)	|◄- - -HC- - - - - -Ar- - HN - Kr- - -HN- - ►| 655
AO (acridine orange)	|◄- - - - - HC - - - - -Ar►| 522 (AO-DNA) 650 (AO-ssRNA)

Physiological probes

Indo-1	|◄- HC - Ar - - ►405 (Indo-1Ca^{2+}) 485 (free Indo-1)
DiOCn (cyanine dyes)	|◄-HC - - - -Ar- - - ►|530
BCECF (2',7-bis-carboxyethyl-5,6,-carboxyfluorescein)	|◄-HC- - - - -Ar- - - -►|530

Excitation spectra (|◄- - - -►|) of various fluorochromes followed by emission peak wavelength in bold (nm).
Major excitation line from different excitation sources within the excitable ranges (optimal or suboptimal) are indicated in abbreviations:
Ar (argon ion laser): 488 nm (blue), 514 nm (blue–green); needs special coated mirror to emit UV at 350 nm.
Kr (krypton laser): 568 nm (orange), 647 nm (red).
HN (helium–neon laser): 543 nm (green), 594 nm (yellow–orange), 633 nm (red)
HC (helium–cadmium laser): 325 nm (UV), 441 nm (blue–violet).
Dye (dye laser): wavelengths are dye-dependent (rhodamine 6G dye laser emits 570-620 nm).

Table 30.2 – Theoretical bases of selected flow cytometric applications.

Ca²⁺ influx

- **Indo-1** (Molecular Probes, Eugene, OR, USA) is a hydrolyzable probe. When excited by UV light (330 nm), Ca^{2+}-bound Indo-1 emits violet (405 nm); free Indo-1 emits blue (485 nm). Thus violet/blue ratio shift reflects $[Ca^{2+}]i$ variation.

- **Fluo-3** is non-fluorescent unless bound to calcium, thus the fluorescene intensity is cell size (Fluo-3 content)-dependent. When excited by a blue excitation at 488 nm, Fluo-3 emits green (530 nm).

Intracellular pH

- **BCECF** (2',7'-bis-carboxyethyl-5,6,-carboxyfluorescein) is a hydrolyzable probe. When excited by a blue light (488 nm), BCECF emits green (530 nm), the intensity of which correlates with the cytoplasmic pH value, thus green (530 nm) /red (620 nm) ratio reflects pH level.

- **DCH** (2,3-dicyanohydroquinone) is a hydrolyzable probe. When excited by a UV light, its violet (425 nm)/green (540 nm) emission ratio reflects pH level.

- **SNARF-1** (carboxy-SNARF-1) is a hydrolyzable probe. When excited at 488 nm, SNARF-1 emits dual emission wavelengths. The emission at 587 nm is a maximal under acidic conditions; while the emission at 636 nm is maximal under alkaline conditions.[15] Thus 640 nm/580 nm ratio increases with increasing pH.

Membrane potential

- **Cyanine dyes**, e.g. $DiOC_6$ (3,3'-dihexyloxacarbocyanine) are lipophilic dyes, permitting free membrane passage. These cationic dyes accumulate in cell interiors. Depolarization causes release of the dyes while hyperpolarization causes uptake of the dye. When excited at 488 nm, $DiOC_6$ emits green (530 nm).

DNA–RNA content/cell cycle progression/cell viability

- **PI** (propidium iodide): Cells are permeabilized to allow PI entry, which intercalates into double-stranded (ds) nucleic acid and becomes fluorescent. Thus cells need to be RNase-treated to remove dsRNA. When excited by a blue excitation at 488 nm, PI–DNA emits orange–red (615 nm). Without permeabilization, PI can only enter cells with impaired membrane, thus PI staining is used to identify dead cells.

- **EB** (ethidium bromide): Cells are permeabilized to allow EB entry, which intercalates into ds nucleic acid. When excited by a UV or blue–green light (510 nm), EB–DNA (or RNA) emits orange–red light (595 nm).

- **FITC-anti-BrdUrd antibody**: BrdUrd is incorporated into cells actively synthesizing DNA, and detected by FITC-anti-BrdUrd antibody.

- **HO dyes** (Hoechst 33258, 33342, 33378, and 33662) can be taken up by living cells, and bind to A–T regions in DNA for stoichiometric DNA stainings. When excited by UV (350 nm), free HO emits at blue–green (500 nm), while HO–DNA emits at blue (460 nm). However, its UV-excited blue flourescence drops when it binds to A–BrdUrd, thus cells in S phase (DNA synthesis) show significant BrdUrd/Hoechst flourescence-quenching.

- **DAPI** (4', 6-diamidino-2-phenylindole; Boehringer Mannheim) is similar to Hoechst dyes, but is cytotoxic and non-sensitive to BrdUrd.

- **MI** (mithramycin; Pfizer, Groton, CT, USA): Cells are permeabilized to allow MI entry, which binds to G–C regions in DNA. When excited at blue/violet wavelength (e.g. He–Cd 441 nm), its green–yellow fluorescence (575 nm) is stoichiometric to DNA contents, and provides a reference level for measuring the BrdUrd/Hoechst fluorescence-quenching.[15, 26]

Table 30.2 – continued

- **7AAD** (7-amino-actinomycin D; Sigma): Cells are permeabilized to allow 7AAD entry, which intercalates into G–C regions in DNA. When excited (e.g. Argon 488 or He–Ne 633 nm), the dye emits fluorescence predominantly red (655 nm).

- **AO** (acridine orange) is a lipophilic, metachromatic dye that accumulates in cell interiors. When excited at 488 nm, AO–DNA intercalation emits green (520 nm). For differential staining of DNA versus RNA, dsRNA are converted by acid denaturation to single-stranded RNA (ssRNA). AO–ssRNA emits red (650 nm).

- **PY** (pyronin Y; Polysciences, Warrington, PA, USA): Cells are permeabilized to allow PY entry, which mainly intercalates and detects dsRNA. The dye is used after dsDNA have been occupied (partially) by dsDNA intercalating dyes. When excited by a blue (488 nm) excitation, PY–dsRNA emits orange (565–574 nm).

Cellular proliferation history and intercellular conjugate formation

- **PKH** (Zynaxis Cell Science, Malvern, PA, USA) are lipophilic dyes that stain plasma membranes. When cells are dividing, daughter cells receive one-half of the dye. Thus its fluorescent intensity can be used to calculate the number of divisions. When excited at 488 nm, PKH-1 and PKH-2 emits green (525 nm), PKH-26 emits red (575 nm).

Hypoxic cell

- **NITP** 7(-)[4'-(2-nitroimidazol-l-yl)-butyl]-theophylline) becomes bioreductively metabolized and binds to cellular macromolecules in the absence of oxygen. NITP can be detected by FITC-anti-theophylline or FITC-avidin when biotinylated.

Peroxidase activity

- **HE** (hydroethidine or dihydroethidium; Molecular Probes) is a chemically reduced dye. Cytoplasmic HE emits blue but changes to ethidium and emits orange–red after intracellular peroxidase catalysed oxidative reaction.

Apoptosis

- **FITC–SA** (fluoroscein isothiocyanate-streptavidin conjugate): DNA strand breaks are dUTP-biotin-end-labelled by the action of TdT (terminal deoxynucleotidyl transferase), and detected by FITC–SA. When excited at 488 nm, FITC emits at green (575 nm).

Tandem dyes for immunofluorescence

- **Duochrome** (PE-Texas Red tandem) is a complex of PE and Texas Red. When excited at 488 nm, PE absorbs the blue light and emits predominantly orange–yellow light, which is in turn absorbed by Texas Red to emit orange–red light (600–640 nm).

- **Cychrome** (PE-Cy5.18 tandem) works analogous to the energy transfer in Duochrome. Blue (488 nm) excitation is absorbed by PE, whose emission is in turn absorbed by Cy5.18 to emit red light (~670 nm). Thus spectral overlap with PE is less than that of Duochrome.

The emission wavelength shown in parentheses indicates the emission peak or the wavelength the emission is measured at. When a fluorochrome is said to emit red, its fluorescence emission is predominantly red.

(Biowhittaker, Walkersville, MD) containing 10% (v/v) fetal calf serum (FCS), 0.05 M β-mercaptoethanol, 25 mM N-[2-hydroxyethyl]piperazine-n'-[2-ethane sulphonic acid] (HEPES), 0.01% (w/v) collagenase (Worthington Biochemical, Freehold, NJ, USA) and 0.01% (w/v) DNase (Boehringer Mannheim, Indianapolis, IN, USA). The suspension is passed through a glass wool column. Cells are pelleted through a Percoll gradient to recover LPL. Lymphocytes from Peyer's patches can be isolated by similar methods. Alternatively, 1.5 mg/ml Dispase neutral protease (Boehringer Mannheim) can be used in Joklik-modified medium (GIBCO, Gaithersburg, MD, USA).[17]

Cells can be further purified by immunomagnetic bead, panning, or fluorescence-activated cell sorting. For example, Percoll-fractionated EC are incubated with anti-CD45 (pan-leukocyte antigen) monoclonal antibody (mAb)-coated magnetic Dynabeads M-450 (Dynal, Great Neck, NY, USA) to remove contaminating IEL cells;[18] while Percoll-fractionated IEL are depleted of EC by incubating with anti-epithelial antigen mAb BerEP4-coated beads and unbound cells are recovered.[19] Cells can also be sorted by fluorescence-activated cell sorting on the basis of dual-light scattering, CD3+, CD45+ or a specific surface marker.[20,21] Alternatively, the contaminating EC can simply be excluded from data collection by light-scatter, CD3+ or CD45+ gate during flow cytometric analysis.[1]

Phenotypic analysis and correlations

Cell surface marker staining and correlations

Cells are preincubated at 4°C for 10 min in phosphate buffered saline (PBS), 0.5% (w/v) bovine serum albumin (BSA), 0.1% NaN₃ containing 20% (v/v) FCS or anti-FcR mAb culture supernatant to block FcR and nonspecific binding sites. For direct stainings using mouse IgG antibodies, 20 mg of purified mouse IgG (Sigma) can be used to ensure effective blocking. For indirect stainings, however, blocking reagents that the secondary antibody recognizes should be avoided. One option is to use a blocking antibody or serum from the species of animal in which the secondary antibody was raised. For example, if goat anti-mouse IgG is used as secondary antibody, 20 μg of goat IgG (Sigma) can be used as a preblock.

Direct stainings for single- or multiple-colour analysis

One million cells are incubated in 0.1 ml of saturating concentration (optimized by titration) of fluorescein isothiocyanate (FITC)-conjugated mAb (whole molecule or Ig F(ab')₂ fragment) in PBS, 0.5% (w/v) BSA, 0.1% (w/v) NaN₃ at 4°C for 30 min, with frequent mixing. For dual- or multiple-colour analysis, cells are incubated simultaneously with a mixture of conjugates (e.g. FITC-, R-phycoerythrin (PE)- and Tri-Colour labelled mAbs) washed and subjected to flow cytometric analysis. Dead cells are excluded from analysis based on dual-light scatter gate or propidium iodide (PI, Sigma) staining (cells are resuspended in buffer containing 2 μg/ml PI in 0.1% (w/v) sodium citrate at 4°C for 10 min). PI exclusion is feasible only when the orange-red detector is reserved. An isotype-matched fluorochrome-coupled irrelevant mAb is used as control to set background gates. For dual- or multiple-colour analysis, the spectral overlaps (cross-contributions) between dyes are compensated for based on single-stranded controls. Data are acquired in list mode and analysed by software programs such as CELLQuest, Lysis II (Becton Dickinson, Mountain View, CA, USA) and Immunocount (Ortho, Raritan, NJ, USA).

For instruments with a single argon ion 488 nm blue excitation source, such as FACScan, FACSort and FACSTrak (Becton Dickinson), Coulter Epics Profile (Coulter, Hialeah, FL, USA), or Ortho Cytoron Absolute (Ortho), FITC-conjugated antibody has been standard for single-colour analysis. FITC (peak emission at 530 nm green) and PE (580 nm orange) are common combination for two-colour analysis. FITC, PE, and one of the conjugates that fluoresces in the red of far-red spectrum, such as PerCP, Cychrome or Tri-Colour (tandem PE-Cy5.18) or Duocrhome (tandem PE-Texas Red) are used for three-colour analysis.

Three-colour analysis can also be performed by dual-laser systems with FITC-, PE- (excited by an argon laser at 488 nm) in combination with APC (allophycocyanin)- or Texas Red- (excited by a dye laser operated at 615 nm) labelled antibodies. Emissions are collected using 525, 575 and 660 bandpass filters.[22,23]

Four-colour analysis can be successfully performed using FITC, PE, PerCP (excited by a 488 nm argon laser) and APC (excited by a krypton-ion laser at 647 nm or a helium-neon laser at 633 nm).[24-26] The APC and PerCP spectral overlap is resolved due to the spatial and electronic separation of their sequential excitation beams. Flow cytometers such as FACStar, FACS Vantage (Becton Dickinson), Coulter EPICS 752, 753, Elite (Coulter) are equipped with dual or multiple laser beams, e.g. argon, krypton, He-Ne,

He-Cd or dye lasers, for flexible multiple-parameter analytical capabilities.

Indirect staining for one-colour analysis

Indirect staining amplifies signals and is suitable for detecting rear antigenic sites. 1×10^6 cells are incubated in 0.1 ml titred excess of unconjugated primary mAb (e.g. mouse mAb) in PBS, 0.5% (w/v) BSA, 0.1% (w/v) NaN_3 at 4°C for 30 min. Either purified mAb or unpurified culture supernatant can be used. The cells are washed and detected in a second step with affinity-purified FITC-conjugated anti-mouse Ig F(ab')$_2$ fragments (e.g. rabbit or goat anti-mouse IgG or IgM). Irrelevant primary mAb is used followed by FITC-conjugated anti-mouse Ig F(ab')$_2$ fragments as control. Cells are washed and subjected to flow cytometric analysis as described above.

Combination of direct and indirect staining in multiple-colour analysis

The above FITC-stained cells are washed and incubated for 10 min with normal mouse serum (1:1000 dilution, Sigma) or 20 mg mouse IgG or IgM (Sigma) to saturate residual binding sites of the secondary antibody. Cells are thereafter stained with PE-conjugated mAb, washed and analysed. Alternatively, biotin-conjugated mAb, followed by R-phycoerythrin-streptavidin (PE-SA, Biomeda, Foster City, CA, USA), Duochrome-SA (Becton Dickinson), Cy5-SA (Pharmingen, San Diego, CA, USA) or Red 613-SA (GIBCO) is used for two- or three-colour staining. mAbs can also be derivatized with hapten (e.g. dinitrophenol (DNP)) and detected with fluorochrome-coupled anti-hapten (e.g. goat anti-DNP (Molecular Probes, Eugene, OR, USA)). When indirect and direct staining are used in combination, the former should be done first.

Correlation of cell-surface marker and intra-cellular antigens

To stain simultaneously for cell-surface markers and intracellular antigens, surface staining should be performed first. Cells are then fixed and permeabilized at 1×10^6 cells/ml with 3:1 methanol/acetone, added and mixed gradually, at 0°C for 10 min, or fixed in 0.5% (w/v) paraformaldehyde in PBS pH 7.2 at 4°C for 10-60 min followed by permeabilization with detergent such as 0.025% (v/v) Tween-20, 0.1% (v/v) Triton X-100, or 0.1% (w/v) saponin in PBS at 4°C (duration needs to be optimized). Fixation preserves surface antigen-antibody complexes, and permeabilizes the cells to permit antibodies or other probes (e.g. SA-conjugates or DNA, RNA probes).

The low molecular weight FITC is the first choice for intracellular staining. If biotin-streptavidin bridging is utilized for intracellular staining, incubate permeabilized cells with 10 mg/ml streptavidin (GIBCO) to block endogenous biotin. Cells are then incubated with biotin-conjugated primary mAb, followed by fluorochrome-conjugated streptavidin, washed and analysed as described above.

IEL have been found to produce lymphokines after antigen exposure that may activate various mucosal immunological defence mechanisms and lead to pathological effects in the gut.[20] Flow cytometric intracellular staining is an alternative to enzyme-linked immunospot (ELISPOT) assay or enzyme-linked immunosorbent assay (ELISA) for detecting cytokine production. Cells are stimulated with agonist in the presence of 2 μM monensin (Calbiochem) to cause intracellular cytokine accumulation. Cells are then permeabilized with 4% (w/v) paraformaldehyde and 0.1% (w/v) saponin, followed by the staining for intracellular cytokines directly or indirectly with various anti-cytokine mAbs. Multicolour staining can assess multiple cytokine profiles at a single cell level.[13,27]

Metabolic activity assays

Cell activation is a process that elicits a cascade of cellular biological responses. Flow cytometry addresses several activation-induced metabolic events, such as intracellular calcium mobilization, cytoplasmic pH and membrane potential change, activation antigen expression, DNA/RNA synthesis and cell division. All of these are related to the development and differentiation of immunological and pathological effects of a variety of cell types.

Analysis of intracellular calcium[2,28,29]

Measurement of intracellular ionized calcium concentration ([Ca^{2+}]i) is of particular interest because Ca^{2+} is a mediator of transmembrane signalling pathways. Elevation in [Ca^{2+}]i, either from intracellular calcium stores or extracellular calcium influx, is a messenger that regulates diverse cellular metabolic processes. To measure [Ca^{2+}]i, cells are loaded with membrane-permeant Ca^{2+} indicator Indo-1 penta-acetoxymethyl ester (Indo-1 AM, Molecular Probes). Intracellular esterases cleave the AM group and trap the dye, which can chelate Ca^{2+} (see Table 30.2 for the theoretical basis of Indo-1 staining).

Specifically, cells are resuspended at 1×10^7 cells/ml in

HBSS containing 1 mM $CaCl_2$, 1 mM $MgCl_2$ and 1% (v/v) FCS. Indo-1 AM is added to a final concentration of 2-5 μM and incubated at 24°C for 45 min, washed and stored at 22°C. Analysis is done with the UV line form of argon laser as the excitation source, configured with bandpass filters centred on 410 nm (violet) and 485 nm (blue). Indo-1 cannot be loaded by dead cells, thus the violet intensity gate could effectively gate out dead cells. The gain setting is used to position the blue signals in the upper end and the violet signals in the lower end of the scale, allowing subsequent violet/blue shifts to remain on scale. Real-time analog violet/blue ratios for each cell are calculated. Once ratio baseline is established, cells can be treated with stimuli and the violet/blue shift documented. Results are displayed as a bivariate dot plot of violet/blue ratio for each cell as a function of time.

Cytosolic pH changes[30,31]

Since cytosolic enzyme activities are frequently pH-dependent, the level of intracellular pH could be of considerable importance to the metabolic state of cells. Flow cytometry can be used to measure cytosolic pH by loading cells with one of the hydrolyzable pH probes, e.g. 2',7'-bis-carboxyethyl-5,6-carboxyfluorescein (BCECF, Molecular Probes), which becomes fluorescent within the cytoplasm, with a peak emission of 530 nm (green). Since the emission intensity at 530 nm is pH-dependent, while the emission around the red region is pH-independent, a ratiometric analysis of green (530 nm)/red (620 nm) value will reflect the pH level.

Cells are suspended at 1×10^6/ml in PBS. The acetoxymethylester form BCECF-AM is added to a final concentration of 1 μM, and cells are incubated at 37°C for 15-60 min. Calibrations and measurements are done with 488 nm excitation and emission measured at 530 nm and 620 nm. Results are displayed as a bivariate dot plot of green/red ratio for each cell as a function of time. Calibrations are performed with aliquots of loaded cells in KH_2PO_4/K_2HPO_4 buffer adjusted to different pH (pH 6.0-7.6), containing 10 μM ionophore nigericin (Molecular Probes), which depolarizes the cells and equalizes the internal/external pH value. The relationship between ratio value and pH value is fitted to a calibration curve.

Cellular membrane potential changes[32,33]

The cyanine dyes $DiOC_n$ are lipophilic, permitting free membrane passage, and become positively charged as the cytoplasm is negative. Depolarization

(decrease in the potential difference) of cells that are equilibrated with the dye will cause release of the dye while hyperpolarization (increase in the potential difference) causes uptake of the dye.

Cells are equilibrated with cyanine dye by incubating in 5×10^5 cells/ml in serum-free medium containing 10 μM 3,3'-dihexyloxacarbocyanine ($DiOC6$, Molecular Probes) at 37°C for 10-30 min. Cells are treated with stimuli (e.g. ionophores or receptor cross-linking antibodies) and are subjected to flow cytometric analysis by a single laser excitation at 488 nm (e.g. FASCan, Coulter Epics Profile) for green (530 nm) fluorescence emission. To measure correlatively cell surface phenotype and membrane potential, PE-labelled antibody is used for surface staining followed by $DiOC_6$ staining.

DNA content analysis and cell cycle staging

PI is the most commonly used probe for DNA content analysis. Since PI intercalates into double-stranded (ds) nucleic acid, cells are permeabilized and RNase-treated to remove dsRNA before PI staining. Cells for the analysis can be from fresh isolated tissues, solid tumours or nuclei from archival paraffin-embedded tissue specimens. Solid tumour cells are prepared by mincing and enzymatic dispersion with 2.5 mg/ml trypsin, 0.5 mg/ml type II collagenase and 20 μg/ml DNase I (Sigma) in PBS at 37°C for 1 hour. Nuclei from paraffin-embedded tissue specimens are prepared by dewaxing a section of the tissue with xylene and rehydrating sequentially by addition and aspiration of 100, 95, 75 and 50% (v/v) ethanol and distilled water. Tissue cells are then incubated in 0.5% (w/v) pepsin A (Sigma) at 37°C for 30 min, washed, resuspended at a concentration of 1×10^6 cells/ml and the RNase (see below) then follows directly.[10,34,35]

Specifically, 1×10^6 cells are washed in Ca^{2+}, Mg^{2+}-free PBS, fixed in 1% (w/v) paraformaldehyde containing 0.001% (v/v) Tween-20 at 4°C overnight. Alternatively, cells are fixed with 70% (v/v) ethanol at 4°C for at least 24 hours. After two washes, cells are treated with 0.5 mg/ml RNase (Sigma) at 37°C for 30 min and then stained with 20-50 μg/ml PI (Sigma) in 0.1% sodium citrate, pH 8.4 at room temperature for 30 min. Cells are then subjected to analysis by 488 nm laser excitation. The red (DNA-PI) signal of individual cells is collected and analysed. Cell numbers are plotted as a function of DNA content and the percentage of cells in the G_o/G_1, S-phase and G_2/M phase is calculated using CellFIT Cell-Cycle Analysis Software (Becton

Dickinson), PARA-1 (Coulter) or Multicycle 2.53 Software (Phoenix, San Diego, CA, USA). Tumour ploidy is expressed by the DNA index (DI) = modal G_0-G_1 peak of the aneuploid population/modal G_0-G_1 peak of the diploid population.

Analysis of dynamic cell cycle progression[36,37]

5-bromo-2'-deoxyuridine (BrdUrd, Sigma)-incorporation indicates cells actively synthesizing DNA, thus detection of BrdUrd incorporation in combination with DNA quantitation permits the analysis of cell kinetic parameters such as cell cycle time. Cells are labelled with BrdUrd and boiled or DNase-treated to partially denature DNA. This allows FITC-conjugated anti-BrdUrd antibody to gain acess to the incorporated BrdUrd. Cells are then stained with PI.

Specifically, cells are cultured under conditions (e.g. cytokine treatment) that may affect the progression of the cell cycle. BrdUrd incorporation is performed 2 hours before harvesting by adding BrdUrd to a final concentration of 5-20 μM. Cells are then washed with PBS and fixed at 4°C overnight in 1% (w/v) paraformaldehyde containing 0.01% (v/v) Tween-20. The cells are then washed and incubated with 4 μg/ml bovine pancreatic DNase I (Sigma) in Ca^{2+},Mg^{2+}-containing PBS at 37°C for 30 min. Cells are then washed and incubated with 0.5 μg FITC-conjugated anti-BrdUrd mAb (Caltag, San Francisco, CA, USA) at 37°C for 45 min followed by staining with PI (see above). Samples are subjected to a laser excitation of 488 nm for 620 nm PI-fluorescence (DNA content) and 520 nm FITC-fluorescence (BrdUrd incorporation). Bivariate dot plots are prepared and cell-cycle statistics are calculated with software as described for PI staining.

Identification of apoptotic cells

Cells can be triggered to undergo apoptosis by diverse physiological, pathological and pharmacological stimuli. In contrast to necrosis, which is a nonspecific mode of cell death caused by toxic agents or cellular stress, apoptotic cells are engaged in controlled activation of processes that break down cellular components, most notably internucleosomal DNA fragmentation. Various antitumour treatments induce apoptosis of tumour cells and therefore a rapid and accurate way to detect apoptotic cells is essential to the study of the impact of apoptosis on cancer development and therapy.

Cells undergoing apoptosis have reduced DNA stainability, probably due to DNA conformational change, lowering its accessibility to DNA-staining dyes.[38] Thus flow cytometric identification of apoptotic cells primarily uses DNA staining dyes, such as PI, to identify cells with reduced stainability. Cells are fixed in 70% (v/v) ethanol, resuspended in 5 μg/ml PI in PBS, 1% (w/v) BSA and subjected to flow cytometric analysis.

Another approach is to end-label and detect DNA strand breaks. Flow cytometric analysis based on the terminal deoxynucleotidyl transferase (TdT)-mediated dUTP-biotin nick end-labelling (TUNEL) can be used.[39,40]

Cells can first be stained for cell surface markers before being fixed with 0.5% (v/v) formaldehyde, 0.05% (w/v) saponin at 4°C for 12 hours. Cells are then washed with PBS, resuspended in 20 μl TdT reaction buffer (0.5 M cacodylic acid, pH 6.8, 1 mM $CoCl_2$, 0.5 mM DTT, 0.05% (w/v) BSA, 0.15 M NaCl; a commercial kit is available from Boehringer Mannheim), 4-12 U TdT (Boehringer Mannheim or Promega, Madison, WI, USA), 1 mM biotin-16-dUTP (Boehringer Mannheim), and incubated at 37°C for 30 min. Cells are then incubated with FITC-streptavidin (SA) at room temperature for 30 min. End labelling can also be done with digoxigenin-conjugated dUTP and detected by FITC-conjugated anti-digoxigenin antibody (ApopTag kit, Oncor, Gaithersburg, MD, USA). By employing multiparameter analysis including phenotypic labelling, it is possible to study apoptosis in specific cell subsets within a heterogenous population.

Application to animal studies

The flow cytometric applications described above can be adopted, without major modifications, to any laboratory animal model. Among these, mouse and rat systems are well established and studied. Some useful mAbs for mouse studies are H57-597 (anti-TCR alpha/beta), 145-2C11 (anti-CD3) and 53.6-72 (anti-CD8) (Pharmingen). Some useful mAbs for rat studies are MRC OX-1 (anti-leukocyte common antigen), MRC OX-8 (anti-CD8), MRC OX22 (anti-CD45RC), MRC OX-33 (anti-CD45, B cell form) (Serotec, Raleigh, NC, USA). Secondary antibodies frequently used are FITC-conjugated goat anti-rat Ig F(ab')$_2$ or anti-hamster Ig F(ab')$_2$ (Caltag).

Results and discussion

Flow cytometers can analyse large numbers of cells and can gate and collect events based on particular characteristic, e.g. the expression of a particular cell surface marker.[41,42] This enables the detection of specific cell subsets from a heterogeneous cell population and has been utilized extensively to identify several intestinal IEL subsets and their functional roles.[1,20,43-46] Since multiple markers may be needed in concert to define a discrete subset, multicolour analyses (e.g. three- or four-colour) are often necessary.

When doing multicolour analyses, several considerations are critical. First, the excitation wavelength should not overlap with the emission wavelengths of dyes used. Secondly, spectral overlaps (spill-over) exist between any dye combinations. For example, the predominantly green FITC emission can cross-contribute some red signal (the red tail of FITC[46]) to the PE detector, which needs to be corrected. Thirdly, energy transfer or 'quenching' occurs when two dyes bind close together and the emission of one overlaps with the absorption of the other dye (e.g. mithramycin (MI) and ethidium bromide (EB), FITC and PE).

Spectral overlap can be compensated electronically or resolved by spatial separation by using two excitation sources (e.g. UV and 488 nm argon lasers) separated by a small distance at the sample stream, such that UV and blue excited emission signals are collected at different times. Alternatively, a filter centred farther away from the contaminating signal can be used. The adverse effect of quenching can be minimized by labeling the more abundant antigenic sites with the donor (e.g. FITC) and the less abundant sites with the acceptor (e.g. PE) fluorochrome.

Simultaneous detection of both cell-surface markers and intracellular antigens allows analysis of functional subsets of cells for the presence or absence of intracellular effector molecules, cytokines, cell cycle regulating proteins or intracellular pathogens.[13] The extent of fixation/permeabilization for probe entry depends on the subcellular location of the antigen (e.g. cytosolic or nuclear).[26,48] Care also should be taken when fixation is involved, as FITC, PE, Texas Red and Duochromes are not affected by fixation, but APC can be destroyed by fixation. PerCP fluorescence also can be lost after permeabilization.[46]

Flow cytometric DNA analysis is used to follow tumour progression and to study the effects of drugs, chemotherapy or radiation of tumour cell cycle perturbation. DNA ploidy pattern, DI, and S-phase fraction obtained from isolated tumor cells or archival samples, when correlated with other diagnostic parameters, are often of prognostic significance (although sometimes no prognostic value can be found). For example, the cases of colorectal cancer,[35,49] metachronous colorectal adenoma,[34] gastric carcinoma,[50,51] and smooth muscle tumours of the gastrointestinal tract[52] have been documented using flow cytometric analysis.

To correlate DNA content with cell surface markers or intracellular antigens (e.g. proliferation-associated nuclear antigen), cells are stained for surface marker, or permeabilized to stain for intracellular antigen with FITC-labelled mAb, respectively, prior to PI staining.[21,53-55] Cells are then subjected to laser excitation of 488 nm. The gate can be set on green (FITC-'trigger') to include only the subset of interest, whose red (DNA-PI) signal is collected and analysed.

Flow cytometric quantitation of BrdUrd incorporation allows the assessment of drug effects on blockage or deceleration of cell cycle progression. To correlate these effects with a cell phenotype, surface staining should be done first with PE-labelled antibody. Cells are then fixed, permeabilized and DNase I treated, as described above. To measure an additional surface parameter, Duochromes or APC can be used, since this permeabilization procedure preserves APC staining. This method is also suitable for evaluating the proliferative status of subsets following stimulation.[37]

To make correlations between phenotyping and DNA/RNA content or S-phase cells, there are various possibilities for fluorochrome combinations. The selection of fluorochromes should take factors such as spectral overlap and the availability of equipment (laser source, optical filter) into consideration (Tables 30.1 and 30.2). For example, Hoechst dye and DAPI (4',6-diamidino-2-phenylindole) (both for DNA staining) are optimally excited by UV light and require a dual laser for the simultaneous measurement of FITC- and PE-stained immunological properties. On the other hand, a single 488 nm excitation can probe for S-phase fraction (FITC-anti-BrdUrd green 525 nm), DNA content (DNA-7AAD (7-amino-actinomycin D) red 655 nm) and surface phenotype (PE orange 570 nm) simultaneously.[56] Acridine orange (AO) and AMCA (7-amino-4-methylcoumarin-3-acetate), but not FITC, are used in combination for cellular antigen and DNA/RNA analysis.[57] Another example of multiparameter staining using single 488 nm excitation source is the simultaneous staining for hypoxia, proliferation and DNA content using FITC (detecting NITP (7(-) [4'-(2-nitroimidazol-1-yl)-butyl]-theophylline), see Table 30.2), PE (detecting BrdUrd incorporation) and 7AAD, respectively.[38]

Flow cytometry is a powerful methodology because of its correlated analysis capability. It will play a more and more important role in clinical and experimental studies with the rapid introduction of new probes, which will make many novel antigenic, biochemical and biophysical applications possible.

Acknowledgement

We would like to thank Ms Elim Pu for her help in the preparation of the manuscript.

References

1. Lefancois L. Phenotypic complexity of intraepithelial lymphocytes of the small intestine. *J Immunol* 1991; **147**: 1746-1751.

2. Sarnacki S, Begue B, Jarry A, Cerf-Bensussan N. Human intestinal intraepithelial lymphocytes, a distinct population of activated T cells. *Immunol Res* 1991; **10**: 302-305.

3. Offit PA, Dudzik KI. Rotavirus-specific cytotoxic T lymphocytes appear at the intestinal mucosal surface after rotavirus infection. *J Virol* 1989; **63**: 3507-3512.

4. Rajasekar R, Sim GK, Augustin A. Self heat shock and gamma delta T-cell reactivity. *Proc Natl Acad Sci USA* 1990; **87**: 1767-1771.

5. Taguchi T, Aicher WK, Fujihashi K *et al.* Novel function for intestinal intraepithelial lymphocytes. Murine CD3⁺, gamma/delta TCR⁺ T cells produce IFN-gamma and IL-5. *J Immunol* 1991; **147**: 3736-3744.

6. Lundqvist C, Baranov V, Soderstrom K *et al.* Phenotype and cytokine profile of intraepithelial lymphocytes in human small and large intestine. *Ann N Y Acad Sci* 1995; **756**: 395-399.

7. Schieferdecker HL, Ulrich R, Hirseland H, Zeitz M. T cell differentiation antigens on lymphocytes in the human intestinal lamina propria. *J Immunol* 1992; **149**: 2816-2822.

8. Bandeira A, Mota-Santos T, Itohara S *et al.* Localization of gamma/delta T cells to the intestinal epithelium is independent of normal microbial colonization. *J Exp Med* 1990; **172**: 239-244.

9. Haas W, Pereira P, Tonegawa S. Gamma/delta T cells. *Annu Rev Immunol* 1993; **11**: 637.

10. Hedley DW, Friedlander ML, Taylor IW, Rugg CA, Musgrove EA. Method for analysis of cellular DNA content of paraffin-embedded pathological material using flow cytometry. *J Histochem Cytochem* 1983; **31**: 1333-1335.

11. Kelleher D, Murphy A, Lynch S, O'Farrelly C. Adhesion molecules utilized in binding of intraepithelial lymphocytes to human enterocytes. *Eur J Immunol* 1994; **24**: 1013-1016.

12. Chardes T, Buzoni-Gatel D, Lepage A, Bernard F, Bout D. Toxoplasma gondii oral infection induces specific cytotoxic CD8 alpha/beta + Thy-1 gut intraepithelial lymphocytes, lytic for parasite-infected enterocytes. *J Immunol* 1994; **153**: 4596-4603.

13. Elson LH, Nutman TB, Metcalfe DD, Prussin C. Flow cytometric analysis for cytokine production identifies T helper 1, T helper 2, and T helper 0 cells within the human CD4⁺CD27-lymphocyte subpopulation. *J Immunol* 1995; **154**: 4294-4301.

14. Madrigal L, Lynch S, Feighery C, Weir D, Kelleher D, O'Farrelly C. Flow cytometric analysis of surface major histocompatibility complex class II expression on human epithelial cells prepared from small intestinal biopsies. *J Immunol Methods* 1993; **158**: 207-214.

15. Darzynkiewicz Z, Robinson JP, Crissman HA. Flow cytometry. In: *Methods in Cell Biology*, 2nd edn. Academic Press, San Diego, 1994.

16. Lundqvist C, Hammarstrom ML, Athlin L, Hammarstrom S. Isolation of functionally active intraepithelial lymphocytes and enterocytes from human small and large intestine. *J Immunol Methods* 1992; **152**: 253-263.

17. Mega J, McGhee JR, Kiyono H. Cytokine- and Ig-producing T cells in mucosal effector tissues: analysis of IL-5- and IFN-gamma-producing T cells, T cell receptor expression, and IgA plasma cells from mouse salivary gland-associated tissues. *J Immunol* 1992; **148**: 2030-2039.

18. Jarry A, Cerf-Bensussan N, Brousse N, Selz F, Guy-Grand D. Subsets of CD3⁺ (T cell receptor alpha/beta or gamma/delta) and CD3-lymphocytes isolated from normal human gut epithelium display phenotypical features different from their counterparts in peripheral blood. *Eur J Immunol* 1990; **20**: 1097-1103.

19. Elson CO, Holland SP, Dertzbaugh MT, Cuff CF, Anderson AO. Morphologic and functional alterations of mucosal cells by cholera toxin and its B subunit. *J Immunol* 1995; **154**: 1032-1040.

20. Barrett TA, Gajewski TF, Danielpour D, Chang EB, Beagley KW, Bluestone JA. Differential function of intestinal intraepithelial lymphocyte subsets. *J Immunol* 1992; **149**: 1124-1130.

21. Yamamoto M, Fujihashi K, Beagley KW, McGhee JR, Kiyono H. Cytokine synthesis by intestinal intraepithelial lymphocytes. Both gamma/delta T cell receptor-positive and alpha/beta T cell receptor-positive T cells in the G1 phase of cell cycle produce IFN-gamma and IL-5. *J Immunol* 1993; **150:** 106-114.

22. Hardy RR, Hayakawa K, Parks DR, Herzenberg LA, Murine B cell differentiation lineages. *J Exp Med* 1984; **159:** 1169-1188.

23. Loken MR, Lanier LL. Three-color immunofluorescence analysis of Leu antigens on human peripheral blood using two lasers on a fluorescence-activated cell sorter. *Cytometry* 1984; **5:** 151-158.

24. Grogan WM, Collins JM. *Guide to Flow Cytometric Methods*. Marcel Dekker, New York, 1990.

25. Shapiro HM. *Practical Flow Cytometry*, 3rd edn. Wiley Liss, New York, 1995.

26. Jacquemin-Sablon A. Flow cytometry: new developments. In: *NATO ASI Series*. North Atlantic Treaty Organization Scientific Affairs Division, Berlin, 1993.

27. Sander B, Andersson J, Andersson U. Assessment of cytokines by immunofluorescence and the paraformaldehyde-saponin procedure. *Immunol Rev* 1991; **119:** 65-93.

28. Liddle RA, Misukonis MA, Pacy L, Balber AE. Cholecystokinin cells purified by fluorescence-activated cell sorting respond to monitor peptide with an increase in intracellular calcium. *Proc Natl Acad Sci USA* 1992; **89:** 5147-5151.

29. Matsuyama T, Yamada A, Deusch K *et al.* Cytochalasins enhance the proliferation of CD4 cells through the CD3-Ti antigen receptor complex or the CD2 molecule through an effect on early events of activation. *J Immunol* 1991; **146:** 3736-3741.

30. Reynolds JE, Li J, Craig RW, Eastman A. BCL-2 and MCL-1 expression in Chinese hamster ovary cells inhibits intracellular acidification and apoptosis induced by staurosporine. *Exp Cell Res* 1996; **225:** 430-436.

31. Musgrove E, Rugg C, Hedley D. Flow cytometric measurement of cytoplasmic pH: a critical evaluation of available fluorochromes. *Cytometry* 1986; **7:** 347-355.

32. Petit PX, Lecoeur H, Zorn E, Dauguet C, Mignotte B, Gougeon ML. Alterations in mitochondrial structure and function are early events of dexamethasone-induced thymocyte apoptosis. *J Cell Biol* 1995; **130:** 157-167.

33. Zamzami N, Marchetti P, Castedo M *et al.* Sequential reduction of mitochondrial transmembrane potential and generation of reactive oxygen species in early programmed cell death. *J Exp Med* 1995; **182:** 367-377.

34. Griffioen G, Cronelisse CJ, Verspaget HW *et al.* Association of aneuploidy in index adenomas with metachronous colorectal adenoma development and a comparison. *Cancer* 1992; **70:** 2035-2043.

35. Tang R, Ho YS, You YT *et al.* Prognostic evaluation of DNA flow cytometric and histopathologic parameters of colorectal cancer. *Cancer* 1995; **76:** 1724-1730.

36. van Laar T, Schouten R, Jochemsen AG, Terleth C, van der Eb AJ. Temperature-sensitive mutant p53 (ala 143) interferes transiently with DNA-synthesis and cell-cycle progression in Saos-2 cells. *Cytometry* 1996; **25:** 21.

37. Carayon P, Bord A. Identification of DNA-replicating lymphocyte subsets using a new method to label the bromo-deoxyuridine incorporated into the DNA. *J Immunol Methods* 1992; **147:** 225-230.

38. Webster L, Hodgkiss RJ, Wilson GD. Simultaneous triple staining for hypoxia, proliferation and DNA content in murine tumours. *Cytometry* 1995; **21:** 344-351.

39. Lund-Johansen F, Frey T, Ledbetter JA, Thompson PA. Apoptosis in hematopoietic cells is associated with an extensive decrease in cellular phosphotyrosine content that can be inhibited by the tyrosine phosphatase antagonist pervanadate. *Cytometry* 1996; **25:** 182-190.

40. Telford WG, King LE, Fraker PJ. Comparative evaluation of several DNA binding dyes in the detection of apoptosis-associated chromatin degradation by flow cytometry. *Cytometry* 1992; **13:** 137-143.

41. Nicholson J, Kidd P, Mandy F, Livnat D, Kagan J. Three-color supplement to the NIAID DAIDS guideline for flow cytometric immunophenotyping. *Cytometry* 1996; **26:** 227-230.

42. Goodman TG, Chang HL, Esselman WJ, LeCorre R, Lefrancois L. Characterization of the CD45 molecule on murine intestinal intraepithelial lymphocytes. *J Immunol* 1990; **145:** 2959-2966.

43. Ohteki T, MacDonald HR. Expression of the CD28 costimulatory molecule on subsets of murine intestinal intraepithelial lymphocytes correlates with lineage and responsiveness. *Eur J Immunol* 1993; **23:** 1251.

44. Robijn RJ, Bloemendal H, Jainandunsing S *et al.* Phenotypic and molecular characterization of human monoclonal TCR gamma/delta T-cell lines from jejunum and colon of healthy individuals. *Scand J Immunol* 1993; **38:** 247-253.

45. Tregaskes CA, Kong FK, Paramithiotis E *et al.* Identification and analysis of the expression of CD8 alpha beta and CD8 alpha alpha isoforms in chickens reveals a major TCR-gamma delta CD8 alpha beta subset of intestinal intraepithelial lymphocytes. *J Immunol* 1995; **154:** 4485-4494.

46. Coligan JE, Kruisbeek AM, Margulies DN, Shevach EM, Strober W. *Current Protocols in Immunology*. National Institutes of Health. John Wiley & Sons Inc, New York, 1994.

47. Fraker PJ, King LE, Lill-Elghanian D, Telford WG. Quantification of apoptotic events in pure and heterogeneous populations of cells using the flow cytometer. *Methods Cell Biol* 1995; **46:** 57-76.

48. Francis C, Connelly MC. Rapid single-step method for flow cytometric detection of surface and intracellular antigens. *Cytometry* 1996; **25:** 58-70.

49. Kimura O, Sugamura K, Kijima T, Kurayoshi K, Makino M, Kaibara N. DNA index as a significant prognostic indicator of colorectal cancer. *Gan To Kagaku Ryoho* 1996; **23:** 118-124.

50. Victorzon M, Roberts PJ, Haglund C, von Boguslawsky K, Nordling S. Ki-67 immunoreactivity, ploidy and S-phase fraction as prognostic factors in patients with gastric carcinoma. *Oncology* 1996; **53:** 182-191.

51. Baretton G, Gille J, Oevermann E, Lohrs U. Flow-cytometric analysis of the DNA-content in paraffin-embedded tissue from colorectal carcinomas and its prognostic significance. *Virchows Arch B Cell Pathol* 1991; **60:** 123-131.

52. Chou TS. Smooth muscle tumors of the gastrointestinal tract: analysis of prognotic factors. *Surgery* 1996; **119:** 171-177.

53. Rapi S, Caldini A, Fanelli A, Berti P, Lisi E, Anichini E, Caligiani R, Sbernini F, Taddei G, Amorosi A, Villari D, Susini T. Flow cytometric measurement of DNA content in human solid tumors: a comparison with cytogenetics. *Cytometry* 1996; **26:** 192-197.

54. Baez A, Torres K, Tan EM, Pommier Y, Casiano CA. Expression of proliferation-associated nuclear autoantigens, p330d/CENP-F and PCNA, in differentiation and in drug-induced growth inhibition using two-parameter flow cytometry. *Cell Prolif* 1996; **29:** 183-196.

55. Yokogi H. Flow cytometric quantitation of the proliferation-associated nuclear antigen p105 and DNA content in patients with renal cell carcinoma. *Cancer* 1996; **78:** 819-826.

56. Toba K, Winton EF, Koike T, Shibata A. Simultaneous three-color analysis of the surface phenotype and DNA-RNA quantitation using 7-amino-actinomycin D and pyronin Y. *J Immunol Methods* 1995; **182:** 193.

60. Aubry JP, Durand I, De Paoli P. 7-amino-4-methylcoumarin-3-acetic acid-conjugated streptavidin permits simultaneous flow cytometry analysis of either three cell surface antigens or one cell surface antigen as a function of RNA and DNA content. *J Immunol Methods* 1990; **128:** 39.

31

Three-dimensional analysis of epithelial cell proliferation

Peter W Hamilton and Kate E Williamson

Summary

This chapter describes a new technique for the three-dimensional visualization and quantitation of glandular epithelial cell proliferation in gastrointestinal mucosa. The tissue used is colorectal biopsy tissue infiltrated *in vitro* with bromodeoxyuridine (BrdUrd). However, the method can be applied to tissue obtained from any gastrointestinal site labelled with any specific marker for cell proliferation. Over 100 serial sections, each 5 μm thick, are cut from colorectal biopsies. All sections are immunohistochemically stained to identify BrdUrd positive cells. Complete colorectal glands are identified by examining sequential sections within the series. Each microscopic image of the sectioned gland is orientated, digitized and stored using a computerized image analysis system. On each of the stored images, the crypt profile is traced and the positive cells and negative cells interactively marked and digitally stored. Using three-dimensional (3D) reconstruction software, the basement membrane of the crypt, the total positive and the total negative fractions can be reconstructed and viewed in three dimensions. The total BrdUrd positive cell number can be automatically calculated for the complete crypt or alternatively, a quantitative compartmental analysis of the labelling index within the crypt can be obtained. This represents a powerful technique: it does not require tissue orientation, it can be carried out on complex glandular structures and is not affected by the biases involved in measuring labelling indices from single tissue sections.

Introduction

The analysis of cell proliferation in gastrointestinal epithelium is important in assessing early growth changes in hyperplasia and neoplasia. However, as gastrointestinal epithelium is composed of distinct glandular units which show distinct variations in proliferation along the length of the gland (e.g. in the normal colon the proliferating compartment occupies the lowest third of the crypt), the measurement of proliferation is not easy. Conventional methods of assessing proliferation in gastrointestinal glands require the tissue to be orientated to ensure longitudinal sectioning of complete glands where the base, middle and mouth of the gland are in the same plane of section.[1] While it is often difficult to obtain complete axial glandular sections, this is vital to ensure that the proliferation profile of the entire cross-sectioned gland is assessed.

Measurement of proliferation is usually carried out by the calculation of a labelling index for a particular marker (number of positively labelled cells/total number of labelled and non-labelled cells). Ratios in biological analysis are, however, notoriously problematic and can be misleading[2,3] as concurrent changes in the denominator (total cell population) can confuse the result. For example, in dogs with gastric hyperplasia induced by prostaglandins, it has been shown that while an increase in the number of proliferating cells within gastric glands does occur, this change is masked when measured as a ratio of total glandular cell number, due to a concurrent increase in the number of non-proliferating cells.[4]

As cell proliferation in gastrointestinal mucosa occurs in distinct glandular units, the gland compartment can be used as the denominator and labelling indices expressed as the number of labelled cells per gland. This can be carried out on well orientated, axially sectioned glands and morphometric measurement of glandular dimensions (e.g. column length and crypt diameter) can provide an index of the gland cell population size.[5] Alternatively, a method has been described which involves the microdissection of glands, squash preparation and the counting of mitoses (positive fraction) per whole gland.[6-8] More recently, confocal laser scanning miscoscopy has been used to visualize small intestinal crypts using optical sectioning.[9] Whole gland analysis has a number of advantages over sectioned tissue: (i) longitudinal orientation of samples is not necessary and (ii) possible axial migration of mitotic cells[10] does not introduce errors into the calculations.[9] Such techniques are, however, largely limited to regular appearing, normal or near-normal epithelial glands.

This chapter describes an alternative method of measuring proliferating cells within the whole gland structure in colorectal mucosa using computerized image analysis and three-dimensional (3D) reconstruction.

Methods

Patients

The colonic mucosal samples used in this study were obtained at colonoscopy from patients in high-risk groups for colorectal cancer and in low-risk controls.

Bromodeoxyuridine incorporation

After removal each biopsy is placed into Dulbecco's modified Eagle medium (DMEM, Gibco, England) at 37°C for 2 min. Excess fluid is removed from the biopsy with filter paper before orientation using a dissecting microscope. The sample is placed onto nitrocellulose paper on dental wax with the submucosa next to the paper and the crypts uppermost. Surplus nitrocellulose paper is cut away. The biopsy is placed into a 1 cm × 1 cm metal processing basket of which the bottom and lid are meshed allowing access to medium. This basket is set on a metal grid suspended immediately above 15 ml DMEM containing 1.5 ml fetal calf serum, 915 µl stock bromodeoxyuridine 5 mg/ml (Sigma B-5002; Sigma, Poole, Dorset, UK) and 180 µl L-glutamine 200 mM in a glass beaker in a 37°C water bath. An inlet filter placed beneath the grid bubbles 95% O_2/5% CO_2 through the medium for the 60 min incubation period. During this incubation the biopsy is constantly in contact with bubbles of medium. Biopsies are then removed from the medium and fixed in 70% alcohol for 4 hours prior to routine processing through ascending alcohols and toluene to paraffin wax. Biopsies are again orientated before embedding in paraffin wax.

Serial sections and immunohistochemistry

Serial sections of the mucosa are carefully cut at 5 µm thickness. Although the number varies, at least 100 serial sections can be cut from a single block at one time.

Each section is then immunostained using a standardized procedure. Briefly, after dewaxing, the DNA is denatured in 1 M HCl at 37°C for 12 min. After thorough rinsing in phosphate buffered saline (PBS, 17 g NaCl, 2.14 g Na_2HPO_4 (anhydrous), 0.72 g NaH_2PO_4 ($2H_2O$) in 2000 ml distilled water final pH 7.0 - 7.2), the sections are sequentially incubated with monoclonal mouse anti-BrdUrd (M744, Dako, High Wycombe, Bucks) (Bu20a), diluted 1:50 in PBST (PBS with 0.05% Tween 20); biotinylated rabbit anti-mouse (Fab')2 antibody (E413, Dako) diluted 1:200 in PBST containing 4% human serum and finally streptavidin-biotin-peroxidase complex (K377, Dako). Diaminobenzidine tetrahydrochloride (Sigma) is applied to give a brown end-product for visualization and the slides are counter-stained with haematoxylin, dehydrated and mounted in synthetic resin.

Section orientation and image capture

A Kontron VIDAS image analysis system (Imaging Associates, Thame, UK) is used for image storage and reconstruction. This comprises a simple IBM PC with a 386DX processor, frame grabbing board and attached digitizing tablet. Image capture, processing, analysis and 3D reconstruction are carried out using Kontron VIDAS v2.1 and the Kontron 3D reconstruction v2.0 software packages. A user application program in Kontron VIDAS macro language has been developed to facilitate the procedure. Digital images are stored on a read/write DPL Optistore 650 Mbyte optical disk drive.

The serial sections are previewed on a standard microscope to identify glands which are complete within the sectioned volume. Each slide in the series is orientated and the image of the sectioned gland digitally stored as a 512 × 512 pixel colour image. Orientation is carried out by video alignment with the previous section using the closest fit of the gland in question and the surrounding structures. Sequential aligned histological images are stored on the optical disk drive for later retrieval and analysis.

3D reconstruction

Each image in the series is recalled from disk and analysed for subsequent 3D reconstruction. For each image (Fig. 31.1a), the basement membrane of the chosen gland is interactively traced using an on-line cursor overlaying the image (Fig. 31.1b). The tracing is then stored digitally as a binary image. Next, BrdUrd-positive cells are highlighted and their positions stored (Fig. 31.1c). Finally, BrdUrd-negative cells are marked and stored as before (Fig. 31.1d). As the original histological images are stored digitally, this allows direct comparison between sequential pairs of sections to ensure that the same cells are not counted twice.

The binary images of basement membrane, positive and negative cell positions are automatically analysed by the 3D reconstruction software and each is entered as a level in the reconstruction. After all images are entered, the completely reconstructed gland can be stored to disk.

Several means of viewing reconstructed images are available. Images can be viewed on the computer screen and rotated to any angle for examination (Fig. 31.2). Data for basement membrane, negative and positive cell co-ordinates are registered in different channels allowing separate or combined analysis of reconstructed images (Fig. 31.3). Colours can be linked to the different channels improving the analysis of positive- and negative-BrdUrd fractions within the crypt. Fig. 31.3 shows a hyperplastic gland from a patient with a family history of colorectal cancer and

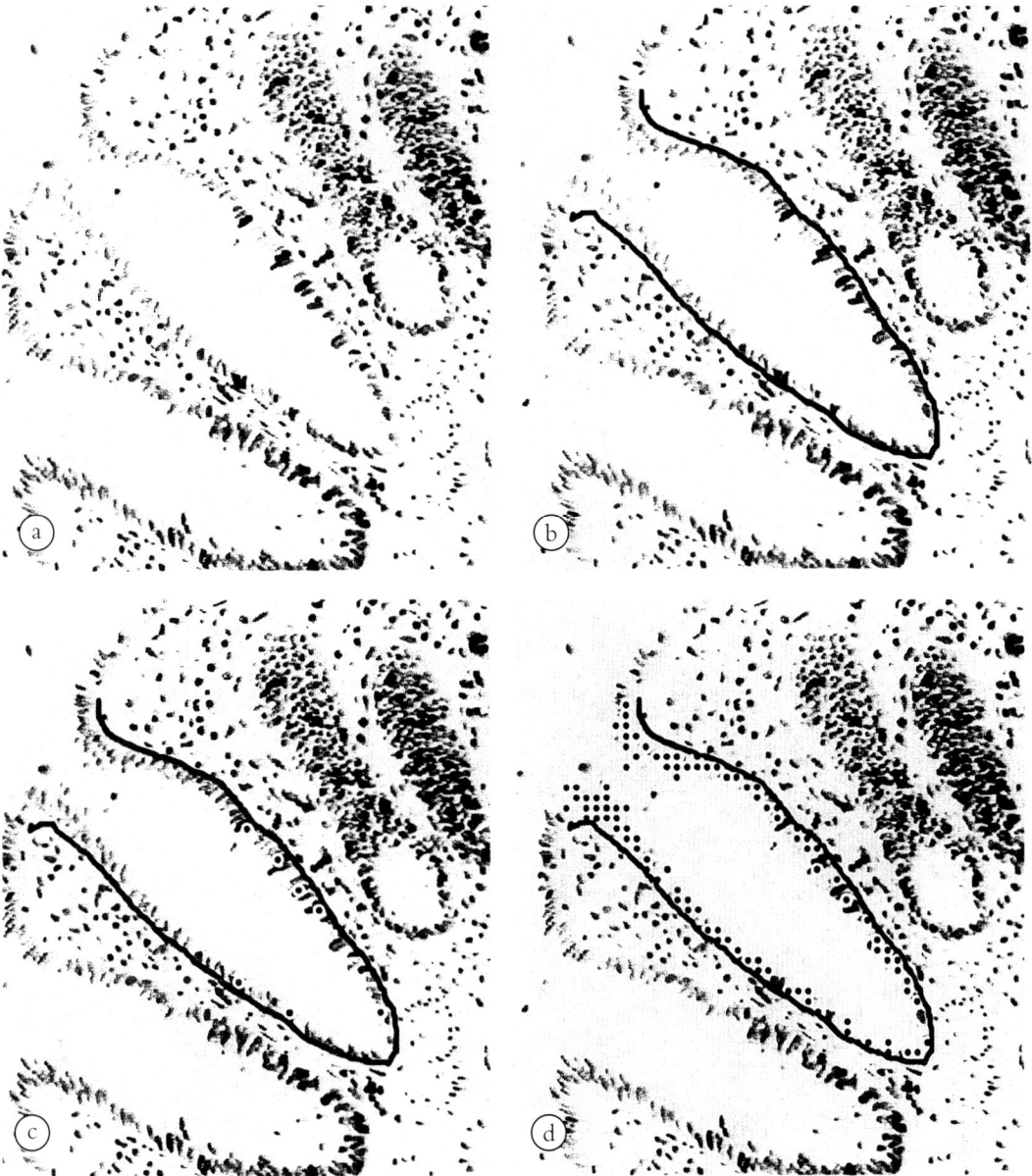

Figure 31.1 – (a) One section in the series used to reconstruct the central gland. (b) The basement membrane of the gland is traced using the computer-linked drawing device. In the same way the positions of the BrdUrd-positive (c) and BrdUrd-negative (d) cells are marked. This is carried out on all sections in the series, the positional information stored by the computer and entered as levels into the final 3D reconstruction.

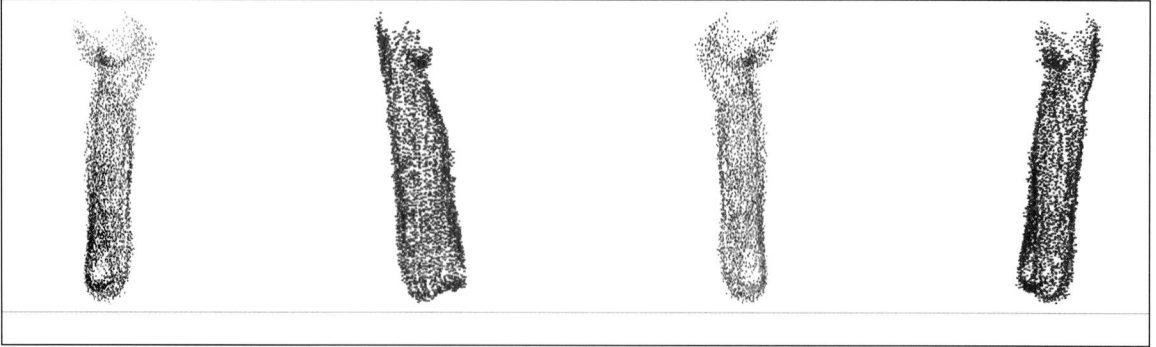

Figure 31.2 – A reconstructed colorectal gland showing all (BrdU-negative and –positive) cell positions. The image can be rotated in 3D space around its longitudinal axis. Four different views of the same gland are shown.

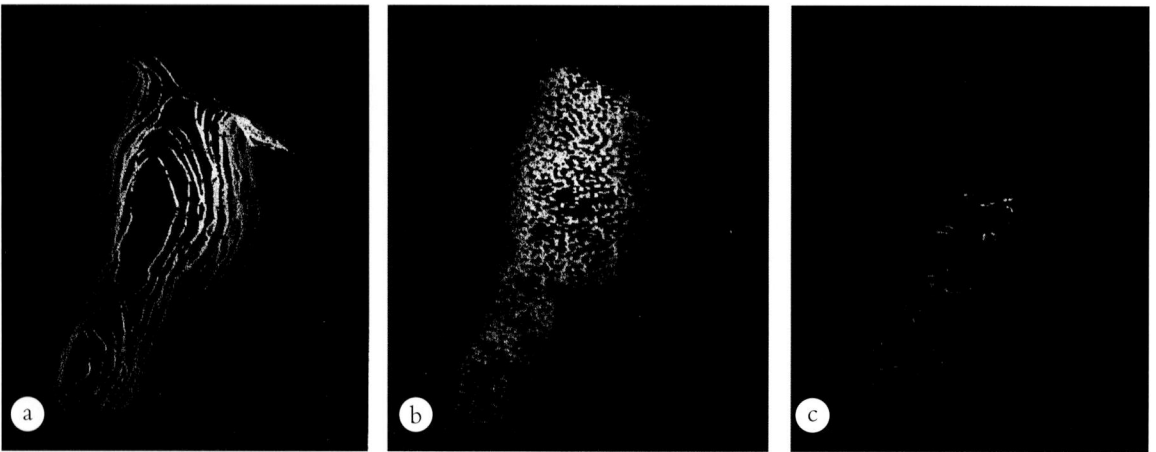

Figure 31.3 – A colorectal gland from a patient with a family history of cancer showing evidence of cell proliferation alterations. (a) Reconstruction of the basement membrane only. (b) Reconstructed image showing all the BrdU-negative epithelial cells. (c) Image showing only BrdU-positive cells which clearly extend into the upper two-thirds of the crypt.

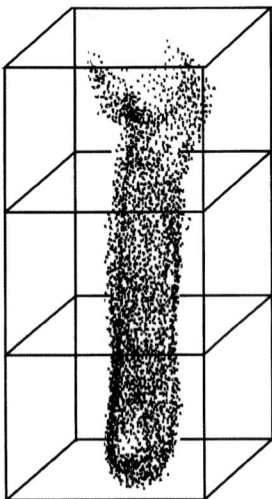

Figure 31.4 – This demonstrates the use of 3D windows to identify gland compartments from which compartmental BrdU-labelling indices can be calculated.

Table 31.1 – Features calculated from proliferation data for the complete gland.

Total number of BrdUrd positive cells per gland

Total BrdUrd labelling index (positive/negative + positive cells) per gland

Compartmental labelling indices

---

consequently at high risk from developing the disease. In addition, the gland can be viewed rotating on the screen through the use of image animation.

Quantitative assessment of the 3D gland proliferation

The binary images used to reconstruct colonic glands can also be subjected to automated quantitative analysis of proliferating cells. From each binary image in the series, the number of positive- and negative-BrdUrd cells which had been recorded are counted by the image analysis software. This allows the features listed in Table 31.1 to be computed. Compartmental analysis of the gland is achieved by the definition of 3D windows (boxes) which can be interactively positioned (Fig. 31.4). The glands can be divided into thirds or fifths on the basis of gland cell numbers counted from the base to the mouth on the most central longitudinal section from the gland.

Application to animal studies

Many animal models of chemically-induced colon cancer have been used to study development, pathogenesis and modulation of this common disease. Some colonic carcinogens act directly while others require metabolic activation.[11] Dimethylhydrazine (DMH) and its metabolites need to be oxidized in the liver to form an active carcinogen *in vivo* which is then transported in the blood to the colon and other organs. These metabolites, in turn, react with cellular macromolecules to form products with target tissue DNA. Methyl radicals have been demonstrated during the metabolism of DMH *in vivo*.[12]

The susceptibility to colon carcinogenesis depends on the species, strain and sex of the animal. The induction of large bowel tumours by DMH is dose-related and the tumour number increases with dose and duration of administration. Nearly all experimental animals develop colon cancer following 20 weekly subcutaneous injections of DMH 20 mg/kg. The earliest morphological change, detectable with scanning electron microscopy, is the appearance of discrete protuberant surface epithelium.[13] There is a decrease in goblet cells and hyperplasia after 5-12 weeks of treatment, focal atypia is evident after 10-15 weeks and severe atypia or carcinomas *in situ* are present after 14-16 weeks. Finally, adenocarcinomas are macroscopically identified in the majority of animals after 20 weeks of treatment.

DMH-induced colon tumours in the rat have been shown to be epithelial in origin with a similar histology to human colonic tumours. A further advantage of DMH-induced carcinogenesis is its specificity for the large bowel. The incidence of cancer in the small bowel is very low. Distal rat colon is more susceptible to DMH than the proximal colon. This is not unexpected because the structure and function of the mucosa of proximal and distal colon differ in both experimental animals and humans. The progressive nature of the DMH model also permits statistically relevant investigations into therapeutic and dietary modulations of colon cancer. This model is therefore appropriate for the 3D study of colorectal carcinogenesis.

Results and discussion

The method is time consuming but provides valuable data on the spatial distribution of proliferation within a gland and on the number of proliferating cells in relation to the entire gland unit. The quantitative data obtained for the gland in Fig. 31.1 is listed in Table 31.2. This shows a high overall proportion

Table 31.2 – Labelling characteristics for the reconstructed gland shown in Fig. 31.3. This shows an increased overall labelling index and a shift in S-phase cells into the upper compartments of the gland.

Total cells in gland	5854
Total BrdUrd-labelled cells per gland	618
Total labelling index	11%
Compartmental labelling indices	
Bottom third	19%
Middle third	13%
Top third	1%

---

of labelled cells in the gland and increased numbers of labelled cells in the middle third of the gland. These changes are indicative of early hyperplasia and are a good marker of risk in patients with a family history of cancer.

The numbers of glands necessary to calculate a representative proliferative value for a particular case is difficult to predict as gland-to-gland variation will depend on the tissue and the nature of the disease being studied. An examination of 10 colonic glands from normal low-risk control patients gave a mean number of labelled cells per gland of 115 (confidence interval 99–131).

Interpretation of reconstructed images is greatly facilitated by colour coding different image components and by rotation of images. This is difficult to convey in a static 2D medium such as a book chapter (examples of images can be found on the internet World Wide Web site:

http://quan7.pt.qub.ac.uk/3d/index.htm

The study of tissues has been for many years based on tissue section analysis which provides a (mostly) 2D view of a 3D structure. This reduction from three to two dimensions invariably results in lost information and leads to observations which are biased.[14] This is almost certainly the case in many studies examining cell proliferation in gastrointestinal mucosa from tissue sections.

It is clear, therefore, that a 3D approach to the analysis of cell proliferation in gastrointestinal epithelium is necessary, not only in the quantitative analysis of gland cell proliferation but also in understanding the spatial relationship between proliferating cells and gland architecture. The gland microdissection technique[6-8] represents a powerful method for examining the total gland cell population. Also, confocal microscopy has offered a novel approach to 3D imaging of microscopic objects,[15-18] including crypts.[9] Relating the number of cells to the gland compartment in this way is much more sensitive to proliferative changes than the calculation of a labelling index.

The method described here, in contrast to the microdissection approach, does not require fresh tissue samples and it can be used to examine glandular changes in stored paraffin-embedded tissue. In addition, the method can be applied to analysis of any marker for glandular proliferating cells that can be identified on tissue sections, e.g. mitotic figures, Ki67, MIB1, BrdUrd and proliferating cell nuclear antigen

(PCNA) immunohistochemistry. In essence, the spatial distribution of any marked cell within gastrointestinal glands can be examined in 3D using the methodology outlined here. This method would provide a more accurate means of assessing related features such as apoptosis, cell differentiation, gene expression and other genotypic and phenotypic markers in relation to the gland unit. Deciphering the intricate cellular organization seen within the gastrointestinal gland in 3D is fundamental to our understanding of a variety of gastrointestinal diseases, including neoplasia.

An important addition to the software is the ability to calculate compartmental indices provided both the labelled and non-labelled cells are counted. This permits a more accurate measure of alterations in the spatial distribution of proliferating cells along the length of the gland and this in combination with a 3D visual perspective represents a valuable analytical tool in the study of gastrointestinal disease.

The number of glands required to obtain a statistically meaningful result depends on the variation in labelled cells between glands. In glands from normal controls this is shown to be quite high although this depends on how small a change is to be detected. Variation is likely to increase in diseased colorectal glands. Goodlad et al[8] report counting 15-20 glands per case using the microdissection technique. This would be possible using the current method but could take as long as 6 hours after serial sections are cut. This method is therefore more suitable as an analytical and quantitative research tool. The effort involved in reconstructing glands can be reduced by counting only the positively labelled cell population and expressing this as number per gland. This, however, precludes the calculation of compartmental indices unless the gland is divided on the basis of its length or volume and positive cells expressed as a number per compartment.

Visualization of 3D changes in glandular architecture and shape is important and using serial sections, possible changes introduced by removal of the gland from its surrounding tissue are avoided. Previous workers have shown that the examination of glandular structure in 3D provides useful information in the study of gastrointestinal neoplastic lesions.[19-21] The current approach, however, allows glandular architecture to be examined in association with cell proliferation and this may provide additional insight into the proliferative and structural development of gastrointestinal neoplasia from its early stages. A major potential use of the 3D technique, therefore, lies in the analysis of tortuous or branching glands which are not easily microdissected.[8] Such glands are found in hyperplastic and adenomatous colorectal mucosa and reconstruction techniques might provide a valuable insight into the structural and proliferative characteristics of such lesions in so far as the glands can be followed in 3D space on serial sections. This method should also be of use in the analysis of proliferation in gastric fundal glands whose complexity makes microdissection difficult.[8]

Future work should examine ways to increase the speed of serial section analysis either by automated image analysis or through the use of confocal laser scanning microscopy (CLSM).

Acknowledgments

This work has previously been presented in *British Journal of Cancer* 1994; **69**: 1027-1031. The study was funded by the Ulster Cancer Foundation, Medical Research Council, Action Cancer, Royal College of Surgeons of Edinburgh, The Queen's University of Belfast and the Royal Victoria Hospital, Belfast.

References

1. Wright N, Alison M. *The Biology of Epithelial Cell Populations*, Vol 2. Clarendon Press, Oxford, 1984.

2. Sokal RR, Rohlf FJ. *Biometry. The Principles and Practice of Statistics in Biological Research*. WH Freeman and Company, New York,1981.

3. Braendgaard H, Gundersen HJG. The impact of recent stereological advances on quantitative studies of the nervous system. *J Neurosci Meth* 1986; **18**: 39-78.

4. Goodlad RA, Madgewick AJA, Moffatt MR, Levin S, Allen JL, Wright NA. Prostaglandins and gastric epithelium: effects of misoprostol on gastric epithelial cell proliferation in the dog. *Gut* 1989; **30**: 316-321.

5. Wright NA, Carter J, Irwin M. The measurement of villus cell population size in the mouse small intestine in normal and abnormal states: a comparison of absolute measurements with morphometric estimators in sectioned immersion-fixed material. *Cell Tissue Kinet* 1989; **22**: 425-450.

6. Clarke RM. Mucosal architecture and epithelial cell production rate in the small intestine of the albino rat. *J Anat* 1970; **107**: 519-529.

7. Ferguson A, Sutherland A, MacDonald TT, Allan F. Technique for microdissection and measurement in biopsies of human small intestine. *J Clin Pathol* 1977; **30**: 1068-1073.

8. Goodlad RA, Levi S, Lee CY, Mandir N, Hodgson H, Wright N. Morphometry and cell proliferation in endoscopic biopsies: evaluation of a technique. *Gastroenterology* 1991; **101**: 1235-1241.

9. Savage TC, Walker-Smith JA, Phillips AD. Novel insights into human intestinal epithelial cell proliferation in health and disease using confocal microscopy. *Gut* 1995; **36**: 369-374.

10. Tannock IF. A comparison of the relative efficiencies of various metaphase arrest agents. *Exp Cell Res* 1967; **47**: 345-356.

11. Rogers AE, Nauss KM. Rodent model for carcinoma of the colon. *Dig Dis Sci* 1985; **30**: S87-S102.

12. Fiala ES. Investigations into the metabolism and mode of action of the colon carcinogens 1,2-dimethylhydrazine and azoxymethane. *Cancer* 1977; **40**: 2436-2445.

13. Filipe MI. Mucin histochemistry in the detection of early malignancy in the colonic epithelium. *Adv Exp Med Biol* 1977; **89**: 413-422.

14. Howard V. Stereological techniques in biological electron microscopy. In: Hawkes PW, Valdre U (Eds) *Biophysical Electron Microscopy*. Academic Press, London, 1990, pp. 479-508.

15. Agard D. Optical sectioning microscopy: cellular architecture in three dimensions. *Ann Rev Biophys Bioeng* 1984; **13**: 191-219.

16. Baak JPA, Thunnissen FBJM., Oudejans CBM *et al*. Potential clinical uses of laser scanning microscopy. *Appl Opt* 1987; **26**: 3413-3416.

17. Brakenhoff GJ, van der Voort HTM, van Spronsen EA, Nanninga N. Three-dimensional imaging of biological structures by high resolution confocal scanning laser microscopy. *Scanning Microsc* 1988; **2**: 33-40.

18. Kett P, Geiger B, Ehemann V, Komitowski D. Three-dimensional analysis of cell nucleus structures visualised by confocal scanning microscopy. *J Microsc* 1992; **167**: 169-179.

19. Takahashi T, Iwama N. Architectural pattern of gastric adenocarcinoma. A 3-dimensional reconstruction study. *Virchows Archiv (Pathol Anat)* 1984; **403**: 127-134.

20. Takahashi T, Iwama N. Atypical glands in gastric adenoma. Three dimensional architecture compared with carcinomatous and metaplastic glands. *Virchows Archiv (Pathol Anat)* 1984; **403**: 135-148.

21. Campbell F, Garrahan NJ, Deverell MH, Whimster WF, Williams GT. Application of a computer aided design system to the 3 dimensional reconstruction of colonic crypts. *J Pathol* 1992; **168** (Suppl): 125.

32

In vitro uptake of nutrients by human duodenal biopsies with special reference to iron

KB Raja and RJ Simpson

Summary

This chapter describes a well-characterised *in vitro* technique that can be used to ascertain the rate and kinetics of uptake of not only iron, but also other nutrients, by human intestinal biopsies. The method allows measurements to be made independently from factors (e.g. hormonal, neural. motility, pH) which are difficult to control *in vivo*, and is thus useful in ascertaining the intestinal defect(s) in the transport of nutrient(s) in patients with clinical disorders. The method can be equally applied to investigating intestinal transport of nutients in animal models.

Introduction

The gastrointestinal tract functions not only as an effective barrier against intraluminal pathogens (bacteria, toxins and antigens) but also controls nutrient absorption. The latter function is performed primarily by the small intestine which extends from the pylorus to the ileocaecal junction and is divided anatomically into three regions namely duodenum, jejunum and ileum. The surface area of the small intestinal mucosa is greatly enhanced by the abundance of finger-like projections (villi). The epithelial lining of the small intestine is a rapidly renewing system: cell turnover takes 48–72 hours with the newly formed cells attaining the characteristics of mature functional cells as they progressively migrate along the villus.[1]

The rate of absorption of nutrients, especially trace metals, is dependent not only on body requirements but also on their bioavailability. Iron is the most important metal in the body and unlike other metals, the levels of iron in the body are maintained primarily by controlling intestinal absorption. Luminal iron is present in both haem and non-haem forms and absorption from the latter is markedly dependent on the intraluminal environment.

Following the introduction of radioactive iron in 1938, major advances have been made not only in the methods used to measure absorption, but also the accuracy of the measurements. The methods are either *in vivo* or *in vitro*, depending on the presence or absence of a systemic blood supply, respectively. Two *in vivo* approaches include the disappearance of iron from the intestinal lumen or the appearance of it in the blood/tissues. Although useful, the *in vivo* methods do have major drawbacks: they provide no information about the site of absorption or details of the kinetics of transport, and interpretation of the data is difficult if steady-state conditions do not prevail within the body.

One obvious advantage of the *in vitro* technique is its independence from effects such as intestinal motility, luminal constituents and pH, neural and hormonal effects, all of which are difficult to control *in vivo*. Attempts to study intestinal iron transport *in vitro* have utilized various methods including everted sacs,[2] isolated segments,[3] isolated enterocytes[4] and brush-border membrane vesicles.[5] However, as the amount of intestinal tissue that can be obtained non-surgically from man is limited, it is difficult to apply the above techniques to study iron absorption *in vitro* in humans.

This chapter describes a well characterized *in vitro* method[6] for ascertaining uptake (and with recent developments, the reduction) of iron by human intestinal tissue. Mucosal uptake represents the first cellular step in iron absorption and is thus a suitable point for studying the interaction between cell biochemistry of iron absorption and the nutritional chemistry of dietary iron. The *in vitro* method satisfies the criteria set by Sallee *et al*[7] for valid measurement of unidirectional uptake into intestinal tissue.

Methods

Intestinal mucosal fragment(s) taken with standard biopsy forceps or a Watson capsule, from overnight fasted subjects undergoing endoscopic examination, are, where necessary, cut into smaller fragments (1-5 mg), rinsed in oxygenated (95% O_2/5% CO_2) physiological buffer (125 mM NaCl, 3.5 mM KCl, 1 mM $CaCl_2$, 10 mM $MgSO_4$, 10 mM D-glucose in 16 mM N-(2-hydroxyethyl)piperazine-N'-2-ethanesulphonic acid (HEPES)-NaOH, pH 7.4; reagents from BDH Merck Ltd, Poole, Dorset, UK) and gently blotted on tissue paper, to remove any adherent food particles and mucus. The fragment(s) are then briefly pre-incubated at 37°C in a similar buffer (2 ml) containing 5 µM cyanocobalamin (Duncan Flockhart Co Ltd. Greenford, UK). It has been shown that isolated intestinal tissue fragments are capable of regenerating ATP levels following incubation in oxygenated glucose-containing medium.[8] The tissue sample(s) are thereafter transferred (periodically if more than one incubation performed) to 2.6 ml of physiological buffer (Fig. 32.1) containing [^{59}Fe]-radioiron (5-10 µCi; NEN Du Pont, Stevenage, Hertfordshire, UK; specific activity 0.185-2.78 TBq/g), as a ferric chelate of a low molecular weight ligand such as nitrilotriacetate (NTA)(Sigma-Aldrich,

Poole, Dorset, UK), citrate[9] (Sigma-Aldrich) or ascorbate[10] (Sigma-Aldrich), to maintain the iron in a soluble, bioavailable form.

The use of low molecular weight complexes of iron to study intestinal iron absorption is justifiable since Glover & Jacobs[11] have shown that a substantial proportion of iron in a test meal is bound to low molecular weight compounds during digestion in the human proximal intestine. In most of our studies NTA has been used (Fe:NTA, 1:2) as it is well characterized,[12] and it forms a relatively stable and bioavailable complex with iron.

[57]Co-cyanocobalamin (0.3-0.5 μCi: Life Screen Ltd, Watford, Hertfordshire, UK; specific activity 0.5-1.0 MBq/nmol), 5 μM, is also included in the medium as an extracellular fluid (ECF) marker to correct for adherent medium and non-specific permeation of the metal complex. The distribution volume of the ECF marker gives a sensitive measure of intestinal permeability[13] and thus of mucosal integrity. Alterations in the ECF volume and thus in intestinal permeability have been reported in coeliac disease[13] and in alcoholic enteropathy.[14]

Following a short incubation (5-6 min), with tissue oxygenation throughout (Fig. 32.1), the uptake reaction is stopped by blotting the tissue and rinsing in 1 ml ice-cold physiological buffer. A rinse time of 3-4 seconds is suitable. More prolonged rinsing leads to a loss of tissue-associated radioactivity.[8] After reblotting and weighing, the radioactivity in the tissue and in an aliquot of the medium is measured using a twin channel gamma-counter. The ^{59}Fe and ^{57}Co counts are determined separately by channel ratio analysis. After correction for ^{57}Co counts, the uptake rate is expressed as pmol/mg wet weight/min (see below). Where more than one fragment has been inserted into an incubation medium, each fragment can be analysed separately to ascertain the uptake rate.

$$\text{Uptake} = \frac{\textbf{cpm A}}{\text{std A}} - \frac{\textbf{cpm B}}{\text{std B}} \times \frac{\textbf{[Fe]}}{\text{W} \times \text{T}}$$

where:

cpm A = tissue ^{59}Fe, corrected for background;

std A = medium ^{59}Fe, corrected for background/μl;

cpm B = tissue ^{57}Co, corrected for background;

std B = medium ^{57}Co, corrected for background/μl;

[Fe] = medium iron concentration (μM or pmol/μl);

W = wet weight of tissue fragment (mg);

T = incubation time (min).

The fact that multiple incubations can be performed simultaneously with tissue fragments from the same

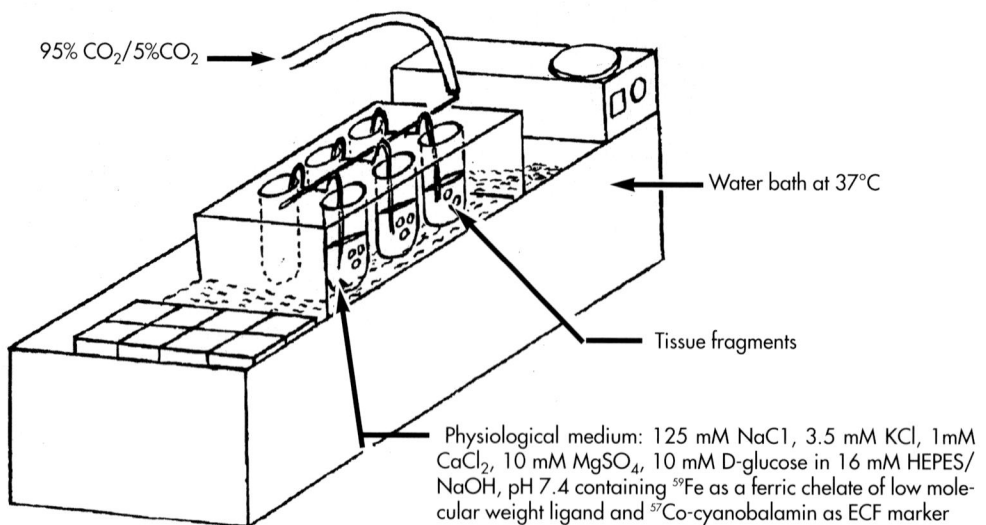

95% CO$_2$/5%CO$_2$

Water bath at 37°C

Tissue fragments

Physiological medium: 125 mM NaCl, 3.5 mM KCl, 1mM CaCl$_2$, 10 mM MgSO$_4$, 10 mM D-glucose in 16 mM HEPES/ NaOH, pH 7.4 containing ^{59}Fe as a ferric chelate of low molecular weight ligand and ^{57}Co-cyanobalamin as ECF marker

Figure 32.1 – In vitro method for determining uptake of iron by intestinal tissue fragments.

individual (Fig. 32.1) allows critical evaluation of the effects of manipulating the medium constituents on iron uptake by intestinal tissue. Thus, we have recently been able to demonstrate that uptake requires prior reduction of Fe(III), the predominant form of iron in the diet, to the ferrous, Fe(II) form.[15]

Determination of intestinal Fe(III) reducing activity

Reduction of iron can be studied *in vitro* in parallel with uptake by including ferrozine (1 mM; Sigma-Aldrich), a very specific Fe(II) chelator,[16] in the incubation medium. Ferrozine is added to the incubation medium (with or without the presence of ^{59}Fe and ^{57}Co) just before the addition of tissue fragments. Fe(II) forms a highly stable, coloured, Fe(II)-(ferrozine)$_3$ complex with a molar absorptivity at 562 nm of 28 600 l/cm/mol,[17] and allows quantitation of tissue-associated Fe(III) reduction rates.

Transfer of fragments from the pre-incubation medium to the incubation medium, as above, is staggered if more than one incubation is being performed (Fig. 32.2). Aliquots (100 μl) of incubation medium removed immediately after the addition of tissue (t = 0 min) and thereafter periodically to the

end of the incubation (Fig. 32.2), are diluted with a known volume of deionized water, and read at 562 nm. At the end of the incubation period, the tissue is blotted and weighed (Fig. 32.2).

The total amount of ionizable iron in one or more of the aliquoted samples is thereafter determined by complete reduction of the sample with excess ascorbic acid and subsequent re-monitoring at 562 nm. This value allows calculation of the total quantity of medium iron reduced by the incubated tissue sample(s). After correction for dilution, the Fe(III) reducing activity is expressed as pmol/mg/min.

$$\text{Fe(III) reducing activity (pmol/mg/min)} = \frac{A \times \text{dilution factor} \times D}{\text{tissue wet weight (mg)} \times B}$$

where:

A = change in absorbance over the incubation period (OD units/min);

dilution factor includes correction for the total volume of the incubation medium;

B = absorbance reading for fully reduced aliquot sample;

D = medium iron content (pmol/100 μl).

Ferrozine in the incubation medium containing ^{59}Fe and ^{57}Co will allow simultaneous determination of tissue Fe(III) reduction and uptake rates. In such circumstances, the tissue fragment(s) post-incubation are processed as for the uptake experiment described above. The inhibitory effect of ferrozine on *in vitro* ^{59}Fe uptake supports the proposition that reduction precedes uptake.

Application to animal studies

This *in vitro* method has been used to investigate the mechanism(s) and regulation of intestinal iron absorption in mice,[18] rats,[19] and rabbits,[20] and can be applied to other species. Extensive studies in mice have revealed that the major route of entry of iron into the intestinal mucosa is via an active, carrier-mediated, electrogenic, membrane-potential dependent pathway.[21] Moreover, any adaptive changes in iron uptake due to changes in body iron requirements occurs via this pathway. This method has also been used to study the uptake of other nutrients, e.g. glucose.[21,22]

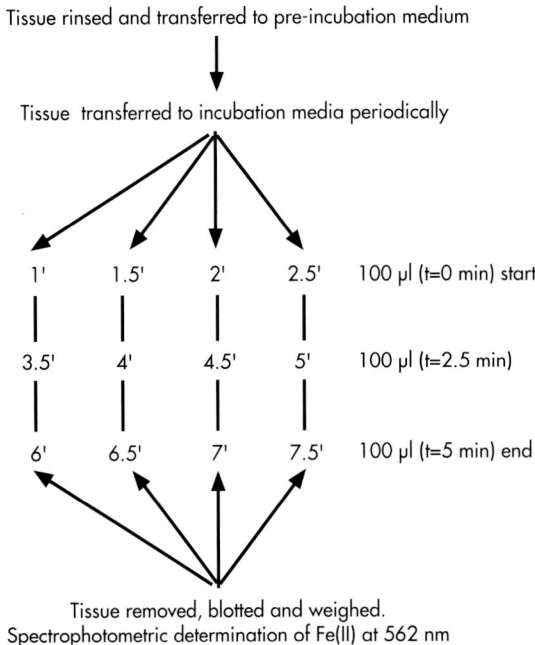

Tissue rinsed and transferred to pre-incubation medium

Tissue transferred to incubation media periodically

1'	1.5'	2'	2.5'	100 μl (t=0 min) start
3.5'	4'	4.5'	5'	100 μl (t=2.5 min)
6'	6.5'	7'	7.5'	100 μl (t=5 min) end

Tissue removed, blotted and weighed.
Spectrophotometric determination of Fe(II) at 562 nm

Figure 32.2 – Steps in the Fe(III) reduction assay.

Table 32.1 – Effect of cations on ^{59}Fe uptake by human duodenal biopsy samples

Medium	Uptake (% contol)
Normal medium	100 (7)
Low Na$^+$/high K$^+$	57.0 ± 20.0 (4)
Replace Na$^+$ with Rb$^+$	64.0 ± 24.0 (3)

Data: Mean ± SD for (n) determinations. Freshly obtained duodenal samples were incubated in either control medium or in experimental medium. Medium Fe^{3+}, 250 μM; NTA, 500 μM. Incubation period = 5 min. Uptake by fragments incubated is expressed as a percentage of the value obtained in control medium.

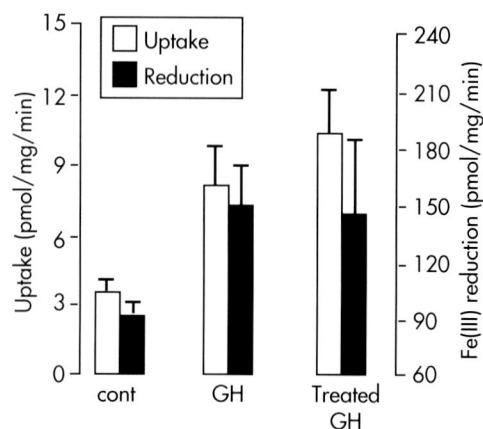

Figure 32.3 – In vitro uptake and reduction of medium iron by human duodenal mucosal tissue obtained from control subjects (cont), patients with genetic haemochromatosis (GH), with and without treatment. Data are given as mean ± SE for 5–10 subjects in each group.

Results and discussion

Table 32.1 shows that iron uptake by human duodenal tissue is significantly reduced by substituting medium Na$^+$ by either K$^+$ (depolarization) or Rb$^+$. These findings demonstrate, as in rodents, the existence of a membrane potential-dependent pathway for iron uptake by human intestinal tissue.

In addition, reduction of medium Fe(III) is a prerequisite for uptake as uptake rates are markedly reduced by the presence in the medium of ferrozine and ferricyanide (1 mM), a non-permeable oxidizing agent, but not by ferrocyanide.[15] Ferrozine itself induces no change in colour in the medium in the presence or absence of iron, which supports previous findings.[23] The non-specific reduction of Fe^{3+}(NTA)$_2$ by ferrozine reported by Cowart *et al*[24] may be attributable to photoreduction reactions.[25] The rate of reduction of medium iron, though not rate-limiting for uptake, is proportional to the incubation period and is not due to the release of reducing factors from tissue fragments.[15]

Previous *in vitro* studies have shown that the uptake of ^{59}Fe by human intestinal tisssue is dependent on the concentration of Fe^{3+}:ligand complex,[9,10] suggesting that the intact complex interacts with some yet unknown protein(s) prior to donating the iron: the intact complex is excluded from cell entry.[9] The hyperbolic dependence of uptake on medium iron concentrations can be subsequently used to determine the apparent kinetic parameters for transport, namely K_m (affinity constant) and V_{max} (maximal uptake

capacity). As to whether the reduction and uptake processes work in unison or are separate entities remains unknown. Teichmann & Stremmel[26] demonstrated the presence of a 160 kDa protein (a trimer of 54 kDa monomers) in human intestinal mucosa and have shown using an antibody against the 54 kDa subunit that uptake of iron by human microvillus membrane vesicles (prepared from material obtained at autopsy or resectioning) is markedly affected (>50% inhibition). *In vitro* incubation of freshly isolated human duodenal mucosa from control subjects in the presence of the antibody, however, only revealed small inhibitory effects on iron uptake [6.0±5.6% (3)] and reduction [25.5±12.3%(3)], respectively. As to whether the incomplete inhibition is due to partial inaccessibility of the antibody, or due to another protein required for the uptake/reduction processes, warrants further investigations.

This chapter describes an *in vitro* method that is invaluable for studying the kinetics and adaptive changes of iron uptake by the intestinal mucosa. Although the physiological responses occuring in the intestine of the organism are difficult to mimic *in vitro*, important knowledge can be gained from using *in vitro* techniques. Indeed, application of the *in vitro* method to samples from laboratory animals and humans has enabled major advances in the understanding of the mechanism and regulation of intestinal iron absorption, which would not have been possible with *in vivo* methods. The method can also be used to ascertain intestinal defects in the uptake of iron (or other nutrients) in patients with clinical disorders. We have shown that there is a selective abnormality in the reduction and uptake of iron by duodenal tissue from patients with genetic haemochromatosis (GH), an inherited disorder of iron metabolism.[15,27] The defect was still evident in GH patients who had undergone treatment (regular venesections) to normalize body iron stores (Fig. 32.3), thus indicating a metabolic abnormality at the intestinal level. Another example is the demonstration of increased passive permeation of iron by duodenal biopsies from chronic alcohol misusers, which may contribute to the iron overload in these subjects.[28]

Acknowledgements

We thank Dr D Pountney for his contribution, Dr W Stremmel for the generous gift of the antibody and Prof. TJ Peters for helpful comments. This chapter is a contribution from King's College Centre for the Study of Metals in Biology and Medicine.

References

1. Gordon JI. Intestinal epithelium differentiation: new insights from chimeric and transgenic mice. *J Cell Biol* 1989; **108**: 1187-1194.

2. Sheehan RG. Unidirectional uptake of iron across intestinal brush border. *Am J Physiol* 1976; **231**: 1438-1444.

3. Forth W, Rummel W. Iron absorption. *Physiol Rev* 1973; **53**: 724-792.

4. Johnson G, Jacobs P, Purves LR. Iron binding proteins of iron absorbing rat intestinal mucosa. *J Clin Invest* 1983; **71**: 1467-1476.

5. Simpson RJ, Peters TJ. Studies of Fe^{3+} transport across isolated intestinal brush-border membrane of the mouse. *Biochim Biophys Acta* 1984; **772**: 220-226.

6. Cox TM, Peters TJ. Uptake of iron by duodenal biopsy specimens from patients with iron-deficiency anaemia and primary haemochromatosis. *Lancet* 1978; **i**: 123-124.

7. Sallee VL, Wilson FA, Dietschy JM. Determination of unidirectional uptake rates for lipids across the intestinal brush-border. *J Lipid Res* 1972; **13**: 184-192.

8. Raja KB, Simpson RJ, Peters TJ. Comparison of $^{59}Fe^{3+}$ uptake in vitro and in vivo by mouse duodenum. *Biochim Biophys Acta* 1987; **901**: 52-60.

9. Cox TM, Peters TJ. The kinetics of iron uptake *in vitro* by human duodenal mucosa: studies in normal subjects. *J Physiol* 1979; **289**: 469-478

10. Duane P, Raja KB, Simpson RJ, Peters TJ. *In vitro* uptake of iron from iron-ascorbate by human duodenal biopsies from control subjects and patients with idiopathic haemochromatosis. *Eur J Gastroenterol Hepatol* 1992; **4**: 661-666.

11. Glover J, Jacobs A. Observations on iron in the jejunal lumen after a standard meal. *Gut* 1971; **12**: 369-371.

12. Sillen LG, Martell AE. *Stability Constants of Metal-Ion Complexes*. Special Edition no. 25. Chemical Society, London, 1971.

13. Bjarnason I, Peters TJ. *In vitro* determination of small intestinal permeability: demonstration of a persistent defect in patients with coeliac disease. *Gut* 1984; **25**: 145-150.

14. Bjarnason I, Ward K, Peters TJ. The leaky gut of alcoholism: possible route of entry for toxic compounds. *Lancet* 1984; **i**: 170-182

15. Raja KB, Pountney D, Bomford A *et al*. A duodenal mucosal abnormality in the reduction of Fe(III) in patients with genetic haemochromatosis. *Gut* 1996; **38**: 765-769.

16. Stookey LL. Ferrozine. A new spectrophotometric reagent for iron. *Analyt Chem* 1970; **42**: 779-781.

17. Gibbs CR. Characterisation and application of ferrozine iron reagent as a ferrous iron indicator. *Analyt Chem* 1976; **48**: 1197-1201.

18. Raja KB, Bjarnason I, Simpson RJ, Peters TJ. *In vitro* measurement and adaptive response of Fe^{3+} uptake by mouse duodenum. *Cell Biochem Funct* 1987; **5**: 69-76.

19. O'Riordon DK, Simpson RJ, Taylor E *et al*. Hypoxia causes hyperpolarization of isolated rat duodenal brush-border membrane and increased iron absorption. *J Physiol* 1995; **489**: 124P.

20. Cox TM, O'Donnell MW. Studies on the control of iron uptake by rabbit small intestine. *Br J Nutr* 1982; **47**: 251-258.

21. Raja KB, Simpson RJ, Peters TJ. Membrane potential dependence of Fe(III) uptake by mouse duodenum. *Biochim Biophys Acta* 1989; **984**: 262-266.

22. Banerjee AK, Raja K, Peters TJ. Effect of insulin induced hypoglycaemia on *in vitro* uptake of 3-O-methyl glucose by rat jejunum. *Gut* 1989; **30**: 1348-1353.

23. Chindambaram MV, Reedy MB, Thompson JL, Bates GW. *In vitro* studies of iron bioavailability. Probing the concentration and oxidation-reduction reactivity of Pinto Bean iron with ferrous chromogens. *Biol Trace Elem Res* 1989; **19**: 25-40.

24. Cowart RE, Singleton FL, Hind JS. A comparison of Bathophenanthrolinedisulfonic acid and ferrozine as chelators of iron (II) in reduction reactions. *Analyt Biochem* 1993; **211**: 151–155.

25. Mueller S, Simpson RJ. Photoreduction of iron at physiological pH; effect of biological buffers. *Biochem Soc Trans* 1993; **22**: 93S.

26. Teichmann R, Stremmel W. Iron uptake by human upper small intestine microvillous membrane vesicles. Indication for a facilitated transport mechanism mediated by a membrane iron-binding protein. *J Clin Invest* 1990; **86**: 2145–2153.

27. Cox TM. Haemochromatosis. *Blood Rev* 1990; **4**: 75–87.

28. Duane P, Raja KB, Simpson RJ, Peters TJ. Intestinal iron absorption in chronic alcoholics. *Alcohol Alcohol* 1992; **27**: 539–544.

33

The future direction of pathology:
Personal perspectives

KB Raja, RJ Simpson, RR Watson and VR Preedy

Pathology deals with all aspects of diseases i.e. nature, causes and development of the abnormal condition, especially the structural and functional changes in the tissues and organs in the body. This branch of medicine encompasses disciplines such as microbiology, cell biology, biochemistry, physiology, genetics, immunology and haematology. Included in these are specialist areas, such as animal experimentation, cytopathology, specific viral diseases such as hepatitis or HIV, *in vitro* testing, transplantation, cancer treatments, diabetic neuropathy, gene therapy, parasitology and arthritis, to name but a few. It is noteworthy that the above-mentioned areas are not distinct entities but have considerable overlap. The ultimate aim of investigations into pathology is to effectively prevent or cure diseases and reduce harm to the individual or groups of individuals.

This book contains a number of useful, well-characterized techniques that are applicable to investigating the pathophysiology of the gastrointestinal tract, including the functional aspect, in both human and animal models. The book does not however, provide an exhaustive list of all techniques that can be used in GI research. In the first chapter, attention was drawn to the possible artifacts that may arise when following particular experimental protocols or procedures. To a certain extent, this depends on the technical advancements in the prevailing experimental methods. As exemplified in Chapter 1, absorption studies performed recently in chronically-catheterized non-restrained animals have demonstrated major differences in not only the manner but also the rate of glucose absorption, as compared to data obtained previously in anaesthetized, perfused (used as the gold standard) animals.

The purpose of this chapter is to briefly speculate on what the medium-term future holds for biomedical research. This is, however, an extremely difficult and almost impossible task. As Gordis[1] recently implied, in his speculation on the future of alcohol research, the guess of the reader or audience is probably as good, or better than that of the author(s) or speaker.

One possible approach in trying to predict the direction of future research is to ascertain popular trends [research tools] by reviewing scientific literature over the last 5-10 years. In the UK, the number of biology and biochemistry-related publications has shown only a moderate increase over the past decade (i.e. 15% increase in 1996 compared to 1986), whilst the number of articles involving molecular biology has shown more spectacular changes (i.e. over 70% increase in 1996 compared to 1986). It thus comes as no surprise that Medical Science today is dominated by the overwhelming force of this new approach.

One area of research discussed in Chapter 1, namely iron metabolism, has over the last decade seen a major shift in emphasis from basic functional studies with cells/tissue/membranes (of both human and animal origin) to studying biological processes at the molecular level (i.e. the cloning of genes and studies of gene inheritance and expression, with a view to ascertaining molecular defects in various clinical conditions). The molecular approach has helped to elucidate not only the basis for post-translational control of the synthesis of proteins involved in iron metabolism in vertebrate cells (two cytoplasmic RNA-binding proteins, iron-regulatory protein 1 and 2, respond to intracellular iron levels and co-ordinate accordingly the levels of two iron-binding proteins, namely ferritin and transferrin receptor, via specifically binding to particular hairpin structures in their respective mRNA's) but has also identified a specific mis-sense mutation, Cys282Tyr, in a novel HLA class-I molecule in a large proportion (>80%) of patients with Hereditary Haemochromatosis:[2] This recessive condition, which is very common in northern Europeans (carrier frequency of 10%), is accompanied by unregulated absorption of iron at the intestinal level, despite massive iron-overload. More recently, the molecular approach has identified a candidate for the long sought -after intestinal brush border membrane iron carrier protein. [3]

It is possible, in principle at least, to clone, sequence and analyze the thousands of functional genes in the human genome with the existing technology, and in due course determine the gene aberrations responsible for all known inherited conditions. This goal is now achievable within the foreseeable future. Identification of genes *per se* should not however, detract from the fact that physiological studies are necessary to determine the functional role of the isolated gene(s). A more challenging goal is that which underlies all analytical biology (including pathology), namely, the translation of observable phenomena into other terms which allow understanding and prediction of the behaviour of living systems.

We thus anticipate that the molecular approach to diseases will continue to be a dominant trend, certainly over the next 5-10 years. Some of the areas of current research which should help to contribute to achieve those goals can be summarized under the following topics:

- **Physical mapping of genes:** Many inherited-disease genes have been mapped and identification of mutations has become a routine diagnostic tool.
- **Genetic basis of diseases:** Genes conferring susceptibility to diseases e.g. cancer, diabetes and heart disease, are rapidly being identified. The precise usefulness of this information for medicine is less obvious and carries with it thorny social and moral issues. Nevertheless, the expansion in knowledge of processes underlying disease will have long term benefits for the development of therapies.
- **Identification of gene function:** Some useful information can be derived from the above two approaches. In many cases, however, the defective gene does not bear any obvious relationship to the disease phenotype.
- **Creation and study of transgenic animals:** Currently of major importance to ascribing function to genes and identifying functional consequences of gene mutations. Also very useful for elucidation of fundamental physiological mechanisms.
- **Developmental regulation of gene function**
- **Control of gene expression**
- **Molecular basis of cellular differentiation:** These three approaches are all related to the elucidation of fundamental mechanisms in biology. It is anticipated that advances arising from these areas will become major forces in pathology in the future.

Role of immune system in diseases: Many diseases involve aberrant or damaging responses of the immune system. The function of the immune system as a protection against disease places it at the heart of both the causes and possible cures for the major diseases including cancer, diabetes and infectious diseases.

There will remain, however, the problem of integrating knowledge gained by reductionist approaches. We anticipate that functional studies of whole cells, tissues and organisms will continue to be necessary and that these combined with the developing research area, Computational Biology, will help our understanding of the complex processes operating within living systems.

Acknowledgments

The authors are grateful for helpful information from Dr King (ISI, USA).

References

1. Gordis E. Alcohol research: celebrating the past, building the future. *Alcoholism: Clin Exp Res* 1996; **20:** 32A-37A.

2. Feder JN *et al.* A novel MHC class I-like gene is mutated in patients with hereditary haemochromatosis. *Nat Genet* 1996; **13:** 399-408.

3. Gunshin H, Mackenzie B, Berger U V, *et al.* Cloning and characterization of a mammalian proton coupled metal ion transporter. *Nature* 1997; **388:** 482-488.

Index